Handbook of Diagnostic
and Structured Interviewing

Handbook
of Diagnostic
and Structured
Interviewing

Richard Rogers

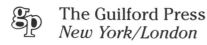

The Guilford Press
New York/London

© 2001 The Guilford Press
A Division of Guilford Publications, Inc.
72 Spring Street, New York, NY 10012
www.guilford.com

Printed in the United States of America

This book is printed on acid-free paper.

Last digit is print number: 9 8 7 6 5 4 3 2 1

Library of Congress Cataloging-in-Publication Data

Rogers, Richard, 1950–
    Handbook of diagnostic and structured interviewing / Richard Rogers.
      p. ; cm.
    Includes bibliographical references and index.
    ISBN 1-57230-678-5 (cloth : alk. paper)
    1. Interviewing in psychiatry. 2. Mental illness—Diagnosis. I. Title.
    [DNLM: 1. Interview, Psychological—methods. 2. Mental Disorders—
diagnosis. WM
141 R728d 2001
RC480.7.R64 2001
616.89′075—dc21   2001033139

About the Author

Richard Rogers, PhD, ABPP, is Professor of Psychology at the University of North Texas, Denton, Texas. His previous academic appointments were in both psychology and psychiatry at Rush University, Chicago, Illinois, and the University of Toronto, Ontario. Formerly Director of Clinical Training at the University of North Texas, Dr. Rogers has an established expertise in diagnostic and clinical assessment. A prolific writer, he has published more than 50 articles devoted to assessment issues. During the 1980s, Dr. Rogers grew to realize the importance of structured interviews for the assessment of differential diagnoses, malingering and other response styles, and forensic issues. In 1992, he and several colleagues authored the Structured Interview of Reported Symptoms, generally regarded as the premier measure for feigned mental disorders. In 1995, he wrote the first professional text devoted to diagnostic and structured interviewing. His contributions to forensic assessment have been recognized by awards from the American Psychiatric Association and the American Academy of Forensic Psychology.

Acknowledgments

I would like to thank my doctoral students for their gentle honesty and direct feedback on early drafts of this book. I would also like to express my appreciation to Jennipher Roman, who worked tirelessly in the library gathering hundreds of articles. Finally, my gratitude to my family for understanding my passion for writing and supporting me in this endeavor.

Contents

I

Introduction

1

Nature of Diagnostic
and Structured Interviewing

Mental health professionals are increasingly challenged to demonstrate the validity of their diagnostic and clinical conclusions. Health maintenance organizations and other third-party payers explicitly demand empirically based methods of assessment. Less overtly, clients and their families express concerns about the fallibility of clinical conclusions, namely, missed diagnoses and misdiagnoses. As part of the solution, structured interviews provide an important method of standardizing evaluations and demonstrating their diagnostic validity.

What are structured interviews? Briefly, structured interviews provide a systematic evaluation by standardizing (1) the specific language of clinical inquiries, (2) the sequencing of these inquiries, and (3) the quantification of responses. Their systematic appraisal of relevant symptoms is likely to reduce misdiagnosis. Likewise, their standardized coverage is likely to reduce missed diagnoses. Before examining the components of structured interviews in detail, I address common misassumptions about structured interviews.

MISASSUMPTIONS ABOUT STRUCTURED INTERVIEWS

Either/Or Fallacy

I occasionally encounter resistance to structured interviewing, especially from more seasoned clinicians. When voiced, their objections are frequently encapsulated in the question, "What is wrong with traditional interviews?" This question is likely based on a faulty premise in forcing an unnecessary choice between structured and unstructured interviews. I refer to this premise as the "either/or" fallacy. The question is best reframed as "Under what circumstances will diagnostic and structured interviewing assist me in meeting my

3

objectives?" Strict adherence to *traditional* interviews is likely to constrain the standardization and systematic coverage of clinical inquiries. Strict adherence to *structured* interviews is likely to damage rapport and limit the relevance of any clinical conclusions because the relationship of symptoms to the patient's current functioning and circumstances remains unexplored.

Routinization

One criticism of structured interviewing is that the process routinizes the interview process. In unskilled hands, structured interviews may impersonalize the interview process and damage rapport. At the very worst, questions piled upon questions can pummel the client. The critical issue is not the structured interviews per se, but their unskilled use. In contradistinction to the misuse of structured interviews, the achievable goal is for the standardized inquiries to become subapparent in the interview process. A useful metaphor is a performance of classical music. In the hands of an inexperienced musician, its formal structure becomes painfully obvious and destroys the music's harmony and flow. In the hands of a professional musician, technical aspects of metrics and notes are barely perceptible. With structured interviews, an optimal performance is an engaging and smooth process that is unimpeded by its standardization.

An issue related to routinization is that the mental health professionals will become "protocol-bound" and miss other important clinical data (see Ruegg, Ekstrom, Dwight, & Golden, 1990). The underlying error in clinical judgment is "premature closure." Inexperienced clinicians are sometimes predisposed to accept their diagnostic impressions readily, without a careful examination of alternative or additional diagnoses. A key consideration is premature closure, which may occur with both standardized (e.g., structured interviews) and nonstandardized (e.g., traditional interviews) methods.

THE RATIONALE FOR STRUCTURED INTERVIEWS

Structured interviews require both additional time and advanced training. What is the justification for their selective use? The rationale is twofold: a reduction of unnecessary variability and concomitant improvements in diagnostic agreement.

Reduction of Unnecessary Variability

The basic rationale for structured interviews is the minimization of needless variability in interviewer-based evaluations. The simplest way to understand structured interviews is to examine sources of diagnostic variability. In a seminal work, Ward, Beck, Mendelson, Mock, and Erbaugh (1962) concluded that most diagnostic variability is a product of the evaluations and *not* the patients. As summarized in Table 1.1, most variability results from (1) idiosyncratic questioning or "information variance" (32.5%), and (2) idiosyncratic rating of responses or "criterion variance" (62.5%). In contrast, very little variability is the result of changes in patients' status (5.0%).

Structured interviews reduce the sources of needless variability. These sources are outlined as follows:

- *Idiosyncratic questions.* The wording of clinical inquiries may affect their understandability and the patients' responses. For instance, questions with negative affect (e.g., "Are you worried about your loss of sleep?" or "Are you bothered by unusual thoughts?") are more likely to measure general dysphoria than specific symptoms (Clark & Watson, 1995). In addition, questions may have an untoward effect on the evaluation if expressed with either a pejorative (e.g., "Do you still have those strange ideas about the police?") or incredulous (e.g., "Do you *really* believe your spouse is out to get you?") tone.

- *Idiosyncratic coverage.* Less than complete coverage is likely to result in underdiagnosis. As described by Rogers (1986), most clinicians subscribe to a hypothesis-testing diagnostic model. In other words, they follow their intuitive hypotheses based on clinical presentation and past history. This non-systematic approach is likely to miss important symptomatology. It is also prone to primacy bias (see Borum, Otto, & Golding, 1993), with individual clinicians overemphasizing their first hypotheses. Moreover, clinicians may also miss important symptoms. Because clinicians rarely have an encyclopedic knowledge of DSM-IV criteria, symptoms beyond the minimum criteria for a targeted disorder are likely to be overlooked in traditional interviews.

- *Idiosyncratic sequencing.* Variability is likely to be magnified by the atypical sequencing of clinical inquiries. A basic assumption of clinical interviews is that ordering of diagnostic questions is likely to influence patients' re-

TABLE 1.1. Why Do Clinicians Disagree? A Distillation of Ward et al. (1962)

Percentage	Sources of disagreement
32.5%	*Information variance:* Variations among clinicians in what questions are asked, which observations are made, and how the resulting information is organized.
62.5%	*Criterion variance:* Variations among clinicians in applying standards for what is clinically relevant (e.g., when does dysphoric mood qualify as depression?) and when the diagnostic criteria are met.
5.0%	*Patient variance:* Variations within the same patient that result in substantial differences in clinical presentation and subsequent diagnosis.

Note. For further discussion, see Ward, Beck, Mendelson, Mock, and Erbaugh (1962); Murphy, Woodruff, and Herjanic (1974); Rogers (1986). Spitzer, Endicott, and Robins (1975a) elaborated on Ward's model, perhaps unnecessarily, by subdividing patient variance into "subject variance" (e.g., different disorders at different times) and "occasion variance" (e.g., different stages of the same disorder at different times).

sponses. As a general rule, both Axis I and Axis II interviews begin with less threatening topics and progress to topics that ask for potentially intrusive information. More specifically, structured interviews initially avoid questions that ask patients to disclose either odd (e.g., psychotic symptoms) or nonconforming (e.g., antisocial behavior) experiences. Research by Rogers, Bagby, and Dickens (1992) suggests that more specific ordering of clinical inquiries significantly affects responses.

• *Idiosyncratic recording.* Clinicians vary remarkably in their depth and style of recording patients' statements. Rarely do clinicians make notations about how the question was asked or whether the information was observed or disclosed by the patient. With an emphasis toward psychopathology, some clinicians report only symptoms and associated features but fail to mention areas of adjustment (e.g., lack of depression or sustained interest in social activities). In addition, unusual or unique data are likely to be given disproportionate attention (see Borum et al., 1993).

• *Nonexistent ratings.* A major source of variability is whether a symptom is clinically relevant. The majority of patients experience dysphoria. At what point does this dysphoria warrant classification as anxiety or a depressed mood? Structured interviews provide an opportunity to classify symptoms as "absent," "subclinical," and "clinical." Some interviews, such as the Schedule of Affective Disorders and Schizophrenia (SADS; Spitzer & Endicott, 1978a), offer gradations of severity beyond the basic trichotomy.

Improvements in the Diagnostic Assessment

Structured interviews provide an unparalleled opportunity to categorize mental disorders and quantify symptoms and associated features. Because of this standardization, clinicians may examine the reliability of individual symptoms and their stability across the course of the disorder. In addition, uniformity can be achieved for examining the consistency of a patient's report and the level of agreement from collateral sources. As described in the previous section, the relative comprehensiveness of the diagnostic coverage vastly improves diagnostic assessment. Moreover, the absence of a diagnosis (e.g., a personality disorder) is established systematically rather than simply inferred.

Reliability

The scientific underpinning of clinical assessment is the reproducibility of its results. Without established reliability, the trustworthiness of clinical observations is not ascertainable. The key indices of reproducibility are (1) agreement between independent observers (i.e., interrater reliability) and (2) consistency of symptoms across brief intervals (i.e., test–retest reliability). Depending on the organization of specific structured interviews, clinicians can determine the reliability at several levels: individual symptoms, dimensional ratings of symptom constellations, and diagnoses.

Test–retest reliability must be differentiated from "temporal stability." Symptoms are not expected to remain identical for long periods of time. Rather, symptoms are likely to change (1) because of the natural course of the disorder, (2) in response to treatment efforts, or (3) as a result of environmental changes. Test–retest reliability is established for designated intervals, typically ranging from 1 to 4 weeks. In contrast, "temporal stability" is a term applied to the chronicity of the disorder. A high level of temporal stability over extended periods (e.g., 6 or 12 months) reflects an unchanging clinical presentation.

Levels of Measurement

Part of the scientific foundation for the diagnostic assessment is its precision of measurement. In psychology and allied disciplines, this precision is categorized by "levels of measurement." To review briefly, levels of measurement may be "nominal" (i.e., present or absent), "ordinal" (i.e., present to a greater or lesser degree), or "interval" (i.e., present as measured in uniform gradations). In psychological assessment, many clinical constructs (e.g., intelligence) are treated as "interval" measurements, despite being fundamentally ordinal in nature.[1] Structured interviews may be used to demonstrate an ordinal level of measurement, comparable to other areas of psychological measurement.

Aligned with level of measurement is the notion regarding clinical thresholds. The mere presence of *any* dysphoria has little diagnostic relevance. As previously noted, the central issue is whether a particular symptom reaches a level of clinical significance. Ward et al. (1962) found that nearly two-thirds of diagnostic disagreement (62.5%) results from a lack of precision in establishing clinical thresholds. To illustrate, when is depression considered *clinical* depression? To clarify this issue, most structured interviews make explicit distinctions between subclinical ("normal") and clinical ("psychopathological") levels.

Systematic Comparisons

By reducing needless variability, structured interviews allow clinicians to make well-defined and methodical comparisons. Examples of salient clinical issues that can be addressed by systematic comparisons are as follows:

1. *Across collateral sources, do others see the patient differently?* Evaluating the degree of correspondence across sources serves two useful purposes. First, it provides additional data to confirm–disconfirm a diagnosis. Second, it

---

[1]As illustrated by Rogers and Shuman (2000), not even IQ scores can be considered interval measurements. Systematic differences (e.g., 15 points) on the Wechsler Adult Intelligence Scale—III (WAIS-III; Wechsler, 1997) cannot be equated. The quantum of intelligence between 115 and 130 bears no resemblance to corresponding comparisons at the low-average (e.g., between 85 and 100) or mentally challenged (e.g., between 55 and 70) ranges.

affords an opportunity to understand multiple perspectives of the client. For example, the Child Assessment Schedule (CAS) allows the clinician to understand both the mother's and the child's perspective of the child's problem areas. Areas of agreement become the foundation for future treatment interventions. Areas of disagreement often provide a useful treatment framework for examining different perspectives.

2. *Across time, what changes have occurred in the patient?* Especially for patients involved in treatment, a vital issue is the mediating effect of changes occurring in the patient as a result of treatment and environmental modifications. The gradual nature of most clinical changes combined with limited insight often militate against patients' awareness of subtle but important changes in their symptomatology and concomitant functioning. Repeat administrations provide valuable data about patient changes.

3. *Across clinicians, do specific practitioners manifest potential biases?* The informal application of an interrater reliability paradigm allows professionals within a clinical setting to test for outliers. For instance, some clinicians may have a relatively high threshold before considering symptoms sufficiently severe as to warrant major depression. Cross-comparisons provide ready access to this information. Of equal importance, such cross-comparisons provide an invaluable training tool to minimize potential biases.

4. *Within the same patient, how much variability in self-reporting should be expected?* Marked inconsistency in self-reporting is sometimes viewed as either evidence of feigning or severe impairment. The retesting of patients within a short interval (e.g., < 2 days) provides useful data on variations typically found in patient populations. Without such normative data, the meaning of inconsistencies cannot be easily discovered.

5. *Within settings, do certain diagnostic patterns emerge?* Without the systematic application of structured interviews, clinical settings often focus only on primary diagnoses. This focus neglects other valuable diagnostic patterns, including Axis II disorders and substance abuse.

6. *Within diagnoses, do specific treatments produce superior results?* The primary goal of treatment is the reduction of targeted symptoms. Structured interviews provide a unique advantage in being able to assess changes in symptom severity. In contrast, symptom checklists (e.g., the Symptom Checklist-90—Revised) place the patients themselves in the role of experts.

Comprehensiveness

Traditional interviews are often focused on presenting problems and key symptoms that form the basis for successive hypothesis generation (Rogers & Shuman, 2000). Once a diagnostic hypothesis is confirmed, the diagnostic process is viewed as completed. Therefore, clinicians tend to stop the diagnostic investigation after the first mental disorder is established (Harkness, 1992; Zimmerman & Mattia, 1998b). In light of this process, we should not be surprised to find that traditional interviews often miss additional diagnoses

(Wyndowe, 1987), particularly among disorders that occur infrequently (Ford, Hillard, Giesler, Lassen, & Thomas, 1989).

Undiagnosed disorders are assumed to be absent. An important source of undiagnosed disorders is implicit assumptions by health care providers regarding whether a patient is "well-functioning." In such cases, many disorders remain uninvestigated (see Jones, Badger, Ficken, Leeper, & Anderson, 1988). The standardized administration of structured interviews substantially removes this "hit or miss" approach to diagnosis. It ensures that major diagnostic categories are not omitted irrespective of clinicians' working hypotheses or their assumptions about patients' level of functioning.

THE VALIDITY OF MENTAL DISORDERS

The validity of diagnostic interviewing is inextricably tied to the validity of diagnosis itself. Sole reliance on the convergence between diagnostic criteria and structured diagnostic interviews is hardly more than a tautological exercise. In the vein of Szasz (1960), how do we know that mental disorders are nothing more than pejorative judgments enshrining social mores and reflecting arbitrary distinctions? Past controversies (e.g., homosexuality as a disorder; American Psychiatric Association, 1968) underscore the conflation between socially defined deviance and diagnostic validation. How can diagnostic validity be addressed? The following section examines Syndeham's criteria for diagnostic validity.

Syndeham Criteria and Diagnostic Validity

Syndeham was credited, in 1753, with the definition of disease in operational terms (see Murphy, Woodruff, Herjanic, & Fischer, 1974). He stated that a disorder is composed of the following three necessary elements: inclusion, exclusion, and outcome criteria:

- *Inclusion criteria.* What are the core characteristics of a disorder?
- *Exclusion criteria.* How does the disorder differ from related disorders? Exclusion criteria are essential for differential diagnosis.
- *Outcome criteria.* What is the likely course of the disorder? The challenge for outcome criteria is the prediction of a singular, if not unique, outcome.

Modern theorists have added little to Syndeham's criteria. Prominent investigators (e.g., Feighner et al., 1972; Murphy et al., 1974; Robins & Guze, 1970) have suggested that the validity of a disorder could be enhanced through external correlates, such as laboratory and familial studies. While theoretically interesting, such correlates are not essential for diagnostic validity.

Researchers have also expanded upon the conceptualization of outcome criteria. With essentially a longitudinal perspective, clinical researchers can also focus on necessary antecedent conditions as evidence of outcome criteria. For example, Cloninger, Martin, Guze, and Clayton (1985) focused on the pathogenesis of specific disorders in order to understand their outcome. Recent work on developmental psychopathology (e.g., Lynam, 1996; psychopathy/conduct disorder as a precursor to antisocial personality disorder) also addresses outcome criteria from a retrospective viewpoint. For purposes of simplicity, etiological criteria are subsumed under outcome criteria.

The understanding of diagnostic validity is pivotal to structured interviews. Therefore, the next several pages examine the three components of Syndeham's model. Current constraints on diagnostic validity are illustrated with two mental disorders: schizophrenia and antisocial personality disorder (APD).

Inclusion Criteria

Cloninger et al. (1985) elaborated on the nature of inclusion criteria in the diagnosis of mental disorders. They argued that the inclusion criteria should represent an intercorrelated group of symptoms that remain constant across time (stability) and within diagnosis (homogeneity). How correlated should inclusion criteria be? Obviously, if high correlations are achieved, then item redundancy is unduly complicating diagnosis (Clark & Watson, 1995). Alternatively, if symptoms are uncorrelated, then it is difficult to argue that they constitute a single entity such as a syndrome or disorder. Intuitively, clinicians want symptoms that "hang together" and are likely to give greater weight to correlated than uncorrelated symptoms (Medin, Altom, Edelson, & Freko, 1982).

The issue of correlated items is further complicated by the current emphasis on polythetic diagnosis. The implicit assumption with polythetic diagnosis is the interchangeability of inclusion criteria (e.g., any combination of three inclusion criteria is equivalent to any other three inclusion criteria; see Rogers, Duncan, & Sewell, 1994). Given the assumption of interchangeability, some item redundancy is likely to be necessary. We have not come to grips with (1) what constitutes the optimal level of intercorrelated symptoms and (2) the ramifications of correlated symptoms for diagnosis.

How do we establish the inclusion criteria for a mental disorder? Broughton (1990) presented a compelling argument for the use of prototypical analysis to establish the core features of mental disorders. Based on the work of Rosch (1973, 1978; see also Osherson & Smith, 1981), categories can be established by the most representative or cardinal features of specific disorders. Livesley (1985a, 1985b, 1986) has championed this approach to diagnosis and conducted an extensive, if partially flawed,[2] prototypical analy-

---

[2]Despite the large sample of North American psychiatrists, the total symptoms/characteristics used for each diagnosis greatly outnumbered the participants involved in prototypical ratings.

sis of North American psychiatrists (Livesley & Jackson, 1986; Livesley, Reiffer, Sheldon, & West, 1987). A singular advantage of prototypical analysis is its simplicity in establishing prototypical symptoms and examining their underlying dimensions.

An important distinction must be made between *core characteristics* and *common features* of a mental disorder. Core characteristics represent distinctive elements that distinguish a particular disorder from others. Common features are prevalent but not necessarily distinctive elements of a disorder. In establishing inclusion criteria, the critical issue is the establishment of core characteristics. Problems occur when diagnoses attempt to rely on common features. As a case in point, "social withdrawal" characterizes many diagnoses including schizophrenic disorders, schizoid and avoidant personality disorders, depression and dysthymic disorders, social phobias, and agoraphobias. A symptom such as social withdrawal does not represent a distinguishing characteristic of any specific disorder and thus has limited value as an inclusion criterion.

Core characteristics of a mental disorder are likely to reflect underlying dimensions. Millon (1991) observed that factor-analytic procedures may assist in establishing the central features of a disorder. Studies have yielded mixed findings on this point, because these dimensions appear to overlap with related disorders. As an example from Clark and Watson (1991), factor-analytic studies of anxiety and depression often yield a nonspecific dimension of "distress" as their first factor, with other dimensions more closely related to the respective disorders. Researchers have also found stable dimensions within disorders. What are the implications of these dimensions to diagnostic validity? They suggest that a simple polythetic model may neglect important dimensions of a diagnosis. A straightforward solution would be the use of a "nested polythetic model" (i.e., specified number of inclusion criteria for each dimension). For example, the DSM-IV diagnosis of posttraumatic stress disorder (PTSD; American Psychiatric Association, 1994) postulates three dimensions of inclusion criteria: (1) reexperienced trauma, (2) avoidance or numbing to trauma-related stimuli, and (3) increased arousal. In the nested polythetic model for PTSD, inclusion criteria for each dimension must be established.

The following subsections illustrate problems with inclusion criteria by focusing on two disorders, namely, schizophrenia and APD.

Inclusion Criteria for Schizophrenia. Historically, inclusion criteria for schizophrenia have served as the flashpoint for acrimonious debates between the Kraeplin conceptualization of schizophrenia as an irreversible illness resulting in a generalized state of "psychic weakness" and the Bleuler model with its cardinal features: loosening of associations, blunted affect, autism, and ambivalence (see Kendell, 1985). Conflict over the core characteristics of schizophrenia have not abated over time, as observed with the emergence of Schneider's symptoms of first rank (e.g., auditory hallucinations, thought insertion, thought withdrawal, thought broadcasting, bizarre sensations, delusional perceptions, and delusions of control). Changes in inclusion criteria have produced dramatic results; the transition from DSM-II to DSM-III decreased the diagnosis of schizophrenia by approximately 50% (Carson, 1991). Comparisons of inclusion criteria for schizophrenia (e.g., research diagnostic criteria (RDC), New Haven, Feighner, Schneiderian, and DSM-III; see Kendell, 1985; Stephens, Astrup, & Carpenter, 1982) demonstrate the marked differences in the application of inclusion criteria. These models produced an average concordance of only 61.7%.

Cloninger et al. (1985) evaluated approximately 500 clinical variables and found five inclusion criteria and one exclusion criterion that differentiate schizophrenia from other disorders. The inclusion criteria were composed of persecutory delusions, delusions of control, firmly fixed mood-incongruent delusions, and auditory hallucinations. Several observations emerge. First, DSM-IV criteria are poorly represented (i.e., omitted criteria include disorganized speech, grossly disorganized or catatonic behavior, and negative symptoms). Second, the analysis of 500 variables to produce these six significant variables increases the likelihood of spurious findings (i.e., Type I error).

Inclusion Criteria for APD. Pervasive problems in establishing inclusion criteria are well illustrated with APD (see Rogers & Dion, 1991; Rogers, Dion, & Lynett, 1992). DSM-II formulations of inclusion criteria (American Psychiatric Association, 1968) emphasized character defects that lead to irresponsibility, impaired social relationships, and an incapacity to conform to societal expectations. In marked contrast, DSM-III inclusion criteria (American Psychiatric Association, 1980) were based on overt behavioral disturbances and dyssocial behavior. More recently, DSM-III-R (American Psychiatric Association, 1987) has refocused inclusion criteria on violent delinquent behavior. Nor has the matter of inclusion criteria been resolved; DSM-IV (American Psychiatric Association, 1994) has introduced further changes in APD inclusion criteria. Given these successive and fundamental changes the number of possible combinations of inclusion criteria are truly numbing. Rogers and Dion (1991) estimated the number of diagnostic variations for only DSM-III and DSM-III-R at roughly 27 trillion. DSM-IV dramatically increases the diagnostic variations; Criterion C (conduct symptoms) multiply from 4,017 in DSM-III-R to 32,647 in DSM-IV.

Given the bewildering array of APD inclusion criteria, two important considerations include the simplification of criteria via factor analysis and the identification of prototypical symptoms. In this regard, Rogers and his colleagues (Rogers, Dion, & Lynett, 1992; Rogers, Duncan, & Sewell, 1994; Rogers, Salekin, Sewell, & Cruise, 2000) conducted a series of prototypical analyses on APD and psychopathy criteria. In a study of 331 forensic psychiatrists, Rogers et al. (1994) identified four underlying factors: F_1, *unstable self image, unstable relationships, and irresponsibility;* F_2, *manipulation and lack of guilt;* F_3, *aggressive behavior;* and F_4, *nonviolent delinquency.* Importantly,

F_2 and F_3 were highest in prototypical ratings, remaining highest in prototypicality even when examined for a large inmate sample (Rogers, Salekin, Sewell, & Cruise, 2000). In rethinking APD, some inclusion criteria (e.g., nonviolent delinquent symptoms within Criterion C) may be common but not core (i.e., distinguishing) characteristics of APD. These studies also suggest the possibility of a nested–polythetic model that requires inclusion criteria for (1) manipulation and lack of guilt and (2) aggressive behavior.

In light of ongoing controversies, the unambiguous conceptualization of APD inclusion criteria is essential. Unfortunately, DSM-IV has further muddled this matter in its attempt to equate APD inclusion criteria and the clinical construct of psychopathy (American Psychological Association, 1994, p. 645). This attempt fails on both conceptual and empirical grounds (see Hare, 1998b; Rogers, Salekin, Sewell, & Cruise, 2000). Germane to the current discussion, APD and psychopathy are markedly dissimilar in their use of inclusion criteria: APD focuses on behavioral criteria, requires both developmental (conduct) and adult symptoms, and utilizes a polythetic perspective. The prevailing view of psychopathy (Hare, 1991) focuses on both trait and behavioral criteria, requires only adult criteria, and aggregates criteria into a composite score.

Exclusion Criteria

The hallmark of differential diagnosis is the careful application of exclusion criteria. For differential diagnosis to be effective, clinicians must be able to classify a disorder by what it is (inclusion criteria) and what it is not (exclusion criteria). For purposes of diagnostic clarity, clear exclusion criteria at the symptom level are optimal. As a hypothetical example, avoidant personality disorder could be augmented by two exclusion criteria at the symptom level.

Avoidant personality disorder is not diagnosed if the following two symptoms are present:

1. Capacity to form a long-term, intimate relationship that the individual views as mutually positive.
2. Capacity to select an occupational environment that meets the individual's need for limited interpersonal contact and a predictable repertoire of work behavior.

The logical argument against these hypothetical exclusion criteria is that they are broadly covered under the general diagnostic criteria for personality disorders (see American Psychiatric Association, 1994, p. 633). The persuasive arguments for these hypothetical exclusion criteria are that (1) they provide specific guidelines for when not to invoke this disorder, and (2) they present a more balanced perspective about what is and is not a particular disorder.

DSM-IV eschews exclusion criteria at the symptom level in favor of more complex decisions. Most DSM-IV exclusion criteria fit into the following categories:

- *Explanatory.* Clinicians are asked to exclude a disorder if it is "better accounted for by another mental disorder" (see, e.g., American Psychiatric Association, 1994, p. 7). Explanatory criteria are invoked "when there are particularly difficult differential diagnostic boundaries" (p. 7). This statement is a frank admission that no explicit exclusion criteria were established. Instead, practitioners are explicitly exhorted to use their own "clinical judgment." Such explanatory exclusions founder on two points: (1) the ambiguity of the standard (i.e., "not better accounted for" defies operationalization) and (2) the complexity of the task (numerous diagnoses might be sequentially considered).
- *Etiological.* Clinicians are asked to determine whether a disorder is "not due to the direct physiological effects of a substance (e.g., a drug of abuse, a medication) or a general medical condition" (American Psychiatric Association, 1994, p. 7). The crux of this determination is "direct physiological effects." The comorbidity of substance abuse and chronic mental disorders militates against clear boundaries. In addition, a panoply of medications have potential side effects that could conceivably affect mood and other symptoms. Unless an unmistakably clear and repetitive pattern can be established, the etiological criteria are especially vulnerable to the post-hoc-ergo-propter-hoc fallacy.
- *Coextensive.* Clinicians are asked to determine whether a particular disorder "does not occur exclusively during the course" of a second disorder (American Psychiatric Association, 1994, pp. 6–7). The coextension of episodes, especially if multiple episodes have occurred, is an especially complex judgment to render.
- *Historical.* Clinicians must evaluate whether "criteria have never been met" for another disorder. If adequate history is available, this criterion appears useful.

In reviewing DSM-IV exclusion criteria, the etiological type is more prevalent for Axis I disorders. The implicit assumption of such exclusion criteria is the rather tenuous supposition of unicausality. Whether this assumption is justifiable must be determined on a case-by-case basis. On the one hand, a convincing argument can be made that alcoholic hallucinosis is etiologically related to chronic alcohol abuse (Mirin & Weiss, 1983). On the other hand, certain organic delusional disorders are likely to be multidetermined, with "functional" and other predispositional factors playing direct although unexplained roles.

DSM-IV has accentuated this diagnostic use of differential etiology by the introduction of "substance-induced" disorders. For example, substance-induced anxiety disorder (American Psychiatric Association, 1994; p. 443) must demonstrate either a temporal relationship (i.e., symptoms develop within a month of substance intoxication or withdrawal) or be etiologically related. With chronic drug users, the first subcriterion appears to be difficult, if not impossible, to apply. The second subcriterion ("known" etiology) appears to beg the question it purports to answer. Further attempts to specify substance-induced anxiety (Criterion C) also involve temporality (i.e., symptoms precede drug use or continue after acute withdrawal) and likewise pose a daunting task in cases of chronic drug use.

Exclusion Criteria for Schizophrenia. Cloninger et al. (1985) found that the *absence* of manic spending sprees provides one of the highest standardized canonical coefficients for the classification of schizophrenic patients. Introduction of specific exclusion criteria at the symptom level would likely improve the homogeneity of mental disorders. In light of Cloninger et al.'s success, researchers should be encouraged to examine systematically the role of specific, symptom-based exclusions in improving diagnostic validity.

DSM-IV exclusion criteria for schizophrenia (American Psychiatric Association, 1994, p. 285) give greater weight to mood than psychotic symptoms. Episodes of mood disorders (major depression, manic and mixed episodes) preempt the diagnosis of schizophrenia unless the duration of mood symptoms has been "brief relative to the duration of the active and residual periods" (p. 286). Even in single episodes of major depression, the issue of duration is clouded by the extended use of maintenance treatment (American Psychiatric Association, 1996). It is difficult to consider a nonsymptomatic patient maintained on an antidepressant regimen to be in full remission. Therefore, levels of improvement (partial vs. full remission) and intervention (acute vs. maintenance treatment) complicate both the duration of mood and schizophrenic episodes. Furthermore, if a depressive episode remains in full remission, then the diagnosis may subsequently change a mood disorder with psychotic features to a schizophrenic disorder as the proportion of overlap decreases to a relatively brief period.

Exclusion Criteria for APD. DSM nosology has made successive attempts to differentiate the merely "bad" (APD) from those who are also mentally disordered. For example, DSM-III excluded APD as a disorder when "due to" severe mental retardation, schizophrenia, or manic episodes (American Psychiatric Association, 1980, p. 321); DSM-III-R and DSM-IV excluded antisocial behavior that occurs "exclusively during the course of schizophrenia or a manic episode" (American Psychiatric Association, 1994, p. 650). These exclusion criteria are ill-considered. Given the early onset for APD (e.g., conduct symptoms prior to age 15), and typically later onset for schizophrenia, this exclusion criterion is unlikely to be applicable (Rogers & Dion, 1991). Likewise, manic episodes typically have a later onset than APD and a relatively short duration (i.e., few weeks to several months; American Psychiatric Association, 1994). Therefore, the criterion of "exclusively during a manic episode" is simply irrelevant.

Outcome Criteria

The longitudinal dimension of mental disorders, encapsulated in the concept of outcome criteria, is the sine qua non of diagnosis. If the course of a disorder cannot be accurately charted, then its validity is unavoidably vitiated. Description for description's sake (i.e., inclusion and exclusion criteria alone) says next to nothing about the course of a disorder or its etiology. Likewise, treatment efficacy can only be understood in terms of outcome criteria.

Outcome criteria are examined from four related perspectives: (1) chronicity, (2) course of the disorder, (3) etiology, and (4) treatment response. As with previous sections, schizophrenia and APD serve as diagnostic examples.

Chronicity. DSM-IV occasionally includes outcome criteria in its diagnostic nomenclature. Unfortunately, the distinction between inclusion and outcome criteria sometimes becomes blurred because of diagnostic circularity (Tsuang & Loyd, 1985). With an acute psychotic episode, how do clinicians differentiate between schizophreniform and schizophrenic disorders? The unpalatable answer is "wait 6 months." A better model would be an empirical validation of specific symptoms that differentiate the outcome of the two disorders. For example, DSM-IV (American Psychiatric Association, 1994, p. 290) articulates good prognostic features (e.g., sudden onset, confusion, and good premorbid functioning) that are likely correlated with rapid recovery (i.e., schizophreniform outcome). In contrast, negative symptoms (e.g., flat affect and poor motivation) are associated with a chronic course and limited treatment response (i.e., schizophrenia outcome; American Psychiatric Association, 1997).

Use of chronicity as an outcome measure is not limited to the schizophrenic disorders. Within dysthymic and cyclothymic disorders, an explicit outcome criterion is imposed: The disorders must remain chronic for at least 2 years. When dysthymia is present for 6 months, how is a dysthymic disorder diagnosed? The unpalatable answer is "wait 18 months." Clearly, a pressing need exists for inclusion criteria that predict outcome criteria.

Chronicity of a disorder is an important dimension of outcome criteria. With the amassing of diagnostic studies, our diagnostic nomenclature would be immensely enriched by the explicit addition of outcome criteria as a formal component of mental disorders. At present, the intrusion of chronicity into the inclusion criteria is likely to obscure rather than elucidate the core characteristics of mental disorders.

Course of the Disorder. In establishing outcome criteria, DSM-IV has paid relatively little attention to documenting successive phases of specific mental disorders. Important exceptions include schizophrenic disorders with three well-defined phases (i.e., prodromal, active, and residual) and APD with two distinct phases (i.e., developmental and adult). The establishment of specific phases would augment our current diagnoses with explicit outcome criteria.

Defining the course of the disorder is particularly troublesome for personality disorders, since risk factors for most Axis II disorders are general and an invariant trait model has been posited (Panzetta, 1974). This view is not universal. Loranger (1988) in the development of the Personality Disorder Examination (PDE), provided for two alternatives: (1) late onset and (2) past disorders. Moreover, the chronicity of personality disorders is assumed rather than investigated. As described in Chapter 3, several APD studies question the chronicity of this disorder.

Etiology. The origin or "cause" of mental disorders can also provide a relevant model for outcome criteria. If the etiology of a particular disorder can be reliably demarcated and a predictable course identified, then the validity of a disorder appears to be well established (Cloninger et al., 1985). The problem with etiology lies in the multiplicity of factors that appear to play small but significant roles in the pathogenesis of mental disorders. As noted by Coie et al. (1993), contributions to mental disorders are multifaceted based on (1) their manifestations in multiple dysfunctions, (2) cumulative effects, and (3) salience at different developmental periods. Because of this complexity, etiological explanations are often difficult to delineate.

Risk factors are sometimes utilized as indirect evidence of etiology. Without establishing the pathogenesis, risk factors reflect the increased probabilities that a disorder will occur based on well-defined characteristics. For schizophrenia (see Murphy & Helzer, 1985), increased risk has been established based on family history of schizophrenia, perinatal factors (e.g., birth complications and seasonality), age (i.e., higher risk between 15 and 45), and gender (greater risk for males). With reference to APD, risk factors include gender (6:1 ratio of males to females), urbanization (2.4:1 ratio of urban to rural), and age (see Robins, 1985). For the purposes of diagnostic validity, risk factors are simply insufficient to establish etiology. To illustrate with the previous example, any assertion about the etiology of APD based on risk factors (i.e., young urban male) is comical. Moreover, risk factors cannot be properly understood without taking into account protective factors, moderator effects, and mediating effects (Rogers, 2000).

The etiology of certain disorders has been well established in a few instances and implicitly assumed in others. In some instances, a compromise of cognitive functioning can be clearly linked to a single etiological factor, such as mental retardation resulting from Down syndrome or dementia secondary to encephalitis (American Psychiatric Association, 1987, 1994). In other cases, the etiology is implicit in the diagnosis. For example PTSD and brief reactive psychosis both assume that the disorder would not have occurred without the trauma. These diagnoses elude the troubling issue of why certain individuals become symptomatic and others do not.

Treatment Response. To employ treatment response as an outcome criteria, investigators must demonstrate a specific treatment outcome linked to a particular disorder. Otherwise, we cannot hope to establish the uniqueness of the particular disorder on a longitudinal dimension. Since psychosocial treatments tend to be relatively effective (or ineffective) with a wide range of disorders, we must turn our attention to biological treatments. However, attempts to use treatment response to drugs designed to treat specific disorders are also thwarted. Kaplan and Sadock (1988) observed that drugs from a specific class often alleviate symptoms from other disorders (e.g., lithium for impulse disorders) and tend to be effective across disorders. While differentiating response rates are found across diagnoses (e.g., electroconvulsive therapy and major depression), research has generally lacked a disorder-specific response to the degree that such findings could be used as outcome criteria for diagnostic validity.

Outcome Criteria for Schizophrenia. Beyond schizophreniform disorders, chronicity poses additional problems in establishing outcome criteria for schizophrenia and distinguishing it from schizoid and schizotypal personality disorders. Symptoms of either Axis II disorder could constitute the prodromal phase of schizophrenia. Only with knowledge of the outcome criteria (i.e., an active phase of schizophrenia) can a diagnosis be confirmed. In recognition of the blurred lines between these personality disorders and the prodromal phase of schizophrenia, DSM-IV (American Psychiatric Association, 1994, pp. 641, 645), allows dual diagnoses. In these instances, the clinician must speculate that the schizoid or schizotypal disorders preceded the prodromal phase and are considered a "premorbid" condition.

The outcome criteria for schizophrenia do not appear to predict the course of the disorder (Endicott, Nie, Cohen, Fleiss, & Simon, 1986). Perhaps the explanation for this lies in four distinctive patterns that have emerged to describe the course of schizophrenia (Kendell, 1985): (1) one episode with full recovery; (2) multiple episodes, with full recovery between episodes; (3) multiple episodes, with residual impairment between episodes that becomes more pronounced; and (4) continuation of a single episode with a chronic and deteriorative pattern.

What are the implications of these outcomes for diagnostic validity? If we were to remain true to the Syndeham criteria, then subtypes of schizophrenia should be based on outcome criteria, such as the course of the disorder. Inclusion and exclusion criteria would be selected on the basis of their ability to predict the course of the disorder from rapid recoveries (similar to schizophreniform disorders) to chronic and deteriorative patterns.

Outcome Criteria for APD. The diagnosis of APD assumes that conduct disorders are a necessary antecedent condition that has etiological significance. However, investigators (see Robins, 1966; Rogers & Zinbarg, 1987) have long known that many youth with conduct disorders do not subsequently develop APD. From an etiological perspective, understanding the key differences between conduct-only and conduct–APD disorders would assist in the establishment of validated outcome criteria. Recent research suggests that specific developmental pathways differentiate adolescent-limited from chronic antisocial behavior (Moffit, 1993) and that gender plays an important role in these pathways (Silverthorn & Frick, 1999). Etiological models for conduct problems have implicated hyperactivity, impulsivity, and attention difficulties (see Lynam, 1996, 1998; Vitacco, Rogers, Neumann, Durant, & Collins, 2000). These research efforts are promising in their efforts to separate time-limited conduct problems from chronic APD.

Outcome criteria for APD must also be considered for middle-aged and older adults. Clearly, some individuals with APD will experience a remission or "burnout" of symptoms by the age of 40 (see Hare, McPherson, & Forth, 1988; Robins, 1966, 1985). It is likely that further remissions occur at older ages. If discriminating variables could be established as inclusion criteria, then outcome criteria could differentiate active and residual APD in older patients. Again, the usefulness of APD lies in its ability to predict accurately the course of this disorder.

Commentary of Syndeham Criteria

The Syndeham criteria provide an invaluable template for understanding the validity of mental disorders. At present, DSM-IV emphasizes inclusion criteria, with comparatively less attention to exclusion and outcome criteria. As illustrated by schizophrenia and APD, practitioners bear a heavy responsibility in applying diagnoses to disordered patients. This understanding includes an appreciation of complex differential diagnoses and an acknowledgment of predictive frailties based on available outcome criteria. Unlike their academic colleagues, practitioners must directly apply diagnostic criteria to clinical cases. For example, they must decide what to disclose to concerned parents of an adolescent exhibiting very odd behavior. Exclusion and outcome criteria for relevant disorders (e.g., schizophrenia, schizophreniform disorder, schizoid disorder, and schizotypal disorder) leave much to be desired in discussing chronicity and impairment.

Researchers face their own struggles in applying Syndeham criteria to mental disorders. The nosological framework, like most scientific enterprises, is inherently conservative. In evaluating diagnostic criteria for DSM-IV, the stated objective was to "maximize empirical input and to minimize subjectivity and bias" (Widiger, Frances, Pincus, Davis, & First, 1991, p. 286). In practice, however, acceptance of DSM-IV criteria appeared to be more influenced by their alignment with earlier DSM diagnoses than any empirical effort (see, e.g., Hare & Hart, 1995; Widiger & Corbitt, 1995). Researchers are urged to overcome nosological inertia in pressing for empirically validated exclusion and outcome criteria.

DSM-IV Diagnostic Model

The integral elements of DSM-IV are its combined emphases on a polythetic, categorical, and atheoretical diagnostic system. In addition, DSM-IV posits a multiaxial system that attempts to integrate Axis I and Axis II disorders with medical conditions (Axis III) and quantifiable ratings of psychosocial stressors and global impairment (Axes IV and V). Although elegant discussions of these elements are available (see Barlow, 1991), I distill and discuss the most salient features of DSM-IV.

Polythetic Diagnosis

Diagnosis based on polythetic models rests on the intrinsic assumptions that all inclusion criteria should be accorded equal weight and that any combination of symptoms that exceeds a predetermined cut score is sufficient to warrant the diagnosis of a mental disorder. With reference to major depression, repeated suicidal attempts and life-threatening weight loss are diagnostically equivalent to chronic fatigue and indecisiveness.[3] An untoward effect of the polythetic model is a conceptual blurring of what constitutes the prototypical features of a mental disorder. In this respect, a myriad of diagnostic combinations occur, with no notion of what constitutes a classic or prototypical example. As illustrated by APD, the number of diagnostic variations reaches millions for each successive DSM version (DSM-III, DSM-III-R, and DSM-IV; Rogers & Dion, 1991; Rogers, Salekin, Sewell, & Cruise, 2000). Lest mental health professionals view APD as a solitary outlier, other disorders also yield unwieldy numbers. When considered across prodromal, active, and residual phases, the diagnostic variations of schizophrenia exceed 9 million for DSM-III-R. For DSM-IV, the numbers are also gargantuan but unknowable because of the decision not to delineate prodromal and residual symptoms.

Diagnostic simplification is essential to diagnostic validity. For example, DSM-IV criteria for schizophrenia could be reduced by eliminating redundant and nondiscriminating symptoms. Subtyping inclusion criteria (negative vs. positive symptoms) might be conceptually justifiable and also achieve diagnostic simplification.[4] Simply pretending that diagnostic complexity does not exist is not a viable solution. In this regard, the DSM-IV decision to avoid explicit prodromal and residual criteria is a reversion to diagnostic subjectivity and contrary to stated goals of empirically validated disorders.

Categorical Diagnosis

Diagnosis within the DSM paradigm is categorical and based on nominal measurements (presence or absence) of inclusion and exclusion criteria. The chief advantage of categorical diagnosis is that clinical attention is paid to pa-

---

[3]After the diagnosis is generated, these symptoms will have a differential effect on estimates of severity.

[4]Four symptoms could be construed as "negative" (i.e., social isolation, decreased vocational efforts, blunted affect, and decreased initiative).

tients' most salient characteristics, which allow for the rapid assessment of many diverse patients (Millon, 1991). Interestingly, DSM-III-R disavowed the very basis of a categorical model (American Psychiatric Association, 1987, p. xxii): "There is no assumption that each mental disorder is a discrete entity with sharp boundaries (discontinuity) between it and other mental disorders, or between it and no mental disorder." DSM-IV (American Psychiatric Association, 1994, p. xxii) echoed this position while changing "sharp boundaries" to "absolute boundaries."

The chief alternative to the categorical model is the use of dimensional diagnoses in which severity ratings (most likely ordinal measurements) are theoretically or empirically derived to compose diagnoses. An obvious advantage of dimensional diagnoses is that discontinuity is not a necessary precondition to diagnostic validation. Interestingly enough, the DSM-IV model is not purely categorical but also includes dimensional components in several forms: (1) direct quantification, as in the case of mental retardation; (2) explicit subtyping of certain disorders on the basis of severity; and (3) presentation of severity ratings for Axes IV and V.

Frances (1982, 1985) provided a useful introduction to dimensional diagnoses. From his perspective, dimensional diagnoses provide more accurate descriptions of psychopathology and minimize the pressure to force an atypical patient into one or another diagnosis. He worries, however, that the very complexity of dimensional diagnosis may be its undoing. Could clinicians make meaningful decisions when faced with an array of dimensional ratings? As noted by Millon, several additional advantages of the dimensional approach include capturing more precise information and representing psychopathologies as continua from normality to abnormality. Dimensional models are also amenable for testing diverse models of psychopathology and include defining diagnostic-specific interpersonal styles (Clark, 1996; Pincus & Wiggins, 1990; Widiger & Frances, 1985) and circumplex models of enduring traits associated with particular disorders (Kiesler, 1983, 1986). Such multidimensional perspectives of diagnosis are likely to enrich both our descriptive and explanatory models of mental illness.

Views of categorical versus dimensional diagnoses are partly attributable to professional training (Blashfield & Livesley, 1991). Psychiatrists are typically trained to assess systematically signs and symptoms; this model corresponds to categorical diagnosis. In contradistinction, psychologists are generally steeped in psychometrics, with its emphasis on dimensional scales and ratings. Their training corresponds to dimensional diagnosis. These differences in professional training have relevance to both current assessments by multidisciplinary teams and future DSM revisions.

The adoption of a dimensional model carries unknown consequences. At present, it has not been systematically tested with respect to outcome criteria and shown to be superior to simpler categorical diagnoses. As noted by Frances (1982), the diagnostic permutations of this admittedly more sophisticated approach may thwart even the most valiant efforts at diagnostic validity. Multivariate models implicit in dimensional diagnoses still require extensive external validation (Skinner & Blashfield, 1982).

Atheoretical Diagnosis

DSM-III, DSM-III-R, and DSM-IV have attempted to circumvent strongly held and potentially divisive theoretical underpinnings (e.g., psychodynamic and biological schools) by promoting a common language and sidestepping theoretical considerations. As noted by Carson (1991, p. 306), the current atheoretical stance is likely a backlash against "the almost regal and at times arrogant dominion enjoyed by psychoanalysis in the approximately three decades after World War II." Whether DSM-III-R or DSM-IV has actually achieved its atheoretical stance differs by professional discipline: 91% of psychiatrists versus 72% of psychologists believed that this objective was achieved (Maser, Kaelber, & Weise, 1991). Faust and Miner (1986) observed that the theoretical influences are submerged but still present, and continue to inform diagnoses.

Morey (1991a) enunciated cogent arguments for the retention of theory in our current nosology. According to Morey, theory provides the underlying principles that, if empirically tested, may inform diagnosis and provide an understanding of common properties underlying different but related disorders (see also Murphy & Medlin, 1985). He cautioned against equating theory with etiology and suggested that theory may play other important roles, such as specifying determinants of treatment responsiveness.

To ignore theory is to be ignorant of it. The placement of each disorder in DSM-IV implies a conceptual framework with implicit etiological factors. Recent debates over the determinants of factitious disorders with predominantly psychological signs and symptoms (FDPS; see Cunnien, 1988; Rogers, Bagby, & Rector, 1989) centered on the production of Ganser-like symptoms. In the end, Ganser syndrome was moved from FDPS in DSM-III to dissociative disorders in DSM-III-R and DSM-IV. Likewise, the theoretically defensible home for PTSD is open to question, with nosological candidates of anxiety, depressive, and dissociative disorders (Davidson & Foa, 1991).

Multiaxial Diagnosis

DSM-IV classifies all mental disorders on Axes I and II. Axis II disorders are distinguished from Axis I largely on the basis of early onset and a stable but chronic course of the disorder (American Psychiatric Association, 1994). Within this framework, developmental and personality disorders are deemed as Axis II and all other clinical syndromes as Axis I. From an empiricist perspective, this framework demands validation. If we accept, for the sake of argument, that onset and course are the preeminent features of mental disorders, then large clinical samples could be sorted by these two principal variables (age of onset and chronicity of the syndrome). I seriously doubt whether the resulting categorization would approximate the current Axis I–Axis II dichotomy.

An important consideration is whether the four most relevant Axes (I, II, IV, and V) constitute discrete dimensions of diagnosis. Would nonoverlapping criteria from each form orthogonal dimensions when large clinical samples are subjected to factor analyses? Do these dimensions predict outcome criteria? We might also speculate regarding the interrelationships among these Axes. For example, I would hypothesize that episodes of Axis I disorders, congruent with the prevailing stress–diathesis model, would likely to be more closely related to Axis IV's psychosocial stressors than would long-standing Axis II disorders. Moreover, it would be interesting to predict overall impairment (i.e., Axis V) by regressing severity ratings on Axes I, II, and IV. Implementing a longitudinal perspective would be useful in demarcating the relative contributions of these axial ratings to Axis V impairment during subsequent episodes.

Axis IV underwent a quiet revolution between DSM-III-R and DSM-IV. DSM-III-R utilized dimensional ratings of psychosocial stressors on a 6-point scale, from none to catastrophic. Importantly, these environmental circumstances were considered "stressors" because of their contributory role in the development of a mental disorder, recurrence of a prior mental disorder, or exacerbation of an existing disorder. In stark contrast, DSM-IV dispensed with the dimensional ratings. Instead, potential problems were simply enumerated in nine broad categories; their relationship to mental disorders remains unaddressed.

What accounts for this reversionary change in Axis IV classification? The American Psychiatric Association (1991) reported problems with DSM-III-R, namely, that it was not commonly used and had apparent problems with reliability and validity. The DSM-IV draft criteria (American Psychiatric Association, 1993) adopted the simple enumeration of problems described in DSM-IV. Unwittingly, the drafters of DSM-IV have perpetuated the problems they sought to address. The reliability and validity of DSM-IV Axis IV disorders were not satisfactorily addressed. Moreover, the emphasis on only problems (i.e., potentially unrelated to mental disorders) rather than psychosocial stressors (i.e., contributors to mental disorders) reduces the clinical relevance of Axis IV.

Axis V is designed to measure global impairment, irrespective of the particular diagnosis or its clinical presentation. DSM-IV has presented the Global Assessment Functioning scale (GAF) to assess overall dysfunction; this global rating scale was borrowed, almost verbatim, from the Global Assessment Scale (GAS; Endicott, Spitzer, Fleiss, & Cohen, 1976). Although intended as a nonspecific measure of impairment, certain themes are apparent with psychosis and violence (self- and other-directed), representing key criteria for those with severe impairment. In addition, Appendix B of DSM-IV includes provisional global ratings for the assessment of relationships and social–occupational functioning.

The notion of impairment, which is implicit in nearly all diagnoses, may be conceptualized from multiple perspectives. As previously noted, Axis V has taken a symptomatic viewpoint in which certain symptoms are perceived as critical. This approach appears to obscure important facets of symptomatology, such as severity and frequency of symptoms. An apparent disparity occurs with Axis II disorders. According to DSM-IV (American Psychiatric Association, 1994), personality disorders can be diagnosed in the absence of impairment, if the patient reports subjective distress. In other words, a patient could be completely well functioning in all areas of his or her life but be unhappy about certain symptoms or characteristics and be defined as mentally ill.

What constitutes impairment resulting from a mental disorder? Table 1.2 outlines four perspectives (retrospective, prospective, normative, and individualistic) represented to varying degrees by DSM-IV Axis V. For developmental disorders, prospective and normative perspectives appear especially salient. For adult Axis I disorders, the retrospective perspective is predominant. For adult Axis II disorders, normative and individualistic perspectives are paramount. Clearly, more theoretical and empirical work is needed in articulating perspectives of impairment by DSM-IV diagnostic categories.

Building on this knowledge of assessment and diagnosis, the next section provides a critical overview of structured interviews. An understanding of this section is essential prior to application of structured interviews in professional practice or applied research.

AN OVERVIEW OF STRUCTURED INTERVIEWS

Structured interviews attempt to maximize the reliability and validity of their measurements by systematizing the assessment process. A major emphasis is

---

TABLE 1.2. Multiple Perspectives on the Definition of Impairment

A. Retrospective view
   Deterioration: The patient has evidenced an observable decline since the onset of the disorder.

B. Prospective view
   Expectations: The patient or his or her family anticipated that he or she would be better adjusted or have greater accomplishments.

   Potential: Earlier observations (e.g., intelligence or achievement testing in early grades) suggest that the patient has not optimized his or her abilities.

C. Normative view
   Deficit: On standard comparisons, the patient falls short of the average or some other accepted standard.

D. Individualistic view
   Distress: The patient experiences negative affect regarding his or her current abilities and adjustment.

the reduction of diagnostic disagreement by exerting control over information and criterion variance. As reviewed in Table 1.1, lack of standardization in clinical inquiries (information variance) and subsequent ratings (criterion variance) are enduring problems in traditional interviews. Through standardization, structured interviews minimize both information and criterion variance.

Characteristics of Structured Interviews

Structured interviews vary greatly in their focus, depth, and coverage. In addition, they can be viewed on a spectrum for ease of use from simple self-explanatory measures to more elaborate interviews. Associated with ease of use is a very different construct of "transparency," namely, the extent to which the purpose of clinical inquiries is obvious to the evaluatee. Finally, structured interviews differ in the complexity and flexibility of clinical inquiries. These characteristics are outlined below.

Breadth versus Depth

Structured interviews are confronted with the "breadth versus depth" dilemma, otherwise known as the bandwidth-fidelity issue (Widiger & Frances, 1987). Interviews with the greatest breadth (e.g., Structured Clinical Interview for DSM-IV) tend to conserve time by (1) minimizing the number of clinical inquiries and (2) screening to rule out certain disorders. In contrast, other interviews are more circumscribed in their coverage, which allows for a more in-depth coverage. For example, the Schedule of Affective Disorders and Schizophrenia (SADS) focuses primarily on psychotic and mood disorders; it devotes multiple questions to each rating and examines associated features of mental disorders. Even more focused are the single-disorder structured interviews, such as the Diagnostic Interview for Borderlines—Revised (DIB-R), which provide comprehensive coverage, but with a very narrow focus. In choosing among structured interviews, clinicians will need to weigh competing demands for depth and breadth in their selection of the most appropriate measure.

Ease of Use versus Transparency

Structured interviews vary substantially in their ease of use (also referred to as "user friendliness"; Nussbaum & Rogers, 1992). Interviews such as the Structured Clinical Interview for DSM-IV—Axis II Disorder (SCID-II) make a concerted effort to simplify administration and scoring. Listed below are three characteristics of simplified interviews, emphasizing ease of use:

1. *Criterial questions.* Do the questions only reflect the specific content of DSM-IV criteria?

2. *Unidimensional scoring.* Do affirmative answers always reflect psychopathology?
3. *Symptom clusters.* Are the symptoms organized by diagnoses? Are symptoms presented in the same order as found in DSM-IV?

Adoption of these three characteristics simplifies administration and scoring. Such ease of use is achieved at the cost of transparency. The patient has a very clear idea about the purpose of questions and is comparatively free to modify his or her responses accordingly. Transparency is not simply an abstract notion; research on psychotherapy (Shadish & Sweeney, 1991) suggests that response patterns are likely affected by the transparency of the measures used.

Structured versus Semistructured Interviews

The key difference in structured versus semistructured interviews is the flexibility allowed the clinician conducting the interview. In a structured interview, all questions must be asked verbatim. In semistructured interviews, clinicians are allowed to ask their own questions when diagnostic issues remain unresolved. Table 1.3 provides a succinct summary of clinical inquiries:

1. Structured interviews utilize standard questions and optional probes.
2. Semistructured interviews utilize standard questions, optional probes, and unstructured questions.

The advantage of structured interviews is that a high level of standardization is ensured. For example, the Diagnostic Interview Schedule (DIS) requires that interviewers follow the prescribed questions, because many interviewers have only modest clinical training. The limitation of structured interviews is that the strict adherence to formulated questions cannot cover all eventualities. For instance, a DIS interviewer may believe that a client is confused about the meaning of a question but has no means to inquire about this confusion. The comparative advantages between structured and semistructured interviews can be examined in terms of information and criterion variance.

TABLE 1.3. Types of Clinical Inquiries Used in Structured Interviews

Type of inquiries	Definitions
Standard questions	Key questions asked of all respondents
Optional probes	Clarifying questions asked if ambiguity occurs in how responses meet criteria
Unstructured questions	Nonstandardized questions formulated by the clinician to assist in the rating of responses

- Structured interviews optimize information variance, occasionally at the expense of criterion variance.
- Semistructured interviews optimize criterion variance, occasionally at the expense of information variance.

Structured Interviews and Inconsistent Data

Mental health professionals have a comparatively easy time in evaluating consistent data from the client and collateral sources. Diagnostic problems arise when significant discrepancies are noted either in the client's own reporting or between the client and collateral sources.

Discrepancies in Clinical Data

Clinicians are often confronted with seemingly inconsistent and discrepant clinical data. With traditional interviews, the problem lies in how to interpret these inconsistencies and discrepancies. Do they represent imprecision in the form and types of questions asked? Do they represent inaccuracies in recording responses? Do they represent deliberate attempts to distort the clinical presentation? Do they represent a fluctuating clinical state?

As previously noted, standardized clinical inquiries can substantially reduce information variance by minimizing variability in the structure of questions. Likewise, the standardized ratings minimize variability in recording responses and establishing clinical significance.

Clinical Presentation and Response Styles

A long-standing concern is that the clinical inquiries elicit accurate and complete information. Clinicians are concerned about patients that deliberately distort their presentations (see Rogers, 1997), either by fabricating symptomatology (malingering and factitious disorders) or denying the existence of psychological problems (defensiveness). Moreover, many patients either overemphasize or underplay their symptoms and the consequences (impairment and distress) arising from these symptoms. Early literature (e.g., Liberty, Lunneborg, & Atkinson, 1964) suggests that patients can be divided into two groups on the basis of their willingness to acknowledge psychological problems to themselves and others:

- Repressors have high threshold before acknowledging psychological difficulties.
- Sensitizers have low threshold before acknowledging psychological difficulties.

While recent studies have not grappled with the validity of these constructs, patients clearly have different thresholds for reporting symptoms of mental disorders.

Other response styles may affect the accuracy and completeness of patients' self reports. Much research interest has been generated in the examination of social desirability and acquiescence (e.g., Couch & Keniston, 1960; Wiggins, 1962), which suggests that patients are less likely to be forthright when seeking social acceptance or approval. Interestingly, when subjects are asked to be honest, they may show less willingness to disclose their symptoms and psychological problems (Goldberg & Miller, 1966). Substantial progress has been made in the assessment of social desirability (e.g., Paulhus, 1998).

Some patients may foil the assessment process by assuming a different role (e.g., a marginally employed male patient may try to present himself as a successful businessperson). Such role taking may distort the clinical presentation in subtle but important ways (see Kroger & Turnbull, 1975).

Minimizing the Effects of Response Styles

An important issue arises regarding the face validity of clinical inquiries and their order of presentation in the structured interview. Questions with high face validity have an increased liability that patients will distort their responses. Ideally, standardized clinical inquiries should not be susceptible to social desirability. If inquiries promote a response bias, then their standardization may unwittingly promote systematic disinformation.

Most diagnostic interviews are designed to be unidirectional. As previously noted, endorsement of nearly every question signifies psychopathology. The problem with this approach is that patients can easily fall into response set (e.g., denial of most psychological problems). Counterbalancing questions so that both negative and positive answers are indicative of psychopathology is one logical method of addressing response sets, such as those found with acquiescence and social desirability.

The following types of clinical inquiries minimize response sets:

1. *Neutral questions* are open-ended inquiries that do not suggest a particular response. An example from the SADS to address dysphoric mood is the following: "How have you been feeling?" Compared to a typical leading question (e.g., "Are you depressed?"), neutral questions require clients to generate their own descriptions of their moods.

2. *Counterbalanced questions* provide two alternatives that are roughly comparable in social desirability. For example, "Do you tend to take what people say on faith or do you tend to look for hidden meanings?" In this example, both alternatives might be viewed as positive or negative.

Use of corroborative data may serve two-related purposes. If the patient is aware that corroborative interviews will be used, then this knowledge may influence his or her self-reporting. Preliminary data on alcoholics (Graber & Miller, 1988) suggest that such knowledge may "keep alcoholics honest."

One possibility is for clinicians to ask for permission to contact others *prior* to conducting interviews.

A second and more common use of corroborative data is substantiation of the patient's account. Use of collateral interviews, for this purpose is a common feature of structured interviews especially for the assessment of children and Axis II disorders. Unfortunately, systematic rules for how to integrate collateral and interview data are rarely available.

How are discrepancies between self-reporting and corroborative sources resolved? Some clinicians appear to give greater weight to reports from clinical staff than from the patients themselves. The danger of this practice is the perpetuation of misinformation. Indeed, if the clinician routinely accepts the professional version, we might ask what purpose is served by reevaluating the patient? Similarly, informants (e.g., family members) are sometimes viewed as more credible, particularly when the patient is an adolescent or involved in legal proceedings. The implicit and often inaccurate assumption is that family members can be objective and do not have "their own ax to grind."

Clinicians must make decisions about discrepant material on a case-by-case basis. They are confronted with three basic alternatives. First, the clinician may judge one version to be so lacking in plausibility that it is readily discarded. Second, he or she clinician may seek further information and clarification from some combination of sources, including the patient, the informant, and others who know the patient. Third, the clinician may interpolate between the two versions and assume some intermediary position (e.g., both describe a loss of appetite and decreased eating but different levels of food intake). In the absence of guidelines from structured interviewing, clinicians must be (1) explicit about how they resolve discrepancies and (2) able to justify their conclusions to colleagues.

Reducing the Criterion Variance

Structured interviews typically include standardized ratings for reducing criterion variance. For instance, the SADS offers ratings that include descriptors and prototypical examples. Sometimes the descriptors are simply a gradation of severity (e.g., "mild," "moderate," "severe," or "extreme"); at other times, they offer either a brief characterization (e.g., "frequent obsessions or compulsions with some impairment in social or occupational functioning or daily routine") or some form of quantification (e.g., concerning weight loss, "5–10 pounds," "10–15 pounds," "15–25 pounds," or over "25 pounds"). Standardized ratings are likely to improve reliability and assist in clinical judgments (Dawes, 1979). In addition, the use of prototypical examples is likely to improve the assessment process (Blashfield, 1992).

Structured interviews also vary in the simplicity of diagnostic decision making. Interviews, such as the SCID, were designed to correspond directly to DSM-IV disorders. In contrast, other measures are more complicated in their scoring and conclusions. For example, the Psychopathy Checklist—Revised

(PCL-R) has a complex scoring system (see Rogers, Salekin, Hill, et al., 2000) because (1) criteria are tied to specific clinical inquiries, and (2) clinicians are expected to consider multiple subcriteria from several sources in rendering a single rating. The complexity of scoring introduces more opportunity for error.[5]

Psychometric Characteristics of Structured Interviewing

In the standardization of structured interviews through an examination of their psychometric properties, the usefulness of specific interviews can be evaluated in terms of reliability and validity. In addition, the clinical applicability of structured interviews is sometimes considered in light of their utility estimates. This section provides a brief overview of psychometric concepts as a template for subsequent chapters.

Reliability

A key issue in the validation of structured interviews is the establishment of their reliability, especially interrater and test–retest reliability. Reliability provides estimates regarding the consistency and reproducibility of clinical findings.

Interrater Reliability. Interrater reliability forms the most fundamental reliability measure for structured interviews. If independent clinicians cannot achieve comparable results in applying a standardized interview to the same patients, then the whole assessment is in jeopardy. How is interrater reliability established? Most commonly, two or more clinicians observe the same interview, live or through videotapes, and make independent ratings of the patient. With some measures (e.g., the PCL-R), case materials are distilled and made available to these clinicians; this procedure may inflate the level of agreement, because this standardization of documentation is not typically available in clinical practice.

For interrater reliability, categorical diagnosis is typically represented by one of three estimates:

1. Kappa coefficients (Cohen, 1960) are the most commonly used statistic; it measures the proportion of agreement corrected for observed base rates. With very low base rates, the diagnoses must be able to exceed the decision never to consider the diagnosis. For example, Grove, Andreasen, McDonald-Scott, Keller, and Shapiro (1981) demonstrated that very high accuracy (i.e., 95%) results in a kappa of .81 at 50% base rate but only .14 at 1% base rate.

2. Yule's Y is rarely used, although it has been recommended for low

---

[5]The PCL-R does produce very reliable total scores. What remains less investigated is whether the criteria and factors can be reliably assessed.

base rates (see Spitznagel & Helzer, 1985). Although not entirely independent of base rates, Yule's Y has greater stability over kappas with low to medium base rates. As an argument against Yule's Y, Shrout, Spitzer, and Fleiss (1987) observe that it is a nonlinear function, which markedly constrains its interpretability.

3. Intraclass coefficients (ICCs) are also commonly used as a measure of diagnostic reliability when more than two raters are employed (see Andreasen et al., 1981; Keller et al., 1981). These coefficients are calculated on the basis on the total variance in clinical ratings that is attributable to differences among clinicians. According to Fleiss and Cohen (1973), ICCs are equivalent to weighted kappas when used with substantial samples.

Test–Retest Reliability. Test–retest reliability involves the readministration of structured interviews after a specified interval. An important consideration is that these evaluations be independent. More specifically, it would be improper to use the same interviewer for both administrations; we could not discern whether consistent results reflected (1) the memory of the interviewer or (2) the test–retest reliability of the measure.

Test–retest reliability is far less common than interrater reliability in the validation of structured interviews (Endicott & Spitzer, 1978) but has a singular advantage of estimating the consistency across styles of questioning (i.e., information variance) as well as ratings (i.e., criterion variance). The interval between administrations may result in changes in the evaluatee (i.e., patient variance) that may potentially confound results.

Attenuation, an important phenomenon affecting test–retest reliability, reflects a tendency of evaluatees to report less symptomatology on successive interviews. Attenuation has been documented across a range of measures (e.g., Loranger, Lenzenweger, et al., 1991; Jensen, Roper, et al., 1995). In addition to attenuation, Robins (1985) observed that test–retest reliabilities may be affected by patients' attempts either to be (1) overly consistent (i.e., to remember and repeat their earlier responses) or (2) innovative (i.e., to avoid repetitiveness and offer novel information). Because of these combined influences, test–retest reliability estimates are generally lower than estimates of interrater reliability.

Test–retest reliability must be differentiated from temporal stability. The crucial difference is the interval between administrations. For test–retest reliability, the interval is relatively short, typically less than 1 month. The rationale for a short interval is the minimization of patient changes that could contaminate results. For temporal stability, the key issue is the stability of symptoms and chronicity of the disorder. Therefore, the interval is typically substantial (e.g., 6–12 months). One exception to this difference in intervals occurs when researchers are interested in establishing lifetime disorders and the interval for test–retest reliability is sometimes extended. For this type of research, Rogers (in press) has recommended a "time-lapse" model, in which the same period of time is covered by both interviews.

Internal Reliability. Some structured interviews organize items into formal scales. In these instances, the internal reliability of the scale is important. Internal consistency, most often represented as alpha coefficients, provides a partial measure of homogeneity (Clark & Watson, 1995). Many structured interviews measure clinical constructs (e.g., DSM-IV polythetic diagnosis) that are not considered formal scales. Therefore, the relevance of internal consistency to structured interviews varies markedly by the measure and its purpose.

Validity

Structured interviews rely heavily on criterion-related and construct validity. These concepts are discussed briefly.

Most structured interviews rely on a form of criterion-related validity called *concurrent validity.* Ideally, concurrent validity utilizes a "gold standard" (i.e., a well-validated and generally accepted measure) against which to validate diagnoses and other clinical constructs. Unfortunately, gold standards are rarely found in the diagnosis of mental disorders. The alternative is referred to as "bootstrapping," whereby one imprecise measure is used to validate a second measure (Robins, Helzer, Croughan, & Ratcliff, 1981). In the validation of the DIS, the structured interview was compared to traditional diagnostic interviews conducted by highly skilled clinicians.

A second form of criterion-related validity is *predictive validity,* which addresses the issue of whether some key behaviors or traits can be prognosticated. For example, does the presence of certain conduct disorder symptoms predict APD? A direct application of predictive validity for a disorder is Syndeham's criteria. As previously discussed, Syndeham's pivotal facet is outcome criteria. Simply, do the inclusion and exclusion criteria allow clinicians to predict accurately the course and outcome of the disorder/syndrome?

Construct validity examines the theoretical and empirical relationships among similar (i.e., convergent) and dissimilar (discriminant) concepts. The relationship among these variables is hypothesized as a nomological net (Cronbach & Meehl, 1955). In its application to structured interviews, construct validity is generally characterized in terms of convergent validity, convergent–discriminant validity, and discriminant validity:

1. Convergent validity addresses the relationship between similar constructs. It differs from concurrent validity in the degree of similitude: Convergent validity measures *similar* constructs, whereas concurrent validity measures nearly *identical* constructs. As a concrete example, major depression on the SADS and on the Minnesota Multiphasic Personality Inventory—2 (MMPI-2) Scale 2 (depression) are similar constructs (convergent validity); major depression on the SADS and on the DIS are nearly identical constructs (concurrent validity).

2. Convergent–discriminant validity is based on the Campbell and Fiske (1959) model of construct validity. A construct (e.g., depression) must demonstrate a stronger relationship with similar constructs (e.g., suicide) than dissimilar constructs (e.g., intelligence).[6] For example, Rogers, Sewell, Ustad, Reinhardt, and Edwards (1995) demonstrated the convergent–discriminant validity of the Schedule of Affective Disorders and Schizophrenia—Change Version (SADS-C) for schizophrenia, depression, and bipolar disorders.

3. Discriminant validity, a distinct type of validation, is separate from convergent–discriminant validity. Often based on contrasted groups design, discriminant validity refers to the ability of one or more measures to discriminate accurately between criterion groups. In the development of the Structured Interview of Reported Symptoms (SIRS; Rogers et al., 1992), different detection strategies were tested for their ability to discriminate between feigners and genuine patients.

Utility Estimates

Structured interviews concentrate on reliability and validity. In some cases, however, utility measurements are provided as measurements of an interview's accuracy. These utility estimates are typically based on independent groups that are established by clinical criteria (e.g., depressed group vs. psychotic group). Utility estimates allow clinicians to evaluate the usefulness of a measure with a specific cut score to classify different criterion groups accurately.

In the absence of gold standards for most diagnoses and clinical constructs, utility estimates are not often used to test the accuracy of structured interviews per se. Instead, they are often used for screening purposes. For example, clinicians are likely interested in knowing what cut score on the Beck Depression Inventory would justify the administration of the SADS or SCID. Utility estimates could provide clinicians with highly useful data on the best cut score, depending on the clinical setting and other relevant variables.

Table 1.4 provides a summary of the commonly used utility estimates. As a simple guide, the following issues should be considered:

- What is the meaning of a score to an individual case? If above the cut score, positive predictive power (PPP) estimates the likelihood that the person has the disorder/condition. If below the cut score, negative predictive power (NPP) estimates the likelihood that the person does not have the disorder/condition.
- Is this measure generally useful? *Sensitivity* estimates the proportion of persons with the disorder/condition that will be correctly identified by

[6]The terminology for construct validity includes the following: (1) Convergent validity is determined by "monotrait–heteromethod" (i.e., correlations of similar constructs from different measures) coefficients; (2) discriminant validity is determined by "heterotrait–monomethod" (i.e., intercorrelations within the same measure) and "heterotrait–heteromethod" (i.e., correlations between dissimilar constructs across measures) coefficients.

TABLE 1.4. Utility Estimates of Diagnostic Validity

A. Schematization of the tested measure against the "gold standard"

"Gold standard" determination

Measure to be tested	Present	Absent
Present	(a) True positives	(b) False positives
Absent	(c) False negatives	(d) True negatives

B. Common utility estimates

Utility estimate	Definition with algebraic notation in parentheses
Positive predictive power (PPP)	True positives ÷ the sum of true and false positives ($a \div a + b$)
Negative predictive power (NPP)	True negatives ÷ the sum of true and false negatives ($d \div c + d$)
Sensitivity	True positives ÷ the sum of true positives and false negatives ($a \div a + c$)
Specificity	True negatives ÷ the sum of true negatives and false positives ($d \div b + d$)
Hit rate	True positives + true negatives ÷ total number ($a + d \div a + b + c + d$)

the cut score. *Specificity* estimates the proportion of persons without the disorder/condition that will be correctly identified by the cut score.

ORGANIZATION OF THE CHAPTERS

Structured interviews have enjoyed a phenomenal if uneven growth during the last several decades. As a result, some structured interviews are well established, with a major body of empirical literature. Other structured interviews are less well developed but offer promising research. To accommodate this unevenness, the subsequent chapters also vary in their depth and breadth. Some chapters are devoted to single interviews, when justified by their clinical significance and empirical research. Other chapters provide greater coverage, with less depth of different interviews.

The general format for structured interviews has three major components:

1. The *Overview* section includes a description of the interview and its development.
2. The *Validation* section examines clinical data on the interview's reliability, validity, and generalizability.
3. The *Clinical Applications* section summarizes how clinicians can apply this structured interview in their practices.

TABLE 1.5. Standardized Format for Reliability Studies

Study (year)	N	Setting In/Out/Com/ Corr/Univ	Dx	Raters Lay/Prof	Reliability Inter/Retest (interval)	Reliability estimates Sx/Cur-Dx/ Life-Dx/Other

Glossary of key concepts

- Study (year) = an abbreviated citation for the study; the full cite is included in the references.
- N = the total number of participants included in the reliability portion of the study.
- For the setting: In = inpatient; Out = outpatient; Com = community; Corr = correctional facility; Univ = university. Multiple checks means that the reliability sample was taken from more than one setting.
- Dx = the number of diagnoses used in the reliability portion of the study.
- For raters: Lay = nonprofessional raters; Prof = professionals with graduate training.
- For reliability: Inter = interrater reliability; Retest = test–retest reliability; Interval = lapsed time between first and second administrations.
- For reliability estimates: Sx = symptoms; Cur-Dx = current diagnosis; Life-Dx = lifetime diagnosis; Other = other composite scales for summarizing data.

Interrater and test–retest reliability are the sine qua non in the validation of structured interviews. To ensure uniformity in the review of structured interviews, interrater and test–retest reliability are presented in a standardized format. Table 1.5 presents a model of this format, with a glossary of key concepts.

The chapters are organized logically into four major sections. The first two sections address Axis I and Axis II interviews, respectively. The third section examines specific application of structured interviews. The fourth and final section comprises summary chapters that integrate earlier chapters and address overarching issues of professional practice and clinical research.

2

Historical Foundations for Structured Interviews: Mental Status Examinations (MSEs)

The historical foundation of structured interviews can be traced to one predominant source, namely, mental status examinations (MSEs), which were first introduced into American psychiatry by Adolf Meyer in 1917 (Tilley & Hoffman, 1981). Beyond their historical importance, MSEs continue to influence the standardization of clinical assessment and diagnostic decision making. This chapter briefly outlines the development of MSEs and their impact on current structured interviews.

As an overview, an MSE is a heterogenous construct that encompasses both standardized and nonstandardized observations and inquiries of the patient. Within standardized formats, the content and structure of MSEs can also vary significantly. For instance, in his survey of psychiatric training programs, Engel (1979) found that 56 different MSEs were in use. These measures can be divided into *comprehensive* and *cognitive* MSEs.

- "Comprehensive" MSEs are designed to (1) measure both cognitive impairment and psychopathology, and (2) provide a template for diagnosis. Examples include the Mental Status Evaluation Record (MSER; Spitzer & Endicott, 1970) and the Missouri Mental Status (MMS; Sletten, Ernhart, & Ulett, 1970).
- "Cognitive" MSEs provide a standardized evaluation of memory and other intellectual functions. Examples include the Mental Status Questionnaire (MSQ; Kahn, Goldfarb, Pollack, & Peck, 1960), the Short Portable Mental Status Questionnaire (SPMSQ; Pfeiffer, 1975), the Mini-Mental State Examination (MMSE; Folstein, Folstein, & McHugh, 1975), the Cognitive Capacity Screening Examination (CCSE; Jacobs, Bernhard, Delgado, &

Strain, 1977), the Cambridge Cognitive Examination (CAMCOG; Roth et al., 1986), and the Neurobehavioral Cognitive Status Examination (NCSE or COGNISTAT; Schwamm, VanDyke, Kiernan, Merrin, & Mueller, 1987).

Comprehensive and cognitive MSEs are reviewed in separate sections. The main objective is a straightforward analysis of their development and contributions to structured interviews. A secondary objective with cognitive MSEs is a practice-oriented synopsis of their current clinical applications.

COMPREHENSIVE MSEs

Dissatisfaction with traditional interviews and nonrigorous diagnoses led to the development of comprehensive MSEs. For example, the MSER and MMS were devised in conjunction with state mental health programs as methods of standardizing relevant clinical data. Despite large-scale efforts, the MSER and MMS did not achieved widespread acceptance among psychiatrists and other clinical staff. While these measures clearly had limitations, a compelling hypothesis is that their nonacceptance and, occasionally, outright rejection reflects fears of encroachment on the otherwise unquestioned domain of seasoned diagnosticians. The very notion of standardization was perceived an affront to clinicians' acumen and diagnostic/dynamic insight. While essentially muted in recent years, negative reactions to standardized assessments continue, at least implicitly. As a concrete example, the majority of clinicians find reasons *not* to use Axis II interviews despite major accomplishments in the last decade. This implicit rejection of Axis II interviews constitutes a general parallel to the widespread rebuffing of comprehensive MSEs.

Mental Status Evaluation Record (MSER)

Development

Spitzer and Endicott (1970) developed the MSER. A primary emphasis of the MSER is the systematic reporting of clinical data in New York state facilities. Contentwise, the MSER furnishes operational definitions of the criteria and concomitant ratings of symptomatology on five gradations: "none," "slight," "mild," "moderate," and "marked." Of these clinical ratings, 50 are deemed essential for all patients in assessment of key symptoms and features. Altogether, clinical ratings are rendered for a total 392 descriptors organized into 172 clinical characteristics. The MSER was intended to provide highly systematized, extensive clinical description of patients. Its data served clinical purposes in facilitating diagnosis and research objectives via standardized symptom ratings.

A distinguishing characteristic of the MSER is its emphasis on observational data. Nearly one-half of the MSER can be completed simply through detailed clinical observations. For example, MSER clinical ratings address the following:

- Physical appearance (e.g., apparent deformities, posture, and dressing and grooming).
- Psychomotor behavior (e.g., tremors, tics, and posturing).
- Interpersonal behavior (e.g., facial expressions and eye contact).
- Speech and thought disturbances (e.g., volume, rate, productivity, incoherence, circumstantiality, loosening of associations, and concreteness).
- Mood in terms of both type (e.g., depression, and anxiety) and quality (e.g., flatness, inappropriateness, and lability).

The MSER is designed to provide systematic ratings of psychopathology, with an emphasis on psychotic symptoms (delusions and hallucinations, bizarre or atypical ideation), somatic functioning and concerns, and interpersonal characteristics (overall attitude and behavior). Symptoms of mood disorders are embedded in a variety of categories, including (1) nonpsychotic thoughts, (2) somatic functioning, and (3) mood and affect. Comparatively less attention is paid to cognitive deficits, although the sensorium (e.g., orientation, recent and remote memory, and clouding of consciousness), attention, distractibility, and a gross estimate of intellectual functioning are evaluated. Consideration is also given to overt expressions of anger and any prior suicide attempts.

Reliability and Validity

Validation of the MSER relied predominantly on psychometric methods developed for traditional testing. Endicott, Spitzer, and Fleiss (1975) evaluated the internal consistency and reliability of the MSER. On the initial sample of 2,001 inpatients, a median alpha of .83 was established, with a comparable estimate of internal consistency (median alpha = .78) on an additional sample of 1,000 psychiatric patients. On a smaller sample, MSER interrater reliabilities for 90 patients ranged from .36 to 1.00, with a median ICC of .75. Test–retest reliabilities for three closely related studies (total N = 119) were generally modest, with median ICC for the three studies of .35, .36, and .50. As the authors suggested, changes in clinical status might explain these results, with an interval between new admissions and retesting as long as 2 weeks.

Endicott et al. (1975) addressed the MSER construct validity on 2,001 inpatients. From 152 clinical variables, they extracted a total of 20 factors that covered a broad spectrum of psychopathology. Factor loadings, variance accounted for, and eigenvalues were not reported for each factor. Moreover, six of the 20 factors appeared to have poor representation with three or fewer items. A reanalysis of these data with confirmatory factor analysis (CFA) would be instructive; it is unlikely that a 20-factor solution explains the underlying dimensions of the MSER.

Endicott et al. (1975) reported additional validity studies. They contrasted inpatients with psychiatric outpatients and patients' relatives. Not surprisingly, they found differences on many of the 20 scales in the expected direction. More stringent tests of the MSER's clinical utility yielded meaningful differences between paranoid and nonparanoid schizophrenics, and organic and nonorganic elderly patients. Furthermore, Endicott et al. were able to document clinical changes in psychiatric patients following inpatient treatment.

In summary, the MSER provides a fairly comprehensive review of symptomatology and clinical observations. As with all measures, the clinical utility of the MSER is highly dependent on how it is used and the available alternatives. In clinical settings where the standard of practice had been idiosyncratic evaluations of varying quality, the MSER offered an incremental improvement in standardizing the assessment and offering a basis of comparison for diagnoses and treatment outcomes.

Contributions of the MSER to Structured Interviews

The MSER was an ambitious attempt to classify and rate Axis I symptomatology. While its influence on the subsequent development of the SADS is obvious from authorship, the MSER appears instrumental in the development of Axis I interviews in general. Three key points are summarized:

1. The MSER attempted to reduce information variance by specifying the clinical coverage needed for a comprehensive assessment of Axis I symptoms and features. Subsequently, structured interviews further decreased information variance by the specification of clinical inquiries.
2. The MSER attempted to reduce criterion variance by defining key terms, offering clear examples, and providing gradations. Besides definitions and examples, structured interviews have added crucial descriptors and examples for their gradations.
3. The MSER attempted to validate empirically its conceptualization of psychopathology. Its investigations sought to evaluate underlying dimensions in the form of scales and to investigate their internal consistency. Several Axis I interviews have also sought to develop summary scales and test them empirically.

The MSER is also instructive for further development of structured interviews. In the last several decades, structured interviews have deemphasized clinical description. The thoughtful combination of clinical description and clinical inquiries is likely to provide the most comprehensive assessment of mental disorders. In addition, the clinical description of the patient's responses to clinical inquires is likely to be productive. For example, increased suspiciousness or reticence following questions about paranoid ideation may be diagnostically significant.

The MSER's efforts to establish homogeneous scales should not go unnoticed by investigators of structured interviews. Although many structured interviews are closely related to DSM and International Classification of Diseases (ICD) diagnoses, the homogeneity of specific disorders is worthy of investigation. Research could benefit both diagnoses and structured interviews, especially in studies of near-neighbor comparisons (e.g., schizophrenia and schizotypal personality disorder) that utilize several interview-based measures.

Missouri Mental Status (MMS)

Description

Beginning in 1966, the Missouri mental health system began to standardize and automate a group of seven clinical measures that included the MMS (Sletten & Evenson, 1972). Conceptualized as an integrated system, the Missouri program followed the inpatient and outpatient interventions on more than 180,000 patients with computer-based approaches to psychological testing, patient histories, treatment, and community adjustment (Altman, Evenson, Hedlund, & Cho, 1978). As a comprehensive system, less attention was paid to each of the specific measures such as the MMS.

The MMS is composed of 120 clinical ratings presented in a single-page format. As with the MSER, most of the attention was paid to the rating of symptomatology (i.e., "none," "mild," "moderate," and "severe") rather than to the provision of clinical inquiries. Its first four sections are devoted to clinical observations regarding appearance (e.g., facial expression and dress), motor activity (e.g., amount of activity, tremors and tics, repetitive acts), speech (e.g., amount, rate, and volume), and interview behavior (affect-based behavior toward the interviewer). One section is dedicated to mood and affect, while two sections address disturbances in thinking as characterized by formal thought disorders (e.g., circumstantiality, perseveration, and loosening of associations) and thought content (e.g., suicidal ideation, obsessions, sexual preoccupation, delusions, and hallucinations). Cognitive abilities are subsumed under two sections: sensorium (e.g., orientation, concentration, and memory) and intellect (e.g., serial 7's, abstraction, vocabulary, and overall ability).

Sletten, Ernhart, and Ulett (1970) attempted to establish the interrater reliability of the MMS with only modest success. The great majority of the individual ratings have poor ICCs (< .40) based on 18 videotaped interviews. Moreover, given the MMS's lack of standardization for clinical inquiries, the videotaped format, with all the questions remaining identical, is likely to provide an *overestimate* of the MMS's reliability. Sletten et al. regrouped MMS items into symptom clusters that make conclusions regarding the reliability of specific MMS sections difficult to apply.

Hedlund, Evenson, Sletten, and Cho (1980) summarized 10 validity studies that employ the MMS in establishing psychiatric diagnosis, predicting response to treatment, and evaluating management problems. Key findings are summarized as follows:

- The MMS has only modest success as a diagnostic measure. Cross-validated results on 3,278 outpatients revealed a concordance rate of approximately 55% (Altman, Evenson, & Cho, 1976).
- The MMS was moderately successful at predicting treatment issues. In particular, multivariate models classified the types of medication administered (Altman, Evenson, & Sletten, 1973; Evenson, Altman, Sletten, & Cho, 1973; Evenson, Altman, Cho, & Sletten, 1974a, 1974b; Sletten, Altman, Evenson, & Cho, 1973) and length of hospitalization (Altman, Angle, Brown, & Sletten, 1972).
- The MMS has mixed success in predicting aggressive behavior toward self and others (Altman, Evenson, & Cho, 1977; Hedlund, Sletten, Altman, & Evenson, 1973). In a cross-validation on 2,762 patients, researchers were able to rule out suicidal attempts in nearly all cases (95.7%) but were less successful at identifying those with prior attempts (44.9%). From the MMS, suicidal thoughts, hypochondriasis, flat affect, and the absence of persecutory delusions contributed to these classifications. Similarly, researchers were able to rule out nearly all patients who did not have a past history of physical aggression (95.9%) but correctly identified only about one-third (34.4%) of aggressive patients. Items from the MMS that contributed to this prediction were assaultive ideas, angry outbursts, impulsive behavior, and nonacceptance of hospitalization. These classification rates reflect the challenges of attempting to predict infrequent multidetermined behavior.

Contributions of the MMS to Structured Interviews

The MMS, like the MSER, attempts to reduce information and criterion variance through the standardization of symptoms and ratings. In addition, the MMS offers the following two contributions to structured interviews:

1. The MMS has set a rigorous standard in its insistence on extensive cross-validation with large diverse samples.
2. The MMS has provided a template for criterion-related validation of diagnostic measures. Rather than be content with several closely related criteria, the MMS has evaluated a broad array of relevant clinical variables via sophisticated multivariate methods.

The MMS has been instrumental in the development of other assessment methods. As a salient example, the MMS was utilized in an impressive study of MMPI correlates, with clinical characteristics validated and cross-validated on monumental samples (> 10,000) for each phase (Gynther, Altman, & Sletten, 1973). The rigor and magnitude of this MMS correlate research remains unmatched.

The MMS also illustrates two competing goals of assessment measures: (1) condensation of the instrument versus (2) comprehensiveness in describing clinical constructs and criterion-based ratings. Although a typographical feat (120 ratings on a single page), the MMS sacrifices easily accessible descriptions for its implementation. As a recent parallel, the Psychopathy Checklist: Screening Version (PCL:SV; see Chapter 11) was strikingly simplified by the removal of descriptors and subcriteria from its answer sheet. While these valuable guides are available in the test manual, the question remains whether the condensation of the PCL answer sheet was achieved at the expense of comprehensiveness and accuracy.

Conclusions Regarding Comprehensive MSEs

Today, comprehensive MSEs have more historical importance than clinical relevance. Both the MSER and the MMS have been subjected to extensive research as methods of standardizing the assessment of psychopathology and improving clinical diagnosis. Research on the MSER laid the crucial groundwork for the subsequent development of the SADS. Studies with the MMS and its family of related measures provided a useful paradigm for the diagnosis, treatment, and community adjustment of persons with severe mental disorders.

Comprehensive MSEs set the stage for the later development of structured interviews. They provided a model for the systematic coverage of psychopathology and made advances in the reduction of information and criterion variance via increased standardization. The resulting measures (e.g., MSER and MMS) were tested extensively with respect to their reliability and validity.

COGNITIVE MSEs

Cognitive MSEs were developed during the last four decades to screen patients for possible cognitive dysfunction and organic involvement. Cognitive MSEs are steeped in tradition; many test items are included more out of tradition and convention than for their diagnostic value. For example, the use of serial 7's, originated by Kraepelin in 1907, and has been incorporated with several variations into cognitive MSEs. As noted by Smith (1967), however, more than 40% of normals make at least one error, and approximately one-fourth (24.2%) make 3–12 errors. Keller and Manschreck (1981) have questioned the use of serial 7's because of their poor discriminant validity. The interpretation of proverbs is another example of tradition rather than empiricism. Proverbs are included on cognitive MSEs as a measure of abstract thinking. Although proverbs typically embody a generalization, accurate interpretation of proverbs is unlikely to assess abstract reasoning. In many instances, the correct interpretation of a proverb is based on overlearned, conventionalized thinking (Lancker, 1990). For example, the meaning of "look before you leap" is typically learned at an early age. Additionally, proverbs are likely to be culturally dependent, thereby limiting their clinical applicability (Tancredi, 1987). Finally, the scoring of proverbs as customarily employed in MSEs is often unreliable (Andreasen, 1977).

The following sections briefly review the development of cognitive MSEs and their parallels to structured interviews. Unlike comprehensive MSEs, cognitive MSEs appear to have only a marginal influence on the later emergence of structured interviews. Still, cognitive MSEs may provide instructive examples for the further development and clinical application of structured interviews. First-generation cognitive MSEs (i.e., MSQ, SPMSQ, MMSE, and CCSE) are very brief measures with considerable item overlap. Nelson, Fogel, and Faust (1986) provide a masterful overview of their development and initial validation. The second generation of cognitive MSEs (i.e., CCSE, CAMCOG, and NCSE) has more extensive measures that cover a wider range of cognitive functions.

First-Generation Cognitive MSEs

Mental Status Questionnaire (MSQ)

Description. Kahn et al. (1960) recognized a major problem with misdiagnoses that affected thousands of elderly patients and resulted in their indefinite institutionalization in nursing and other health care facilities. They observed that many elderly patients with obvious cognitive problems were automatically assumed to suffer from dementia with an underlying progressive disease. As an alternative, they found "pseudodementia," in which cognitive difficulties are sequelae of depression. Once the patients were treated for depression, the cognitive deficits were largely resolved. The brilliance of Kahn et al. lay in their recognition of a crucial diagnostic issue and their straightforward efforts to address it.

Kahn et al. (1960) sought to identify simple items that discriminate between true dementia and pseudodementia. They identified 10 items related to orientation, personal information, and general knowledge. These items were tested with institutionalized elderly.

Reliability and Validity. MSQ research has established excellent reliability for its total score. For example, Foster, Sclan, Welkowitz, Boksay, and Seeland (1988) found very high interrater reliability ($r = .99$) on 40 psychiatric patients for both psychiatrists and research assistants. In addition, Lesher and Whelihan (1986) administered the MSQ and seven other MSE measures to 36 nursing home residents in a test–retest design at 2- to 4-week intervals. They found that the MSQ had excellent overall reliability as evidenced by internal consistency (alpha = .81), split-half reliability ($r = .82$), and test–retest reliability ($r = .87$).

Kahn et al. (1960) performed the original validation on 1,077 institutionalized patients from state mental hospitals, nursing homes, and homes for the aged. Nearly all patients with no errors on the MSQ had mild or no cognitive impairment; conversely, nearly all patients that completely failed the MSQ had moderate to severe impairment. However, middle-range scores were apparently less discriminating, although these percentages were not reported. With respect to concurrent validity, Fillenbaum (1980) reported a sensitivity of 55% and a specificity of 96% for diagnosis of organic mental disorder in a community sample of 83 elderly persons.

Researchers also evaluated the MSE's convergent validity. Key findings are summarized as follows:

- Lautenschlaeger, Meier, and Donnelly (1986) found high rates of agreement between the MSQ and the MMSE for both severely impaired and unimpaired participants, but poor agreement for moderately impaired individuals.
- Lesher and Whelihan (1986) found a generally high correlation ($Mr = .90$) between the MSQ and seven other MSE measures, including the SPMSQ and lesser-known MSE measures.
- Reid, Tierney, Zorzitto, Snow, and Fisher (1991) conducted a large clinical study of the MSQ with 162 patients with dementia (i.e., Alzheimer's, Parkinson's, and other etiologies) and 102 neurologically normal participants. They found that the MSQ had a moderately high correlation ($r = -.79$) with the London Psychogeriatric Rating Scale (Hersch, Kral, & Palmer, 1978) and significantly predicted organic diagnosis.

Short Portable Mental Status Questionnaire (SPMSQ)

Pfeiffer (1975) developed the SPMSQ based on the MSQ. The SPMSQ differs from the MSQ by the addition of three items: telephone number, mother's family name, and serial 3's. The SPMSQ evaluates orientation to time (day of the week and date) and place (name of the place and street address), memory of personal (birth date, age, telephone number, and mother's family name) and public information (current president and his predecessor), and concentration (serial 3's). Pfeiffer proposed four classes of intellectual functioning based on SPMSQ scores and educational levels: intact functioning, and mild, moderate, and severe impairment.

One cause for concern in the initial normative sample ($N = 939$) was pronounced differences in individual-item failure rates for Anglo Americans ($M = 11.1\%$) and African Americans ($M = 21.8\%$). Similar differences were observed in a subsequent clinical study of 141 patients, in which three times more African American than Anglo American patients had seven or more errors. To account for these differences, Pfeiffer proposed a cut score one point lower for African Americans. Unfortunately, he did not offer an explanation for this scoring modification.

Reliability and Validity. Pfeiffer (1975) conducted the original test–retest reliability (4-week interval) of the SPMSQ on two small samples of elderly participants and found moderately high correlations of .82 and .83. In a previously cited study, Lesher and Whelihan (1986) reported high overall reliability for the SPMSQ with respect to internal consistency (alpha = .83), split-half reliability ($r = .95$), and test–retest reliability ($r = .82$).

Pfeiffer (1975) evaluated the concurrent validity of the SPMSQ on elderly patients and elderly participants residing in institutions. Most patients (92.3%) with moderate to severe impairment on the SPMSQ were diagnosed with organic brain syndrome (OBS). The SPMSQ was much less effective with the institutional sample; only 7 of 27 patients with OBS (25.9%) had low scores on the SPMSQ. Nelson et al. (1986) summarized early validity studies with the SPMSQ that revealed differences in SPMSQ scores for cognitively intact and impaired participants. Christensen, Hadzi-Pavlovic, and Jacomb (1991) conducted a meta-analysis of three SPMSQ studies and found a mean effect size that was slightly lower than other MSEs (2.39 vs. 2.73) but superior to many neuropsychological tests and subtests (i.e., their *M* effect size = 1.84).

Studies have also addressed the convergent validity of the SPMSQ. Key findings are summarized as follows:

- Foreman (1987) examined the intercorrelations of three MSEs on 66 elderly medical inpatients. For the SPMSQ, correlations were high with the MMSE ($r = .83$) and moderate with the CCSE ($r = .63$).
- Dalton, Pederson, Blom, and Holmes (1987) in a study of 40 Veterans Administration (VA) patients found that performance on the SPMSQ did not correlate significantly with either clinical diagnosis (phi = .20) or neuropsychological data (phi = .24).
- Skurla, Rogers, and Sunderland (1988) found that the SPMSQ was correlated with severity of dementia ($r = .60$), but unrelated to daily living tasks ($r = .14$).

Like the MSQ, the SPMSQ has relatively modest sensitivity and generally acceptable specificity. In other words, low scores on the SPMSQ typically signal organic impairment. In contrast, participants with mild dementias are unlikely to be detected by the SPMSQ. As observed by Dalton et al. (1987), clinicians should avoid drawing conclusions from "normal" scores on the SPMSQ alone, because of the very real possibility of undetected cognitive impairment.

Mini-Mental State Examination (MMSE)

Folstein et al. (1975) devised the MMSE for the quantitative assessment of cognitive performance. They described the MMSE as "mini" because of its exclusion of psychopathology, but believed it constituted a thorough review of cognitive functions. Based on earlier work (see, e.g., Shapiro, Post, Lofving, & Inglis, 1956), they constructed the MMSE in two sections, with the first requiring only verbal responses and the second necessitating reading and behavioral responses. The MMSE consists of 11 items that entail the following: orientation (time and place), naming of objects, serial 7's, remembering objects, following directions, writing a sentence, and copying a geometric figure. Rovner and Folstein (1987) provided detailed instructions on its administration.

Reliability and Validity. The overall reliability of the MMSE is consistently high. With one exception (i.e., Olin & Zelinski, 1991), studies of both interrater and test–retest reliabilities (Bird, Canino, Rubio-Stipec, & Shrout, 1987; Dick et al., 1984; Folstein et al., 1975; Foster et al., 1988; Uhlmann, Larson, & Buchner, 1987) exceed .80 when administered to neurological patients, patients with mental disorders, and community samples. The exception (Olin & Zelinski, 1991) found a poor test–retest reliability. However, these results can be explained by the use of nondemented participants whose MMSE scores (1) were unimpaired (first testing, $M = 28.08$; second testing, $M = 27.68$) and (2) reflected small differences (i.e., 82% of the sample had differences ≤ 1). Nelson et al. (1986) summarized the early concurrent validity studies that found MMSE differences among criterion groups (dementia, nonorganic disorders, and normals), although the use of specific cut scores may produce significant misclassifications. For example, the recommended cut score (< 24) resulted in high numbers of false positives for those with less than an eighth-grade education (Anthony, Le Resche, Niaz, Von Korff, & Folstein, 1982) and the very elderly (Bleeker, Bolla-Wilson, Kawas, & Agnew, 1988).

Research has examined the discriminability of MMSE scores in differentiating dementia from other disorders. For individual MMSE items, Rosen and Fox (1986) examined discriminant validity for patients with dementia and those with other diagnoses (i.e., depressive, bipolar, schizophrenic, and substance abuse disorders). Patients with dementia were clearly differentiated from others in terms of orientation, spelling "world" backwards, words recalled and serial 7's. On total MMSE scores, Christensen et al. (1991) performed a meta-analysis on 12 studies of the MMSE. In differentiating between patients with and without dementia, they found slightly higher mean effect sizes for the MMSE than several other MSEs and many neuropsychological measures. Christensen et al.'s data provide strong evidence of discriminant validity for the MMSE, including ratings of severity ("mild," "mild–moderate," and "severe").

Folstein, Anthony, Parhad, Duffy, and Gruenberg (1985), as part of the

NIMH epidemiological studies in Baltimore, examined the MMSE for 810 community participants evaluated by psychiatrists and 34 participants referred for complete neurological assessments. They found no differences in MMSE performance based on race or sex. Very few participants without dementia or delirium scored in the impaired range on the MMSE. They concluded that the MMSE should be employed for screening rather than diagnosis.

Criterion-related validity of the MMSE has also included evidence of neurological impairment, with mixed results with respect to brain lesions and atrophy. The key findings are summarized as follows:

- DePaulo and Folstein (1978) found that MMSE cut scores (< 24) identified only a minority of neurological patients with brain lesions.
- Tsai and Tsuang (1979) found that MMSE differentiated between patients with positive (i.e., pathological) and negative computerized tomographic (CT) scans. On closer inspection, however, the MMSE was effective only when cerebral atrophy occurred, but not with focal lesions alone. Patients with cerebral atrophy were distinguishable from others by their total MMSE scores, orientation, registration, and recall.
- Dick et al. (1984) found that the MMSE differentiated approximately three-fourths of patients with cerebral lesions but was consistently ineffective among patients with right-hemisphere lesions.
- Prohovnik, Smith, Sackeim, Mayeux, and Stern (1989) found a modest positive correlation ($r = .39$) between the loss of grey matter in patients with dementia and scores on the MMSE.
- Using neuroimaging, van Gorp et al. (1999) found that the MMSE traditional cut score (< 24) was approximately 77% accurate in differentiating between patients with dementia and normals; this percentage increased dramatically with a higher cut score (≤ 26).

The convergent validity of the MMSE has also been examined in relationship to intellectual functioning of the Wechsler Adult Intelligence Scale (WAIS). For example, in a small sample of mixed diagnoses, Folstein et al. (1975) found substantial correlations between the MMSE and Verbal (.78) and Performance (.66) IQ. From a sample of Alzheimer's patients, Farber, Schmitt, and Logue (1988) found a high correlation of .83 between the MMSE and the WAIS-R Full Scale IQ. In a study of 37 neurological patients, Dick et al. (1984) found somewhat lower correlations for Verbal ($r = .45$) and Performance ($r = .58$) IQs. Overall, these results are very positive considering that many cases of dementia do not affect all facets of patients' intellectual functioning.

Research on the MMSE in relationship to neuropsychological testing has been less encouraging. Faustman, Moses, and Csernansky (1990) employed the Luria–Nebraska Neuropsychological Battery as a criterion measure for evaluating the efficacy of the MMSE. They found that the MMSE only identified approximately 20% of inpatients with clear evidence of cognitive impairment. McBride-Houtz (1993) administered the MMSE and two other MSEs (i.e., CCSE and NCSE) to geriatric patients, with the Halstead–Reitan Neuropsychological Test Battery as the criterion measure. A moderate correlation of −.60 was found between the MMSE and the global performance score of the Halstead–Reitan (i.e., General Neuropsychological Deficit Scale; Reitan & Wolfson, 1988). However, categorizations of impaired and unimpaired participants yielded a disappointing sensitivity of 20% for the MMSE. All mildly impaired patients were missed by the MMSE. One major constraint of the study was that nearly every patient was impaired (i.e., 50 of 52); therefore, estimates for specificity were inadequately represented.

The MMSE has also been used to document progressive decline in patients with dementia. A large-scale study by Clark, Sheppard, et al. (1999) found that substantial variations in MMSE scores for sequential administrations obscured differences in cognitive functioning for patients with probable Alzheimer's disease. Over extended periods ($\geq$ 3 years), the expected decline was observed.

In summary, the MMSE is a brief and highly reliable screen for cognitive functions. Although influenced by educational status (Uhlmann & Larson, 1991), validity data would suggest the MMSE may be effective in screening patients with moderate to severe dementia. The danger with the MMSE, as with other first-generation cognitive MSEs, is the assumption that "normal" scores are, by themselves, evidence that patients are cognitively intact.

Spanish Translation. Several studies have investigated the clinical utility of a Spanish MMSE translation. The MMSE was originally translated as part of the Epidemiological Catchment Area program (ECA; Karno, Burnam, Escobar, Hough, & Eaton, 1983). Escobar et al. (1986) administered the MMSE to 1,244 Mexican Americans. They found that three orientation items (season, state, and county), two memory and calculation items (serial 7's and spelling "world" backwards), and one language item (repeating a sentence) appeared ethnically biased.[1] Bird et al. (1987) modified the MMSE to make it more appropriate to the Puerto Rican culture, addressing seasons of the year, orientation (i.e., Puerto Rico has no states or counties), and several linguistic changes.

Several Diagnostic Interview Schedule (DIS; see Chapter 3) studies incorporating the MMSE evaluate its psychometric properties. Burnam, Karno, Hough, Escobar, and Forsythe (1983) suggested a high test–retest reliability for OBS on Spanish–Spanish administrations (kappa = .88) and English–English administrations (kappa = .79), but low levels of agreement for Spanish–English administrations (kappa = .32). These results reflect only indirectly on the MMSE, since other components of the DIS also address organic-

---

[1]Items were deemed to be ethically biased if Spanish-speaking respondents scored significantly lower than English-speaking participants. Of course, other factors (e.g., unknown sampling biases) could contribute to these differences.

ity. More germane is a study by Canino et al. (1987b) in which cognitive impairment was reevaluated (Spanish–Spanish administrations), resulting in a moderate reliability (kappa = .69).

Community surveys reveal small but statistically significant differences. Combining three surveys of older persons, Mungas, Reed, Marshall, and Gonzalez (2000) found slight decrements ($M = 2.9$) in Spanish compared with English MMSEs, which may be partially attributable to educational differences. The variability of MMSE scores was much greater for the Spanish ($SD = 4.1$) than the English ($SD = 2.5$) administrations.

Cognitive Capacity Screening Examination (CCSE)

Description. Jacobs et al. (1977) developed the CCSE as a more extensive MSE than its predecessors (MSQ, SPMSQ, and MMSE). While the CCSE covered similar cognitive tasks (orientation, concentration, serial 7's, repetition, verbal concept formation, and short-term recall), it placed a greater emphasis on the recall of numbers (forwards and backwards) and simple calculations. Patients were also questioned regarding three antonyms and three similarities. Although the CCSE is described as a 30-item MSE, sequential subtractions for serial 7's are counted as six items. One major difference between the CCSE and other cognitive MSEs is that the CCSE does not include any items from long-term memory based on either personal history or common knowledge.

Reliability and Validity. The original study by Jacobs et al. (1977) simply reported the overall concordance of three clinicians on 6 participants. More recently, Haddad and Coffman (1987) reported excellent test–retest reliabilities ($r = .87$) on 49 elderly participants at 1-week intervals. In a previously cited study, Foreman (1987) found a high internal consistency for the CCSE (alpha = .97).

A brief report by Carnes, Gunter-Hunt, and Rodgers (1987) on 27 elderly patients documented variations in the CCSE when readministered by the same clinician after a 2-hour interval; nearly every patient manifested changes in scores on both short-term memory (88.9%) and calculation tasks (100.0%). This lack of stability in CCSE scores, while possibly reflecting diurnal variations in the elderly, does raise questions regarding test–retest reliability. Unfortunately, Carnes et al. do not provide any formal estimates of reliability.

For concurrent validity, most studies have employed utility estimates in comparing CCSE results with clinical diagnoses. The following summary of key findings is provided:

- Jacobs et al. (1977) found a high sensitivity (95.8%) and specificity (98.5%) for the CCSE among patients with organic disorders compared with other patients and hospital staff.

- Nelson et al. (1986) summarized three additional studies of the CCSE's validity that evidence moderate to excellent specificity. Greater variability was found for sensitivity, ranging from 48.8% (Webster, Scott, Nunn, McNeer, & Varnell, 1984) to 72.7% (Kaufman, Weinberger, Strain, & Jacobs, 1979) and 100.0% (Omer, Foldes, Toby, & Menczel, 1983). Consistent with research on the MMSE, they found the CCSE to be ineffective with right-hemisphere lesions.
- Several more recent studies (e.g., Haddad & Coffman, 1987; Hershey, Jaffe, Greenough, & Yang, 1987) have evidenced excellent sensitivity and moderate specificity.

Several studies have compared the diagnostic efficacy of the CCSE in comparison to other MSEs. While highly correlated with the MMSE ($r = .85$; Strain et al., 1988), Foreman (1987) concluded that the CCSE was superior to MMSE and had a perfect agreement with clinical diagnosis. Interestingly, Schwamm et al. (1987) found that the CCSE was inferior to the NCSE in accurately classifying 30 neurological patients (i.e., 43.3% vs. 93.3%). Their results must be tempered by the fact that the NCSE was developed rather than cross-validated on these results.

McBride-Houtz (1993) conducted the only study of the CCSE in comparison to a neuropsychological test battery (Halstead–Reitan). In her previously cited study, she reported a moderate correlation of –.62 between the CCSE and a global measure of impairment on the Halstead–Reitan. As with the MMSE, she found a very modest sensitivity rate of 22%. A higher cut score (≤ 24) improved the sensitivity to 56%.

In conclusion, the CCSE appears to be a worthwhile screening measure, with validity comparable to the MMSE. The CCSE offers a broader sampling of verbal abilities than previously described MSEs, although these additional items do not appear to add incremental validity. Psychologists may feel comfortable using either the MMSE or the CCSE in a brief screen for cognitive impairment. As previously noted, the absence of observed deficits cannot be equated with normal functioning given the variable sensitivity rates.

Relevance of First-Generation MSEs to Structured Interviews

The MSQ made a highly significant contribution to clinical assessment in its recognition of a critical question in differential diagnosis. Importantly, the MSQ sought to address the differential diagnosis by the straightforward identification of discriminating items. This elegantly simple approach could easily be applied to structured interviews. For example, with adolescents, the diagnostic picture is often clouded in youth between attention-deficit/hyperactivity disorder (ADHD), conduct disorder (CD), and impulsivity (Vitacco et al., 2000). Given many similarities in behavioral manifestations, the issue of differential diagnosis becomes essential.[2] With adults, what are the differentiating characteristics between schizophreniform disorder and schizophrenia? Although general correlates have been observed, the lack of any standardized assessment based on discriminating items is very apparent.

First-generation cognitive MSEs are enlightening to structured interviews because of their unadorned simplicity. An understandable impulse would be to dismiss these measures as simplistic. However, the meta-analysis by Christensen et al. (1991) suggests that simple methods are likely to have comparable, if not superior, effect sizes to much more elaborate approaches. These MSEs attempt to crystallize the differences between disorders. In this line of thinking, the crucial issue is not common characteristics but distinguishing characteristics (Rogers & Cruise, 2000).

The SPMSQ is informative to structured interviews in its honest attempts to address moderator effects. Should diagnostic results be interpreted blithely, without consideration of background (e.g., education) or cultural identification (e.g., self-described ethnicity)? While we are likely to quarrel with its solution (i.e., simply adjusting scores among ethnic groups to achieve comparable proportions), the objective of evaluating moderator effects is often neglected with structured interviews. For example, high scores on psychopathy as measured by the PCL (see Chapter 12) are likely to have different meanings based on gender and ethnicity.

An important lesson can also be learned from the MMSE. While a valuable screening measure, the MMSE tends to eclipse all other cognitive MSEs in terms of its general acceptance. Is this ascendancy deserved? On empirical grounds, the MMSE is better validated than other first-generation MSEs. However, this does not appear to justify its status as "the most widely used mental status examination in the world" (Salmon, 2000, p. 426). The term "diagnostic canonization" was coined to describe the elevated status of uncritical acceptance that is achieved by the MMSE. Clinicians and researchers must cautiously reevaluate any assessment measure that has attained this elevated status.

Second-Generation Cognitive MSEs

Cambridge Cognitive Examination (CAMCOG)

Description. Roth et al. (1986) devised a comprehensive assessment of the elderly (i.e., the Cambridge Mental Disorders for the Elderly Examination, or CAMDEX) through diagnostic interviews, collateral interviews, medical procedures, and a structured interview for cognitive dysfunctions referred to as the CAMCOG. The CAMCOG incorporated 11 items from the MMSE, with 43 additional items to address other elements of cognitive dysfunction.

---

[2]Alternatively, an argument could be made for comorbidity, but the magnitude of the diagnostic overlap argues against this approach, meeting Syndeham's criteria for exclusion and outcome criteria.

These items address orientation, language, memory, praxis, attention, abstract thinking, perception, and calculation. Greater coverage is given to cognitive abilities such as language, abstract thinking, and calculation. One goal of the CAMCOG was the creation of a measure that could accurately evaluate mild dementias that are often missed by first-generation MSEs (see Reisberg, Ferris, De Leon, & Crook, 1982). Generally, the cut score for dementia is < 80 of 107 total points.

Reliability and Validity. The original reliability study by Roth et al. (1986) on 40 geriatric patients suggested high concordance rates for dementia (95.7%), with exceptionally high interrater reliabilities for individual items (median phi coefficient = .90). When fine distinctions were attempted with respect to subcategories of dementia, a moderate level of agreement (phi coefficient = .63) was achieved.

Hendrie et al. (1988) also found a high interrater reliability in a videotaped study of 40 elderly patients with mental disorders and 15 age-matched controls. Phi coefficients for the CAMCOG ranged from .50 to 1.00, with most (78.3%) of individual items exceeding .75. The overall correlation between CAMCOG ratings was also high ($r = .88$).

In validity studies, the CAMCOG appears to be highly accurate in distinguishing dementia from depression, with 92% sensitivity and 96% specificity. Hendrie et al. (1988) found significant differences in CAMCOG scores among dementia, depression, and elderly controls. O'Conner (1990) concluded that the CAMCOG should be utilized for mild dementia because of its diagnostic accuracy. Beyond dementia, the CAMCOG has been utilized to evaluate Down syndrome and cognitive decline found in older patients (Hon, Huppert, Holland, & Watson, 1999).

Cultural influences on the CAMCOG have not been adequately explored. Nearly all the research has been conducted on British populations, although Hendrie et al. (1988) found comparable results on an American sample.

In summary, the CAMCOG appears to be a superior MSE for the evaluation of cognitive dysfunction in English-speaking patients. In cases where depression is suspected, the entire CAMDEX can be administered to improve diagnostic accuracy. Although further validation would be welcome, the CAMCOG appears to have a high level of interrater reliability and sufficient criterion-based validity to warrant its clinical application.

Neurobehavioral Cognitive Status Examination (NCSE or COGNISTAT)

Kiernan, Mueller, Langston, and Van Dyke (1987) developed the NCSE as a cognitive MSE to assess mental abilities in five areas: language, constructions, memory, calculations, and reasoning. Recognizing the relatively low sensitivity rates of the MMSE and the CCSE, the NCSE was designed to measure specific abilities on items of graded difficulty. With screening items, the NCSE consists of 64 items, most of which are scored as passed–failed. Unlike other

MSEs, the NCSE includes a subtest called "Design Constructions," which is an analogue to the WAIS—III block designs. The NCSE was devised to screen for specific cognitive dysfunctions plus those of mild severity that might otherwise be overlooked by the first generation of cognitive MSEs (Schmidtt, Ranseen, & DeKosky, 1989). These items are divided into 10 scales: orientation, attention, comprehension, repetition, naming, constructions, memory calculations, similarities, and judgment. Each scale begins with a difficult screening item, that is failed by approximately 20% of the normal population. If this item is failed, then the patient is administered the complete scale.

Kiernan et al. (1987) provided the original standardization data on 60 unimpaired adults (age range 20–66) and 59 geriatric volunteers (age range 70–92) that yielded slight decrements in functioning for the elderly. Unfortunately, Kiernan et al. did not report whether differences occurred due to education, race, or gender. More recently, data are available on 800 inpatients with mental disorders (Salmon, 2000). Patients evidenced cognitive deficits that appear to increase gradually with age.

Reliability and Validity. Studies of interrater and test–retest reliability are limited to hospital settings. According to Salmon (2000), the evidenced NCSE moderate interrater (kappa = .57) and moderately high (kappa = .69) test–retest reliability when applied to inpatient samples. Mitrushina, Abara, and Blumenfeld (1994) found little variation in NCSE scale scores for inpatients with mental disorders in a test–retest format (interval = 10 days). Three NCSE scales yielded positive but variable results (Spearman rhos from .52 to .81). In general, the NCSE has only moderate reliability that does not compare favorably to other cognitive MSEs.

Schwamm et al. (1987) conducted the original validation study of the NCSE on 30 patients with documented central nervous system lesions. In optimizing the classification, Schwamm et al. found that 28 of the 30 patients (93.3%) were correctly identified by the NCSE. The scoring criterion was any low score on the 10 scales. These results were generally confirmed by van Gorp et al. (1999), who found that failure on at least one or two subtests accurately differentiated 96% of dementia and nondementia cases.

Several studies have compared the NCSE with neuropsychological test batteries. Key findings are summarized as follows:

- Meek, Clark, and Solana (1989) examined test results for the Luria–Nebraska, the Trail-Making Test, and the NCSE on 34 inpatient substance abusers. Using the screening test of the Luria–Nebraska as a point of comparison, the NCSE had a sensitivity of 84.6% and a specificity of 47.4%. However, these percentages are likely to be misleading because the complete Luria–Nebraska was not administered.
- McBride-Houtz (1993) examined the clinical usefulness of the NCSE in comparison to the MMSE and CCSE in a sample of 52 older adults with suspected cognitive impairment. Employing the General Neuropsychological

Deficit Scale from the Halstead–Reitan as a criterion measure, she found that the NCSE outperformed both the MMSE and CCSE. More specifically, she found that the NCSE correlated with the overall impairment at –.67 and had a sensitivity of 82%. As previously noted, the availability of only two unimpaired participants militated against establishing specificity.

• Marcotte, van Gorp, Hinkin, and Osato (1997) compared individual NSCE scales to specific neuropsychological measures and WAIS-R subtests, and produced very positive correlations (median = .64; range from .40 to .83) as evidence of convergent validity.

In conclusion, the NCSE appears to be a highly effective screen for dementia and other forms of cognitive impairment. Its strength lies in its substantial validation with both structural (imaging) and functional (neuropsychological) criteria.

Relevance of Second-Generation Cognitive MSEs to Structured Interviews

Second-generation cognitive MSEs were developed in the mid-1980s, years after the emergence of major Axis I structured interviews. Although the basic structure and standardization of structured interviews had already evolved, an examination of these cognitive MSEs continued to be instructive. Three areas are of particular relevance: focus on individual characteristics, utilization of screening criteria, and the establishment of gold standards.

The CAMCOG highlights the importance of individual characteristics in the assessment of clinical conditions. In diagnostic assessment and subsequent treatment interventions, the focus typically extends beyond the diagnosis to specific symptoms/features. The CAMCOG exemplifies the importance of establishing the reliability of individual criteria on which clinical changes can be documented regarding both the course of the disorder (e.g., gradual cognitive decline) and treatment response (e.g., specific treatment gains). Optimally, a reliable and highly detailed assessment becomes the preliminary framework for later treatment.

The NCSE provides an instructive example on the use of screening criteria to streamline the assessment process. While Axis I interviews (e.g., the SADS and SCID) tend to rely on cardinal symptoms to screen for specific disorders, the NCSE proposes a very different approach: Screening items are selected based on their low but still appreciable frequency (i.e., 20%) in normal populations. To apply this model to Axis I interviews, rather than the use of hallucinations and delusions to screen for psychotic symptoms, clinical inquiries would focus on less severe psychopathology observed in nonclinical samples. For instance, depersonalization and illusions might serve as sensitive screens for psychotic symptomatology.

The NCSE is distinguished from most assessment measures by its selection of a biologically based gold standard. The use of brain lesions as an external criterion for the original validation provides a rigorous standard. Like all gold standards, brain lesions have important limitations in establishing their presence and significance. Still, structured interviews would clearly benefit from this level of analysis. For the substance abuse sections of structured interviews, laboratory tests, such as hair analysis, may play an instrumental role in establishing a gold standard independent of self-reporting (Rogers & Kelly, 1997). In summary, the NCSE underscores a critical issue for structured interviews and most diagnostic methods; namely, that their heavy reliance on self-reported symptoms becomes a major obstacle to establishing truly independent criteria for external validation.

Clinical Applications of Cognitive MSEs

Mental health professionals must screen clinical populations for memory problems and other forms of cognitive impairment. In a compelling review, Herrmann (1982) found virtually no relationship between reported memory problems and actual memory impairment. More recent research (e.g., Zelinski, Gilewski, & Anthony-Berstone, 1990) has established, at best, a small association between these two facets of memory. In other words, clinicians can take little comfort in a patient's assertion that his or her memory is intact. Use of a cognitive MSE might well be considered the first step in the investigation of potential memory dysfunction. Box 2.1 provides a summary of sources for accessing MSEs.

Studies have found cognitive MSEs to be useful screens for changes in

---

BOX 2.1. Sources for Cognitive MSEs

- CCSE is available in Haddad and Coffman (1987, Figure 1, p. 5).
- CAMCOG is available commercially as part of the CAMDEX-R through Cambridge University Press on the internet, *www.cup.org;* by phone, (914) 937-9600; by fax, (800) 872-7423; or by mail, 110 Midland Avenue, Port Chester, NY 10573.
- MMSE is available in the Appendix of the Folstein et al. (1975, pp. 196–198) original article.
- MSQ is available in Kahn et al. (1960, p. 326).
- NCSE (recently marketed as COGNISTAT) is available commercially from Northern California Neurobehavioral Group, Inc., by phone, (800) 922-5840, or by mail, P.O. Box 460, Fairfax, CA 94978. It is also distributed by Psychological Assessment Resources (PAR), by phone, at (800) 331-8378; on the internet, *www.parinc.com,* or by mail, P.O. Box 998, Odessa, FL 33556.
- SPMSQ is available in Pfeiffer (1975, Table 1, p. 434).

cognitive status, although these measures are likely to have a ceiling effect in treatment outcome research. Investigations have documented in patients the natural course of a disorder (e.g., Folstein et al., 1975; McHugh & Folstein, 1988), need for institutional placement (e.g., Fisk & Pannill, 1987; Knopman, Kitto, Deinar, & Heiring, 1988), and response to treatment regimens (e.g., Denicoff, Joffe, Lakshmanan, Robbins, & Rubinow, 1990; LaRue, Spar, & Hill, 1986; Thal, Salmon, Lasker, Bower, & Klauber, 1989). Because of their limited range, cognitive MSEs should only be used to document cognitive changes in individuals with moderate to severe dementias. In addition, patients must be screened for functional disorders that may confound these measures (see, e.g., Haddad & Coffman, 1987).

Stonier (1974), who offered several interesting observations that may reduce the specificity of cognitive MSEs, found that cognitively intact patients with low MSE scores often display dramatic improvements on repeat administrations. In other words, cognitively intact patients evidence learning on MSE items that they previously missed. In contrast, patients with dementia typically evidence negligible to small ($\leq$ 4 points) improvements after multiple administrations (Doraiswamy & Kaiser, 2000). In applying these findings, clinicians may be able to improve their overall accuracy simply through the readministration of a cognitive MSE.

First-Generation Cognitive MSEs

The selection of a cognitive MSE is dependent upon several factors: (1) the purpose of the assessment, (2) the use of other clinical measures, and (3) the availability of professional resources. Clinicians must decide whether to use brief, first-generation or more comprehensive, second-generation MSEs. Because of their brevity and user-friendly format, first-generation measures, particularly the MMSE, have gained wide acceptance among practitioners. Among the second-generation MSEs, both the CAMCOG and NCSE have distinguished themselves because of their range of clinical data and diagnostic accuracy.

The first-generation MSEs are highly intercorrelated (e.g., Baldelli, Toschi, Motta, Marra, & Muratori, 1991; Herst, Voss, & Waldman, 1990; Lautenschlaeger, Meier, & Donnelly, 1986; Lesher & Whelihan, 1986). This finding is not surprising given the considerable item overlap among the MSQ, SPMSQ, MMSE, and CCSE. All four measures have good reliability, although substantially more research has been conducted with the MMSE than with the other measures.

The MMSE is likely to be chosen as a first-generation MSE for three reasons. First, the MMSE appears to have slightly better clinical utility than other first-generation measures (see, e.g., Christensen et al., 1991). Second, the MMSE has wider applications; it is unrestricted by age and is available in a Spanish version. Third, normative data are available for both English and

Spanish versions based on large-scale epidemiological studies. If only 5 minutes are likely to be allotted to screen for moderate to severe dementia, then the MMSE is likely to be the measure of choice. The MMSE is readily available (see Box 2.1).

As a brief screening measure, clinicians may find the cut score (< 24) on the MMSE to be a useful first step. In a recent review, Salmon (2000) found that the large majority of studies utilize this cut score, although higher and lower cut scores have been proposed. Many participants who perform below this score are likely to have moderate to severe dementia. However, many elderly patients with scores in the 24–27 range may also be cognitively impaired (see Jackson & Ramsdell, 1988).

One recommendation with the MMSE is that clinicians pay closer attention to actual performance on individual items than to any single score. Extrapolating from Rosen and Fox (1986), the following should signal the need for further investigation: (1) any problems with orientation, (2) marked problems with serial 7's (two or fewer correct responses), (3) inability to spell "world" backwards, or (4) very poor recall (failure to remember more than one of the three words). Gross failures on any one of these cognitive tasks are likely to differentiate between cognitively impaired patients and those with major mental illness.

The next step in the clinical evaluation of patients with poor performance on first-generation MSEs is dependent on the assessment issues. When the emphasis is on the patients' cognitive abilities, the use of intellectual and neuropsychological testing would be useful to document specific impairments and indicate organic involvement (see Lezak, 1983). When differential diagnosis is paramount, referrals for neurological and neuropsychological consultations are advised.

Second-Generation Cognitive MSEs

Both second-generation MSEs deserve our attention as screening measures for cognitive impairment; Box 2.1 provide information on obtaining these measures. The CAMCOG is designed for use with elderly populations and provides a systematic approach to assessment that includes the evaluation of functional disorders and medical conditions. The CAMCOG appears to have excellent reliability even at the symptom level. Since the CAMCOG incorporates the MMSE, clinicians may make comparisons of MMSE scores with treatment response and outcome data. The CAMCOG provides a thorough screening of cognitive capacities and should be useful in the assessment of elderly.

The NCSE differs from the other MSEs in its development of 10 specific scales. Inspection of these scales may signal potential impairment that needs further investigation. The NCSE's reliability is certainly adequate, although lower than that of the MMSE and CAMCOG. Importantly, several studies (e.g., McBride-Houtz, 1993; Schwamm et al., 1987) suggest that the NCSE has superior discriminability in distinguishing between patients with mild cognitive impairment and those who are cognitively intact. Anecdotally, Mueller (1988) reported that the systematic use of the NCSE as a screening measure approximately doubles the cognitive dysfunction detected by psychiatrists in their consultations with medical and surgical patients. The NCSE could be improved by the establishment of specificity rates for diverse, nonhospitalized populations.

II

Differential Diagnosis
for Axis I Disorders

3

Diagnostic Interview
Schedule (DIS)

OVERVIEW

The Diagnostic Interview Schedule (DIS) is a highly structured diagnostic interview designed to enable professional and nonprofessional interviewers to assess current and lifetime diagnoses of common mental disorders (Helzer & Robins, 1988). Much of the validation research occurred with Version III (DIS-III; Robins et al., 1985) and Version III—Revised (DIS-III-R; Robins, Helzer, Cottler, & Goldring, 1989). The DIS-IV (Robins, Cottler, Bucholz, & Compton, 1995) was published in 1995 with several minor revisions in January, 2001.

The DIS-IV is an extensive diagnostic interview organized into 19 diagnostic modules. Because the DIS-IV is intended to be used by both professionals and nonprofessionals, it utilizes a structured rather than semistructured format. Clinical inquiries are read verbatim; unlike semistructured interviews, no latitude is provided for unstructured questions initiated by the interviewer. A Probe Flow Chart indicates how optional probes should be implemented to ensure accurate clinical ratings. Clinicians are also provided with a detailed training manual on how to code reliably the clinical ratings of specific items (Robins, Cottler, & Keating, 1991).

Many clinical ratings are composed of multiple questions and some (particularly substance abuse items) require the completion of subcriteria. DIS-IV items are scored in a complex format that combines clinical relevance and possible etiology:

1 = denial of symptom
2 = subclinical (i.e., so mild as not to require professional help or interfere with functioning)
3 = clinically relevant symptoms, with etiology caused by medication, drugs, or alcohol

4 = clinically relevant symptoms, with etiology caused by physical illness or injury

5 = clinically relevant symptoms, with etiology likely due to a psychiatric disorder

Interviewers are asked to make additional ratings concerning the onset and recency of symptoms.

The DIS differs fundamentally from most other diagnostic interviews on three important parameters. First, the DIS attempts to identify any organic etiology either through exogenous substances (e.g., alcohol or drugs) or medical conditions (see, e.g., Splenger & Wittchen, 1988). Second, the DIS incorporates a formal assessment of cognitive impairment via the MMSE (Folstein, Folstein, & McHugh, 1975, see Chapter 2). Third, the DIS has retained criteria from other systems: earlier DSM versions, Feighner criteria (Feighner et al., 1972), and Research Diagnostic Criteria (RDC; Spitzer, Endicott, & Robins, 1978). This feature allows researchers to make direct comparisons across diagnostic systems (see Robins, Cottler, & Keating, 1991).

The original purpose of the DIS was to assess the current episodes and lifetime prevalence of selected mental disorders (Robins, Helzer, Croughan, & Ratcliff, 1981). It was designed as a research instrument for extensive epidemiological studies to ascertain the prevalence and incidence of mental disorders throughout the United States, through a monumental undertaking by the Epidemiologic Catchment Area Program (ECA; Regier et al., 1984). Given the breadth of the ensuing studies, with nearly 10,000 subjects from three research sites alone (Robins et al., 1984), the ECA program was compelled to use lay interviewers with modest training in clinical interviews. Because of this, the DIS emphasizes clarity in its structured questions and detailed instructions regarding its administration. Beyond its original intent, the DIS has been used in a variety of clinical and research settings by both clinicians and lay interviewers (Helzer & Robins, 1988).

DIS-IV diagnoses focus on substance abuse and dependence (i.e., alcohol, barbiturates, opioids, cocaine, amphetamines, hallucinogens, cannabis, and tobacco), schizophrenia, mood disorders, anxiety disorders, and a small selection of other disorders. DIS-IV expanded the coverage from DIS-III-R to include four diagnoses arising in childhood (i.e., ADHD, separation anxiety disorder, oppositional defiant disorder, and CD). Diagnostic subtyping was added to pain disorder, specific phobia, and depression. Finally, the diagnosis of dementia with the MMSE was augmented from the Blessed, Tomlinson, and Roth (1968) assessment of dementia. Box 3.1 provides a summary of DIS-IV highlights and the source for securing copies.

The initial development of the DIS involved the creation of clinical inquiries that closely parallel the DSM-III inclusion and exclusion criteria (for a full review of its development, see Robins, 1987; Robins & Helzer, 1991). In generating clinical inquiries, the authors modeled questions after those asked by experts (Helzer et al., 1985). Diagnostic interviews were transcribed and

---

BOX 3.1. Highlights of the DIS-IV

- *Description:* A structured diagnostic interview that covers DSM-IV disorders the DIS-IV provides detailed information about onset, duration, and recency of symptoms.

- *Administration time:* The required time is highly variable depending on the patient and the coverage. Estimated time is 1½ to 2 hours.

- *Skills level:* College-level interviewers can be trained to administer the DIS-IV in a 1-week period. Training materials are only available to clinicians that enroll in a 5-day training course; tuition for training is $1,100.

- *Distinctive features:* The DIS (especially earlier versions) is unmatched in its cross-cultural applications. An important feature is its Spanish translation, with research on Puerto Rican, Mexican, and Mexican American versions. The DIS should also be considered for evaluations when the onset, duration, and possible etiology of symptoms are needed.

- *Cost:* Price list on 3/1/2001 for DIS-IV = $25.00 for a single sample copy; $500 for the DIS-IV package of expanded materials.

- *Source:* Lee Robins, PhD, by phone, (314) 362-2469, by fax, (314) 362-2470, or by mail, Deptartment of Psychiatry, Washington University School of Medicine, Campus Box 8134, 4940 Children's Place, St. Louis, MO 63110-1093. Also available on the internet, *epi.wustl.edu/dis/dishome.htm.*

---

effective phrasings were gleaned for the DIS inquiries. Moreover, optional probes were fashioned to assess severity and nonpsychiatric reasons for symptom endorsement. Revisions of the DIS inquiries involved pretesting on patient and nonpatient samples, and subsequent refinement of problematic questions. These modifications resulted in Version II, on which initial comparisons were made between psychiatrists and lay interviewers (Robins et al., 1982). Additional alterations in the DIS, implemented to improve the clinical inquiries and resulted in Versions III (Robins et al., 1985) and III-A (Robins, Helzer, Cottler, & Goldring, 1989), which incorporated minor changes in wording and allowed interviewers to evaluate the recency of symptoms. DIS-IV (Robins et al., 1995) was introduced to parallel DSM-IV modifications.

Several computerized versions of the DIS have been developed to provide either patient- or interviewer-based administrations. One argument favoring patient-based administrations (see Blouin, Perez, & Blouin, 1988) is the reduction of information variance by the elimination of clinician variability in the rating of responses.[1] Several variations (see Blouin et al., 1988; Griest et al., 1984; Mathisen, Evans, & Meyers, 1987) are interactive programs that

---

[1] Of course, the counterargument is that the self-administered DIS must rely upon the patient's interpretation of questions, which may also confound information variance.

provide the necessary branching and probes in response to patients' answers. An important limitation of these programs is that they do not cover all DIS diagnoses. For interviewer-based programs, Wyndowe (1987) provides lay interviewers with questions and ratings presented on the screen.

An abbreviated paper-and-pencil version of the DIS (DISSA, or DIS—Self-Administered; Kovess & Fournier, 1990) is also available which covers depressive disorders, anxiety disorders, and alcoholism. The justification for this very circumscribed version of the DIS is that the selected disorders are those most frequently found in nonreferred community samples. As discussed below, the DISSA may have clinical value in screening community subjects for undiagnosed mental disorders.

One notable advantage of the DIS-IV is that it has been translated into Spanish and Chinese. Of particular interest in the Spanish versions is a cultural awareness of the heterogeneity of Hispanic patients, with systematic comparisons of Mexican Americans, Mexicans, and Puerto Ricans (see Anduaga, Forteza, & Lira, 1991). The cross-cultural applications of the DIS will be discussed below, with reference to its generalizability.

VALIDATION

An important facet of the DIS is its concerted attempt to establish clinical utility with nonprofessional or lay interviewers. This emphasis, inherited from its epidemiological origins, places a singular burden on the DIS's validation particularly with respect to its diagnostic reliability.

Diagnostic Reliability

Most reliability studies with the DIS serve two, related purposes. The concordance between two (typically one lay and one professional) interviewers is compared for interrater and test–retest reliability. Utilizing the same data, lay interviewers is compared to professional interviewers as a test of concurrent validity. As a result, data are lacking on reliability studies with similarly trained interviewers. We might assume that two mental health professionals would have the same or higher levels of agreement than lay–professional pairs. However, empirical data would be helpful in confirming this assumption.[2]

DIS reliability studies are summarized in Table 3.1. An important consideration is the version of DIS used in reliability studies. The early studies (e.g., Hesselbrook, Stabenau, Hesselbrock, Mirkin, & Meyer, 1982; Robins et al., 1981) employed Version II. Later studies employed Versions III, III-A, or III-R. None of the studies reported in Table 3.1 test the reliability of the most recent

---

[2]The alternative hypothesis is that clinicians may feel less obligated to follow the DIS format diligently, thereby reducing reliability.

TABLE 3.1. Reliability Studies of the Diagnostic Interview Schedule (DIS)

Study (year)	N	Setting		Dx	Raters		Reliability		Reliability estimates		
		In/Out	Com/Univ		Lay	Prof	Inter/Retest	(interval)	Sx/Cur-Dx/Life-DX		Other
Robins et al. (1981)	216	✓	✓	18	✓	✓	✓	(NA)			.66
Hesselbrook et al. (1982)	42	✓[a]		9	✓		✓				.95
Burnam et al. (1983)[b]	61	✓		12	✓	✓		✓ (1 wk)			.50
Helzer et al. (1985)[c]	370		✓	11	✓	✓		✓ (6 wk)			.49[d]
Bird et al. (1987)[b,e]	189		✓	1	✓	✓		✓ (<1 day)		.69	.57
Canino et al. (1987b)[b]	189		✓[g]	15	✓	✓		✓ (<1 day)		.60	
Wells et al. (1988)[f]	230		✓	2	✓	✓		✓ (3 mo)	.49[h]	.57[h]	
Wittchen et al. (1989)[i]	20	✓	✓	5	✓	✓		✓ (1–3 days)		.82[i]	
Bushnell et al. (1990)[b]	259	✓	✓[k]	3	✓	✓		✓ (1 mo)		.66[l]	
Anduaga et al. (1991)[b]	15		✓	??	✓	✓	✓			.89[m]	
Vandiver & Sheer (1991)	486		✓	NA	✓[o]			✓ (9 mo)		.46[n]	.43[n]
Cottler et al. (1998)	453	✓	✓	1	✓	✓		✓ (10 days)	.54[p]	.53[p]	

Note. According to the general design, lay interviewers were compared to professional interviewers. The agreement between the DIS administration was considered reliability; the extent to which the lay interviewers approximated the professional interviewers was considered concurrent validity. See Table 1.5 (p. 35) for a glossary of terms and abbreviations. Unless otherwise noted, reliability estimates are the following: symptoms are correlations; diagnoses are kappa coefficients; others (summary scales) are intraclass coefficients (ICCs).

[a] Inpatients on an alcoholic unit.

[b] Spanish translation.

[c] Community participants were selected on the basis of their diagnoses. While many may not be involved in treatment, the "outpatient" designation appeared the most appropriate.

[d] Weighted kappas produced lower coefficients (median kappa = .28).

[e] The study assessed only cognitive impairment on the Mini-Mental State Examination (MMSE).

[f] Modified procedure with a standard DIS interview compared to a telephone DIS interview.

[g] Participants were preselected to ensure that 50% had depressive symptoms.

[h] Depression only.

[i] Abbreviated German translation covering five diagnoses.

[j] ICCs addressing the onset of the episode only.

[k] Participants were preselected for possible depression, alcoholism, or bulimia.

[l] Yule's Y for bulimia only.

[m] ICCs.

[n] The study eliminated disorders believed to be uncommon; as a result, kappa coefficients may be inflated.

[o] Interviewers are simply described as trained and experienced, without mention of their professional status.

[p] Kappa coefficients; the study only addressed antisocial personality disorder and conduct disorder in substance abusers.

revision: Version IV. Given the rewriting of clinical inquiries and addition of diagnoses, the relative lack of reliability data on DIS-IV is a serious constraint.

Setting, Diagnoses, and Interviewers

DIS reliability studies have been conducted in a range of clinical and community settings. As reported in Table 3.1, data on inpatients are generally combined with other samples. Therefore, comparisons between inpatient and outpatient settings are not possible. In general, higher reliabilities are reported when diagnoses are more focused in the reliability sample.

A potential concern with DIS reliability is its diagnostic coverage. If we impose two limits on DIS studies, namely, a relatively recent revision (at least Version III) and language (English), the maximum coverage in any single study is 11 diagnoses. Reliability data are not available on the majority of DIS-III-R or DIS-IV diagnoses. To be precise, clinicians should not characterize the DIS-III-R or DIS-IV as reliable interviews. Rather, they should discuss the reliability of diagnostic categories (e.g., mood disorders) or specific diagnoses.

What is the relevance of the DIS's limited diagnostic coverage to practitioners? The answer depends on the setting and the diagnostic issues. The most common diagnoses in most clinical settings are covered by the reliability studies. For specialized settings or less common disorders, the diagnostic coverage for reliability is likely to become more salient.

Most DIS reliability studies combine lay and professional interviewers. The current data suggest a moderate level of reliability employing this research paradigm. As mentioned previously, reliability estimates might increase if studies were limited to professional interviewers.

Symptom and Diagnostic Reliability

The reliability of symptoms on the DIS is largely overlooked. The reproducibility of symptom ratings is indispensable in providing an accurate description of symptomatology and in measuring changes due to the course of the disorder or response to a treatment regimen. In one of the primary studies, Helzer et al. (1985) examined the level of agreement for the total number of symptoms associated with specific disorders. While interesting, these data do not address symptom reliability. Agreement on the number of symptoms offers little assurance that clinicians will agree on particular symptoms (e.g., paranoid delusions or auditory hallucinations).

Subsequent studies have focused on specific diagnoses. Wells, Burnam, Leake, and Robins (1988) found that many depressive symptoms were reliably assessed; although four symptoms were particularly problematic (i.e., kappas < .40). Cottler, Compton, Ridenour, Abdallah, and Gallagher (1998) examined symptoms of APD in substance-abusing samples. She and her colleagues found moderate kappas for APD, with greater agreement on adult than on developmental symptoms.

The DIS focuses primarily on test–retest reliability of diagnoses, which is likely to produce lower estimates than interrater reliability because of patient variance and attenuation of symptom reporting on repeat administrations (see Chapter 1). On this point, the sole interrater reliability study (Hesselbrock et al., 1982) found almost perfect agreement (*M* kappa = .95) based on videotapes of 42 inpatients on an alcohol treatment unit. Although the kappas may be somewhat inflated because of the foreknowledge of alcohol abuse/dependence, these estimates are still impressive.

Test–retest reliability studies of lifetime diagnoses have produced mixed results. Although Robins et al. (1981) were able to achieve a moderate level of reliability (median kappa = .67) for lifetime diagnoses on Version II, subsequent investigators have been much less successful in establishing test–retest reliability. In the Helzer et al. (1985) and Vandiver and Sheer (1991), studies, median kappa coefficients were modest (< .50). However, the Vandiver and Sheer study is limited by the long interval between administrations (i.e., 9 months) and the use of a university sample. Interestingly, Helzer et al. (1985) found that much of the disagreement involved borderline cases in which the patient marginally met or did not meet the diagnostic criteria. In other words, psychologists should have much greater confidence in their diagnostic reliability when the patient substantially exceeds the minimum inclusion criteria.

English-language test–retest reliability studies of current episodes tend to be focused on a narrow band of diagnoses. The Vandiver and Sher (1991) study addressed only common diagnoses; other studies were limited to single diagnoses, such as depression (Wells et al., 1988), bulimia (Bushnell, Wells, Hornblow, Oakley-Brown, & Joyce, 1990), and APD (Cottler et al., 1998). Overall, this coverage is disappointing for clinicians who want to address current episodes.

Reliability of Self-Administered Versions

Although not structured interviews per se, self-administered DISs are important to clinicians who may wish to use these versions for screening purposes. Blouin et al. (1988) administered a computerized DIS for test–retest reliability with a 1-week interval. In a mixed sample (80 patients and 20 community participants), they achieved a modest median kappa of .49 for current diagnoses. Kovess and Fournier (1990) tested a self-administered version limited to six disorders. In comparison to standard administrations, they found modest median reliabilities for professional (.45) and lay (.40) interviewers. Clearly, the magnitude of these kappa coefficients argues for the circumscribed use of self-administered DIS versions as possible screens.

Reliability of DIS-IV

No published studies of DIS-IV reliability were found. Dr. Robins (Lee N. Robins, personal communication, February 23, 2000) forwarded the first reliability data (Horton, Compton, & Cottler, 1998). Horton et al. examined test–retest reliability at 10-day intervals for 140 substance abusers. For life-time diagnoses, good agreement was achieved for four substance abuse diag-noses (median kappa = .61). For nine other adult disorders, the agreement was more variable (.20 to .63; median kappa = .43). Horton et al. also report reliabilities on nine symptoms or symptom constellations; these yielded a moderate level of agreement (median kappa = .47).

Reliability of Non-English DIS Versions

Burnam et al. (1983) conducted an elegant study of a Spanish DIS translated and validated primarily for a Mexican American population. For test–retest reliability, the DIS was administered on two occasions (1-week intervals) to monolingual outpatients. The kappa estimates were in the low-moderate range (median = .50). Anduaga et al. (1991) made minor modifications in a Spanish DIS for use in Mexico. This version appeared to have good interrater reliability (ICC = .89) for current diagnoses. When compared to clinical diag-noses, it demonstrated relatively low sensitivity (8–63%; median of 39%), but high specificity (78–99%; median of 93%).

Canino et al. (1987b) carried out a separate translation of the DIS for use with Puerto Rican samples. Two translators were employed independently to resolve any disparities in comprehension and usage. The resulting DIS was administered twice in the same day, with a median kappa of .60 (see Table 3.1), to a mixed sample of psychiatric patients and community participants. The Bird, Canino, Rubio-Stipec, and Shrout (1987) DIS MMSE was found to be culturally bound. With substantial modifications, Bird et al. produced moderately reliable classifications on the MMSE (kappa = .69).

Preliminary data (Wittchen et al., 1989) are available on a German trans-lation of the DIS. With a sample of 20 patients, Wittchen and his colleagues focused on the onset of disorders and were able to achieve a high level of agreement. More data are needed on the diagnostic reliability of the German DIS.

In summary, the Spanish DIS offers comparable reliability to the English DIS version. Importantly, research had address within-minority differences by creating Mexican and Puerto Rican translations. In contrast, the German DIS has yet to be sufficiently validated.

Diagnostic Validity

DIS validity studies concentrate on concurrent validity via systematic compar-isons of DIS to clinical diagnoses by experienced psychiatrists. As observed in Chapter 1, this practice, called bootstrapping (Robins et al., 1981), uses one imprecise method (psychiatric interviews) to establish the classificatory accu-racy of the DIS. Other validation studies have sought to demonstrate predic-tive validity of specific disorders, with a focus on their onset (e.g., etiology

TABLE 3.2. Concurrent Validity Studies of the Diagnostic Interview Schedule (DIS) for Major Diagnostic Categories

Study (year)	Version	N	Agreement with external diagnoses (kappas)				
			Mood	Psychotic	Anxiety	Substance	Overall
Robins et al. (1982)	II (E)						.22
Burnam et al. (1983)	II (E)	65	.37	.45	.38	.60	.37
	II (S)	61	.43	.56	.32	.59	.33
Anthony et al. (1985)	II (E)	810	.17	.19	.10	.35	.14
Helzer et al. (1985)[a]	III (E)	370	.36		.34	.60	.38
Hwu, Yeh, & Chang (1986a)	II (C)	287	.75	.54	.31	.53	.54
Canino et al. (1987)[a]	III (S)	189	.30	.29	.49	.45	.46
Erdman et al. (1987)[b]	III (E)	210	.26	.15	.05	.06	.07
North et al. (1997)	III (E)	97	.30	.53		.69	.53

Note. These kappa coefficients are intended only as general estimates. In most cases, they represent the unweighted median kappa coefficients for reported disorders within a diagnostic category. In other instances, data were already grouped by diagnostic category. Concurrent validity studies focus on Versions II and III; no data are available on Versions III-R or IV. The language used in the concurrent validation is included in parentheses: E = English; S = Spanish; C = Chinese.
[a]Comparisons of lay interviewers' diagnoses with clinical diagnoses by psychiatrists who had administered the DIS and conducted additional interviewing.
[b]Reported for current episode. Kappas are generally comparable for lifetime diagnosis except for substance abuse (.24).

and risk factors) and outcome criteria (e.g., course of the disorder). Less attention has been paid to construct validity (i.e., convergent or convergent–discriminant validity).

Concurrent Validity

Concurrent validity studies often produce only moderate kappa coefficients (.40 to .50 range) even for well-established Axis I disorders (e.g., major depression and schizophrenia). As summarized in Table 3.2, the DIS is no exception. In reviewing the overall kappa coefficients across eight major studies, more than half the studies do not reach this benchmark, and several have very modest median kappas (i.e., < .30).

Concurrent validity was also examined for broad diagnostic groups. The rationale for this organization is twofold: (1) Most studies covered at least some disorders within each diagnostic category; and (2) clinicians selecting measures are interested in general diagnostic groups but rarely have sufficient information to focus on a single diagnosis.[3] As summarized in Table 3.2, substance abuse disorders appear the most robust, with the majority of studies

[3]If the clinician is confident that only one disorder needs to be addressed (e.g., social phobia), then the reason for administering a comprehensive Axis I interview is obscure.

reporting kappas exceeding .50. Psychotic disorders (predominantly schizophrenia) also fared relatively well, with kappas > .40 in four of seven studies. Data on concurrent validity are decidedly more mixed for mood and anxiety disorders. In the latter case, the number of anxiety disorders being addressed militated against high kappa coefficients.

One challenge to establishing concurrent validity is that the majority of studies utilized community rather than clinical populations. Reliance of community samples decreased the prevalence of specific disorders within the validation studies. Kappa coefficients are strongly affected by low proportions (see Chapter 1). Therefore, Helzer and Robins (1988) recommended the use of Yule's Y for estimating agreement. As a specific example, Helzer and Robins applied Yule's Y to the Helzer et al. (1985) study. Instead of a modest kappa (median = .38; see Table 3.2), Yule's Y produced a mean estimate of .64 (see Helzer & Robins, 1988, p. 10). However, Yule's Y is difficult to interpret because it is a nonlinear function (Shrout et al., 1987).

Two major studies of concurrent validity were conducted by the authors of the DIS (Robins et al., 1982; Helzer et al., 1985). Both studies compared data from lay interviewers to clinical interview data from psychiatrists. Because the psychiatrists had already administered their own DIS interviews, these results are likely influenced by their knowledge of DIS responses. Therefore, results of these studies should be interpreted cautiously in light of this methodological limitation.[4]

Anthony and his colleagues (1985; see also Folstein, Anthony, et al., 1985) conducted an elegant study of DIS concurrent validity. As a gold standard, they employed four research psychiatrists who independently administered the Present State Examination (PSE; Wing, Cooper, & Sartorius, 1974), which was augmented to include DSM-III diagnoses. Beyond standardized PSE ratings, the psychiatrists were free to make their own clinical inquiries and observations. The DIS interviews were administered to 810 community participants by 77 lay interviewers who had completed an 8-day training program. Anthony et al. (1985) found very low rates of agreement for the eight most common diagnoses (i.e., kappas from –.02 to .35, with a median of .14). Sensitivity was very low (median for disorders = .18) and specificity was extremely high (median = 1.00).

Two general observations emerge from the concurrent validity studies. First, most studies confirm the findings of Anthony et al. (1985), with high to very high specificity estimates and modest sensitivity estimates. In general, practitioners can have greater confidence in establishing the absence than the presence of a DIS diagnosis. Second, the studies summarized in Table 3.2 clearly demonstrate that Spanish and Chinese translations of the DIS have comparable concurrent validity to the standard English versions.

Beyond general studies, DIS studies of concurrent validity have focused

---

[4]This limitation only affects concurrent validity, not interrater reliability. For concurrent validity, the external measure should be completely independent of the measure being validated.

on substance abusing populations. Overall, these studies have yielded very modest results except for substance abuse disorders:

- Hasin and Grant (1987a, 1987b, 1987c), in a study of 120 substance-abusing patients (mostly alcoholics), compared the DIS DSM-III and the SADS—Lifetime Version RDC diagnoses. A comparison of DSM-III and RDC criteria produced very low kappas. When DSM-III inclusion criteria were applied to both measures, however, the kappa coefficients were moderately high (median = .85).
- Griffin, Weiss, Mirin, Wilson, and Bouchard-Voelk (1987) compared DIS and clinical diagnoses on 124 drug-abusing inpatients. Kappas were modest (i.e., .40) for common Axis I disorders (major depression and panic disorders) but improved for alcohol abuse/dependence (.57) and drug abuse/dependence (.89).
- Ford et al. (1989) produced dismal kappa coefficients (–.08 to .23) on 75 inpatients from a substance-abuse treatment unit.

In conclusion, substance-abusing patients pose special challenges to diagnostic evaluations. Such patients are often poor historians and may be motivated to dissimulate their substance abuse history (Rogers & Kelly, 1997). In general, these data raise questions about the accuracy of DIS Axis I disorders for diagnoses unrelated to substance abuse.

Predictive Validity

DIS predictive validity studies have concentrated on Syndeham's outcome criteria (see Chapter 1), namely, forecasting the natural course of specific disorders. A major research effort involves large-scale follow-up studies for the vast ECA studies in the early 1980s. After extended intervals (typically 10–15 years), community participants were recontacted and systematically evaluated. Key results from major studies are summarized below:

1. Major depression appears to follow a general pattern, with prodromal symptoms predicting major depression (see Eaton et al., 1997). A bimodality of onset was evidenced for both females (30 and 55 years) and males (40 and 55 years). In community samples, the duration of episodes was relatively short (8–12 weeks).
2. Precursors of panic disorders were identified (Eaton et al., 1998). In general, the incidence of panic disorder was reduced significantly with age. However, the ability to predict recovery was thwarted by the heterogeneity of the disorder and its course.
3. Obsessive–compulsive disorder (OCD) does not appear to be a stable diagnosis; this variability with DSM-III OCD (Nestadt, Bienvenu, Cai, Samuels, & Eaton, 1998; see also Nelson & Rice, 1997) may not apply to DSM-III-R or DSM-IV OCD.

4. Alcohol abuse and dependence remained relatively stable over a 10-year period (Demalle, Cottler, & Compton, 1995). Specific symptoms predicted new cases of alcohol abuse/dependence: desire to stop or control drinking, or physiological effects (i.e., shakes) as a result of drinking. Interestingly, respondents appeared to be relatively inconsistent in reporting lifetime use.

ECA studies for the course of specific disorders have considerable value in establishing the predictive validity of the DIS and the concomitant DSM diagnoses. In general, these studies offer some empirical support for specific disorders. The notable exception appears to be the DIS-III/DSM-III OCD, which manifested substantial instability.

Breslau and her colleagues (Breslau, Davis, Peterson, & Schultz, 1997; Breslau et al., 1998; Chilcoat & Breslau, 1998) conducted programmatic research on DIS-IV diagnoses of PTSD and specific predictors. Breslau et al. (1998) found that specific risks of PTSD were associated with (1) gender and background, and (2) the type of trauma (e.g., PTSD in 20.9% of those exposed to assaultive violence[5] vs. 2.2% of those learning about others' trauma). In addition, PTSD and substance abuse appear to have a bidirectional effect: PTSD increases the risk of drug abuse, and drug abuse increases the risk of PTSD following a trauma. Regarding gender differences, exposure to traumatic events did vary significantly by sex; however, women, especially those traumatized at an earlier age, were more susceptible than men. Preexisting anxiety and major depression were substantial risk factors for both genders.

A large body of research has examined the DIS in relationship to prodromal symptoms, risk factors, and outcome criteria. Major findings include the following:

- Bland, Newman, and Orn (1997) found substantial remission rates in a large community sample for Axis I disorders and APD; these patterns varied by age and gender. The data suggest that the outcome criteria in nonreferred samples are generally positive, including disorders typically considered difficult to treat (e.g., substance abuse disorders).
- Although APD predicts criminality, CD symptoms appear to have a predictive role beyond adult APD criteria (Cacciola, Rutherford, Alterman, & Snider, 1994).
- A temporal relationship was found between cocaine abuse and prior diagnoses of mood and anxiety disorders (Halikas, Crosby, Pearson, Nugent, & Carlson, 1994).
- Although certain disorders are sometimes linked with violence (e.g., APD or schizophrenia), a large-scale DIS study (Swanson, Borum,

---

[5]See also North, Smith, and Spitznagel (1997) who reported DIS diagnoses following a mass shooting.

Swartz, & Monahan, 1996) found that substance abuse combined with a major mental disorder had the most predictive value.

- Unemployment is a predictor of depression, but depression is not a predictor of unemployment (Dooley, Catalano, & Wilson, 1994).
- Lifetime diagnoses are moderately stable, with "borderline" cases evidencing considerable instability (Vandiver & Sheer, 1991).

Construct Validity

Construct validity studies with the DIS have focused predominantly on convergent validity. This section summarizes several major studies with both Anglo American and Hispanic samples. These general studies are followed by more specific research that is organized by specific diagnoses.

Rubio-Stipec, Shrout, Bird, Canino, and Bravo (1989) performed an elegant factor analysis that compared a Puerto Rican sample (i.e., Canino et al., 1987b) with Mexican American (Burnam et al., 1983) and Anglo American samples from Los Angeles (Burnam, Hough, Karno, Escobar, & Telles, 1987). They examined five symptom groups associated with alcoholism, psychotic disorders, mood disorders, phobias, and somatization disorders. Of these, four factors (all but somatization) yielded very high congruence coefficients for both the Mexican American and Anglo American samples. Scales based on these factors evidenced good internal consistencies (alphas ranging from .58 to .90, with a median of .82). The results of Rubio-Stipec et al. (1989), with the exception of somatization disorder, support the construct validity of the DIS across Hispanic and Anglo cultures.

Fantoni-Salvador and Rogers (1997) examined the convergent validity for four common DIS diagnostic categories (i.e., alcohol dependence and depressive, anxiety, and schizophrenic disorders) for unilingual Hispanic patients. As evidence of convergent validity, they found moderate correlations between DIS symptoms and corresponding clinical scales on two multiscale inventories: PAI (Personality Assessment Inventory) and MMPI-2. Diagnostically, the hit rates were in the moderately high range, with an overall average of .72 for the PAI and .64 for the MMPI-2.

An important focus of the DIS is the convergent validity of specific disorders. With a focus on large-scale studies, the key findings are distilled as follows:

- A high level of convergence has been established for major depression. In a large-scale study (N = 613), Zimmerman and Coryell (1988) found a high concordance (kappa = .80) between DIS major depressive disorder and depression on the Inventory to Diagnose Depression (IDD; Zimmerman & Coryell, 1987). Whisman et al. (1989) compared specific symptoms of DIS depression with an interview version of the Hamilton Depression Rating Scale (HDRS; Hamilton, 1960).

Even with a 2-week interval, the convergence was very high (median ICC = .89).

- Convergent validity was also established for substance abuse disorders. Studies (Gavin, Ross, & Skinner, 1989; Ross, Gavin, & Skinner, 1990) examined 501 patients evaluated for substance abuse. For alcohol abuse/dependence, DIS disorders manifested moderate correlations of .65 with the Michigan Alcoholism Screening Test (Selzer, Vinokur, & Van Rooijen, 1975) and .58 with the Alcohol Dependence Scale (Skinner & Horn, 1984). DIS substance abuse disorders also evidenced moderately high correlation of .75 with the Drug Abuse Screening Test (DAST; Skinner, 1982).
- A moderate level of convergent validity was established for DIS psychotic symptoms. Spengler and Wittchen (1988) compared the DIS to two other standardized clinical interviews on 291 inpatients. The DIS-II evidenced high concordance (> 80%) and moderate agreement with the Inpatient Multidimensional Psychiatric Scale (median kappa = .47), and modest agreement with Assessment and Documentation of Psychopathology (median kappa = .31).

Studies without large-scale samples have also addressed convergent validity for specific disorders. Studies with APD (Cooney, Kadden, & Litt, 1990; Perry, Lavori, Cooper, Hoke, & O'Connell, 1987) produce variable results, depending on which convergent measures are used. Promising data are found for symptoms associated with borderline personality disorder (Swartz, Blazer, George, & Winfield, 1990; Swartz et al., 1989). DIS symptoms associated with somatization disorder appear to be associated with unexplained medical symptoms and utilization of health care services (Katon et al., 1991).

Validity of DIS Computerized Versions

Computerized and other self-administered versions of the DIS focus on concurrent validity with standard DIS administrations. Key findings about concurrent validity are summarized by different computerized versions:

- C-DIS (Computerized-DIS; Blouin et al., 1988) addresses all DIS diagnoses with moderate test–retest reliability (mean kappa = .57).
- Griest C-DIS (Griest et al., 1984) is a computerized version that surveys all DIS diagnoses with the necessary branching and probes. Mathisen et al. (1987) found modest agreement with psychiatric diagnosis (median for primary diagnosis, kappa = .40).
- DISSA (DIS—Self Administered; Kovess & Fournier, 1990) is an abridged questionnaire format that covers major depression, generalized anxiety, panic attacks, phobias, and alcoholic disorders. Kovess and Fournier found a moderate level of agreement between physicians' checklists of DSM-III symptoms and the DISSA (median kappa of .51).

- Microcomputerized DIS (Wyndrowe, 1987) provides lay interviewers with questions, probes, and ratings on screen. The results are modest, with 9 of 21 diagnoses confirmed by clinical diagnoses.
- DISSI (DIS Screening Interview; Robins & Marcus, 1987) is available in both questionnaire and computerized formats for use with 11 common disorders. Robins and Marcus cross-validated the DISSI on three additional data sets (combined N's of approximately 12,000) with sensitivity $\geq 75\%$ on 11 diagnoses except for somatization (67.0%) and cognitive impairment (44.3%), and specificity rates $\geq 80\%$, with the exception of cognitive impairment (76.2%). Bucholz et al. (1991) tested the clinical utility of interviewer- and self-administered DISSI versions. Using the traditional DIS as the standard, they found that the self-administered DISSI had generally satisfactory sensitivity and specificity (median for each was .79). Diagnostic agreement with the DIS varied widely with kappas ranging from .34 to .87 (median of .52) for the self-administered version.
- Quick-DIS (Q-DIS) addresses lifetime diagnoses for 25 independent sections. Once minimum criteria are decided,[6] the questions skip to the next section. In a small clinical sample, Bucholz, Marion, Shayka, Marcus, and Robins (1996) found good agreement on most of the 19 disorders that were evaluated (median kappa = .75).

Erdman et al. (1992) compared the traditional DIS to a computerized self-administered DIS and a computerized interviewer-administered DIS. Their results were comparable to earlier research (Griest et al., 1987), with moderate levels of diagnostic agreement (median kappa of .59) between the self-administered and traditional DIS interviews. The computerized interviewer-based interview appeared to offer no real advantage over the self-administered C-DIS and had a comparable level of diagnostic agreement (median kappa of .61) with the traditional DIS.

The Erdman et al. (1992) study examined two additional dimensions of computer-administered diagnostic interviews: reading comprehension and response bias. After excluding participants with very low reading levels from the study (i.e., raw scores of less than 10 on the reading subtest of Wide Range Achievement Test; Jastak, Bijou, & Jastak, 1978), they found no differences in symptoms and diagnoses across reading levels. They found that symptom endorsement was affected by response style, with correlations of −.30 for the traditional format and −.39 for the self-administered version between number of symptoms and a short-form of the Marlowe–Crowne Social Desirability Scale (Greenwald & Satow, 1978). Employing the Q1 scale (Johnson, Williams, Klingler, & Gianetti, 1988) as a screening measure for

---

[6]This occurs when either (1) minimum criteria for the disorder are met or (2) the minimum criteria cannot be met (i.e., even if all unasked criteria were endorsed, the patient would not meet minimum criteria).

unreliable or exaggerated response style, they found positive correlations of .38 for the standard DIS and .65 for the computerized self-administered version. This latter finding would suggest either (1) greater propensity for participants to feign on the self-administered version or (2) greater confusion among patients with major mental disorders, when they are responsible for reading and rating items on their own.

In conclusion, six DIS versions (computerized or questionnaire formats) have produced variable success. For screening purposes, two choices appear particularly viable: the DISSI and the Q-DIS. While slightly dated, the DISSI is based on the more than 12,000 research participants and produces very positive results with both sensitivity and specificity (i.e., for most disorders; kappas > .75). While based on modest samples, results from the Q-DIS are promising.

GENERALIZABILITY AND CROSS-CULTURAL RESEARCH

The continuing epidemiological focus of DIS research has resulted in unparalleled data on its generalizability to specific populations in the United States. DIS studies are often relied upon for clinical data regarding the prevalence of mental disorders based on age, gender, and ethnicity. This reliance begs the question of generalizability: Do observed differences reflect (1) true differences in population or (2) biases or other limits in the DIS? As the pioneering interview for epidemiological research, the DIS is often seen as a de facto gold standard. Whether this is completely warranted cannot be addressed systematically with existing studies.[7] However, it is reassuring that basic sociodemographic differences (e.g., higher prevalence of mood disorders in women) are observed across structured interviews.

Robins et al. (1984) conducted a monumental study on lifetime prevalence of DIS disorders across research sites, gender, age, and ethnicity on 9,543 community participants. The key findings from this ECA are summarized as follows:

- *Research sites.* Although statistical differences were found for nine specific disorders, the magnitude of these differences was generally small (i.e., < 2%). A remarkable exception was phobias, which ranged from 7.8% to 23.3%.
- *Gender.* Expected differences were found for male (i.e., APD and substance abuse) and female (mood and anxiety) predominant disorders. One exception was the diagnosis of panic disorders, which largely failed to demonstrate the predicted differences.
- *Age.* The data on age and prevalence are particularly complex. Some diagnoses (e.g., schizophrenia, major depression, and APD) evidenced

[7]Since these psychiatrists also administered the DIS, these estimates of agreement may be inflated (32.6%), in which case approximately 11% of the diagnoses would not generalize across settings.

an adult lifespan pattern that was consistent across sites. Other diagnoses (e.g., alcohol abuse/dependence and simple phobia) had high, variable age-related patterns across sites.

- *Ethnicity.* Unfortunately, data on ethnicity were dichotomized (African American and others). Relatively few diagnostic differences were found and none were consistent across the three sites. A disturbing trend is the consistent pattern among ethnic groups; invariably, African Americans had higher prevalence rates than others.

Several other studies have employed ECA data. Myers et al. (1984) evaluated 6-month prevalences of common mental disorders. Across the lifespan, substantial gender differences were observed, although phobia and dysthymia were common for both men and women. Subsequently, Eaton et al. (1989) utilized an expanded ECA data set (13,538 community participants) to examine incidences by gender and age. While similar patterns were observed for substance abuse and cognitive impairment, most disorders evidence a gender-specific pattern with considerable intersite variability.

Other large-scale studies in North America were entirely separate from the ECA investigations. Newman and Bland (1998) studied 1,964 Canadian community participants and found marked differences from the Eaton et al. (1989) study, with nearly twice the incidence of major depression and half the rate of phobias. Newman and Bland questioned the reliability of participants to recall lifetime symptoms thus inflating the incidence of major depression. However, they also acknowledged that the risk of depression may also be greater at this site (Edmonton, Canada) than other research sites. Galbaud du Fort, Bland, Newman, and Boothroyd (1998) examined spousal similarities for mental disorders in the Edmonton study. DIS results for 519 married pairs suggested an increased likelihood of similar disorders for mood and substance abuse disorders. More intriguing were the apparent interrelationships between spousal diagnoses of mood, anxiety, and substance abuse disorders. For example, a wife's diagnosis of phobia was associated with an increased likelihood of APD or drug abuse in the husband.

Stout, Steege, Blazer, and George (1986) evaluated prevalence rates for 223 women referred to a premenstrual syndrome clinic. When they compared this sample to female community participants from the ECA Durham site, they found a higher prevalence of dysthymia, anxiety, and substance abuse. However, the Stout et al. findings likely reflect clinical characteristics of this referred sample rather than question the results of previous epidemiological research.

More focused epidemiological research has addressed anxiety and mood disorders. Key findings are summarized as follows:

- In a 10-country study of 40,000 community participants, panic disorder appeared to have generally stable prevalence with the exception of Taiwan, where the overall rate of mental disorders is apparently very low (Weissman et al., 1997; see also Andrade, Eaton, & Chilcoat, 1996). Consistent findings were gender differences (i.e., higher in females) and comorbidity (i.e., agoraphobia and major depression).

- Combat-related PTSD was studied in 2,490 Vietnam veterans, with a 12% prevalence rate (Boscarino, 1995). An important finding was that most correlates were nonspecific. For example, both delinquency and lack of social support were risk factors for not only PTSD but also generalized anxiety, depression, and substance abuse.

- The estimated incidence of social phobias (.004 to .005 per year) appears stable for age, gender, and race over a 13-year follow-up of 1,920 community participants (Neufeld, Swartz, Bienvenu, Eaton, & Cai, 1999). New cases of social phobia appeared secondary to other disorders, especially depressive and panic disorders.[8]

- Prevalence of depression and anxiety appear somewhat lower for Mexican Americans (Hoppe, Leon, & Realini, 1989) than for ethnic groups reported in the ECA studies (see Robins et al., 1984). However, Mexican American males had a moderately high rate of generalized anxiety disorder (11.1%). In predicting prevalence rates, the lack of family cohesiveness and extended family contact appeared to be risk factors.

- Lifetime prevalence of alcohol dependence for Navajo Indians was very high for males (70.4%) and females (29.6%). History of conduct disorders appeared to predict the most severe cases of alcohol- and nonalcohol-related problems.

DIS studies have also examined the prevalence of common mental disorders in correctional settings. As part of the Edmonton study, Bland, Newman, Thompson, and Dyck (1998) compared 6-month and lifetime prevalences for common mental disorder between inmates and the general population. As expected, high rates of APD, alcohol abuse/dependence, and drug abuse/dependence were found. Higher rates than in the general population were also found for mood disorders (21.1% for last 6 months), schizophrenia (2.2% for last 6 months), and, surprisingly, OCD, (8.3% for last 6 months). In contrast, Teplin and Voit (1996) found lower rates of depression and higher rates of schizophrenia for male inmates. They also found that females had high rates of mood disorders and PTSD. Data on older inmates ($\geq$ 50 years) suggest that prevalence rates may increase with age (Koenig, Johnson, Bellard, Denker, & Fenlon, 1995). These studies, taken together, indicate an increased prevalence in current and lifetime diagnoses covering a range from predicted to unexpected mental disorders. Still unknown are (1) the proportion of specific disorders that predated incarceration and (2) the proportion that are the result of incarceration.

---

[8]This finding may hold true for other phobias; see Bienvenu and Eaton (1998) regarding blood–injection–injury phobia.

DIS research has also examined prevalence rates and issues of generalizability in studies outside of the United States. These studies include such diverse countries as Taiwan (Hwu, Yeh, & Chang, 1989; Hwu, Yeh, Yeh, & Chang, 1988), Hungary (Szadoczky, Papp, Vitrai, Rihmer, & Furedi, 1998), Germany (Hill, Rumpf, Hapke, Driessen, & Ulrich, 1998), Iceland (Stefannson, Lindal, Bjornsson, & Guomundsdottir, 1991), and Puerto Rico (Canino et al., 1987a). Common patterns of mental disorders, including gender differences, emerged from these studies. However, lifetime prevalences did evidence considerable differences across cultures.

Chinese DIS

Hwu, Yeh, Chang, and Yeh (1986) are responsible for the DIS—Chinese Modification (DIS-CM) and the subsequent modification of items for greater relevance in Chinese culture. They found a moderate level of agreement between clinical diagnoses and the DIS-CM, with a median kappa = .54. In comparison to U.S. data, Hwu et al. (1986) found much lower prevalences for schizophrenia, and mood and anxiety disorders. As noted by the investigators, such conclusions may be confounded by cross-cultural differences that were not examined. In a follow-up study, Hwu, Yeh, and Chang (1989) found that lifetime prevalence rates were apparently related to both gender and setting (urban, town, or rural). The investigators concluded that these rates may reflect true as well as cultural differences.

Studies of the DIS-CM may have limited relevance to Chinese American populations, since validity studies were based in Taiwan. In comparison to other measures, however, the DIS-CM has received the most validation for Chinese populations.

Spanish DIS

Karno et al. (1983) translated the DIS into Spanish for the evaluation of large Mexican American populations in southern California. As reported previously, Burnam et al. (1983) established moderate test–retest reliabilities in comparisons of English–Spanish and Spanish–Spanish administrations. Across 19 diagnoses, they found far-ranging values for sensitivity (from .00 to .92; median of .50) and excellent specificity (from .69 to .99; median of .89). Anduaga et al. (1991) made minor modifications in the Spanish version of the DIS for use in Mexico. This version appeared to have good interrater reliability (ICC = .89). When compared to clinical diagnoses, it demonstrated modest sensitivity (.08 to .63; median of .39), but high specificity (.78 to .99; median of .93).

Canino et al. (1987b) carried out a separate translation of the DIS for use with Puerto Rican samples. Two translators were employed independently, so that any disparities in comprehension and usage could be resolved. In addition, the DIS's Mini-Mental State Examination was found to be culturally bound and substantially modified (Bird, Canino, Rubio-Stipec, & Shrout,

1987). The resulting DIS was administered twice in Spanish by a psychiatrist and a lay interviewer, with a median kappa of .59 (see Table 3.1). When the DISs administered by lay interviewers were compared to clinical diagnoses, the sensitivity was moderately high (median = .65) and the specificity was superb (median = .91). Canino et al. (1987a) examined the prevalence rates of mental disorders in Puerto Rico in a large-scale epidemiological study of 1,513 community participants; they found prevalence rates comparable to those established in the United States.

Four important conclusions can be drawn from research on the DIS Spanish versions:

1. Spanish versions achieve reliability estimates that are comparable to the DIS standard version.
2. The clinical utility of Spanish versions varies with culture and nationality. Despite minor modifications, the Mexican American version has substantially poorer sensitivity rates in Mexico. Likewise, clinicians that evaluate second- and third-generation Puerto Ricans residing in the United States must choose between the Puerto Rican version, which has culturally specific items but no validation on American samples, and the Mexican American version, which lacks cultural sensitivity and has differences in language usage.
3. The major problem with DIS Spanish versions is the rather modest rates of sensitivity. Anduaga et al. (1991) provide a useful summary of sensitivity and specificity rates for Mexican American and Puerto Rican versions.
4. Despite the aforementioned problems, DIS Spanish versions, validational studies far surpass other structured interviews.

CLINICAL APPLICATIONS

Beyond its obvious value in epidemiological research, the principal advantage of the DIS is that paraprofessionals can be competently trained in its administration. With the increased strains on the public care of the mentally ill, paraprofessionals frequently assume the primary role in assessment and nonmedical treatments. Psychologists can train and supervise paraprofessionals with the DIS and thereby substantially improve the diagnostic assessments offered in many public agencies. Ideally, a diagnostic triage could be implemented for patients who meet, or nearly meet, the diagnostic criteria for mental disorders to be referred to a psychologist or other trained mental health professional.

Evaluations

The primary focus of the DIS reliability and validity studies is the lifetime prevalence of common mental disorders. Moderate levels of diagnostic reliability are established for approximately one-half the disorders covered by the DIS. In terms of breadth and depth, the DIS favors breadth with its extensive coverage of Axis I disorders. The DIS should be considered for evaluations in the following circumstances:

- The clinical focus addresses diagnoses rather than symptoms.
- Systematic attention to etiological issues appears warranted.
- Issues regarding ethnicity and culture are prominent.
- Bilingual clinicians are available to administer Spanish versions.
- Use of paraprofessionals excludes the administration of other Axis I interviews.

An important consideration is the selection of DIS versions. The majority of validity studies employ the DIS-II or some variation of DIS-III. The recently published DIS-IV has an important advantage regarding its compatibility with DSM-IV. At present, the DIS-IV is substantially limited by available validation. For example, the only reliability data appear to be unpublished.

Screening

The need to screen patients systematically for undetected mental illness extends beyond community mental health centers. For example, Jones et al. (1988) found that primary care physicians routinely miss mental disorders. Compared on the DIS, physicians missed (1) most mood (73.9%) and anxiety (80.0%) disorders, and (2) all organic and psychosexual disorders. Clinicians have experimented with screening measures that employ the DIS for a more complete assessment as part of the service delivery to large health maintenance organizations (HMOs; see Berwick et al., 1991).

Screening underserved populations with the DIS can also extend beyond the traditional patients presenting with physical or mental complaints. For example, Teplin (1990) found that approximately two-thirds (62.5%) of detainees with severe mental disorders went undetected and untreated. Although frequently served by social agencies, homeless persons may lack adequate diagnoses and intervention (North, Smith, Pollio, & Spitznagel, 1996; LaVesser, Smith, & Bradford, 1997).

Use of the DIS and DIS-derived screening measures for the identification of undetected disorders requires careful attention in the training and implementation phases. Particularly when using paraprofessionals, psychologists must periodically assess staff members' competence in DIS administrations. As a note of concern, most research studies on the DIS examine interrater reliability shortly after training and do not assess whether levels of diagnostic agreement attenuate over time.

I strongly recommend that subthreshold cases (i.e., almost meeting the inclusion criteria) receive complete evaluations. Helzer et al. (1985) found that most diagnostic disagreements occur in marginal cases (i.e., those just below or just above the threshold). Screening evaluations would likely show improved sensitivity if subthreshold cases (one or two inclusion criteria below the designated threshold) were also comprehensively assessed.

Self-administered DIS versions have a very circumscribed clinical role for several reasons. As previously summarized, the validation of most versions is quite limited. Self-administered versions that have only a modest correspondence with the standard version compound the problems of reliability and validity. Furthermore, the self-administered versions provide only partial coverage of the DIS diagnoses.

The use of the computer-administered DISSI would appear to be advantageous in screening large numbers of patients for possible mental disorders. Another very different application of self-administered versions is *postscreening* assessments, in which measures are employed as a double-check against missed diagnoses. In this regard, even measures with very modest sensitivity rates may be clinically useful. Given that the data suggest generally good sensitivity and specificity, use of the DISSI in this regard is strongly recommended.

Table 3.3 summarizes the three main advantages of the DIS: (1) administration by paraprofessionals, (2) use in screening large samples for undetected mental disorders, and (3) availability of several Spanish versions. In addition, Table 3.3 summarizes important limitations of the DIS.

TABLE 3.3. Advantages and Limitations of the Diagnostic Interview Schedule (DIS) in Diagnostic Evaluations

Advantages

- *Paraprofessionals.* The DIS can be administered by paraprofessionals with only modest levels of training.
- *Spanish version.* The DIS, more than other interview measures, has been translated and validated in Spanish.
- *Self-administered screens.* The DIS has self-administered versions (computerized and paper-and-pencil) that may also be used for pre- and postscreening.[a]

Disadvantages

- *Symptoms.* The reliability of DIS symptoms has been largely neglected because of its emphasis on diagnoses. For practitioners interested in the evaluation of symptoms (e.g., major depression), the DIS has limited value.
- *Etiology versus symptom severity.* Interviewers are asked to make complex decisions regarding the primary causes of specific symptoms. Because of this emphasis on etiology, the DIS pays relatively little attention to symptom severity.
- *Response styles.* Research has consistently demonstrated that the DIS is vulnerable to response styles.

[a]Self-administered versions have a circumscribed role because (1) they cover only a limited number of diagnoses, and (2) they only approximate DIS diagnoses.

Limitations of the DIS in Clinical Practice

As noted in Table 3.3, the DIS focuses on diagnoses rather than symptomatology. Both reliability and validity studies restrict most analyses to the diagnostic level. In clinical practice, changes in symptoms rather than diagnoses are often the benchmark of change, whether positive (e.g., response to treatment) or negative (e.g., decompensation). The use of the DIS for evaluation of treatment cases appears circumscribed to the establishment of common diagnoses rather than to the broader assessment of symptomatology.

The DIS asks clinicians to make determinations regarding the etiology of symptoms. Symptoms are formally rated whether they are the result of exogenous substances or medical conditions. Given the complexity of mental and physical disorders, the likelihood of making these distinctions based on patients' self-reports appears very tenuous. Many Axis I patients have chronic histories of substance abuse that greatly complicate the ascertainment of etiology for other Axis I diagnoses. Simply because a symptom was previously observed in the absence of organic factors (substance abuse or a medical condition) does not preclude a subsequent causal relationship with organic factors. Moreover, this attention to etiology requires substantial time, thereby limiting questions on symptom severity.

The DIS is vulnerable to response styles. Alterman et al. (1996) utilized indicators of feigning and defensiveness on the PAI (Morey, 1991b). Several important findings emerged. First, individuals suspected of feigning were more frequently diagnosed with major depression and agoraphobia. Second, interviewers appeared unaware of response styles. In a more narrow study, Cottler et al. (1998) examined differences between self-acknowledged liars and substance-abusing patients. Not surprisingly, measures of internal consistency were lower for self-acknowledged liars. In general, these data (see also Erdman et al., 1992) indicate that the DIS is vulnerable to response styles. At present, no methods for detecting response styles are available with the DIS.

DIS research suggests that mental disorders in informants may also influence reports. In particular, Chilcoat and Breslau (1997) found that depressed mothers overreport mood and anxiety disorders in their children. When using informants for collateral interviews, practitioners must consider the potential influences of mental disorders and motivation on the accuracy of such interview data.

4

Schedule of Affective Disorders and Schizophrenia (SADS)

OVERVIEW

Description

The Schedule of Affective Disorders and Schizophrenia (SADS; Spitzer & Endicott, 1978a) is an extensive, semistructured diagnostic interview designed primarily for the assessment of mood and psychotic disorders. The SADS is divided into Part I for current episode and Part II (otherwise known as the SADS—Lifetime Version, or SADS-L) for prior episodes. In Part I, individual symptoms are rated twice: the worst period of the current episode and the current time (i.e., the previous week). Through comparative ratings, clinicians are able to assess the severity of the disorder and minimize day-to-day fluctuations in clinical status (Endicott & Spitzer, 1978). Finally, for the assessment of key symptomatology, Spitzer and Endicott (1978b) devised the SADS—Change Version, or SADS-C, that consists of 45 symptoms selected from the SADS Part I.

Box 4.1 highlights the key features of the SADS. As an overview of the SADS, subsequent paragraphs are devoted to its coverage, symptom ratings, and structure of clinical inquiries.

Coverage

An important feature of the SADS is its in-depth examination of specific disorders. Unlike other commonly employed diagnostic measures, the SADS provides highly detailed information regarding the intensity and duration of specific symptomatology. As noted earlier, the SADS also provides comparison within the current episode (worst period vs. current time) and across episodes. The trade-off for this comprehensiveness is the relatively narrow

---

BOX 4.1. Highlights of the SADS

- *Description:* A semistructured diagnostic interview that focuses primarily on mood and psychotic disorders.

- *Administration time:* SADS Part I (current disorders) averages 45–75 minutes; SADS Part II (past disorders) averages 15–60 minutes.

- *Skills level:* Advanced, with clinical sophistication at interviewing and gradational ratings. Extensive training materials are available.

- *Distinctive features:* The SADS offers reliable gradations for evaluating the severity of symptoms. Overall, its reliability is unmatched. It is especially suitable when evaluations consider retrospective diagnoses or when issues of response style (malingering or defensiveness) are likely to be considered.

- *Cost:* Price list on 3/1/2001 for SADS interview booklets = $3.00. Because the SADS was developed on federal funds, copying is permissible.

- *Source:* Jean Endicott, PhD, by mail, Department of Research and Training, New York State Psychiatric Institute, Unit 123, 1051 Riverside Drive, New York, NY 10032; or by phone, (212) 543-5536.

---

spectrum of disorders covered by the SADS. The SADS allows for the diagnosis of 23 disorders and provides subcategories of schizophrenia, schizoaffective disorder, and major depression.

The SADS was developed prior to the final revisions and implementation of DSM-III. Therefore, its coverage of DSM-IV Axis I disorders is not entirely complete. Fortunately, a substantial convergence is observed between the SADS Research Diagnostic Criteria (RDC; Spitzer, Endicott, & Robins, 1975b, 1978) and DSM-IV disorders. However, clinicians must be knowledgeable about the two systems, so that they may supplement the SADS with additional questions required to make DSM-IV diagnoses.

Symptom Ratings

An important feature of the SADS Part I is its emphasis on the degree of impairment. Most mood symptoms and behavioral observations are rated on 6-point scales (0 = no information; 1 = not at all; 2 = slight, an occasional symptom of low intensity; 3 = mild, a common symptom of low intensity; 4 = moderate, a frequent symptom or symptoms of low to medium intensity; 5 = severe, a very frequent symptom or symptoms of at least medium intensity; and 6 = extreme, unremitting symptoms of high intensity). Within these gradations, a rating of at least 3 is required to be "clinically significant." Most gradations are anchored with a description, and some also provide representative examples.

Most other symptoms are rated on 3-point scales (0 = no information; 1 = absent; 2 = suspected or likely; and 3 = definite). Certain psychotic symptoms (i.e., delusions and hallucinations) are rated on a 6-point scale, which is used as a composite rating of impairment. For past episodes, patients often have difficulty in recalling the severity of specific symptoms. Therefore, SADS Part II is rated dichotomously (0 = no information; 1 = no; 2 = yes).

The SADS also provides an overall rating of the patient's level of functioning, typically for the worst period in the current episode and current time. The Global Assessment Scale (GAS; Endicott, Spitzer, Fleiss, & Cohen, 1976) provides a single rating (1 to 100) based on 10 levels of impairment/adjustment:

- GAS scores from 1 to 30 include three levels, reflecting extreme to pervasive impairment.
- GAS scores from 31 to 60 include three levels, reflecting moderate to severe impairment.
- GAS scores from 61 to 80 include two levels, reflecting slight to mild impairment. Impairment at these levels may not require clinical intervention.
- GAS scores from 81 to 100 include two levels, reflecting good to superior adjustment.

An important consideration is that SADS ratings and subsequent diagnoses are based on composite appraisals that combine patient responses with other clinical data (e.g., records and collateral interviews). When additional information is not available, however, SADS interview data are highly useful in establishing lifetime diagnoses (Leckman, Sholomsaks, Thompson, Belanger, & Weissman, 1982).

Structure of Clinical Inquiries

The format of the SADS is semistructured, with three levels of clinical inquiries that include the standard questions asked of each patient. In addition, the SADS also provides optional probes (i.e., questions enclosed in parentheses) that are used to clarify incomplete or ambiguous responses. Finally, as a semistructured interview, the SADS allows the clinician to construct his or her own unstructured questions. Typically, unstructured questions are only used when ambiguities are not resolved by the optional probes.

A general caution applies to the SADS and all other semistructured interviews: clinicians are sometimes tempted to "cheat" on the symptom ratings. The most common form of cheating is to turn the rating criterion into an unstructured question. For example, SADS question 351 addresses diurnal variations in mood; the actual rating criterion could be used as an unstructured question if the clinician asked, "In the morning was your mood mildly worse [i.e., rating of 3] or considerably worse [i.e., rating of 4]?" These types of questions are considered cheating because symptom ratings should reflect the clinician's best estimation based on multiple sources of data rather than the literal response from a mentally disordered person.

Rationale and Development

Studies in the early 1970s paint a rather gloomy picture for the diagnoses of mental disorders. A series of studies by Welner and his colleagues (Liss, Welner, & Robins, 1972; Welner, Liss, & Robins, 1972, 1973) suggests that many patients went undiagnosed and that the implementation of a structured interview and use of standardized diagnostic criteria would substantially reduce both missed diagnoses and misdiagnoses. Studies from the U.S.–U.K. diagnostic project (Cooper et al., 1972) suggest that marked discrepancies across research sites could be greatly decreased by using structured interviews. Finally, Spitzer and Fleiss (1974) found very poor agreement among experienced diagnosticians across six major reliability studies.

During the 1970s, Spitzer and Endicott (1975a) experimented with several psychiatric rating forms and interviewing materials. These measures included the Psychiatric Status Schedule (PSS; Spitzer, Endicott, Fleiss, & Cohen, 1970), the Current and Past Psychopathology Scales (CAPPS; Endicott, & Spitzer, 1972), the Problem Appraisal Scales (Herz, Spitzer, Gibbon, Greenspan, & Reibel, 1974), and the Mental Status Evaluation Record (MSER; Endicott, Spitzer, & Fleiss, 1975; Spitzer & Endicott, 1970; Spitzer, Endicott, Cohen, & Fleiss, 1974; see also Chapter 2). As a culmination of these efforts, they proposed (1) the development of the RDC to control criterion variance, and (2) the creation of the SADS as a comprehensive interview to control information variance.

Development of the RDC and SADS

Feighner et al. (1972) expressed dissatisfaction with the DSM-II diagnoses and developed their own research criteria. These criteria, widely known as the Feighner criteria, achieved a high level of diagnostic concordance for 15 disorders (see Helzer et al., 1977; Matarazzo, 1983). Spitzer et al. (1978) elaborated on these criteria and brought the total number of diagnostic categories to 23. In addition, diagnostic subtyping was developed for many disorders. The reliability of the RDC when employed with traditional interviews appeared high, with a median kappa of .86 (Spitzer et al., 1978).

Zwick (1983) provided a helpful critique of the RDC and its use with schizophrenic, schizoaffective, and depressive disorders. She noted that these criteria, while superior to their predecessors, warranted further refinement and validation. For example, Zwick observed that the RDC minimum period for schizophrenic symptoms (i.e., 2 weeks) is probably too brief, citing research by Helzer, Brockington, and Kendell (1981).

Comparatively little is published about the actual development of the

SADS. It evolved through three editions; the second edition became available in 1975 (Spitzer & Endicott, 1975b) and the third edition was produced in 1978 (Spitzer & Endicott, 1978a). A primary goal of the SADS was to assist in the differential diagnoses between mood and psychotic disorders for the National Institute of Mental Health (NIMH) collaborative study on the psychobiology of depression.

The SADS was designed to be used in conjunction with the RDC (Endicott & Spitzer, 1978). SADS items were organized into eight summary scales: depressed mood and ideation, endogenous features, depressive-associated features, suicidal ideation and behavior, anxiety, manic syndrome, delusions–hallucinations, and formal thought disorder. Very slight modifications were made in the SADS during 1979.[1]

Development of SADS Versions

Fyer, Endicott, Manuzza, and Klein (1985) attempted a further modification of the SADS-L that included anxiety disorders from DSM-III and DSM-III-R. This new version is referred to as the SADS-LA (Lifetime Version, Anxiety Disorders). The SADS-LA has been tested by several investigators (i.e., Leboyer et al., 1991; Manuzza, Fyer, Klein, & Endicott, 1986); their research is summarized in the reliability and validity sections.

Green and Price (1986) experimented with abbreviated versions of the SADS that rely upon truncated "packets," or SADS questions based on initial clinical presentation. Comparisons were made across 72 psychiatric inpatients screened for preselected diagnoses. By concentrating on only five diagnoses, Green and Price achieved moderately comparable results, with kappas greater than .70.

Herzog, Keller, Sacks, Yeh, and Lavori (1992) modified the SADS-L to include eating disorders (i.e., EAT-SADS-L). However, because the reliability and validity of this version have not been reported, use of the EAT-SADS-L should be limited to clinical research.

VALIDATION

More than most other diagnostic interviews, the SADS has paid careful attention to the various elements of reliability (interrater, test–retest, and internal consistency). In the following subsections, I summarize the relevant research with respect to reliability and criterion-related validity.

Diagnostic Reliability

Researchers from the NIMH collaborative study on the psychobiology of depression conducted several major studies of the SADS's reliability (i.e., An-

[1]The more recent version of the SADS is designated as the third edition, 1978–1979.

dreasen et al.,1981; Endicott & Spitzer, 1978; Keller et al., 1981). These studies were focused at three levels: symptoms, summary scales, and diagnoses. In addition, research has focused on either the current episode (SADS, Part I) or lifetime diagnosis (SADS-L). NIMH studies are characterized by large samples, broad range of diagnoses, and very positive findings.

Other investigators have also examined SADS reliability. These studies are much more variable in terms of sample and methodology; they vary substantially in sample size and setting. Attention must also be given to number of diagnoses for reliability estimates (e.g., Rosen, Mohs, Johns, et al., 1984, address only a single diagnosis) and whether the standard SADS was administered.

Table 4.1 summarizes 21 investigations that examine SADS interrater and test–retest reliability. The following subsections distill salient findings that are relevant to both practitioners and researchers.

Setting, Diagnoses, and Interviewers

The SADS was clearly designed to be used with clinical populations. Importantly, reliability studies provide a good representation of both inpatient and outpatient settings. These studies examine both current symptoms and current diagnoses. As is common with most Axis I interviews, reliability studies of community samples focus primarily on lifetime diagnoses.

SADS reliability studies focus on psychotic, mood, and anxiety disorders. This focus is clearly understandable in light of its diagnostic coverage.

Reliability studies of the SADS were conducted almost exclusively with mental health professionals. The one study (Rounsaville, Cacciola, Weissman, & Kleber, 1981) that utilized a combination of lay and professional raters produced the least favorable results for current diagnoses.[2]

The SADS should not be used with nonprofessionals for two reasons:

1. Insufficient studies are available.
2. Available research produces good interrater but inadequate test–retest reliability. Without the presence of professionals (i.e., interrater reliability paradigm), the reliability of the SADS with lay interviewers is questionable.

Symptom and Diagnostic Reliability

Mental health professionals often go beyond simple diagnoses to describe and quantify relevant symptomatology. The key issue is whether a structured interview is sufficiently reliable for the accurate description of symptoms. Reliability data on the SADS strongly support the reproducibility of symptoms in both interrater and test–retest paradigms. Several studies (Andreasen et al.,

[2]However, part of these disappointing results may be explained by the research design. A test–retest interval of 6 months for current episodes is likely to lead to increased patient variance.

TABLE 4.1. Reliability Studies for the Schedule of Affective Disorders and Schizophrenia (SADS)

Study (year)	N	Setting In	Out	Com	Univ	Dx	Raters Lay	Prof	Reliability Inter/Retest	(interval)	Reliability estimates Sx/Cur-Dx	Life-Dx/Other
Endicott & Spitzer (1978)	150	✓				19		✓	✓			.96
	60	✓				17		✓	✓	(1–3 days)		.83
Endicott et al. (1981)[a]	45	✓				NA[b]		✓	✓		.84	
Spitzer et al. (1978)	68	✓				18		✓	✓		.86	
	49			✓		18		✓	✓			.87
	150[c]	✓				19		✓	✓		.91	
	60[c]	✓				18		✓	✓	(1–3 days)	.73	
Mazure & Gershon (1979)[d]	49	✓	✓					✓	✓	(6 mo)		.79
Andreasen et al. (1981)[e]	50	✓	✓			5		✓	✓	(<1 day)	.81	.87
	50	✓	✓			5		✓	✓	(6 mo)	.72	
Keller et al. (1981)[e]	25	✓	✓			4		✓	✓	(<1 day)	.63 .69	.83
Merikangas (1981)	50				✓			✓	✓	(6 mo)		.77
Rounsaville et al. (1981)[f]	40	✓	✓			16	✓	✓	✓		.88	
	20	✓	✓			16	✓	✓	✓	(10 days)	.49	
	117	✓	✓			16	✓	✓	✓	(6 mo)	.32	
Strober et al. (1981)[g]	95	✓						✓	✓		.75	
Andreasen et al. (1982)[b]	8		✓			3		✓	✓		.76	.75
McDonald-Scott & Endicott (1984)[a,e]	50	✓				5		✓	✓		.88	.93
Rosen, Mohs, Johns, et al. (1984)	54	✓	✓			1		✓	✓			.77
Spiker & Ehler (1984)	62	✓	✓	✓		7		✓	✓	(<1 day)	.57	.77

Study	N										
Bromet et al. (1986)[i]	131		✓			3		✓	(18 mo)		.34
Hasin & Grant (1987a)	11	✓	✓			2	✓	✓			.91
Rapp, Parisi, & Walsh (1988)[j]	15		✓				✓	✓		.94	
Fyer et al. (1989)[k]	104		✓			6	✓	✓	(0–2 mo)	.44	
Manuzza et al. (1989)[l]	104		✓			6	✓	✓	(0–2 mo)		.68"
Leboyer et al. (1991)[m]	55	✓	✓	✓			✓	✓	(3 mo)	.65	.71
Kendler et al. (1994)[o]	40		✓			6	✓	✓			.91
Nelson-Gray et al. (1996)	9		✓			2	✓	✓			.92

Note. See Table 1.5 (p. 35) for a glossary of terms and abbreviations. Unless otherwise noted, reliability estimates are as follows: symptoms = intraclass coefficients (ICCs); diagnoses = kappa coefficients; others (summary scales) = ICCs.

[a] SADS-C.

[b] All patients had depressive disorders; other disorders are not reported.

[c] Same samples are used in Endicott and Spitzer (1978).

[d] Mixed sample of patients with mood-disorders, their first-degree relatives, and medical controls.

[e] ICCs for diagnosis.

[f] Opiate addicts (outpatients and untreated addicts).

[g] Adolescents.

[h] Used eight videotapes and 36 clinicians.

[i] SADS-L was administered, although only subsections were readministered. In addition, a serious nuclear accident (Three Mile Island) may have affected the reliability estimates.

[j] Elderly medical patients.

[k] Anxiety symptoms only.

[l] Same sample as Fyer et al. (1989).

[m] French and German translations of SADS-L.

[n] For DSM-III-R diagnoses; estimates are higher for research diagnostic criteria (.76) and DSM-III (.82).

[o] The study appears to be a follow-up of hospitalized patients.

1982; McDonald-Scott & Endicott, 1984; Rapp, Panisi, Walsh, & Wallace, 1988) have produced moderately high to high estimates (i.e., median r's from .76 to .94) for interrater symptom reliabilities. For test–retest reliabilities, the estimates are more variable, although two of three studies (Andreasen et al., 1981; Keller et al., 1981) produced moderate to high reliability coefficients for intervals of less than 1 day (r's of .63 and .81) and 6 months ($r = .72$). For the third study, Fyer et al. (1989) found mostly modest correlations on the SADS-LA in an analysis of anxiety symptoms alone. Interestingly, the lowest correlations were found for 20 symptoms related to generalized anxiety disorder (GAD); symptoms of panic disorders and phobias tended to be in the moderate range. In summary, the test–retest reliability for the SADS produced outstanding results, whereas the results for the anxiety section of the SADS-LA were decidedly mixed.

The SADS-C also has excellent interrater reliability for individual symptoms. Endicott, Cohen, Nee, Fleiss, and Sarantakos (1981) evaluated 45 inpatients with outstanding reliabilities (median ICC = .84). Because patients with schizophrenia or severe manic episodes were excluded, some individual symptoms were not sufficiently represented.

The interrater reliability of the SADS was examined closely for current disorders. In general, the interrater reliability produced good to superb median reliability estimates for current diagnoses. Of eight studies that examined interrater reliability, two studies produced moderate results (median kappas of .75), while six studies produced outstanding results (i.e., median kappas or ICC > .85).

Test–retest reliabilities for current diagnoses were generally in the moderate range when professional raters were employed. The sole study (Rounsaville et al., 1981) that used lay and professional raters yielded unsatisfactory test–retest reliabilities (i.e., .49 for a 10-day interval and .32 for a 6-month interval). Four studies utilized test–retest reliability with professional raters for current diagnosis; three studies produced very similar results (median kappas of .65, .69, and .73, respectively). The fourth study (Spiker & Ehler, 1984) produced only a moderate median kappa of .57; the problem diagnosis in this study was schizoaffective disorder. Overall, these results suggest moderate test–retest reliability when interviewers have professional training.

Test–retest reliabilities were substantially higher for lifetime than for current diagnoses. One explanation for this finding is that the increased prevalences of lifetime disorders exerted a positive effect on reported kappa coefficients. With respect to median kappa coefficients, four of nine comparisons clustered between .77 and .79. In addition, two studies had high median reliability coefficients: .86 (Spitzer, Endicott, & Robins, 1978) and .91 (Hasin & Grant, 1987a), although interpretation of the second study is attenuated by the narrow range of diagnoses. Only one study (Bromet, Bunn, Connell, Dew, & Schulberg, 1986) reported an inadequate test–retest reliability; however, this study is very atypical on several grounds. First, the interval between administrations was exceedingly long (18 months); patient variance may account for some of the differences even in lifetime diagnoses. Second, the same interviewers were often used for both administrations, potentially confounding the results. Third, the readminstration did not follow the standard protocol; only diagnoses of major depression, minor depression, and GAD were considered. As a general conclusion, the SADS appears reliable for lifetime diagnoses when the standard administration is followed and the interval is a reasonable period (≤ 6 months). With a more extended interval, concerns about temporal stability rather then test–retest reliability are raised (e.g., see Simon, Endicott, & Nee, 1987).

Reliability of Summary Scales

Especially in research settings, mental health professionals become interested in dimensional ratings that represent a composite of mood, anxiety, or psychotic symptoms. For these purposes, summary scales were created (Endicott & Spitzer, 1978). These summary scales have outstanding reliability coefficients (ICCs > .80) for both interrater and test–retest reliabilities.

Diagnostic Validity

The SADS's validity was established through studies of criterion-related, convergent, and construct validity. For criterion-related validity, research examined (1) predictive validity, with a focus on outcome criteria, and (2) concurrent validity with other structured interviews.

Predictive Validity

The first validation studies of the SADS were closely tied to RDC diagnoses. They were linked to Syndeham's criteria of diagnostic validity, with an emphasis on exclusion and outcome criteria. The relation of these early outcome studies to RDC criteria is summarized by Feighner et al. (1972) and Spitzer et al. (1978). Since that time, a large body of research has examined the SADS in relationship to outcome criteria. In light of the SADS's original development to study the psychobiology of depression, it is not surprising that mood disorders predominate these outcome studies.

Primary findings from SADS studies of outcome criteria with mood disorders are as follows:

- Endicott and Spitzer (1979) examined differences between endogenous and nonendogenous major depression. With respect to the latter, 2-year outcome data did not support the commonly held notion that endogenous depression had poorer outcomes; indeed, the opposite may be true (see also Gallagher & Thompson, 1983).
- The course of major depression is well documented. Coryell et al. (1994) conducted a multisite NIMH study with the SADS on episodes of ma-

jor depression. Regardless of the number of episodes or referral sources, the course of most episodes was well defined, with recovery for 60% of the cases in 6 months and 80% in 12 months. In medical patients, Kessler, Cleary, and Burke (1985) found that a smaller proportion of cases recovered. This finding is likely attributable to the fact that most cases were undiagnosed and untreated by patients' primary care physicians.

• Outcome research has also examined new cases of major depression. Bromet et al. (1986) studied depression in 391 female community participants over an 18-month period. As expected, persons with few SADS depressive symptoms had a low incidence of subsequent depression when originally tested. In a university sample, Hokanson, Rubert, Welker, Hollander, and Hedeen (1989) found that chronically depressed first-year students had low social contact, anhedonia, and increased stress. However, new cases of depression were less clear with regard to antecedent symptoms, which appeared to be associated with general indices of psychopathology.

• Parental major depression predicts depression in offspring. In a 10-year longitudinal study conducted by Wickramaratne and Weissman (1998), parental depression dramatically increased the likelihood of offspring depression during both adolescence and adulthood. Of particular significance, the earlier age of onset in parents markedly increased the likelihood of depression in offspring, especially during childhood.

• A 15-year SADS follow-up found that nearly two-thirds (63.9%) of hyperactive children were likely to maintain mild to moderate symptoms despite childhood treatment (Weiss, Hechtman, Milroy, & Perlman, 1985).

• Several studies have addressed treatment responsiveness of patients with bipolar disorders. Interestingly, Freeman, Clothier, Pazzaglia, Sesem, and Swann (1992) found that more severe depression on the SADS-C was associated with treatment responsiveness for patients in manic episodes.

Research has also examined the course and treatment responsiveness of other mental disorders. These studies frequently include participants with comorbid disorders. The major findings are summarized as follows:

• For schizophrenic disorders, negative symptoms and delay in treatment appear to predict poor treatment response and a chronic course, although this is not always the case (Rosen, Mohs, Johns, et al., 1984). The addition of antidepressants to antipsychotic medication may produce modest positive changes in SADS negative symptoms (Siris et al., 1991). Loebel et al. (1992) found that delay in treatment was associated with poor treatment outcomes (i.e., time to remission and level of remission).

• Specific SADS symptoms appear to predict treatment noncompliance in schizophrenic patients. Duncan (1995; see also Duncan & Rogers, 1998) found that the severity of anger, delusions, and hallucinations predicted medication noncompliance.

• As expected, comorbidity tends to produce negative outcomes. In the treatment of opiate abusers, Kosten, Rounsaville, and Kleber (1986) found that depression complicated the treatment and outcome of opioid dependence. In predicting the outcome of combat-related PTSD, lifetime diagnoses of depression and GAD were associated with nonrecovery (Engdah, Speed, Eberly, & Schwartz, 1991).

• Overall level of functioning is predictive of treatment response and future hospitalizations. Endicott et al. (1976) found that nearly one-half (48.3%) of patients with low GAS scores (< 40) were rehospitalized within 9 months. Kessler et al. (1985) found that even moderate GAS scores were likely to be associated with chronic disorders. Rogers and Wettstein (1985), in an 18-month follow-up of potentially dangerous outpatients, found that low GAS scores predicted rehospitalization.

Concurrent Validity

Systematic comparisons between structured interviews are relatively uncommon for Axis I disorders. Therefore, this section is relatively brief in its description of concurrent validity. As described in Chapter 3, Hesselbrock et al. (1982) examined the diagnostic concordance for the SADS-L and the DIS (Diagnostic Interview Schedule). They found moderately high kappas (.72 to 1.00, with a median of .76) for four common diagnoses. Farmer et al. (1993) compared the SADS-L to the Schedule for the Clinical Assessment of Neuropsychiatry (SCAN; Wing et al., 1990). For DSM-III diagnoses, the agreement across broad diagnostic groups (no diagnosis; mood, anxiety, and schizophrenic disorders) was excellent, with 89% agreement and a kappa of .81.

Two focused studies of concurrent validity found mixed results with substance abusers. Boyd, Weissman, Thompson, and Myers (1983) compared SADS-L interviews with RDC criteria for alcoholism to DSM-III alcohol abuse (78.8% concordance) and ICD-9 alcohol dependence (64.7% concordance). The SADS-L was more encompassing; it included nearly all DSM-III (96.3%) and ICD-9 (91.7%) diagnoses. Producing more negative results, Hasin and Grant (1987a, 1987b, 1987c; see Chapter 3) compared DIS and SADS-L diagnoses for 120 drug abusers. Although the measures evidenced moderately high agreement for substance abuse, poor kappa estimates (.04–.46) were found for anxiety disorders, depression, and APD.

Construct Validity

Convergent Validity. Dean, Surtees, and Sahsidharan (1983) compared the SADS to a different diagnostic system, namely, the Present State Examination (PSE; Wing, Cooper, & Sartorius, 1974; Wing, Nixon, Mann, & Leff, 1977). From an original sample of 576 female community participants, 80 disordered women were evaluated. Of three common disorders, good agreement was found for major depression, with modest agreement for minor depression, and GAD.

Convergent validity for the SADS has also been examined with reference to the Personality Assessment Inventory (PAI; Morey, 1991b). Rogers, Ustad, and Salekin (1998) found moderate correlations between the SADS and the corresponding PAI scale (*r*'s from .40 to .67); the notable exception was manic symptoms, which were only modestly correlated (*r* = .31). Because many patients have substantial symptomatology associated with several disorders, other significant correlations (e.g., depression and anxiety) were also observed.

The bulk of SADS convergent validity studies compare SADS results to measures of psychopathology. In the original study, Endicott and Spitzer (1978) correlated the SADS summary scales with the Katz Adjustment Scales completed by patients and relatives, and the Symptom Checklist—90 (SCL-90; Derogatis, 1977). The *M* correlations of the SADS summary scales with the Katz Adjustment Scales were .42 for relatives and .40 for patients; similarly, the *M* correlation with the SCL-90 was .47. Although relatively modest, such validity coefficients are typical in the presence of multiple sources of data (Cronbach, 1970). More recently, Rogers, Harris, and Wasyliw (1983) compared SADS-C and SCL-90 administrations across two time periods with forensic outpatients. On 23 comparable symptoms, they found moderate to moderately high correlations (i.e., *M r*'s of .54 for the first and .68 for the second administration). Despite these positive findings, Rogers et al. expressed concern regarding the variability of individual correlates across administrations.

Studies have focused on the convergent validity of the SADS for patients with mood disorders. Convergent validity is amply demonstrated for major depression:

- Endicott et al. (1981) found with 45 inpatients that the SADS and the Hamilton Depression Rating Scale (HDRS; Hamilton, 1960) correlated at .84 with depression syndrome, .80 with endogenous features, and −.69 with the GAS.
- Hurt, Friedman, Clarkin, Corn, and Aronoff (1982) compared comparable items from the HDRS to the SADS-C, with a high correlation for young adults (*r* = .86) and a moderate correlation for adolescents (*r* = .72).
- Myers and Weissman (1980) compared major depression on the SADS to the Center of Epidemiologic Studies—Depression scale (CES-D; Radloff, 1977). Although the overall concordance was high (92.5%), the greatest agreement was found for the absence of depression.
- Johnson, Magaro, and Stern (1986) found that the SADS-C depression scale correlated highly with the Beck Depression Inventory (BDI; .81) and the HDRS (.96).
- With 150 elderly medical inpatients, Rapp and his colleagues (Rapp, Parisi, & Walsh, 1988; Rapp, Parisi, Walsh, & Wallace, 1988) found

moderate correlations for depression between the SADS and (1) the BDI (Beck, Ward, Mendelson, Mock, & Erbaugh, 1961), (2) the Self-Report Depression Scale (Zung, 1965), and (3) the Geriatric Depression Scale (Yesage et al., 1983).

- In elderly outpatients, Hill, Gallagher, Thompson, and Ishida (1988) found that SADS items associated with suicide were predicted by the BDI and the Hopelessness Scale (Beck, Weissman, Lester, & Trexler, 1974).

Familial and genetic correlates were used to examine the construct validity of SADS diagnoses. Maziade et al. (1992) reviewed the major genetic-linkage studies for bipolar disorders; most of these studies (76.7%) with structured interviews used the SADS or the SADS-L. In general, they provide mixed evidence of SADS-based diagnoses. Kendler, Gruenberg, and Kinney (1994) utilized the SADS-L to examine genetic patterns of schizophrenic adoptees. They found a clear genetic pattern for schizophrenia and schizophrenia spectrum disorders in first- and second-degree relatives. More recently, Horwarth et al. (1995) compared genetic patterns on the SADS-LA for proband groups with panic and depressive disorders. They found familial transmission patterns for panic disorders and social phobias.

Convergent–Discriminant Validity. Rogers et al. (1995) evaluated the convergent and discriminant validity of the SADS-C in a clinical sample of jail referrals. With a multitrait–mulitmethod matrix (Campbell & Fiske, 1959), Rogers et al. established the construct validity of the SADS-C for schizophrenic, depressive, and bipolar disorders. The SADS-C demonstrated relatively modest convergent validity but superb discriminant validities.

Discriminant Validity. Using contrasted-groups design, studies have sought to establish differences between diagnostic groups based on SADS data. As an initial study, Endicott and Spitzer (1979) evaluated differences between patients with schizoaffective disorders and psychotic depression. They established logical symptom differences between the two diagnoses. In a large study of inpatients, Secunda et al. (1985) found predicted differences for SADS manic symptoms with the following M scores: 39.6 manic, 21.4 bipolar, 10.2 depressed, and 13.3 schizophrenic. On the SADS-C, Johnson et al. (1986) examined differences in composite scores for schizophrenic, depressed, and manic patients. Marked differences in the expected direction were found for these three diagnoses.

The discriminant validity of the SADS was also examined for response styles. Ustad, Rogers, and Salekin (1998) compared 24 suspected malingerers with 63 genuine patients. Highly significant differences were found on dissimulation scales for both the SADS and SADS-C. A subsequent discriminant function produced high classification rates (> 90%).

GENERALIZABILITY AND CROSS-CULTURAL RESEARCH

Studies of experienced clinicians (Andreasen et al., 1981; Keller et al., 1981) indicate that SADS validity is generalizable across research sites, and inpatient and outpatient populations. The NIMH collaborative studies on the psychobiology of depression from five centers (Boston, Chicago, Iowa City, New York, and St. Louis) yielded highly consistent results.

Epidemiological studies provide indirect data on generalizability, although sociodemographic differences sometimes reflect true differences in lifetime prevalence rates. Weissman, Myers, and Harding (1978; Weissman & Myers, 1980) conducted a longitudinal study of 511 community participants that were systematically evaluated on the SADS at three time periods spanning 8 years. In general, very few differences were found related to age and race. One exception was an overrepresentation of substance abuse among minorities. Several important differences were observed with social class and mood disorders: increased prevalence of bipolar disorder among upper social classes and increased prevalence of depression among lower social classes.

Vernon and Roberts (1982) conducted a large-scale study of current and lifetime SADS diagnoses based on community samples of 219 Anglo Americans, 187 African Americans, and 122 Mexican Americans. Based on the SADS, these investigators found comparable prevalence rates for current episodes of major depression (1.8% Anglo Americans, 2.1% African Americans, and 2.5% Mexican Americans). Interestingly, African Americans (9.6%) had lower lifetime diagnoses of major depression than either Anglo Americans (19.2%) or Mexican Americans (18.9%). Prevalence rates for bipolar and schizoaffective disorders were generally comparable.

Available research on French and German translations of the SADS (see, e.g., Leboyer et al., 1991) indicate a moderate level of symptom and diagnostic reliability. More germane to North America would be Spanish translations of the SADS. Translations and concomitant validation studies have not been found.

In summary, current studies suggest that the SADS is generalizable to a wide range of clinical settings. Regarding ethnicity, relatively few differences were found for three reference groups: Anglo Americans, African Americans, and Hispanic Americans (specifically Mexican Americans). Systematic studies of the SADS with other minority populations are not available.

CLINICAL APPLICATIONS

The hallmark of the SADS is its impressive interrater reliabilities for current episodes. In clinical settings where highly reliable diagnoses are critical for mood and psychotic disorders, practitioners would do well to consider the SADS based on the reproducibility of its results for individual symptoms, summary scales, and diagnoses. The SADS could also be integrated with sections of the SCID to produce a more comprehensive diagnostic framework for Axis I disorders. Table 4.2 includes a summary of SADS advantages and limitations in clinical assessments.

The SADS is the measure of choice when the severity of symptoms is a significant issue. In many clinical contexts, practitioners must do more than simply enumerate symptoms and render diagnoses. Rather, the pivotal question is the degree to which these symptoms are present. For example, researchers on treatment and treatment outcome are especially interested in the change in target symptoms; rarely are symptoms completely resolved. As a further example, forensic evaluations are concerned with gradations of symptoms in addressing a particular psycholegal standard (e.g., Rogers & Shuman, 2000).

Clinical Settings

The SADS is immensely useful in evaluating common Axis I disorders, with comprehensive coverage of mood and psychotic symptoms and adequate coverage of anxiety symptoms. The SADS provides helpful information about as-

---

TABLE 4.2. Advantages and Limitations of the Schedule of Affective Disorders and Schizophrenia (SADS) in Diagnostic Evaluations

Advantages

- *Reliability.* The SADS, more than any other diagnostic measure, has outstanding interrater reliabilities for current episodes that extend from individual symptoms to summary scales and diagnoses. In addition, the SADS compares favorably to other measures on lifetime diagnoses.

- *Symptom severity.* The SADS provides severity ratings for many symptoms experienced during the current episode; these ratings allow clinicians to estimate accurately the salience of particular symptoms as well as treatment response.

- *Response styles.* The SADS has clinical guidelines for the assessment of response styles. Especially with feigning, these guidelines serve an important screening function.

Limitations

- *Narrow band of diagnosis.* Although the SADS is designed to cover 23 mental disorders, the majority of its diagnoses are mood disorders and their subtypes. For a comprehensive review of Axis I disorders, clinicians must supplement the SADS with additional clinical interviews.

- *RDC-based diagnosis.* One complication with the use of the SADS is that the clinical inquiries are focused on research diagnostic criteria (RDC) diagnostic criteria, rather than DSM-IV criteria. Although the diagnostic systems are often very close, clinicians must be aware of the differences and augment the SADS with additional clinical inquiries.

- *Sophisticated training.* As a semistructured diagnostic interview, the SADS requires that clinicians be well versed in diagnosis and have a working knowledge of the SADS's administration and scoring. However, training materials are readily available.

sociated features and clinical correlates that are not covered by other Axis I interviews. In line with the breadth–depth issue, thorough attention is paid to the most common symptoms of mental disorders. The trade-off is that relatively uncommon disorders (e.g., dissociative disorders) are not covered.

The SADS and SADS-C are well suited for documenting changes in clinical status for patients with major mental disorders. For studies that assess either the course of these disorders or treatment response, the SADS and the SADS-C would appear to be the measures of choice. They not only provide severity ratings but also incorporate associated clinical features that may be important markers regarding chronicity and response to specific treatments.

A principal advantage of the SADS over other Axis I interviews is found in the SADS-C. It allows clinicians to evaluate reliably key symptoms or summary scales either as a screen or a follow-up measure. Its screening function is underutilized. In 15–20 minutes, time-pressured practitioners can cover key symptoms and reliably estimate their severity. Because these symptoms and concomitant disorders would need to be covered in any unstructured interview, the SADS-C requires virtually no additional expenditure of time.

Response Styles

Rogers (1984) demonstrated that all psychological measures are vulnerable to feigning and other patient response styles. While his review did not cover structured interviews, subsequent research by Rogers (1997) has amply demonstrated this point. Therefore, practitioners must be prepared to systematically address feigning and defensiveness as potential response styles in clinical evaluations.

Rogers (1988) described how the SADS could be employed to assess feigning and response consistency. Clinical methods include comparisons of SADS data with (1) unstructured interviews, (2) repeat administrations of the SADS, and (3) informant SADS reports on the patient. More recently, Rogers (1997) provided descriptive data on how the SADS could be used as a screen for either feigning or defensiveness. As a specific example of the latter, Rogers identified eight very common symptoms (i.e., item numbers 234, 238, 244, 265, 272, 330, 418, and 433). Because most patients (80%) report at least two of these symptoms, the lack of common symptoms can be used as a screen for defensiveness.

Ustad, Rogers, and Salekin (1998) reported data from a contrasted-groups design for the identification of potential feigners. Interestingly, the combination of dissimulation scales proved highly effective at identifying potential feigners on both the SADS and the SADS-C. Despite these positive findings, Ustad et al. concluded that the SADS and SADS-C should only be used for screening potential cases, not for the actual determination of feigning.

Informant interviews are frequently used when the accuracy of a patient's reporting is questioned. A highly original study by Chapman, Mannuzza, Klein, and Fyer (1994) examined the usefulness of family members as informants for 2,193 pairs of participants. Based on SADS-LA diagnoses, they found that family informants were highly variable in their accuracy, being most accurate with alcoholism and least accurate with depression. Compared to the patients, family informants were the most accurate if they had the same disorder, less accurate if they had another disorder, and least accurate if they had no disorder. Reassuringly, family members rarely reported diagnostic data that were not warranted. Specificity was uniformly high (> .85) except that family members with the same disorder had a small tendency to also report other disorders (specificity = .72).

Medical Settings

The SADS has also proven useful in medical settings (Cavanaugh & Wettstein, 1989; Weddington, Segraves, & Simon, 1986). The study by Kessler et al. (1985) has especially important implications for the treatment of primary care patients. Based on the SADS-L, they found that nonpsychiatric physicians in the role of primary health care providers only recognized 20% of *chronic* mental disorders that were present for at least 6 months. Moreover, these same physicians missed nearly every *new* case of mental disorders; they recognized a mere 3% of new cases over the same 6-month period. Use of the SADS, or even the SADS-C, would dramatically improve clinical care for the mentally disordered.

The need for systematic assessments is highlighted by medical care for the elderly. In his SADS study of elderly patients, Rapp, Parisi, and Walsh (1988; Rapp, Parisi, Walsh, & Wallace, 1988) found that medical staff overlook mental disorders. As a stark example, none of the 27 depressed patients were accurately diagnosed. Obviously, treatment interventions are compromised by the inadequacy of diagnoses. The addition of the SADS or SADS-C appears clinically justified.

Forensic Settings

Rogers and his colleagues (Rogers, 1986; Rogers & Cavanaugh, 1981; Rogers & Cunnien, 1986; Rogers & Shuman, 2000; Rogers, Thatcher, & Cavanaugh, 1984) have made a strong argument for the use of the SADS in forensic evaluations. Because of its impressive interrater reliability and adequate test–retest reliability over lifetime diagnoses, the SADS lends itself to the assessment of impairment at specific time periods. For example, insanity evaluations require an assessment of symptomatology/impairment at a discrete time period, namely, the time of the offense. In two related studies, Rogers, Cavanaugh, and Dolmetsch (1981; Rogers et al., 1984) were able to establish significant differences in SADS summary scales and the GAS for patients clinically determined to be sane and insane. The SADS provided clear evidence of pervasive psychotic symptomatology in defendants evaluated as insane.

The SADS also appears to be appropriate for civil forensic cases. Because of its value for retrospective diagnosis and symptom severity, it is useful for establishing multiple time perspectives. For personal injury cases, the SADS may be adapted so that the intensive coverage of Part I is considered at three discrete time periods: (1) just prior to the injury, (2) soon after the injury (e.g., 3 to 6 months), and (3) the present time. This expanded administration of the SADS provides a structure for understanding the acute and long-term effects of the injury. In addition, clinicians can assess whether the reported progress (a) is consistent with other clinical data and (b) fits a typical pattern of treatment response. In summary, the SADS lends itself to a variety of forensic evaluations.

Summary

The SADS is adaptable to a wide range of clinical settings in which reliable, precise measurement is imperative. Because of its versatility, I would argue for the inclusion of the SADS in the clinical training of mental health professionals. For psychologists in particular, an argument could be marshaled that the level of preparation on the SADS be on par with more traditional psychometric approaches.

5

Structured Clinical Interview for DSM-IV Disorders (SCID) and Other Axis I Interviews

OVERVIEW

This chapter features the Structured Clinical Interview for DSM-IV Disorders (SCID; First, Spitzer, Williams, & Gibbon, 1997). During the last decade, the SCID has attracted widespread interest and large-scale research studies. In addition to the SCID, several other Axis I interviews are examined in detail. For example, the Comprehensive Assessment of Symptoms and History (CASH; Andreasen, 1987a) is especially suited for the evaluation of psychotic disorders. In addition, the Present State Examination (PSE; Wing et al., 1974) operationalizes ICD models of diagnoses. While rarely used in North America, the PSE is employed extensively in Europe and other parts of the world. Finally, the Composite International Diagnostic Interview (CIDI) was developed under the auspices of the World Health Organization—Alcohol, Drug, and Mental Health Administration (1987). The CIDI combines the DIS (Chapter 3) with the PSE to create a composite measure for evaluating both DSM and ICD diagnoses.

This chapter also includes brief synopses of other Axis I interviews. These interviews are typically limited in their validation or have circumscribed applications. Recent examples include the Mini-International Neuropsychiatic Interview (MINI; Sheehan et al., 1997) and the Diagnostic Interview for Genetic Studies (DIGS; Nurnberger et al., 1994).

STRUCTURED CLINICAL INTERVIEW FOR DSM-IV DISORDERS (SCID)

Description and Rationale

Spitzer, Williams, Gibbon, and First (1989) described the early development of the SCID, from its initial conceptualization in 1983 to its first draft in

1985. In light of DSM-III and its fundamental changes in diagnoses, the SCID was developed to standardize DSM-III evaluations of mental disorders. Under the aegis of the NIMH, an extensive field trial was carried out in the mid-1980s (see Williams, Spitzer, & Gibbon, 1992). Much of the available research was conducted on the DSM-III-R version (Spitzer, Williams, & Gibbon, 1987a, 1987b) that was subsequently published by the American Psychiatric Press (Spitzer, Williams, Gibbon, & First, 1990b). In 1997, the most recently published version of the SCID incorporated the changes implemented with DSM-IV (First, Sptizer, Williams, & Gibbon, 1997). Box 5.1 provides highlights of the SCID and information on its availability.

The SCID for Axis I disorders is divided into the Clinical Version (SCID-CV) and Research Version (SCID-RV). This review focuses on the SCID-CV because it has received the most research effort; the SCID-RV supplements the SCID-CV with additional disorders and diagnostic specifiers. In addition to these versions, the SCID-II (First, Spitzer, Gibbon, Williams, & Benjamin, 1994) is an Axis II interview designed to assess personality disorders (see Chapter 9).

The SCID-CV comprises an Overview Section (e.g., current problems and symptoms, and treatment history), Summary Score Sheet (i.e., lifetime and current diagnoses, and Global Assessment Functioning scale, or GAF), and nine modules for disorders/syndromes. The organization of mood and psychotic disorders involves two steps: (1) clinical ratings of symptomatology, and (2) integration of symptoms for diagnosis and differential diagnosis.

BOX 5.1. Highlights of the SCID

- *Description:* Successive versions of the SCID evaluate DSM-III, DSM-III-R, and DSM-IV disorders. The purpose of the SCID is to provide adequate coverage of DSM inclusion criteria across a broad range of disorders.

- *Administration time:* Typically, ranges from 1 to 3 hours. The duration is directly related to whether hierarchical screens are employed.

- *Skills level:* The SCID requires administration by mental health professionals skilled in rendering diagnoses. Training materials are available.

- *Distinctive features:* The SCID is distinguished by its direct correspondence with DSM-IV and its breadth of diagnostic coverage. Its focus is on diagnosis rather than symptomatology.

- *Cost:* Price list on 3/1/2001; SCID-1 set (user's guide, administration booklet, and five score sheets) is $77.

- *Source:* HealthSource Bookstore, by phone, (800) 713-7122; on the internet, *www.healthsourcebooks.org;* or by mail, 1400 K Street, NW, Washington, DC 20005-2401.

In comparison, the remainder of the SCID is organized in modules that combine symptoms and diagnoses.

The most complex and challenging module of the SCID-CV is the Psychoactive Substance Use Disorders. Psychologists and other mental health professionals are asked to identify significant substance abuse in eight drug classes: (1) sedatives–hypnotics–anxiolytics, (2) cannabis, (3) stimulants, (4) opioids, (5) cocaine, (6) hallucinogens/phencylidine, (7) other, and (8) polydrug use (i.e., at least three of these categories). Each reported drug class is then rated on as many as 15 symptoms or characteristics.

The organization of the SCID-CV is hierarchical with explicit decision trees for when to discontinue administrations of each module. The advantage of this organization is that the interviewer minimizes unnecessary expenditure of time on symptoms that are unlikely to qualify for a particular disorder. The two disadvantages of this approach are that (1) diagnoses may be occasionally overlooked and (2) ratings of key symptoms are frequently absent. In cases where the review of symptomatology is critical, practitioners may wish to ignore the hierarchical screens and administer complete sections.

The scoring system for individual symptoms is based on a 3-point scale: 1 = absent/false, 2 = subthreshold (i.e., the criterion is nearly met), and 3 = threshold/true (i.e., meets or exceeds the criterion). Nearly all symptoms are rated for the current episode. Interviewers are encouraged to use all sources of clinical data in making their ratings.

Clinical inquiries are organized into standard questions, branching questions, optional probes and unstructured questions. The majority of questions are composed of standard questions that are routinely asked of each patient. In addition, branching questions are occasionally used. These are presented with prefatory instructions that are capitalized, such as "IF YES," "IF UNCLEAR," and "IF NOT ALREADY KNOWN." Finally, optional probes are presented in parentheses and should be used to clarify clinical ratings of diagnostic criteria. One important feature of the SCID-CV is the attention paid to the patient's own description of symptoms. Certain clinical inquiries, particularly those addressing mood states, will specify "OWN EQUIVALENT" as explicit permission to use the patient's own words to describe symptomatology. The SCID-CV is "semistructured" in that the interviewer must augment the SCID inquiries with his or her own clinical inquiries in cases of inadequate or ambiguous information.

The primary purpose of the SCID is to provide comprehensive coverage of most DSM-IV Axis I disorders. The SCID-CV is not exhaustive; seven major diagnostic categories are not addressed (i.e., developmental disorders, organic mental disorders, dissociative disorders, sexual disorders, sleep disorders, factitious disorders, and impulse control disorders). In addition, less common mood, anxiety, and somatoform disorders are also not covered. Nevertheless, the SCID-CV provides the broadest coverage among Axis I diagnostic interviews The SCID-CV distinguishes itself by its formal coverage of DSM-IV diagnostic criteria.

The trade-off for diagnostic interviews, described in Chapter 1, is breadth versus depth. Because of SCID-CV breadth, the majority of diagnostic criteria are evaluated by single inquiries. Clearly, more extensive questioning would unduly lengthen the interview process. Even so, some clinicians are selective in their administration of SCID-CV modules that may introduce additional variability in rendering diagnoses.

Reliability Studies of the SCID

SCID reliability studies (see Table 5.1) have focused predominantly on current diagnoses with the DSM-III-R version. However, results are likely applicable to the SCID DSM-IV version for two reasons. First, many Axis I disorders remain relatively unchanged between DSM-III-R and DSM-IV. With these diagnoses, the SCID modules are nearly identical. Second, studies with DSM-IV SCID (Levin, Evans, & Kleber, 1998; Ventura, Liberman, Green, Shaner, & Minz, 1998; Zimmerman & Mattia, 1998b) produce reliability estimates that are comparable if not higher than those found in DSM-III-R SCID research (see Table 5.1).

Interrater reliability studies for current diagnoses varied from moderately high (kappas > .75) to superb (kappas > .85). These results are impressive given the diversity of cultures and the use of several translated versions. The only exception was a south Indian study translated into Kannada, which yielded only a moderate kappa of .67; both the diverse culture and the translation may have contribution to this decrement in agreement. Although many studies examined targeted diagnostic groups (three or fewer disorders), studies with a range of disorders produced comparable results.

Williams, Gibbon, et al. (1992) conducted the largest test–retest reliability study reported for diagnostic interviews, with 390 clinical and 202 nonclinical participants. The study found moderate reliabilities (mean kappa = .61) for current episodes with clinical participants. Because of a much smaller number of diagnoses, kappa coefficients for nonclinical participants were only modest (mean = .37). A cause of major concern was the marked fluctuations observed across sites even for common disorders. For example, Williams, Gibbon, et al. found dramatic variations: (1) major depression from .37 to .82, and (2) alcohol abuse/dependence (.00 to .73). Several factors may contribute to these fluctuating and lower-than-expected kappas:

- Unlike most studies, interviewers were brought in from other research centers without any prior knowledge of patients.
- The study was international in scope, combining different cultures and two languages (English and German).

Williams, Spitzer, and Gibbon (1992) produced high test–retest reliabilities when they focused on the diagnosis of panic disorders and its subtypes.

TABLE 5.1. Reliability Studies for the Structured Clinical Interview for DSM-IV Disorders (SCID)

| | | Setting | | Raters | Reliability | Reliability estimates |
Study (year)	N	In/Out/Com/Univ	Dx	Lay/Prof	Inter/Retest (interval)	Sx/Cur-Dx/Life-Dx/Other
Riskland et al. (1987)	75	✓	2	✓	✓	.76
Skre et al. (1991)[a]	54	✓✓	13	✓	✓	.85
Williams, Gibbon, et al. (1992)[b]	390	✓✓ ✓	21	✓	✓ (< 2 wk)	.61 .68
	202		16	✓	✓ (< 2 wk)	.37 .51
Williams, Spitzer, et al. (1992)[c]	72	✓✓	1	✓	✓ (< 1 wk)	.87
Sato et al. (1993)[d]	20	✓	1	✓	✓	1.00
Nunes et al. (1996)[e]	31	✓	3	✓	✓ (NA)	.73
Segal et al. (1995)	40	✓	3	✓	✓	.80
Weiss, Raguram, et al. (1995)[f]	80	✓	6	✓	✓	.67
Levin et al. (1998)	30	✓	7	✓ ✓	✓	> .78
Ventura et al. (1998)[g]	6	✓[h]	NA	✓	✓	.77
Zimmerman & Mattia (1998b).	17	✓	12	✓	✓	.94

Note. See Table 1.5 (p. 35) for a glossary of terms and abbreviations.

[a] Norwegian translation; diagnoses limited to those with four or more cases.

[b] English and German SCID versions with raters from different sites.

[c] Study of panic disorders includes 11 countries and several translations.

[d] Study of major depression with a Japanese sample.

[e] A modified SCID to address temporal relationship of substance abuse to other disorders.

[f] Study in south India translated into Kannada.

[g] Study used six SCID videos and 30 raters.

[h] Source of the patients was unspecified.

With the majority of the sample qualifying for this disorder, high levels of agreement are not surprising.

Interestingly, two studies examined the test–retest reliability of lifetime SCID diagnoses. Because of the greater prevalence of lifetime episodes, the Williams, Gibbon, et al. (1992) kappa coefficients were higher than for current episodes alone. Their results were generally comparable to those of Nunes et al. (1996). Overall, the SCID appears to have moderate test–retest reliabilities for lifetime disorders.

Because of the SCID's emphasis on disorders, symptom reliabilities are overlooked. In cases where clinicians are especially interested in measuring symptom changes that are either naturally occurring (i.e., the course of a disorder) or treatment-related, the SCID is not likely to be the measure of choice. Clinicians have no assurance that any observed change in key symptoms does not reflect variability in measurement (i.e., the SCID) rather than variability in the patient (i.e., improvement or deterioration).

SCID studies suggest that experienced clinicians can be trained to render reliable diagnoses. Training programs vary from a formal, 32-hour didactic review (Kidorf, Brooner, King, Chutuape, & Stitzer, 1996) to joint training on 10–15 cases (Maier, Buller, Sonntag, & Heuser, 1986). Ventura et al. (1998), who developed an elaborate training program that included SCID resources, self-instructional materials, and reliability checks, produced highly reliable results.

In summary, the reliability studies consistently demonstrate that the SCID has good-to-superb reliability for the diagnoses of current episodes. For test–retest reliability, moderate levels are found for clinical samples. For reliability at the symptom level, the SCID has not been formally tested.

Validity Studies of the SCID

SCID studies, perhaps because of the SCID's one-to-one correspondence with DSM-III-R and DSM-IV diagnoses, have paid relatively little attention to concurrent validity. Instead, SCID research has focused on convergent validity with psychometric and biological correlates. In addition, SCID research has addressed criterion-related validity in relationship to Syndeham's model. This research has examined Syndeham's inclusion/exclusion criteria (e.g., diagnostic boundaries) and outcome criteria (e.g., etiology and course of disorders).

Concurrent Validity

Several SCID studies have examined concurrent validity via Spitzer's (1983) Longitudinal Expert Evaluation using All Data (LEAD) model. The strength of this model is that it combines all relevant clinical data to achieve composite diagnoses. Its main limitation is criterion contamination; specifically, no measure (e.g., the SCID) is entirely independent of the LEAD standard. Primary results of the studies utilizing the LEAD model are summarized as follows:

1. A high level of agreement (kappa = .83) is found for mood and schizophrenic disorders when SCID data from field interviewers are compared to composite diagnoses by senior psychiatrists (Maziade et al., 1992).
2. SCID diagnosis of major depression appears to be in close agreement with LEAD[1] diagnosis and in moderate agreement with an independent CIDI diagnosis (Booth, Kirchner, Hamilton, Harrell, & Smith, 1998).
3. Shaner et al. (1998) used the LEAD model to evaluate diagnostic uncertainty with the SCID. Importantly, it does not appear to be related to the symptoms per se. Instead, hierarchical exclusion rules (especially ruling out organic disorders) and general characteristics of disorders (e.g., duration of the episode) appear responsible for diagnostic uncertainty.

Duncan (1987) compared SCID diagnoses for schizophrenia and bipolar disorders on 48 outpatients who were also administered the DIS and had their clinical records systematically reviewed. Duncan found that the SCID diagnoses outperformed the DIS and accurately identified 77% of schizophrenic and 85% of bipolar disorders. Both measures evidenced only modest agreement with the record review, which suggests either limitations in record-keeping or constraints of SCID-based diagnosis.

Several studies have examined the concurrent validity of new diagnostic measures while utilizing the SCID as a quasi–gold standard (i.e., bootstrapping). For example, Ross, Swinson, Larkin, and Doumani (1994) evaluated the Computerized DIS (C-DIS) in relationship to the SCID in a sample of substance abusers. Not surprisingly, the level of agreement was moderate (median kappa = .56) for commonly occurring substance abuse disorders. However, mood and anxiety disorders evidenced poor agreement (median kappa = .22). Interestingly, the overall percentage of agreement for individual diagnoses was quite good (median = 83.9%). On the MINI (Sheehan et al., 1997), Sheehan achieved moderate kappas for 15 current (median = .67) and 7 lifetime (median = .73) disorders.

In summary, most SCID studies on concurrent validity conform to either the LEAD model or bootstrapping procedures. Despite their methodological limitations, results fall into the expected ranges for Axis I interviews. Overall, kappas establish a moderate level of diagnostic agreement.

Convergent Validity

The SCID has been compared to a range of specialized scales to evaluate the convergent validity for specific disorders. The following major findings are summarized by diagnostic categories:

---

[1]A limitation of the LEAD model is criterion contamination because SCID data influence the final diagnoses.

1. *PTSD*. Several studies (e.g., Constans, Lenhoff, & McCarthy, 1997; Pitman, Altman, & Macklin, 1989) of combat-related PTSD indicate convergence between the SCID diagnoses and the Mississippi Scale for Combat-Related PTSD (Mississippi Scale; Keane, Caddell, & Taylor, 1988). The SCID PTSD module was compared to the Clinician-Administered PTSD scale for DSM-IV (CAPS; Blake et al., 1990) with moderate convergence (kappa = .75; Hyer, Summers, Boyd, Litaker, & Boudewyns, 1996). One concern about the SCID PTSD module is that it may lead to underreporting in battered women (Weaver, 1998).

2. *Panic disorders*. Two studies of SCID-diagnosed panic disorders yielded only modest evidence of convergent validity. Maier et al. (1986) compared SCID panic disorders with ICD-9 classifications for 97 patients presenting with panic attacks. Although ICD-9 does not diagnose panic disorders per se, only a minority (30.9%) warranted any ICD-9 diagnosis of anxiety disorder. Ganellen, Maturza, Uhlenhuth, Glass, and Easton (1986) found only minor differences between SCID-diagnosed panic and agoraphobic disorders.

3. *Depression*. Through the use of receiver operating characteristics (ROC) analysis, Stuckenberg, Dura, and Kiecolt-Glaser (1990) found that SCID depression and dysthymia could be identified by scales that measure depression: the Hamilton Depression Rating Scale (HDRS; Hamilton, 1960), the Beck Depression Inventory (BDI; Beck et al., 1961), and the Brief Symptom Inventory depression scale (BSI; Derogatis & Spencer, 1982).

4. *Substance abuse*. Kranzler, Kadden, Babor, Tennen, and Rounsaville (1996) found strong convergent evidence for four SCID substance abuse diagnoses and pathological patterns on several scales, including the Addiction Severity Index (ASI; McLellan et al., 1992).

5. *Psychotic disorders*. Cassano, Pini, Saettoni, Rucci, and Dell'Osso (1998) attempted to differentiate between psychotic patients with and without comorbidity. Unfortunately, the heterogeneity of primary diagnoses (psychotic disorders and mood disorders with psychotic features) and the range of comorbid Axis I diagnoses militated against reliable differences. Comorbidity resulted in high SCL-90 scores. In addition, many psychotic patients had elevated scores on the Scale for the Assessment of Negative Symptoms (SANS; Andreasen, 1984a), providing evidence of convergent validity.

A different approach to convergent validity is the examination of biological markers that are postulated as correlates of specific disorders. These studies often provide only general support because of the nonspecificity of laboratory studies. One major exception is substance abuse disorders, for which laboratory tests can provide specific evidence. In this vein, Kidorf et al. (1996) established a positive relationship between (1) urinalysis, and (2) past and present episodes of cocaine dependence and sedative dependence disorders.

SCID research has also examined differences in brain structure and functioning for specific diagnoses. For example, Schwartz, Aylward, Barta, Tune, and Pearlson (1992) found differences in brain structure (i.e., wider Sylvian fissures) between patients with schizophrenia and normal controls but failed to confirm other past results (e.g., increased ventricles). Research by Schramke, Stow, Ratcliff, Goldstein, and Condray (1998) suggests that post-stroke patients are likely to experience distress rather than SCID disorders. In addition, SCID diagnoses did not appear to be affected by the site of the stroke.

Biological markers associated with panic disorders were also examined in SCID research:

- Gaffney, Fenton, Lane, and Lake (1988) found preliminary differences between patients with panic disorders and normal controls on sodium lactate infusion. Although small physical differences were noted, the major effect appeared to be psychological, with panic induced by increased behavioral sensitivity.
- Pecknold et al. (1987) found significant differences in the imipramine-binding sites for patients with panic disorders, major depression, and panic disorder plus major depression. Patients with depression only had lower levels of imipramine-binding sites than normal controls. Interestingly, patients with both panic disorders and panic plus depression evidenced a nonsignificant trend toward higher levels.
- Lesser, Rubin, Lydriard, Swinson, and Pecknold (1987) found a negligible relationship between abnormalities in thyroid function and panic disorders.

In summary, biological markers provide only modest evidence of diagnostic validity. In addition, several studies compare specific disorders to normal controls. In these cases, the data cannot address whether predicted differences are applicable to the diagnoses in question or are shared by a spectrum of mental disorders.

Syndeham and Predictive Validity

As discussed in Chapter 1, Syndeham theorized that specific disorders are predicated on inclusion, exclusion, and outcome criteria. For inclusion and exclusion criteria, the major challenge is establishing clear diagnostic boundaries. For outcome criteria, the focus is on a longitudinal perspective addressing such components as etiology, course, and outcome of the disorder.

Diagnostic Boundaries. Multiaxial diagnoses are based on the premise that comorbidity will commonly occur among patients with mental disorders. However, the key issue is whether this overlap is excessive. When the majority of patients share the same two disorders, then the clarity of diagnostic boundaries is brought into question. This section considers comorbidity from four vantage points: (1) psychotic disorders, (2) substance abuse disorders, (3) mood and anxiety disorders, and (4) Axis I–Axis II interactions.

Several studies have evaluated comorbidity with psychotic disorders. Strakowski et al. (1993) examined diagnostic overlap for patients experiencing their first psychotic episode. Encouragingly, patients with schizophrenic or delusional disorders had relatively little Axis I comorbidity. In contrast, patients having mood disorders with psychotic features, especially bipolar disorders, had substantial overlap. More recently, Cosoff and Hafner (1998) found that substantial proportions of patients with schizophrenic and schizoaffective disorders also warranted anxiety disorders (43.3% and 45.0%, respectively).

Patients with substance abuse disorders frequently experience both Axis I and Axis II disorders. Thevos, Brady, Grice, Dustan, and Malcolm (1993) found that the majority of patients with alcohol or cocaine dependence qualified for other Axis I disorders. Interestingly, marked differences were observed by gender and type of dependence. For example, the prevalence of mood disorders for women with alcohol (73.7%) dependence was nearly twice that for women with cocaine (38.1%) dependence. The Thevos et al. (1993) study illustrates the complexity of comorbidity. In clinical practice, many patients qualify for multiple substance abuse disorders that are further complicated by both gender and an array of comorbid disorders.

The comorbidity between mood and anxiety disorders is well established and clearly transcends any single Axis I interview. Brawman-Mintzer et al. (1993) found that patients with generalized anxiety disorder (GAD) had substantial comorbidity with major depression (42.2%) and other mood disorders (11.0%). More dramatically, Pini et al. (1997) found almost complete overlap of anxiety disorders with bipolar disorder (79.2%), major depression (92.1%), and dysthymia (88.0%), with an overall weighted mean of 87.4% in a mixed sample of outpatients and inpatients. The Pini et al. study raises serious questions about diagnostic overlap between mood and anxiety disorders.

Axis I–Axis II interactions also have implications for diagnostic boundaries. Alnaes and Torgersen (1989) examined comorbidity in a large outpatient sample. Mood disorders evidenced a major overlap (84.6%) with Axis II disorders, especially avoidant and dependent personality disorders. A comparable overlap was found for anxiety disorders (81.0%), although personality disorders appeared more evenly distributed. A study by Shelton et al. (1997) evaluated Axis II disorders in 410 patients with dysthymia. The majority (57.3%) had comorbid Axis II disorders (predominantly Cluster C) in addition to other mood and anxiety disorders. Of even more concern, approximately one-fourth (25.6%) qualified for two or more personality disorders.

Longitudinal Perspectives. The etiology and causal pathways of mental disorders pose a formidable challenge to both the validation and measurement of mental disorders. Several SCID studies have undertaken the arduous task of evaluating antecedent conditions that may contribute to specific disorders:

1. *Parenting.* Carter, Joyce, Mulder, Luty, and Sullivan (1999) found differences in the adequacy of parenting for depressed outpatients. Although differences were ascertained for depression, the most significant relationships were found for Axis II disorders. Carter et al. theorized that parental deprivation might lead to a personality dysfunction which subsequently contributed to Axis I disorders such as depression. Regarding parental history, Buydens-Branchey, Branchey, and Noumair (1989) found dramatic differences in patients with early-onset alcoholism: 73.3% had fathers with alcoholism compared to 12.3% of mothers.

2. *Maturation.* Hayward et al. (1992) found that the emergence of panic attacks peaked in female adolescents and appeared to be related to pubertal maturation.

3. *Genetic contributions.* Kendler et al. (1995), utilizing SCID diagnoses, conducted an outstanding study of 1,030 female–female twin pairs. They established two general genetic influences: (a) phobia, panic disorder, and bulimia nervosa, and (b) major depression and GAD. In contrast, alcoholism appeared to have a specific genetic influence.

SCID research has also investigated the longitudinal perspective of specific disorders by evaluating treatment outcome. In this regard, several research teams have addressed the course and treatment outcome of SCID-diagnosed panic disorders. Noyes et al. (1990) examined 89 patients with panic disorders after 3 years of treatment. Level of initial impairment predicted subsequent adjustment. In an 8-week study of alprazolam, Ballenger et al. (1988) found that the majority of treated patients had a resolution of panic attacks (55%), although nearly one-third in the placebo condition (32%) also experienced a cessation of panic attacks. As a follow-up, Coryell and Noyes (1988) investigated those patients responding to placebo in the Ballenger et al. study. They found that patients with either few panic attacks or concurrent depression were likely to have recoveries under the placebo condition. As a parallel, Lesser et al. (1988) investigated treatment outcome for panic patients with and without secondary depression. Patients treated with alprazolam reported parallel improvements in anxiety and depressive symptoms. In summary, treatment outcome studies of panic disorder do not appear to be diagnosis-specific; rather, improvements extend beyond panic attacks to mood disorders.

SCID studies have investigated treatment outcome beyond panic disorders. Key findings are summarized as follows:

- Severity of cocaine dependence predicts treatment relapse (Weiss, Griffin, & Hufford, 1992).
- Major depression is less likely to respond to treatment with comorbid Axis II disorders, especially from Cluster A (Sato, Sakado, & Sato, 1993).

- Patients with Axis I and Axis II disorders appear to evidence general remission following 2 years of intensive psychodynamic self psychology (Monsen, Odland, Faugli, Daae, & Eilertsen, 1995). While excluding patients with chronic schizophrenia, the remission rate at follow-up approximately 5 years later was impressive for patients with both psychotic and mood disorders.

Clinical Applications

Use of SCID interviews over traditional interviews clearly improves clinical practice. In a comparison of 500 SCID to 500 traditional interviews, Zimmerman and Mattia (1998b) revealed several important findings. In comparison to SCID interviews, traditional interviews missed close to one-half (43.5%) of comorbid Axis I disorders.[2] When comorbid Axis I SCID diagnoses increase (i.e., three or more disorders), traditional interviews miss at least some of the comorbid disorders in most (78.9%) of the cases. Overall, Axis I diagnoses were most likely to be missed for anxiety and somatoform disorders.

SCID diagnoses also have relevance in primary care settings. For patients screened by the Center for Epidemiologic Studies—Depression scale (CES-D; Radloff, 1977), Schwenk, Coyne, and Fechner-Bates (1996) found that primary care physicians did not diagnose the majority of patients warranting SCID diagnoses of major depression. Undetected SCID diagnoses varied by severity: mild (81.6%), moderate (62.1%), and severe (26.7%). The combination of standardized screens and selective SCID interviews would greatly facilitate the accurate identification and effective treatment of mental disorders.

Kobak et al. (1997) investigated the systematic use of a screen in combination with the SCID. They utilized the Primary Care Evaluation of Mental Disorders (PRIME-MD; Spitzer et al., 1994) in two innovative formats: (1) desktop computer and (2) touch-tone telephone with interactive voice response technology. When divided into large diagnostic categories (e.g., mood disorders), both versions of the PRIME-MD exceeded 80% accuracy.

Clinicians may wish to seek collateral interviews and information, especially in the evaluation of psychotic patients. Fennig et al. (1994) evaluated psychotic symptoms in first-admission patients. They found that 13.7% denied all psychotic symptoms, while 33.3% revealed only some of their hallucinations and delusions. No clear pattern was observed based on either demographic variables or initial diagnoses. Therefore, clinicians may wish to proceed with record reviews and collateral interviews when any psychotic symptoms are suspected.

---

[2]Although not randomly assigned to an assessment group (SCID vs. traditional), the samples were derived from the same setting and appear comparable with respect to sociodemographic and self-reported clinical variables.

The SCID interview has been applied to a wide range of mental health and medical settings. In addition, the SCID has been utilized in forensic and correctional settings (see Arboleda-Florez et al., 1995; Stalenheim & von Knorring, 1996). Clinicians should feel comfortable in using the SCID with a broad array of clinical populations. In the following sections, I discuss the advantages and limitations of the SCID.

Advantages of the SCID

The SCID is a well-validated Axis I interview with the following several important advantages:

1. *Diagnostic breadth*. For current diagnosis, the SCID offers the widest coverage of Axis I disorders, with clinical inquiries that parallel DSM-IV inclusion criteria.
2. *Hierarchical approach*. The SCID is designed to screen out Axis I disorders efficiently in order to expedite its administration.
3. *Diagnostic reliability*. For establishing current disorders, the SCID has good-to-superb reliability. Several studies employ stringent designs that may disadvantage SCID reliability estimates in comparison to other Axis I disorders.
4. *Compatibility with DSM-IV*. The SCID is designed so that its ratings have a one-to-one correspondence with DSM-IV. However, the extent to which SCID inquiries elicit DSM-IV inclusion criteria has not been formally tested.

Limitations of the SCID

The SCID has the following important limitations in its applications to clinical practice:

1. *Neglect of symptomatology*. The overall focus of the SCID is to achieve diagnoses, with little attention to key symptoms. Because of this inattention, practitioners cannot be assured whether differences in symptom ratings reflect either (a) the unreliability of the SCID for that symptom or (b) change in the patient. To evaluate treatment changes, practitioners often want to assess changes in symptom severity. The SCID provides only clinical and subclinical gradations.
2. *Depth*. As previously observed, the trade-off between breadth and depth must be considered. For the most part, the SCID interview is designed to evaluate only what is minimally necessary to render a DSM-IV diagnosis.
3. *Transparency*. The SCID is organized by diagnostic categories, with most items worded in the pathological direction (i.e., affirmative responses typically signify impairment). Preliminary data suggest that the SCID is vulnerable to response styles (Rogers, Bagby, & Prendergast, 1993).

In summary, the SCID is a well-validated Axis I interview. It should be given strong consideration in settings in which the emphasis is on current diagnosis rather than symptomatology. The SCID is especially well suited for medical settings in which the classification of mental disorders requires comprehensive coverage. Given the demands on primary care staff, missed diagnoses are not likely to be uncovered if not originally detected during an Axis I consultation.

COMPREHENSIVE ASSESSMENT OF SYMPTOMS AND HISTORY (CASH)

Development and Rationale

Andreasen (1987a) and her colleagues developed the CASH for evaluating signs, symptoms, and history in patients with major psychotic and mood disorders. With a realization of the continuing changes in diagnostic systems, Andreasen developed the CASH to assess symptomatology and biological, psychological, and social correlates of mental disorders. By focusing on symptoms and correlates, Andreasen hoped to avoid the variability and possible arbitrariness of diagnostic standards.

The CASH represents an integration of the SADS and two specialized measures: the Scale for the Assessment of Negative Symptoms (SANS; Andreasen, 1984a) and the Scale for the Assessment of Positive Symptoms (SAPS; Andreasen, 1984b). From a historical perspective, Andreasen (1982) became concerned that negative symptoms were disregarded in the diagnosis of schizophrenic disorders. As a result, she developed the SANS to measure five subscales of negative symptoms: affective flattening or blunting, alogia, avolition–apathy, anhedonia–asociality, and attentional impairment. Initial data on 26 inpatients were very promising. To complement the SANS, Andreasen (1984b) developed the SAPS to evaluate four subscales of positive symptoms: hallucinations, delusions, bizarre behavior, and formal thought disorder. While the wording of some SAPS inquiries is borrowed directly from the SADS, the SAPS differs substantially in both its increased coverage and rating criteria.

Description of the CASH

The CASH is organized into three major sections: present state, past history, and lifetime history. Box 5.2 provides a summary of its key features. In the present state section, the clinician addresses psychopathology during previous last month.[3] Many clinical inquiries are reproduced without modification from the SADS. Unlike the SADS, however, the CASH provides severity rat-

---

[3]An exception to this rule occurs when the current episode is less than 6 months' duration. Under these circumstances, the clinician is instructed to rate each symptom at its worst during that 6-month period.

BOX 5.2. Highlights of the CASH

- *Description:* The CASH, an extensive semistructured Axis I interview, incorporates other validated measures. It includes portions of the SADS and complete versions of two specialized scales of psychotic symptoms: the SANS (negative symptoms) and the SAPS (positive symptoms). It also contains the MMSE and GAS.

- *Administration time:* Typically, approximately 2 hours.

- *Skills level:* The CASH requires extensive training. As with the SADS, clinicians must be knowledgeable of the clinical inquiries and the corresponding criteria.

- *Distinctive features:* The CASH focuses on psychotic and mood disorders, with modules to address substance abuse, handedness, and gross cognitive impairment. For psychotic patients, an alternative to the CASH is the standardized administration of the SADS plus the SANS and SAPS.

- *Cost:* The CASH (also the SANS and SAPS) is available from Dr. Andreasen at no charge.

- *Source:* Copies of the CASH are available by mail from Nancy Andreasen, MD, PhD, 200 Hawkins Drive, Room 2911 JPP, Iowa City, IA 52242; by phone, (319) 356-1553; or by fax, (319) 356-2587.

---

ings on individual psychotic symptoms: (i.e., 0 = not at all; 1 = questionable; 2 = mild; 3 = moderate; 4 = marked; and 5 = severe). Moreover, the CASH differs from the SADS in its extensive clinical observations. Derived from the SANS, the CASH requires extensive observations of formal thought disorder, including circumstantiality, pressured speech, distractible speech, thought blocking, perseveration, and clanging. Like the DIS, the CASH also includes the MMSE as part of its administration.

The past history section summarizes psychopathology for previous episodes of psychotic and mood disorders. Categorical ratings (presence or absence) are required for past symptoms on three facets: (1) ever present, (2) present in the initial 2 years of the disorder, and (3) present much of the time since the onset of the disorder. The lifetime history section addresses substance abuse disorders, prodromal symptoms of schizophrenia, and hypomanic and dysthymic symptoms. Substance abuse symptoms are scored for current and past use, while other symptoms are evaluated as to whether they are premorbid, prodromal, intermorbid, or residual. As with the SADS, the clinician makes overall ratings of social and overall functioning that include the GAS.

Validation of the CASH

A crucial difference between the SADS and the CASH is the latter's greater focus on psychotic symptoms, with its inclusion of the SANS and SAPS. Therefore, I summarize key findings for these specialized scales and subsequently, validity data on the CASH itself.

SANS and SAPS: Validation of the CASH Psychotic Symptoms

Reliability. Table 5.2 summarizes SANS and SAPS reliability studies derived from two primary sources: (1) two studies conducted by Andreasen and her colleagues at the University of Iowa and (2) predominantly unpublished research from European (Spain and Italy) and Asian (Japan and China) countries. Unpublished studies are cited as personal communications (Andreasen, 1990; Andreasen & Grove, 1986). Descriptions lack data on sample sizes, participants' settings, diagnoses, and ratings (see Table 5.2).

Data on interrater reliability produce impressive ICCs for individual symptoms. These estimates range from moderate (.64 and .68) to very high (.81, .86, and .88). Clinicians can employ the SANS and SAPS with confidence that their interview and observational data are highly reproducible. In the three studies (see Table 5.2) that allow direct comparisons, interrater reliability appears similar between the SANS ($M = .76$) and SAPS ($M = .79$). Although infrequently reported, subscales appear to have high levels of interrater reliability. As a summary of the interrater reliability, two observations emerge:

1. For the reliability of individual psychotic symptoms, the SANS and SAPS appear to produce unprecedently high reliability coefficients that appear relatively stable across both cultures and translations.
2. The reliance on unpublished research limits the clinical applicability of these findings. For what settings and which diagnoses should the SANS and SAPS be employed?

The test–retest reliability of the SANS and SAPS has only been examined in study of the CASH per se. With a very short interval (less than 1 day), ICCs dropped substantially. Surprisingly, delusions were the most affected, with dramatic differences between interrater (median ICC = .88) and test–retest (median ICC = .39) reliability. Studies of test–retest reliability with different samples (e.g., outpatient) and longer intervals (e.g., 2–4 weeks) would be highly desirable.

Andreasen (1990) and colleagues examined the internal reliabilities of the SANS and SAPS subscales on 117 inpatients with schizophrenia. They found moderate alphas for SANS (median = .75) and SAPS (median = .74). Given the circumscribed nature of these subscales, the high item-total correlations are understandable.

Validity. An extensive literature examines the validity of the SANS and SAPS:

TABLE 5.2. Reliability Studies for the Comprehensive Assessment of Symptoms and History (CASH) and Its Two Component Scales (SANS and SAPS)

Study (year)	Scale	N	Setting In/Out/Com/Univ	Dx	Raters Lay/Prof	Reliability Inter/Retest (interval)	Reliability estimates Sx/Cur-Dx/Life-Dx/Other[a]	
Andreasen (1982)	SANS	26	✓	NA	✓	✓	.86	.90
Ohta et al.[b]	SANS	NA		NA		✓	.64	
Humbert et al.[c]	SANS	NA		NA		✓	.88	.94
	SAPS	NA		NA		✓	.78	.89
Moscarelli et al.[d]	SANS	NA		NA		✓	.72	
	SAPS	NA		NA		✓	.81	
Phillips[e]	SANS	NA		NA		✓	.77	
Andreasen et al. (1991)[f]	SANS	30	✓	6	✓	✓	.68	
	SAPS	30	✓	6	✓	✓	.79	
	SANS	30	✓	6	✓	✓ (< 1 day)	.59	
	SAPS	30	✓	6	✓	✓ (< 1 day)	.51	
Andreasen et al. (1992)	CASH	30	✓	6	✓	✓	.75	.85
	CASH	30	✓	6	✓	✓ (< 1 day)	.65	.65

Note. All reliability estimates are intraclass coefficients (ICCs), SANS = Scale for the Assessment of Negative Symptoms; SAPS = Scale for the Assessment of Positive Symptoms. See Table 1.5 (p. 35) for a glossary of terms and abbreviations.

[a]Subscale scores for SANS and SAPS.

[b]A Japanese study cited in Andreasen and Grove (1986).

[c]Personal communication of unpublished data from Spain; cited in Andreasen and Grove (1986).

[d]Personal communication of unpublished data from Italy; cited in Andreasen and Grove (1986).

[e]Personal communication of unpublished data from China; cited in Andreasen (1990).

[f]Data collected as part of the CASH.

• Regarding construct validity, Andreasen et al. (1994; Andreasen, Arndt, Miller, Flaum, and Nopoulos, 1995) summarized SANS–SAPS factor-analytic studies, with most utilizing principal components analysis. Despite many variations, the majority of studies (see Andreasen, 1997) support the distinction between negative symptoms and two components of positive symptoms (psychotic symptoms and bizarre behavior).

• Andreasen et al. (1994) summarized imaging studies that generally support the differentiation of negative and positive symptoms based on (1) structural differences on CT scans (e.g., ventricular enlargements with negative symptoms) and (2) blood flow differences on positron-emission tomography (PET) scans. Moreover, differences in cognitive abilities have been observed, with negative symptoms implicated in lower functioning (Andreasen, Flaum, Swayze, Tyrrell, & Arndt, 1990).

• Negative symptoms appear less responsive than positive symptoms to traditional treatment interventions Andreasen, Flaum, Arndt, and Swayze (1991).

CASH Reliability

Andreasen, Flaum, and Arndt (1992) examined the CASH's reliability on a sample of 30 inpatients with schizophrenic or mood disorders. As summarized in Table 5.2, interrater reliabilities were excellent for both symptoms and current diagnoses. Despite limited numbers (three disorders had ≤ 2 participants), the diagnostic estimates were excellent. However, larger diagnostic groups from multiple settings are needed to demonstrate the generalizability of these findings beyond those of the original investigators and their inpatient unit.

Test–retest reliability resulted in lower scores despite the brief interval of less than 1 day. As summarized in Table 5.2, psychotic symptoms appeared to be substantially reduced (see Andreasen et al., 1991) in contrast to symptoms in general (see Andreasen et al., 1992). With the median ICC for individual symptoms at .65, these coefficients compare favorably to most Axis I interviews.

For the accuracy of retrospective evaluations, Andreasen et al. (1992) collected contemporaneous ratings of CASH symptoms and compared them to retrospective reports at 6-month intervals. Although no quantitative data were reported, the investigators described patients as having poor retrospective recall of negative symptoms; conversely, informants had poor retrospective recall of positive symptoms.

CASH Validity

The validity of the CASH appears to be generally assumed rather than rigorously tested. This assumption appears to be based on two considerations: (1) the validity of its component scales (i.e., SADS, SANS, SAPS, MMSE, and

GAS) and (2) content validity with DSM diagnoses. The following paragraphs briefly summarized available CASH studies.

Andreasen et al. (1992) reported preliminary data based a design analogous to the LEAD model. Two raters (patient CASH vs. informant-based CASH) compiled all data to render a "gold standard" diagnosis. Although this model resulted in a high level of agreement (most ICCs >.70), the criterion contamination is likely to inflate these coefficients.

Andreasen (1987b) compared CASH data for inpatients, including 22 manic, 27 major depressive, and 110 schizophrenic episodes. As expected, positive and negative symptoms were more prominent in patients with schizophrenia than in those with mood disorders. However, two unanticipated findings emerged. First, of the three groups, patients with manic episodes rated highest on the subscale "formal thought disorder." Second, two subscales of negative symptoms did not differentiate between the diagnoses: "avolition–apathy" and "attentional impairment." Differences in mood symptoms corresponded to the predicted pattern in the three diagnostic groups. In addition, several discriminant models demonstrated the usefulness of positive and negative symptoms for the classification of schizophrenia but not mood disorders. Finally, patients with schizophrenia evidenced the least progress and longest hospitalizations among the diagnostic groups.

Miller and colleagues (Miller, Flaum, Arndt, Fleming, & Andreasen, 1994; Miller, Perry, Cadoret, & Andreasen, 1994) conducted two CASH studies regarding negative symptoms and treatment. Miller, Flaum, et al. (1994) withdrew 59 patients with schizophrenia from their medications. Although psychotic symptoms remained relatively stable, they observed a modest but significant increase in negative and disorganized symptoms. In the second study, Miller, Perry, et al. (1994) evaluated 34 inpatients whose schizophrenia had not responded to past medication trials. Patients evidenced significant differences on three dimensions (negative symptoms, psychotic symptoms, and disorganization). In particular, negative symptoms evidenced a consistent decrease in severity. Interestingly, negative symptoms were the best predictor of the outcome.

In summary, the CASH appears to be a reliable Axis I interview that draws much of its validation from four earlier measures: SADS, SANS, SAPS, and MMSE. Overall, results are generally positive regarding the pattern of symptoms and their predicted relationships. The next section examines the usefulness of the CASH in clinical settings.

Clinical Applications

The CASH appears to have considerable potential as a measure for reliably assessing Axis I symptomatology. It is characterized by its incorporation of other validated scales, including the SADS, SANS, SAPS, MMSE, and GAS, as well as the development of abbreviated versions for the evaluation of treatment outcome.

The primary application of the CASH is the evaluation of psychotic and mood-disordered patients. Its inclusion of the SANS and SAPS has two important advantages.

1. The SANS and SAPS provide the best documentation of psychotic symptoms on two bases. First, the level of measurement allows practitioners to estimate accurately the severity of psychotic symptomatology. Second, the focus of individual symptoms provides excellent interrater reliability data unmatched by other Axis I interviews.
2. The SANS and SAPS have important implications for documenting treatment progress and outcome in patients with psychotic and mood disorders.

The CASH's interrater reliability for mood disorders appears comparable to the SADS. This finding is not particularly surprising given the substantial overlap between the two measures in evaluating these symptoms. Can SADS data on mood symptoms be used to buttress the modest sample ($N = 30$) for purposes of reliability? Practitioners are likely to be divided on this important issue. Although often minor, many small differences occur between the two SADS and the CASH on mood symptoms. Large-scale reliability studies are needed to examine the reproducibility of the CASH in different settings with different patient populations.

A viable alternative to administering the CASH in its entirety is the standardized administration of the SADS augmented by the SANS and SAPS. This augmented SADS provides two well-validated measures, each of which has been extensively tested. The SADS has outstanding reliability and validity for both symptoms and diagnoses. Its very good coverage of psychotic symptoms could be further augmented by the expanded rating criteria and coverage of the SANS and SAPS. The addition of these two measures allows for a comprehensive coverage of psychotic symptoms and the treatment implications of negative and positive symptomatology.

PRESENT STATE EXAMINATION (PSE) AND THE SCHEDULES FOR CLINICAL ASSESSMENT OF NEUROPSYCHIATRY (SCAN)

This sections addressed two closely aligned measures, namely, the PSE and the SCAN. The PSE, with its rich European tradition, has evolved over the last four decades as the prominent structured interview for the assessment of symptomatology within the ICD framework. More recently, attention has focused on the SCAN, which incorporates the PSE and several ancillary measures. In line with large-scale clinical research, the most recent edition of the PSE (i.e., 10th edition) is reviewed with the SCAN literature. Box 5.3 highlights the important features of both the PSE and the SCAN.

BOX 5.3. Highlights of the PSE and SCAN

- *Description:* Within an ICD framework, the PSE and SCAN focus on clinical characteristics and symptomatology, with a secondary emphasis on diagnosis.

- *Administration time:* 60 to 90 minutes.

- *Skills level:* The PSE may be used by paraprofessionals with extensive training and direct supervision; the SCAN is intended for use by mental health professionals. All interviewers are required to have extensive training prior to administration.

- *Distinctive features:* The PSE and SCAN attempt to provide a comprehensive assessment of clinical phenomena; together, they represent the most commonly used ICD-based interviews.

- *Cost:* Price list for the SCAN (including the PSE-10) on 3/1/2001 = $26.95 for the manual, $24.00 for the glossary, and $21.00 for the code book.

- *Source:* SCAN, including the PSE-10, is available through American Psychiatric Publishing Group, on the internet, *www.appi.org;* by phone, (800) 368-5777; by fax, (202) 789-2648; or by mail, 1400 K Street, NW, Washington, DC 20005-2403. An updated manual is available from Cambridge University Press.

Present State Examination (PSE)

Description and Rationale

The PSE was developed to assist in the classification of psychotic and neurotic symptoms (Wing, 1996). It later represented the "crystallization of Anglo European clinical methods and concepts, much influenced by the phenomenological approach of Jaspers and Schnieder" (Luria & Guziec, 1981, p. 250). While North American practitioners are unlikely to employ the PSE in their professional practices, its clinical applications continue to flourish in Europe and many parts of the world.

The PSE was originally developed to standardize the assessment of psychopathology through the use of accepted clinical inquiries and operationalized definitions (Wing, Birely, Cooper, Graham, & Isaacs, 1967). With its phenomenological emphasis on clinical description, the PSE has organized signs and symptoms into a syndromal structure that is very different from other structured interviews. For example, signs/symptoms of depression may be subsumed in several diverse syndromes, including "delusional and hallucinatory syndromes" and "specific neurotic syndromes."

Wing et al. (1990) described the origins of the PSE in preliminary studies conducted in the late 1950s. After five editions, the first study of the PSE was published (Wing et al., 1967). The 7th and 8th editions were studied extensively in relationship to the U.S.–U.K. Diagnostic Project (Cooper et al., 1972) and the WHO-sponsored International Pilot Study of Schizophrenia (World Health Organization, 1979). Although intended as a descriptive measure, more recent studies have examined its usefulness with ICD-8 and ICD-9 diagnoses. Unlike the gradual evolution found with most structured interviews, recent PSE editions have represented dramatic changes in both structure and ratings:

• The 8th edition (Wing et al., 1974), with approximately 500 items, provides an exhaustive coverage of psychotic and neurotic characteristics. For most symptoms, the interviewer is provided with a standard question and is encouraged to make additional inquiries.

• The 9th edition (Wing, 1976) is a much briefer version with 140 items; many infrequently recorded symptoms were eliminated. As observed by Luria and Guziec (1981) many 9th edition items are relatively complex, with multiple symptoms amalgamated into single ratings.

• The 10th edition (World Health Organization, 1994) substantially expands the coverage by the addition of new sections for cognitive impairment and somatoform, eating, dissociative, and substance abuse disorders. A total of 1,224 items are evaluated. Ratings are augmented by the addition of a "subclinical" level.

Fundamental changes in recent PSE editions strikingly reduce the accumulated evidence of its validation. Specifically, validity studies on one edition have little bearing on other editions. Therefore, practitioners and clinical researchers would be prudent to consider editions as a separate but related measures.

The scoring system for the PSE-9 has three ratings: 0 = symptom absent; 1 = occasional or not severe; and 2 = almost continuous or severely distressing. For PSE-10, different 4-point ratings are used for Parts I and II (see the description of the SCAN). As noted by Cooper, Copeland, Brown, Harris, and Gourlay (1977), clinicians should be conservative in making their ratings; when in doubt, the lower rating should be given. In general, these ratings are limited to the previous 4 weeks, since more extended periods may constrain PSE reliability.

Reliability of the PSE

Early reliability studies conducted by Wing et al. (1967) reported on a series of small studies that employed the 3rd, 4th, and 5th editions of the PSE. These early studies maximized agreement by simply calculating correlations on PSE psychotic sections for only psychotic patients, and PSE nonpsychotic sections for only nonpsychotic patients. The reliability of more recent editions is summarized in Table 5.3; as previously noted, the PSE-10 is presented with-

TABLE 5.3. Reliability Studies for the Present State Examination (PSE)

Study (year)	Ed	N	Setting				Raters		Reliability		Reliability estimates			
			In	Out	Com	Univ	Lay	Prof	Inter/Retest	(interval)	Sx	Cur-Dx	Life-Dx	Other
Wing et al. (1967)	5th	93	✓	✓				✓	✓					$.92^a$
Kendell et al. (1968)	7th	15	✓	✓				✓	✓	(1 wk)				$.82^a$
		37	✓	✓				✓	✓					$.85^a$
		25	✓	✓				✓	✓	(few days)	.41			$.65^a$
Luria & McHugh (1974)	8th	6^b	✓				✓	✓	✓			$.80^c$		$.94^c$
Cooper et al. (1977)	8th	30		✓			✓	✓	✓	(1 wk)				$.76^a$
		26		✓			✓	✓						$.50^a$
Wing, Nixon, et al. (1977)	9th	28			✓		✓	✓				.63		
		95			✓		✓	✓	✓	(1–4 wk)	.39			
Remington et al. (1979)	9th	52^d		✓				✓	✓		$.70^e$			
Rodgers & Mann (1986)	9th	526			✓			✓	✓		$.71^f$			$.96^g$
Mignolli et al. (1988)^h	9th	30	✓	✓	✓			✓	✓		.96			$.98^a$
		30	✓					✓	✓	(4–9 days)	.83			$.94^a$
Lesage et al. (1991)^i	9th	18^d	✓	✓				✓	✓					$.70^j$

Note. Most PSE reliability studies do not address specific ICD diagnoses but rather "cases" (i.e., whether the patient has any major disorder requiring treatment). Ed. = editions. See Table 1.5 (p. 35) for a glossary of terms and abbreviations.

[a]Correlations for PSE sections.

[b]Videotapes for reliability.

[c]For current diagnoses, and PSE sections. W (Kendall's coefficient of concordance) was used instead of kappa.

[d]Combination of videotapes and patient interviews.

[e]For 26 symptom ratings on female participants only.

[f]For 48 symptom ratings.

[g]Correlation for total PSE score.

[h]Italian translation.

[i]French translations.

[j]Kappas for PSE sections.

in the discussion of the SCAN. Three key findings from the 8th and 9th editions are distilled:

1. Current and lifetime diagnoses are deemphasized. The available data suggest a moderate[4] interrater reliability for the 8th and 9th editions. The variability of findings across different translations must be taken into account in deciding whether to use these editions. Test–retest reliability has not been adequately tested for either the 8th or 9th editions.
2. The PSE sections appear to have moderate interrater reliability and adequate test–retest reliability as dimensional ratings of psychopathology.
3. Small subsets of PSE items appear to have good interrater reliability on the 9th edition.

PSE reliability studies are variable with respect to the PSE edition, their completeness (abbreviated or full versions), training and background of the evaluators, and their samples. In brief, the 8th and 9th editions appear to have adequate interrater reliability for syndromes/scales. Much less is known about the interrater reliability of individual symptoms or diagnoses. Similarly, the test–retest reliabilities have not been sufficiently tested and are highly variable even within studies. In summary, clinicians may feel comfortable in their use of the PSE (8th and 9th editions) for the dimensional evaluation of syndromes/scales but should remain circumspect with respect to its other applications.

PSE Validity

Concurrent Validity. The PSE, because of its phenomenological perspective, has devoted relatively little attention to its relationship to independent diagnoses. Available research typically addresses only circumscribed disorders. In addition, the relationships between measures are often expressed simply as percentages of agreement (i.e., concordance rates) that do not correct for chance agreement. With these constraints in mind, characteristic findings for the PSE 9th edition are distilled as follows:

- The PSE 9th edition evidences moderately high (> 75%) concordance rates with clinical diagnoses for depression (Bebbington, Sturt, & Kumakura, 1983; Huxely, Korer, & Tolley, 1987; Maurer, Biehl, Kuhner, & Loffler, 1989).
- The PSE 9th edition has relatively modest concordance rates for schizophrenia, with estimates ranging from 50% (Huxley et al., 1987) to 60% (Maurer et al., 1989).

[4]For the 8th edition, Kendall's W is less stringent than the kappa, which controls for base rates.

In summary, the PSE has focused primarily on the identification of "cases" (any major disorder) rather than specific diagnoses. Available studies on the 9th edition do not address the breadth of Axis I disorders. They appear to offer the best concordance rates for depression. Please note that PSE-10 concurrent validity is subsumed in the SCAN review.

Syndeham and Predictive Validity. Construct validation via Syndeham's criteria addresses the longitudinal perspectives of mental disorders. Watt, Katz, and Shepherd (1983) conducted an early outcome study of the PSE with 121 schizophrenic patients divided into treatment and nontreatment conditions and reevaluated after 1 and 5 years. The study documents differences in outcome, with substantial numbers having either a single episode (16%) or multiple episodes with little residual impairment (32%). More recently, the PSE has been utilized in major studies of Axis I disorders. Recent findings are summarized as follows:

- First episodes of schizophrenia do not appear to be predicted by demographic variables, socioeconomic status, or family history; only a personal history of mental disorders occurred in the majority of cases (Vazquez-Barquero et al., 1996).
- In retrospectively examining the course of paranoid schizophrenia and schizoaffective disorders over nearly two decades, periods of remission and reduction of positive symptoms are commonly observed (Lerner, Bergman, Liberman, & Polyakova, 1999). For those patients evidencing improvement, psychotic symptoms tended to be replaced by mood symptoms. In prospective research (Menezes, Rodrigues, & Mann, 1997), DSM-III-R symptoms better predicted outcome than the PSE nuclear syndrome. Importantly, 23.8% of patients had no PSE psychotic symptoms at 24-month follow-up.
- In establishing relapses of schizophrenia, the PSE demonstrates moderate agreement with clinical assessments and an interview-based Brief Psychiatric Rating Scale (BPRS; Lukeoff, Nuechterlein, & Ventura, 1986) in a 12-month follow-up (Linszen et al., 1994).
- Sociocultural issues appear to affect the course and incidence of psychotic disorders. In Great Britain, the course of psychotic disorders appeared comparable; however, persons of African descent were more likely to be hospitalized and detained by police (Goater et al., 1999). A cross-national study of 10 countries (Susser & Wanderling, 1994) found a much higher incidence of brief psychoses for developing (e.g., India and Nigeria) than for industrialized (e.g., Ireland, Japan, and United States) countries.
- PSE research has also investigated the role of life events and environmental conditions on the onset and course of depression. Nazroo, Edwards, and Brown (1997) examined how the effects of adverse life events differentially affect couples. With the exception of financial and marital problems, women evidence a higher risk of depression, especially with family-related issues. Leenstra, Ormel, and Giel (1995) explored whether a positive life event

(PLE) affects recovery from depression and anxiety. Their data provide only weak evidence of PLE and recovery. Brown and Moran (1997) found that depression is likely in single mothers. Their financial hardships, despite full-time employment, and difficult life events appear to be antecedents of depression.

• The relationship between physical symptoms and subsequent mental disorders was evaluated in an elegant study by Hotopf, Mayou, Wadsworth, and Wessely (1998). In a 7-year follow-up on 3,262 community participants, physical symptoms (e.g., chest pains or headaches) were associated with an increased incidence of PSE symptoms and concomitant disability.

A major strength of the PSE has been the large-scale and sophisticated research addressing the onset and course of specific disorders. In general, these studies provide useful evidence of how PSE-based diagnoses can predict onset, relapse, and recovery. This evidence is especially robust for schizophrenia and other psychotic disorders.

Convergent Validity. PSE studies have placed a major emphasis on convergent validity with the General Health Questionnaire (GHQ; Goldberg, 1978) and other self-report measures. Key findings are summarized as follows:

• Extensive research (e.g., Banks, 1983; Henderson, Duncan-Jones, Byrne, Scott, & Adcock, 1979; Ormel, Koeter, Van Den Brink, & Giel, 1989; Wilmink & Snijders, 1989) with the 30-item GHQ provides strong convergent evidence for the PSE as a general measure of psychological impairment.
• Moderate correlations were found between an abbreviated PSE and the SCL-90-R on samples of diabetic and bulimic patients (Peveler & Fairburn, 1990).
• Studies provide mixed evidence regarding the PSE and measures of social functioning (Sturt, 1981; Sturt & Wykes, 1987).

A number of studies have examined the relationship of the PSE to biological markers. For example, Bachneff and Engelsmann (1983) found meaningful differences on key PSE symptoms and electroencephalograph (EEG) recordings. Psychotic symptoms appear to be associated with increased dimethyltryptamine excretions that decrease as the clinical status improves (see Murray, Oon, Rodnight, Bireley, & Smith, 1979). Similarly, differences in response on the dexamethasone suppression test (DST) documented treatment response on selected PSE items (Smith, Carr, Morris, & Gilliland, 1988).

Generalizability across Cultures

A major strength of the PSE has been its implementation in diverse cultures. With extensive epidemiological research, cross-cultural differences can be examined directly. Disparate findings may reflect (1) diagnostic limitations, (2) constraints on PSE generalizability, or (3) true cultural differences.

Review of the major epidemiological studies (e.g., Hodiamont, Peer, & Sybern, 1987; Lehtinen, Lindholm, Veijola, & Vaisanen, 1990; Mavreas, Beis, Mouyias, Rigoni, & Lysketsos, 1986; Vazquez-Barquero et al., 1987) suggest comparable prevalence rates for males (range from 7.2% to 8.6%) but substantially more variation for females (7.5% to 22.6%). Although cultural influences could affect the prevalence of mental illness, this more than twofold difference between countries with low prevalence (Netherlands and Finland) and high prevalence (Spain and Greece) is cause for concern. Further research with different structured interviews is needed to distinguish between cultural differences and psychometric constraints.

In summary, the PSE 8th and 9th editions were intended to systematize the symptoms and clinical characteristics associated with Axis I disorders. As such, less emphasis has been placed on its relationship to clinical diagnosis. The validational studies focus on "psychiatric morbidity" or the presence of any major disorder rather than the specific symptomatology associated with a particular disorder. North American mental health professionals must take care not to judge the PSE in ethnocentric terms considering that the PSE was constructed with a European tradition. As an important caution, currently reviewed PSE studies can be conceptualized in three major categories: (1) full administration of the 8th edition, (2) full administration of the 9th edition, and (3) highly abbreviated administration (i.e., typically 40 items) of the 9th edition. Generalization across these versions has not been adequately investigated.

Clinical Applications

The PSE, especially the full 8th edition, provides an unparalleled phenomenological review of relevant symptomatology and associated features. In particularly challenging treatment cases, such an exhaustive review may provide a richer and more comprehensive view of the relevant phenomenology than what is typically found in routine DSM-IV diagnoses. For example, a patient with an atypical psychosis may be understood within non-DSM psychopathology with reference to assessment and treatment outcome.

Another important feature of the PSE is its extensive use in international studies with an emphasis on cultural and cross-cultural matters. With assistance from WHO, the PSE has been translated into 40 different languages. Studies have shown its clinical usefulness in European countries (e.g., Garyfallos et al., 1991; Hodiamont et al., 1987; Hout & Griez, 1984; Lesage, Cyr, & Toupin, 1991), English-speaking countries (i.e., Ni Nuallain, O'Hare, & Walsh, 1990; Romans-Clarkson, Walton, Herbison, & Mullen, 1990), and African countries (Gillis, Elk, Ben-Arie, & Teggin, 1982; Katz et al., 1988; Okasha & Ashour, 1981; Orley & Wing, 1979).

The WHO-sponsored study by Katz et al. (1988) illustrates the culturally specific dimensions of mental disorders. Samples of Indian ($n = 86$) and

Nigerian (n = 123) schizophrenics were assessed on the PSE and ICD-9. Katz et al. found differences in the subtypes of schizophrenia as well as symptomatology. For example, Indian patients with schizophrenia possess more systematized delusions and olfactory hallucinations. In contrast, Nigerian patients with schizophrenia have more delusions of control, thought insertion, and visual hallucinations. Swartz, Ben-Arie, and Teggin (1985) found that certain symptoms were culturally bound and therefore difficult to interpret meaningfully. Practitioners who evaluate substantial numbers of patients from other cultural backgrounds may find the PSE a useful adjunct to their assessments.

The limitations of the PSE to North American DSM-based practice are readily apparent. While reliability studies suggest a moderate level of agreement for dimensional ratings of ICD syndromes, studies vary across editions and tend to focus on a limited range of diagnoses. In general practice, most clinicians may feel more comfortable with the SADS or SCID than the PSE because of their diagnostic applications. In epidemiological and community studies, the DIS may have greater relevance than the PSE because of its more extensive reliability and validity studies.

Schedules for Clinical Assessment of Neuropsychiatry (SCAN)

Description and Rationale

The SCAN, developed under the aegis of WHO, "aimed at improving the accuracy and reliability of measurement and classifying of psychiatric disorders" (Wing et al., 1990, p. 589). The core component of the SCAN is the PSE 10th edition. The three objectives of the SCAN, as articulated by Wing (1996), include (1) rigorous clinical observation, (2) common clinical language standardized across different diagnostic systems, and (3) accumulation of clinical knowledge as a result of this standardization.

The SCAN (WHO, 1994) is composed of 27 sections. The PSE is the predominant measure consisting of the first 25 sections. The remaining two sections include the following:

1. The Item Group Checklist (IGC) comprised of 59 ratings defined in PSE-10 terms and based on secondary sources (e.g., records and informants).
2. The Clinical History Schedule (CHS), an optional section of 88 items for the tabulation of childhood data, intellectual functioning, social relationships, adult personality, clinical diagnoses, and physical illness.

The SCAN is a highly detailed semistructured interview that includes both standard questions and optional probes. Symptoms and associated features are rated on a 4-point scale: 0 = absent, 1 = present to a minor degree, subclinical level; 2 = present, clinical level, and 3 = present in a severe form.

For behavioral symptoms, the ratings reflect gradations of frequency: 0 = did not occur, 1 = occurred but probably uncommon or transitory, 2 = occurred on multiple occasions, 3 = present more or less continuously. Optional ratings are provided for attributions regarding etiology (e.g., substance abuse, side effects of medication, and diseases affecting the brain) and lifelong traits.

Some experimentation with a Computer-Administered SCAN (i.e., C-SCAN) has led to less than satisfactory results. Although patients often view the C-SCAN positively (Dignon, 1996), its results are substantially discrepant with the standard SCAN interview (Brugha, Kaul, Gignon, Teather, & Wills, 1996). The C-SCAN is not reviewed because it is (1) self-administered rather than being an interview, and (2) not recommended for clinical practice.

Reliability

Several recent investigations (see Table 5.4) have examined the interrater and test–retest reliability of the SCAN. In outpatient and community samples, research has low-moderate interrater reliability (median ICC = .46; Andrew, Peters, Guzman, & Bird, 1995) and moderate test–retest reliability (median kappa = .52; Brugha, Nienhuis, Bagchi, Smith, & Meltzer, 1999). In contrast to these studies, Wing, Sartorius, and Ustun (1998) reported interrater reliabilities that were high for ICD-10 (median kappa = .83) and moderately high for DSM-III-R (median kappa = .78) current diagnoses. These results are especially noteworthy given the magnitude of the undertaking (N = 440) and compilation of different translations. In addition, Wing et al. (1998) found moderate test–retest reliabilities for ICD-10 diagnoses (median kappa = .71) but with marked variability (kappas from .25 to .81).

More specific applications of the SCAN have been evaluated, focusing on SCAN substance abuse and its reliability with targeted populations. A large-scale study (N = 287) by Easton et al. (1997; see also Ustun et al., 1997) investigated test–retest reliability for substance abuse disorders utilizing English and a Turkish translation. For four disorders (alcohol, opiates, cannabis, and cocaine), they established moderately high reliabilities for both current (median kappa = .79) and lifetime (median kappa = .78) diagnoses. Symptoms related to these disorders were moderately reliable among alcohol abusers (median kappa = .67).

In summary, SCAN studies produced mixed results, from low-moderate to high reliability, for major disorders. Importantly, substance abuse disorders have moderately high reliabilities for both current episodes and lifetime diagnoses. Despite the SCAN's focus on clinical description, the reliability of symptoms and clinical characteristics has been largely overlooked.

Validity

Concurrent Validity. Clinical research has evaluated the concurrent validity of the SCAN in relationship to the SADS, CIDI, and the Clinical Inter-

TABLE 5.4. Reliability Studies for the Schedules for Clinical Assessment of Neuropsychiatry (SCAN), Including the Present State Examination—10 (PSE-10)

Study (year)	N	Setting				Dx	Raters		Reliability			Reliability estimates			
		In	Out	Com	Univ		Lay	Prof	Inter	Retest	(interval)	Sx	Cur-Dx	Life-Dx	Other
Andrews et al. (1995)	29					4		✓	✓				.46[a]	.46[a]	
Easton et al. (1997)[b]	287	✓	✓	✓		4		✓		✓	(<1 mo)	.67	.79[c]	.78	.97[f]
Wing et al. (1998)[d]	440	✓				9		✓	✓				.83[e]		
	236	✓				7		✓		✓	(<2 wk)		.71[g]		
Brugha et al. (1999)	61	✓	✓			5	✓	✓		✓	(<1 wk)		.52		

Note. See Table 1.5 (p. 35) for a glossary of terms and abbreviations.

[a] Intraclass coefficients (ICCs).
[b] Focused on alcohol and drug dependence disorders only with English and Turkish translations.
[c] Ustun et al. (1997) provide additional data on the same sample for substance abuse rather than dependence with a median kappa of .50.
[d] Multiple translations that were tested in 14 countries.
[e] ICD diagnoses; for DSM-III-R, median kappa = .78.
[f] ICC; symptoms organized into seven superordinate categories and summed.
[g] ICD diagnoses; for DSM-III-R, median kappa = .71.

view Schedule—Revised (CIS-R; Lewis, Pelosi, Araya, & Dunn, 1992). The key findings are summarized as follows:

- A moderate level of agreement was observed with the SADS for both a modest inpatient sample (Kendall's tau = .68; Silverstone, 1993) and a mixed sample of psychotic patients and their first-degree relatives (kappa = .81 for DSM-III and .54 for DSM-III-R diagnoses; Farmer et al., 1993).
- CIDI comparisons yielded moderate associations with anxiety and depression (median ICC = .46; Andrews et al., 1995) and substance abuse disorders (median kappa = .56; Farmer et al., 1996). A noteworthy finding in the Farmer et al. study was the moderate agreement at the symptom level (overall median kappa = .50), with considerably less convergence for cannabis (median kappa = .30) than other disorders (see also Compton et al., 1996).
- Negligible agreement (median kappa = −.01; M kappa = .05) was found between the CIS-R and the SCAN ICD-10 for seven diagnoses (Brugha, Bebbington, et al., 1999). Interpretation of these results is constrained by the paucity of validational data on the CIS-R and the relative infrequency of mental disorders in this community sample.

In general, SCAN studies with clinical samples demonstrated a moderate level of concurrent validity for Axis I disorders. In contrast to older, well-established interviews, these results are comparable or possibly stronger than what is typically found in clinical research. The results for substance abuse disorders are especially robust given the difficulty in achieving a satisfactory concordance with this broad diagnostic category.

Other Types of Validity. Construct validation has been examined via Syndeham's criteria, with an emphasis on the course and outcome of disorders. For example, Eaton et al. (1998) examined 35 new cases of panic disorders in a 12-year follow-up on 1,771 participants. They found that demographic differences affect incidence (e.g., more new cases for females and younger persons) and comorbidity diminishes the likelihood of recovery. Studies have also examined outcomes following traumatic brain injury (Deb, Lyons, Koutzoukis, Ali, & McCarthy, 1999), cervical surgery (Taylor, Creed, & Hughes, 1997), and trials of antidepressant medication (Gorenstein, Gentil, Melo, Lotufo-Neto, & Lauriano, 1998; Gormley, O'Leary, & Costello, 1999). In general, these studies offer promising findings about outcome criteria. The lack of large-scale programmatic research militates against any firm conclusions on this component of construct validity.

SCAN studies have evaluated its construct validity with reference to substance abuse disorders. Hapke, Rumpf, and John (1998) found symptomatic differences among those patients with alcohol-related disorders that were detected versus undetected by their primary care physicians. Nelson, Rehm, Ustun, Grant, and Chatterji (1999) established via confirmatory factor analysis (CFA) a single-factor solution for severe substance abusers. Among less-severe substance abusers, two factors emerged that were associated with abuse and dependence, respectively.

Convergent validity studies have examined the SCAN and its relationship primarily with research scales. Research has investigated the SCAN for patients with chronic fatigue syndrome (Farmer et al., 1996), somatization (Fink et al., 1999), psychotic symptoms (Bebbington & Nayani, 1995) and overall functioning (Bebbington, Brugha, Hill, Marsden, & Window, 1999). In most cases, the SCAN was used as the criterion measure for the validation of research scales. Therefore, few conclusions can be drawn from these studies.

Generalizability

Epidemiological studies allow clinical researchers to explore sociodemographic differences in SCAN data. In a study combining the CIS-R and the SCAN, Jenkins et al. (1997b) found differences in Great Britain, with higher prevalences based on residence (urban), region (Wales), work status (unemployed), and ethnicity (Asian). The regional and particular ethnic differences were surprising. In contrast, Vazquez-Barquero et al. (1997) found no differences in age, education, and employment in their epidemiological study of Northern Spain. Predictable gender differences were found, with high prevalences of mood and anxiety disorders for women, and alcoholism and psychosis for men. These studies underscore the need to investigate cultural differences in both the manifestations of psychopathology and their potential effects on Axis I interviews such as the SCAN.

Clinical Applications

The SCAN, building on its PSE tradition, is best conceptualized as an Axis I interview for ICD disorders. As observed by Bebbington (1992), the major thrust of the PSE/SCAN has been a bottom-up approach: "Its primary aim is an objective and comprehensive description of clinical phenomena" (p. 256). Unlike most Axis I interviews that favor a close nexus between symptoms and diagnoses, the SCAN is interested in symptomatology in its own right. Direct comparison with other Axis I interviews is likely to obscure this crucial difference.

Validation of the SCAN, with its phenomenological emphasis, poses special psychometric challenges. Merely demonstrating diagnostic reliability is insufficient for establishing the reliability at the item level. Likewise, criterion-related and construct validity are especially difficult to establish for a vast array of clinical phenomena. Mental health professionals are likely to be divided on whether the SCAN is adequately validated for clinical practice.

The main obstacle to implementing the SCAN as a measure of clinical phenomenology is the dearth of research on the reliability and validity of its symptoms and associated features. With more than 1,200 ratings, its comprehensiveness poses a daunting task to researchers. Therefore, SCAN studies address its validation at predominantly syndromal and diagnostic levels. The major exception is the diagnostic category of substance abuse disorders, which has been examined extensively.

Current recommendations for clinical practice are outlined as follows:

- The SCAN is recommended for substance abuse disorders, both in describing symptomatology and rendering diagnoses.
- The SCAN is recommended in general clinical practice for evaluating current ICD and DSM diagnoses.
- The SCAN is not recommended for the evaluation of symptoms and other clinical phenomena. Except for substance abuse symptoms, the reliability and stability of SCAN items have not been adequately tested.

An additional application of the SCAN would be to compare DSM-IV and ICD-10 diagnoses. The principal alternative is the CIDI (see next section), which has been applied to multiple diagnostic systems. An obvious need is large-scale research in line with Farmer et al. (1996) that investigates the concordance of symptoms, syndromes, and diagnoses with measures from both the ICD (SCAN) and DSM (CIDI) traditions.

COMPOSITE INTERNATIONAL DIAGNOSTIC INTERVIEW (CIDI)

Description, Rationale, and Development

The Composite International Diagnostic Interview (CIDI) Version 1.0 was developed under the auspices of the WHO—Alcohol, Drug, and Mental Health Administration (1987). The original CIDI was based on the DIS—Version III and augmented with questions from the PSE. Therefore, the CIDI included all items from the DIS, although some items were modified to improve their cross-national use (Robins et al., 1988). Because of fundamental differences between the DIS and the PSE, the CIDI provides only broad PSE classification and does not attempt to evaluate PSE syndromes. Box 5.4 provides a description of the CIDI and information on its availability.

The rationale for the CIDI's development was to "serve cross-cultural epidemiologic and comparative studies of psychopathology" (Robins et al., 1988, p. 1069). To achieve this purpose, the CIDI is intended to be a highly structured interview that (1) may be administered by nonprofessionals and (2) is easily translated into different languages.

The CIDI has evolved through multiple versions. As summarized by Janca, Ustun, and Sartorius (1994), the CIDI—1.2 Version (WHO, 1993) was in-

---

BOX 5.4. Highlights of the CIDI

- *Description:* The CIDI is a structured diagnostic interview for evaluating DSM and ICD diagnoses.

- *Administration time:* Time varies with the experience of the interviewer: 1 hour and 45 minutes for newly trained interviewers, 1 hour and 15 minutes for seasoned interviewers.

- *Skills level:* Paraprofessionals with extensive training can utilize the CIDI.

- *Distinctive features:* The CIDI is especially useful for cross-cultural research utilizing multiple diagnostic systems. A weakness of the CIDI is the substitution of CIDI–DIS comparisons for formal reliability studies.

- *Cost:* The CIDI may be downloaded free; contact Dr. Robins for charges to have copies mailed.

- *Source:* Available on the internet, *www.who.int/dsa/cat98/men8.htm;* or from Lee Robins, PhD, by phone, (314) 362-2469; by fax, (314) 362-2470; or by mail, Department of Psychiatry, Washington University School of Medicine, Campus Box 8134, 4940 Children's Place, St. Louis, MO 63110-1093.

---

tended to correspond to DSM-III-R diagnoses. More recently, the CIDI—Version 2.0 (WHO, 1997) was published to address DSM-IV and ICD-10 diagnoses. Beyond the basic CIDI versions (1.0, 1.2, and 2.0), a CIDI—Primary Health Care Version (CIDI-PHC) was developed to address psychological problems that frequently present in medical settings; unlike other CIDI versions, the CIDI-PHC was intended for use primarily by clinicians (see Janca et al., 1994). In addition, the University of Michigan version of the CIDI (UM-CIDI) is utilized in some U.S. studies; it excludes the MMSE and somatoform disorders and includes APD and PTSD. Finally, various CIDI modules were developed to address diagnoses such as substance abuse, PTSD, and APD (Janca et al., 1994).

Validation of the CIDI

The validation of the CIDI is daunting because of (1) its multiple revisions, (2) versions with substantively different content, and (3) translations into more than a dozen languages. Validation is further complicated by variations in administration, with the addition of computer-assisted interviews and the use of different diagnostic standards (e.g., DSM vs. ICD). As a result of this complexity, it is difficult to draw firm conclusions about the CIDI's validity.

For most structured interviews, reliability and validity are addressed in separate sections. This organization did not appear to be feasible with the

CIDI because most "reliability" studies compared the CIDI to the DIS. Are comparisons of the CIDI and the DIS really evidence of reliability? On one hand, all DIS items are included on the CIDI. On the other hand, wording and rating for some individual items were changed. In addition, other items from the PSE were interspersed with DIS items, which may create subtle but important changes in patients' responses.

Reliability

CIDI–DIS comparisons are often used to establish estimates of reliability. These comparisons are really quasi-reliability studies because the measures are not identical in the structure and wording of clinical inquiries. As noted by Wittchen (1994), questions were modified during the field trials to reduce ambiguity and improve cross-cultural understanding. Early representative CIDI–DIS studies include the following:

- Semler et al. (1987) tested Version 1.0 (German translation) with a test–retest paradigm (2-day interval) on 60 inpatients and found moderate agreement on 13 lifetime diagnoses (median kappa = .60).
- Wittchen et al. (1989) provided a further analysis of the Semler et al. study with Version 1.0 (German translation) on 14 symptoms/syndromes. In this small subset, the agreement was high (median ICC = .77).
- Sartorius et al. (1993) tested the CIDI-PHS in multinational studies of 14 countries. With 19 videotaped interviews, they reported an overall reliability coefficient of .92 but did not provide details about the type of cases or the type of reliability coefficient.

Wittchen (1994) compiled all the available WHO research on the CIDI for both interrater ($N = 575$) and test–retest ($N = 158$) reliability. He established exceptionally high interrater reliability (median kappa = .94) across 19 Axis I disorders. In contrast, test–retest reliabilities (< 3-day interval) were in the moderate range (median kappa = .69). Subsets of symptoms were also reported to have good reliability.

Several CIDI reliability studies after Wittchen et al. (1994) have produced moderate results. Peters, Clark, and Carroll (1998) compared the CIDI—Version 1.1 to CIDI—Auto Version 1.1 for patients with anxiety disorders and medical patients. For the eight DSM-III-R diagnoses (six anxiety and two mood disorders), the diagnostic agreement was moderate (median kappa = .61). Heun, Muller, Freyberger, and Maier (1998) examined lifetime episodes of CIDI disorders in a test–retest format and found moderate reliabilities (median kappa = .69) for four common disorders.

The CIDI extends beyond the DIS to address PSE categorizations. With the CIDI—Version 1.0 (English), Farmer, Katz, McGuffin, and Bebbington (1987) examined symptom agreement for PSE items on the CIDI with the PSE itself. Reliability estimates on 30 patients were obtained by three experienced psychiatrists. The estimates were generally low (median kappa = .27) on the 45 symptoms that could be evaluated. For general CATEGO classes, the ratings were moderate (weighted kappa = .55). In summary, these data do not support the use of CIDI–PSE symptoms but provide moderate support for broad classifications.

Validity

Studies address the CIDI's validation with an emphasis on concurrent validity. As previously noted, the complexity of the CIDI versions militate against definite conclusions. Summarized below are the major studies:

- Rosenman, Korten, and Levings (1997) compared the CIDI—Auto Version 1.1 (English) to clinical ICD-10 diagnoses on 126 Australian inpatients. Patients utilized the self-administered computerized version with an observing research assistant. The level of diagnostic agreement was poor (kappa = .23 for general diagnostic class).
- Peters and Andrews (1995) utilized the CIDI—Auto Version 1.0 (English) in a self-administered format with 98 outpatients in treatment for anxiety disorders. Based on a LEAD model for DSM-III-R disorders, kappa coefficients for six anxiety disorders and major depression were generally modest (median kappa = .38).
- Janca and colleagues (Janca, Robins, Bucholz, Early, & Shayka, 1992; Janca, Robins, Cottler, & Early, 1992) administered the CIDI—Version 1.0 (English) to 20 patients. Although moderately high kappas were achieved between CIDI and DSM-III-R diagnoses, the study was flawed by criterion contamination. Psychiatrists rendering the clinical diagnoses either observed or administered the CIDI.
- Lyketsos, Aritzi, and Lyketsos (1994) evaluated 11 CIDI diagnoses compared to clinical evaluations. They found low-moderate agreement (median kappa = .59) for the Greek translation.

Several focused studies were also conducted on CIDI concurrent validity and specific diagnostic categories:

- Booth et al. (1998) compared the UM-CIDI (English) to SCID-III-R diagnoses on 54 medical inpatients. They found low to low-moderate levels of agreement for lifetime (kappa = .46) and current (kappa = .51) depression.
- Cottler et al. (1997) examined substance abuse disorders on the CIDI—Version 1.0 (multiple languages) on current substance abusers from Greece, Luxembourg, and the United States. When compared to the SCAN, diagnoses of alcohol and drug dependence produced moderate agreement (median kappa = .53), while substance abuse diagnoses had negligible agreement (median kappa = .07). Specific symptoms related to dependence criteria

varied substantially (e.g., for alcohol, median kappa = .54; for cannabis, median kappa = .31; for opiates, median kappa = .58).

In summary, the validation of the CIDI for DSM diagnoses has relied primarily on DIS research. The basic assumption is that the validity of the DIS is transferred to the CIDI. The logic of this assumption is attenuated by the multiple versions, differences in content, and various translations. Practitioners must consider diagnostic validity within specific parameters; namely, (1) which CIDI version, (2) which language, and (3) which diagnoses.

Several studies have addressed the prevalence of mental disorders in the United States and other countries. Using the UM-CIDI, Kessler et al. (1994) conducted the National Comorbidity Study with 8,098 noninstitutionalized participants. The major findings are summarized as follows:

- Gender differences followed expected patterns, with an increased prevalence of mood and anxiety disorders for females, and APD and substance abuse disorders for males.
- Regarding ethnicity, lifetime prevalence appeared lower for African Americans than both Anglo Americans and Hispanic Americans. These differences are at variance with the Robins et al. (1984) results, which found few disparities between Anglo Americans and African Americans.
- Communities were also evaluated on population density (urban vs. rural) and regional location. Interestingly, urbanicity accounted for minimal differences. However, some regional differences were observed (e.g., greater prevalence of APD in the western region); it is unclear whether this reflects limits in the CIDI generalizability or true regional differences.

Further analyses by Kessler et al. suggest the complex interrelationships among sociodemographic variables in predicting disorders. Wittchen, Zhao, Kessler, and Eaton (1994) found that an increased prevalence of GAD was not associated with race or income when other factors were taken into account. Rather, gender (female), marital status (separated or divorced), and employment (homemaker) appear to be the most robust predictors. Large-scale epidemiological research is also available on the CIDI for other countries besides the United States (e.g., Canals, Domenech, Carbajo, & Blade, 1997; Lin, Goering, Lesage, & Streiner, 1997).

Clinical Applications

The CIDI is an ambitious WHO project for the validation of an Axis I interview that provides both DSM and ICD diagnoses for cross-national epidemiological research. For practitioners in North America, the CIDI is limited in its clinical usefulness for two primary reasons:

1. Although moderate levels of agreement were found between the CIDI and the DIS, clinicians are cautioned about relying on CIDI–DIS research. As observed by Kesseler et al. (1994), the CIDI differs fundamentally in its questions and probes. As a result, the CIDI classifies disorders much more frequently than does the DIS. Despite this caveat, the Wittchen (1994) compilation does suggest that the CIDI produces highly reliable diagnoses for current episodes, with moderate test–retest reliabilities over short periods (i.e., < 3 days).

2. Many key studies of the CIDI are not directly applicable to North America because of different translations (e.g., German) or cultures (e.g., Australia).

In summary, the CIDI is an important cross-cultural epidemiological measure. For DSM diagnoses, the breadth of psychometric data clearly favors the use of the DIS rather than the CIDI. Still, the synthesis by Wittchen (1994) supports the use of the CIDI for current diagnoses with established reliability. Concurrent validity studies, while variable, offer substantial support for common Axis I disorders.

OTHER STRUCTURED INTERVIEWS FOR AXIS I DISORDERS

This section provides a succinct synopsis of other Axis I interviews (see Box 5.5 for data on accessing these measures). These interviews vary considerably in terms of their validation and clinical applicability; they can be grouped into two general categories:

1. Several structured interviews with a small but well-developed literature appear to have gained clinical acceptance within select research facilities and circumscribed geographical areas. Examples are the Royal Park Multidiagnostic Instrument for Psychosis (RPMIP; McGorry, Kaplan, Dossetor, Copolov, & Singh, 1988) and the Polydiagnostic Interview (PODI; Philipp & Maier, 1986).

2. Other recently developed structured interviews appear to be promising. A prime example is the Mini-International Neuropsychiatric Interview (MINI; Sheehan et al., 1997).

Axis I Interviews with Circumscribed Clinical Focus

Royal Park Multidiagnostic Instrument for Psychosis (RPMIP)

McGorry et al. (1988) constructed the RPMIP as a semistructured diagnostic interview designed to assess functional psychoses from multiple diagnostic perspectives. Besides DSM and RDC diagnoses, other classificatory models of schizophrenia (e.g., Kraepelin, Bleuler, and Schneider) are considered (McGorry, Copolov, & Singh, 1990).

BOX 5.5. Sources for Other Axis I Interviews

Author addresses and other sources are provided for this category of Axis I interviews. These sources are based on information provided in research articles.

- Copies of the CIS-R are available from its first author, Dr. Glyn Lewis, Institute of Psychiatry, De Crespigny Park, London, Great Britain SE5 8AF. Another potential source is Rachel Jenkins, Mental Health Division, Department of Health, Wellington House, 133-155 Waterloo Road, London, Great Britain SE1 8UG.

- The DIGS, including the current version, DIGS code manual, DIGS training manual, and DIGS software, is available on the internet, *www-grb.nimh.nih.gov/gi.html*.

- The MINI is reproduced in the *Journal of Clinical Psychiatry, 59*(Suppl. 20), 34–57. While copyrighted, permission is granted for free copying by clinicians and researchers in nonprofit and publicly owned settings. Complimentary copies of the MINI-Plus and MINI-Kid are available on the internet, *www.medical-outcomes.com*.

- The PDI-R is available through Western Psychological Services by phone, (800) 648-8857, or by mail, 12031 Wilshire Boulevard, Los Angeles, CA 90025-1251.

- RPMIP is authored by Patrick D. McGorry, PhD, The National Health and Medical Research Council Schizophrenia Research Unit, Royal Park Hospital, Private Bag 3, Parkville, Melbourne, Victoria 3052, Australia.

Description. The RPMIP is a semistructured Axis I interview involving both patient and informant interviews. With ratings of 260 items, it includes the following components: overview, duration and onset, alcohol/drug screening, mood disorders, psychotic symptoms, and prodromal/residual symptoms. Symptoms are scored as "true" or "false," with additional categories reflecting the uncertainty or inapplicability of symptoms: ? = unknown; N/E = not elicited; N/A = not applicable. Unlike many Axis I interviews, the RPMIP focuses only on the current episode. It is intended for use by experienced interviewers. Because of its diagnostic complexity, computer scoring is available.

Validation. McGorry, Singh, et al. (1990) conducted an interrater reliability study on 50 inpatients. With the use of two raters, they achieved good reliability for different diagnoses/formulations of schizophrenia (median kappa = .76), schizoaffective disorder (median kappa = .79), and mood disorders (median kappa = .91). More impressively, the reliabilities for individual symptoms were exceptional, with the majority greater than .70. No data were presented on test–retest reliability.

McGorry, Singh, et al. (1990) also tested the validity of the RPMIP utilizing Spitzer's (1983) LEAD model. An inherent limitation of this model is the inclusion of the RPMIP in the establishment of an expert diagnosis based on all available information. This inclusion leads to criterion contamination and is likely to inflate results. For DSM-III diagnoses, the LEAD model resulted in a moderate level of agreement (median kappa = .68), although kappas were highly variable (.19 to 1.00).

More recent research has examined the factor structure of the RPMIP and the diagnostic agreement among its many systems. McGorry, Bell, Dugeon, and Jackson (1998) performed a principal axis factor analysis (PAF) on 92 core items from the RPMIP in a large inpatient sample of first-episode psychoses. A four-factor model identified the following dimensions: manic-based psychotic symptoms, depression-based psychotic symptoms, a Bleurian blend of negative symptoms, and Schneiderian first-rank symptoms. This factor solution provides partial support for multiple dimensions of psychotic symptoms as conceptualized by the RPMIP. Other studies (McGorry et al., 1992, 1995) have explored the relationships between diagnostic systems. Low to moderate levels of agreement among diagnostic formulations may provide modest justification for the RPMIP's inclusion of so many different models.

The RPMIP has also been used to study the course of psychotic and mood disorders. In a very interesting study, Jackson, McGorry, and Dudgeon (1995) examined prodromal symptoms among psychotic inpatients. Although important differences were found for schizophrenia (e.g., odd/bizarre ideation) and psychotic depression (e.g., decreased energy/interests), the study revealed similar patterns among other prodromal symptoms. Symptoms also differed substantially from schizoaffective, delusional, and bipolar disorders. In a second study, the RPMIP was used to study the stability of negative symptoms among inpatients with first-episode psychoses (Edwards, McGorry, Waddell, & Harrigan, 1999).

Clinical Applications. The initial reliability study with the RPMIP produced very promising results. Despite limitations in the LEAD model, RPMIP research offers moderate evidence of concurrent and construct validity. In light of these findings, the RPMIP is likely to have circumscribed clinical applications on research and clinical units specializing in the treatment of psychotic disorders. It is recommended that practitioners and researchers conduct their own reliability studies to provide additional substantiation regarding the reproducibility of their results.

Diagnostic Interview for Genetic Studies (DIGS)

The DIGS (Nurnberger et al., 1994), a collaborative effort produced by the NIMH Genetics Initiative, was designed to evaluate psychotic and mood disorders. With an emphasis on symptomatology, the DIGS combines DSM diagnostic criteria with RDC and Feighner criteria. To ensure comparability with European studies, a checklist of operational criteria is also included. The DIGS is an amalgamation of earlier structured interviews, with items incorporated from the SADS, SCID-III-R, DIS, and CASH.

Description. The DIGS, a semistructured interview that requires considerable clinical judgment in its administration and scoring, is composed of 12 sections: Introduction (MMSE, detailed demographics, and medical history), Somatization, Overview (history of mental health treatment and known past episodes), Mood Disorders, Substance Abuse Disorders, Psychosis, Comorbidity (temporal relationships between disorders), Suicidal Behavior, Anxiety Disorders, Eating Disorders, and Sociopathy. Because of its emphasis of symptomatology, entire sections are administered if any screening items are endorsed. The average administration time is 2½ hours.

Validation. Nurnberger et al. (1994) are responsible for the primary validation of the DIGS. Samples were preselected to address four principal diagnoses: major depression, bipolar disorders, schizoaffective disorders, and schizophrenia. Test–retest reliabilities were examined after a 4- to 10-day interval, using professionals from both the same and collaborating sites. Professionals from the same site produced moderate kappas for the four disorders, with a median of .76 (range from .39 to .84). Unexpectedly, professionals from other sites (i.e., no prior knowledge of patients) produced higher reliability estimates (median kappa = .86; range from .45 to .96). These estimates are likely inflated over what is typically found in clinical practice by (1) strictly limiting the number of diagnoses and (2) ensuring similar proportions of each disorder. Despite the DIGS emphasis on symptoms and clinical descriptions, reliability is only reported at the diagnostic level.

Two more recent studies examined the reliability of the DIGS for translated versions. Presig, Fenton, Metthey, Berney, and Ferrero (1999) evaluated a French version of the DIGS for both interrater and test–retest reliability. Unlike Nurnberger et al., these investigators did not preselect patients by diagnoses. For interrater reliability, the kappas were excellent (median kappa = .86) for five psychotic and mood disorders. After an extended interval of 6 weeks, the test–retest reliability was in the moderate range (median kappa = .62). Deshpande et al. (1998) evaluated the interrater reliability of a Hindi translation of the DIGS. With a modest sample of 20 patients, they achieved only a low-moderate level of agreement (median kappa = .55). On close inspection, two of the three raters were highly concordant, while the third rater produced disparate results.

The validity of the DIGS was evaluated via a bootstrapping operation whereby DIGS diagnoses were compared to clinical diagnoses. As with reliability studies, number of disorders was circumscribed. For three disorders, Nurnberger et al. (1994) found moderately high kappas (.72, .77, and .78). For five disorders, Presig et al. (1999) found low-moderate agreement (median kappa = .54). Deshpande et al. (1998) found low-moderate agreement with clinical diagnoses (median kappa = .56) but excellent agreement with the PSE (median kappa = .80). In addition to these studies of concurrent validity, research has shown promise for the DIGS in identifying sexually dimorphic genetic effects for obsessive–compulsive disorder (Karayiorgou et al., 1999) and differences in bipolar disorders associated with the female reproductive system (e.g., pregnancy, childbirth, and menopause; Blehar et al., 1998).

Clinical Applications. The clinical use of the DIGS is constrained by the focal nature of the existing research. Although designed to evaluate approximately 22 Axis I disorders and six personality disorders, current research has focused on only four to five Axis I disorders. For the English and French versions, moderate to excellent reliabilities have been established for major depression and bipolar disorders, and schizophrenia. Less agreement was observed for schizoaffective disorders. These reliability estimates are likely inflated by the small number of diagnoses and the preselection procedure utilized by Nurnberger et al. (1994). Concurrent validity produces generally positive results; as with reliability, these data address less than 20% of DIGS diagnoses.

Nurnberger et al. (1994) reported that the DIGS is not designed for routine clinical practice. Regardless of its original design, the DIGS is not sufficiently validated to address the spectrum of disorders likely encountered in clinical practice. In specialized settings, the DIGS may prove to be a valuable composite measure, although reliability (both symptom and diagnostic) would likely need to be established.

Mini-International Neuropsychiatic Interview (MINI)

Sheehan et al. (1997, 1998) described the development of the MINI as a brief Axis I interview. Its purpose was to provide a rapid and accurate evaluation of both DSM and PSE criteria as well as subsyndromal variants. For efficient utilization of services, the MINI was intended to be used by trained paraprofessionals that provide standardized data to clinicians in mental health and medical settings.

Description. The MINI exists in four versions. The MINI itself is a semistructured interviews of approximately 15 minutes' duration for use in clinical settings and research. The MINI-Plus is an extended semistructured interview (45–60 minutes) intended for research purposes. The MINI-Screen is a 5-minute structured interview designed for primary care settings. Finally, the MINI-Kid, a measure in its developmental stages, is proposed to assess common disorders in children and adolescents. This review focuses on the original MINI, on which most validity studies have concentrated.

The MINI is organized by diagnoses, with responses coded dichotomously ("yes" or "no") with unidirectional scoring (i.e., "yes" equals psychopathology). Specific disorders are typically screened via several clinical inquiries. Patients responding affirmatively to screening items are administered questions addressing DSM and ICD criteria. Altogether, the MINI is intended to cover 17 disorders in approximately 15 minutes. Developed as an international measure, English and French versions were validated simultaneously.

Validation. Sheehan et al. (1998) provided a useful summary of the MINI's reliability and validity based on several prior studies (e.g., Lecrubier et al., 1997; Sheehan et al., 1997). Combining across 23 current and lifetime diagnoses, reliability estimates were computed on 84 patients for both inter-rater and test–retest (1- to 2-day interval) reliability. Overall, the results were exceptional. The median kappas were .92 for interrater and .78 for test–retest reliability.

Validation studies summarized by Sheehan et al. (1998) produced very positive results. With a large sample of 370 patients, the median kappa for MINI versus SCID-CV diagnoses was .67. Similarly, the MINI versus CIDI diagnoses yielded a moderate level of agreement, with a median kappa of .63. Beyond diagnoses, the MINI appears effective at eliciting psychotic symptoms such as delusions and hallucinations (Amorim, Lecrubier, Weiller, Hergueta, & Sheehan, 1998). Efforts to validate a self-report version of the MINI proved substantially less successful, with a median kappa of .48.

Clinical Applications. A major purpose of the MINI was to provide rapid assessment and quality assurance for the delivery of mental health services within a managed care environment. The available data support the clinical use of the MINI for this purpose. An impressive feature of the MINI is that reliability and validity data were developed concurrently in a binational study of two language versions. As research continues (e.g., Lejoyeux, Feuche, Loi, Solomon, & Ades, 1999), other applications of the MINI are likely to be validated. For example, circumscribed data on social phobia (Boer & Dunner, 1999) suggest that the MINI may have value in detecting undiagnosed disorders in primary care settings. The MINI is not intended to supplant the focus of more extensive Axis I interviews that comprehensively address symptom characteristics and severity.

Clinical Interview Schedule—Revised (CIS-R)

The CIS-R (Lewis et al., 1992) is a semistructured interview intended for use by nonprofessional interviewers. Recent applications have focused on health care and epidemiological research (Jenkins et al., 1997a, 1997b).

Description. The CIS-R, described as a "bottom-up" interview, with its primary focus on describing clinical phenomena (Jenkins et al., 1997b), is composed of 14 symptoms that focus on anxiety and depression. For each symptom endorsed, the interviewers typically ask four additional probes/questions. The answers to the probes ("no" = 0; "yes" = 1) are summed to produce a severity rating (0 to 4). Because of concerns of the ability of nonprofessionals to exercise appropriate clinical judgment, the CIS-R has implemented the following standards: Ratings are (1) highly standardized, (2) restricted to less complicated nonpsychotic symptoms, and (3) limited to the present time.

Validation. Lewis et al. (1992) examined the reliability across interviewers giving separate administrations separated by several minutes. For 100 patients at a general health center, a moderate level of reliability (median kappa = .56; median r = .67) was achieved for individual symptoms. In the determination of "cases" (mental disorders as a category), pairs of psychiatrists were slightly more reliable (kappa = .75) than nonprofessional psychiatric pairs (kappa = .70). Lewis et al. also reported interrater reliability on a Spanish version for 45 patients at a Chilean primary care clinic that produced superb results (median kappa = .88; median r = .95) for CIS-R symptoms.

Clinical Applications. The CIS-R is intended for a broad range of clinical and nonclinical settings. Clinically, the CIS-R is principally employed in general health care settings to screen for common symptoms and possible mental disorders. Given its simplicity, the CIS-R is best considered a reliable screen for common symptoms of anxiety and depression. A primary advantage is its easy implementation by nonprofessionals with minimal training. In nonclinical settings, the CIS-R is a straightforward measure that has been successfully adapted to epidemiological and survey research.

Psychiatric Diagnostic Interview (PDI)

Othmer, Penick, and Powell (1981) constructed the PDI as a structured interview that can be reliably administered by paraprofessionals. Originally intended to evaluate Feighner criteria, the PDI was revised to incorporate DSM-III criteria. Subsequently, a DSM-III-R version was published (Othmer, Penick, Powell, Othmer, & Read, 1989).

Description. Designed as an uncomplicated Axis I interview that can be utilized easily by trained paraprofessionals, the PDI is composed of 15 basic syndromes for current and lifetime diagnoses. Several sections are atypical for Axis I interviews: mental retardation, homosexuality, and transsexualism. For each syndrome, the PDI has a logical organization: Cardinal (core criteria), Social Significance (impact on social, vocational, and family functioning), Auxiliary (associated symptoms), and Time Profile (onset and duration). The items are scored dichotomously in a yes–no format.

Validation. Viatori (1985) summarized the reliability of the PDI as clearly adequate. For example, the test–retest reliability yielded moderate levels of agreement for both current (kappa = .72) and lifetime (kappa = .67) diagnoses. Walters, Chlumsky, and Hemphill (1988) conducted a pilot study for test–retest reliability on 14 inmates after approximately 4 months. The median kappa for lifetime diagnoses on five syndromes was .70.

Weller et al. (1985) examined the concurrent validity of the PDI in comparison to the DIS on 86 inpatients. They found good agreement between the two measures, with an overall kappa of .72. In addition, Powell, Penick, and Othmer (1985) compiled data from several samples to study basic differences in PDI scores for medical patients, and psychiatric inpatients and outpatients. Although cited as discriminant validity, global differences based on patient status provided little evidence of how scales discriminate between specific diagnoses. In addition, four syndromes were poorly represented: obsessive–compulsive disorder, anorexia nervosa, homosexuality, and transsexualism. Finally, the PDI has been employed in different clinical settings with forensic patients (e.g., Walters, Mann, Miller, Hemphill, & Chlumsky, 1988), patients with schizophrenia (Abous-Saleh, Suhaili, Karim, Prais, & Hamdi, 1999) and alcoholism (e.g., Larson & Heppner, 1989; Penick et al., 1994).

The PDI—Revised (PDI-R) was expanded to 17 syndromes plus 4 derived syndromes that correspond to DSM-III-R diagnosis (Othmer et al., 1989). The PDI-R manual reported a study of 53 inpatients that were administered both the PDI and the PDI-R. The percentages of agreement between the two versions were high, ranging from 81.1% to 100.0%; kappas, reported to be significant, were not tabulated. As evidence of content validity, seven experts judged the PDI-R converage of DSM syndromes to be "fair" (12.5%) or "good" (85.7%). Othmer et al. (1989) did not present concurrent validity data on the PDI-R and DSM-III-R diagnoses.

Clinical Applications. The PDI appears to have been overlooked in recent clinical practice. As a straightforward Axis I interview, it provides useful information about DSM diagnoses, with a moderate level of reliability. Professionals are likely to view PDI syndromes, similar to the MINI, as tentative diagnoses to be confirmed by experienced clinicians. A cause of concern in the original PDI is its emphasis on sexual orientation (homosexuality and transsexualism); these were removed in the PDI-R. The PDI and PDI-R also include interview items for OBS and mental retardation; these disorders are better addressed by specific screens and tests of cognitive functioning.

Currently in development, a new version of the PDI, the PDI-IV (personal communication, Susan D. Weinberg, Western Psychological Services, September 24, 2000), will correspond to DSM-IV. The PDI-IV validation will be need to be evaluated once the professional manual is published.

Polydiagnostic Interview (PODI)

Philipp and Maier (1986) developed the PODI as a systematic method for the diagnosis of psychotic and mood disorders. According to M. Phillipp (personal communication, April 14, 1993), the PODI should not be considered a structured interview in its own right but rather a modification of the SCID.

The "polydiagnostic" component of the PODI refers to its focus on multiple diagnostic systems (i.e., DSM-III, RDC, and research models). The PODI stresses reliable evaluation at the symptom/sign level as a way of circumventing the arbitrary conventions provided by any single diagnostic system.

Description. Philipp and Maier (1986) compiled many items on the PODI from existing Axis I measures. For DSM-III diagnoses, they adopted large portions of the SCID, with additional items from the PSE 9th edition. The PODI consists of more than 180 ratings and requires 2–3 hours to complete. For scoring, Philipp and Maier simplified complex diagnostic criteria by dividing them into relevant subcomponents. A computer program is employed to integrate subcomponents and apply different diagnostic criteria.

Validation of the PODI. To investigate interrater reliability, the PODI was administered to 137 psychiatric inpatients. Philipp and Maier (1986) reported that the majority of mood and psychotic criteria had kappas > .80 but did not provide any measure of central tendency. Agreement regarding clinical observations was lower but always above their threshold of moderate consistency ($\geq$ .50). Reliability estimates were only computed for individuals who manifested the disorder (e.g., "expansive mood" was derived solely from the 18 patients with manic episodes). This approach inflates base rates and reliability estimates. A more stringent test of interrater reliability would be to compute reliability coefficients for the full sample.

Philipp and Maier acknowledge the difficulties in establishing the diagnostic validity because the PODI is an amalgamation of measures. Because of this limitation, they assert that the PODI has some evidence of "procedural validity" in its systematic application of subcriteria and criteria to diagnoses. Procedural validity refers to systematized procedures that produce consistent results. Despite its amalgamation of measures, construct- and criterion-related validity are still feasible and desirable.

Clinical Applications. The PODI is an ambitious project for the integration of diagnostic criteria from a wide range of nosological and research models. Strictly speaking, the PODI is not a structured interview but an amalgamation of previously developed measures (SCID and PSE). As such, the emphasis has been on its use as a decision model for comparing different diagnostic systems.

The PODI has not been adequately tested for clinical use. The only available study is flawed by inflated reliability coefficients. No data are currently provided regarding its construct- or criterion-related validity. In the absence of further research, the PODI is not recommended for clinical practice.

6

Axis I Interviews for Children and Adolescents

OVERVIEW

Traditionally, the assessment of psychopathology in children has been achieved by such diverse methods as play therapy and behavioral assessment. Clinicians have often been skeptical of self-reports by children and early adolescents (Herjanic, Herjanic, Brown, & Wheatt, 1975). As summarized by Achenbach (1985), the last two decades have yielded a proliferation of instruments including standardized rating scales and structured interviews. These developments parallel the emergence of the DSM-III and adult diagnostic measures. Following this brief overview of child diagnostic interviews,[1] five diagnostic interviews are featured: (1) the Schedule of Affective Disorders and Schizophrenia for School-Age Children (Kiddie-SADS or K-SADS; Chambers et al., 1985), (2) the Diagnostic Interview Schedule for Children (DISC; Costello, Edelbrock, Dulcan, Kalas, & Klaric, 1984), (3) the Child Assessment Schedule (CAS; Hodges, Kline, Stern, Cytryn, & McKnew, 1982), (4) the Diagnostic Interview for Children and Adolescents (DICA; Herjanic & Reich, 1982), and (5) the Children's Interview for Psychiatric Syndromes (CHIPS; Weller, Weller, Fristad, & Rooney, 1999).

Historically, Rutter and Graham (1968) developed one of the earliest structured interviews for children as a component of the Isle of Wight Inventory, which combined unstructured and structured components. Many questions were unstructured, with the precise wording left to the interviewer's discretion. The interviewer also asked the child to complete standardized tasks that were incorporated into systematic ratings of psychopatholo-

---

[1]For simplicity, I use the term "child" to encompass children and adolescents unless otherwise specified.

gy on 21 categories. As a forerunner of structured interviews, the Isle of Wight Inventory also included a parent interview, with questions extending beyond symptomatology to child–family relationships and marital–family issues.

Herjanic et al. (1975) set the stage for child diagnostic interviews by systematically assessing the reliability of children's (ages 6 to 16) self-reports. With 50 outpatient children, they assessed the completeness and accuracy of self-reports in comparison to parent reports on the same structured interview. Although reported as simple concordance rates, Herjanic et al. found good agreement of factual information and symptoms (> 80%) and moderate agreement of descriptions of behavior (75%) and mental status (69%). These investigators also found good interrater reliability and concluded that structured interviews were likely to assume a significant role in child assessment.

Reliable assessment of children involves the corroboration of self-reporting with standardized observations and collateral interviews by parents, teachers, and mental health professionals. Toward this end, Achenbach, McConaughy, and Howell (1987) performed a classic meta-analysis of 119 studies of children from various settings (e.g., clinics, regular and special classrooms, and facilities for delinquents). They found that informants who had a similar relationship with the child (e.g., both parents or two different teachers) evidenced a moderate level of agreement among themselves (r's ranging from .54 to .64, with a median of .58). In contrast, different sets of informants (e.g., parent vs. teacher) yielded only modest levels of agreement (r's ranging from .24 to .42, with a median of .27). Comparable levels of agreement were found when child ratings were compared to those of informants (r's ranging from .20 to .27, with a median of .25). As might be expected, higher correlations were found for externalized (e.g., hyperactivity and delinquency) than internalized (e.g., social withdrawal and anxiety) problems.

What is the significance of the Achenbach et al. study to child assessment? Clinical data from any single source are unlikely to capture the complex array of psychological problems experienced by many children. For clinicians evaluating children and adolescents, the systematic integration of multiple data sources appears essential to the assessment process.

Child-based diagnostic interviews share important commonalities and differences. As noted by Gutterman, O'Brian, and Young (1987), these interviews share much in common: (1) comparable age groups, parallel interviews (child and parent versions), and (2) general reliance on DSM taxonomy as their gold standard. Significant differences (see Hodges, 1993) also occur in organization, ratings of severity, and training of interviewers. For each measure, a similar framework is used to facilitate cross-comparisons. Each diagnostic interview is organized into three components: description, validation, and clinical applications. This chapter concludes with a synopsis of additional structured interviews for children.

SCHEDULE OF AFFECTIVE DISORDERS AND SCHIZOPHRENIA FOR SCHOOL-AGE CHILDREN (K-SADS)

Description

The K-SADS was originally developed by Puig-Antich and Chambers (1978) as part of an effort to study the parallels between prepubertal and adult depression. Therefore, K-SADS items corresponded with the SADS, so that direct comparisons could be rendered between adult and child symptomatology. W. J. Chambers (personal communication, July 2, 1993) articulated other goals of the K-SADS. First, the K-SADS presents clear definitions of symptoms and behavior. Second, it offers a semiquantitative rating of intensity/severity of symptoms and behavior. Third, the K-SADS is intended to produce clinical judgments by trained clinicians, integrating sources of data and implementing sophisticated estimates of symptom severity.

The K-SADS is designed for sequential administrations with first the parent(s) and then the child. Box 6.1 provides a basic description and information on the availability of the K-SADS. Clinical data from both sources are combined into summary ratings. When marked discrepancies occur, the child

---

BOX 6.1. Highlights of the K-SADS-IV and K-SADS-PL

- *Description:* The K-SADS is an extensive, semistructured interview for the evaluation of child diagnoses; it differs from other child interviews in its emphasis on symptom severity. The K-SADS-IV evolved from earlier versions and is simply updated to meet DSM-IV specifications. The K-SADS-PL differs in structure (more complex, with the inclusion of a screening phase) and ratings (simplified, with fewer gradations).

- *Administration time:* It varies substantially across clinical cases, but parent and child interviews typically require 60–75 minutes each.

- *Skills level:* Like the SADS, the K-SADS-IV and K-SADS-PL require sophisticated interviewers with considerable training.

- *Distinctive features:* With the parent interview administered first, the K-SADS attempts to reconcile disparities by sharing the parent's perspective. The K-SADS-III-R and K-SADS-IV have a solid psychometric foundation. The K-SADS-PL is unique in its attempt to utilize 82 symptoms as a comprehensive screen for DSM-IV disorders.

- *Cost:* Copies are available gratis from the authors of each version.

- *Source:* The K-SADS-IV is available from Paul Ambrosini, MD, by mail, 3200 Henry Avenue, Philadelphia, PA 19129-1137, or by phone, (215) 843-4402. The K-SADS-PL is available from Joan Kaufman, MD, Department of Psychology, Yale University, P.O. Box 208205; by phone, (203) 432-2353, or on the internet, *www.wpic.pitt.edu/ksads*.

is presented with the parent's perspective in an effort to resolve the inconsistency. Like the SADS, ratings are made for the worst period of the last episode and also for the current time (i.e., the previous week).

The interview process begins with a brief, unstructured interview in which the purpose of the assessment is explained and presenting problems are explored. The organization of questions closely parallels the SADS. For example, most of questions on mood disorders use identical wordings and scoring criteria as the SADS. However, additional questions are employed to assess symptoms from the child's perspective. Similar to the SADS, nonpsychotic symptoms are typically rated on a 6-point scale of severity: 1 = not at all; 2 = slight–subthreshold; 3 = mild; 4 = moderate; 5 = severe; and 6 = extreme.

The K-SADS includes several components not found in the SADS. Its broadened coverage includes expanded sections on anxiety disorders, conduct symptoms, and psychotic symptoms. Regarding the latter, extensive inquiries are provided for hallucinations (e.g., command) and their differentiation from other phenomena (e.g., illusions, eidetic imagery, and imaginary companions).

The original K-SADS has been updated in several versions. Importantly, these versions utilize the same core inquiries and ratings but differ in coverage. Key differences are outlined as follows:

- The K-SADS-E (Epidemiological Version; Orvaschel, Puigh-Antich, Chambers, Tabrizi, & Johnson, 1982) added the following diagnostic categories: attention deficit disorder (ADD), alcohol abuse and dependence, drug abuse and dependence, and suicidal behavior.
- The K-SADS-III-R (Ambrosini, Metz, Prabucki, & Lee, 1989) was designed to assess 31 DSM-III-R disorders: 10 mood, 5 anxiety, 5 psychotic, 4 behavioral, 2 eating, and 5 additional disorders. The K-SADS-III-R was subsequently updated (Ambrosini, 1992) with the incorporation of 17 items from the Hamilton Depression Rating Scale (HDRS).
- K-SADS-PL (Present and Lifetime Version; Kaufman et al., 1997) is designed to assess 32 DSM-III-R and DSM-IV child diagnoses. It differs fundamentally from other K-SADS versions in both organization and ratings. The K-SADS-PL is organized into an 82-symptom screen interview followed by five diagnostic sections.
- K-SADS-IV (Ambrosini & Dixon, 1996) closely parallels the K-SADS-III-R in structure, clinical inquiries, and ratings. A small proportion of items were updated to DSM-IV specifications.

This section focuses on the K-SADS-III-R and K-SADS-IV in an examination of their validation and clinical applications. These versions have evolved from the K-SADS and K-SADS-E, which constitute the foundation of this structured interview. In contrast, the K-SADS-PL diverges markedly from other K-SADS versions. While retaining many clinical inquires, the K-SADS-PL differs in its organization (i.e., two phases: screen interview and diagnostic sections) and clinical ratings. Given the paucity of research on this fundamentally different model, the K-SADS-PL is only be briefly summarized.

Reliability

The bulk of reliability studies on the K-SADS was conducted in the 1980s (see Table 6.1). These studies focused on both interrater and test–retest reliability across a variety of clinical and nonclinical settings. The key findings are summarized by three categories: symptoms, diagnoses, and summary scales.

The K-SADS has exceptional reliability at the symptom level. Studies have established excellent interrater reliability on both symptom subsets (Apter, Orvaschel, Laseq, Moses, & Tyano, 1989; Chambers et al., 1985) and the entire K-SADS (Cashel, Rogers, Sewell, & Holliman, 1998; Hammen et al., 1987). As expected, coefficients are lower for test–retest reliability but still in the moderate range. The K-SADS is likely to be the child interview of choice when symptoms are the focal point.

Studies of the K-SADS diagnoses produced good to superb reliabilities (see Table 6.1). For interrater reliability, four studies produced high to very high kappas, ranging from .78 to .86. For test–retest reliability, the kappas were more varied (i.e., .54, .76, and .78) but still in the acceptable range. Interpretation of these very positive findings is tempered by the limited range of diagnoses and the emphasis on mood disorders.

K-SADS summary scales are more relevant to clinical research than to professional practice. Nevertheless, these summary scales appear to possess adequate (r = .72; Chambers et al., 1985) to superb ($kappa_{interrater}$ = .93; $kappa_{test–retest}$ = .84; Apter et al., 1989) reliabilities.

Other studies have addressed other aspects of reliability, including retrospective diagnosis and internal consistency. Key findings are highlighted as follows:

- Ovaschel et al. (1982) studied the retrospective assessment of depressive symptoms with a present-episode administration followed by a retrospective administration covering the same episode after a 12-month episode. Children ranging from ages 6–11 years were accurate in their symptom recall to the extent that retrospective diagnoses were highly consistent (median kappa = .86) for four disorders.
- Ambrosini et al. (1989) found excellent alpha coefficients (median alpha = .82) for five disorders.

Studies have cross-informant consistency, comparing children's self-reporting with their parents' collateral reports. As such, these studies do not formally address reliability because different but related data sources[2] were

---

[2]Sources are not independent because parents often rely on children's reports to inform their own accounts. Likewise, children are often educated about their symptoms by their parents.

TABLE 6.1. Reliability Studies for the Schedule of Affective Disorders and Schizophrenia for School-Age Children (K-SADS)

Study (year)	N	Setting In / Out / Com			Dx	Raters Lay/Prof	Reliability Inter/Retest (interval)	Reliability estimates Sx/Cur-Dx/Life-Dx/Other			
Reliability studies											
Orvaschel et al. (1982)	17		✓		2	✓	✓ (12 mo)				.86[a]
Chambers et al. (1985)	52		✓		4	✓	✓ (< 3 days)	.58[b]	.54		.72[c]
Hammen et al. (1987)	35			✓[d]	NA	✓	✓	.96[e]	.84		
Lahey et al. (1988)[f]	75		✓		9	✓	✓	.86[g]			
Ambrosini et al. (1989)	25		✓		7	✓	✓	.85[h]			
Apter et al. (1989)[i]	70	✓			6	✓	✓ (1 wk)	.72[j]	.78		.93[k]
	70	✓			6	✓	✓	.59[j]	.78		.84[k]
Fendrich et al. (1991)	59		✓		2	✓	✓ (2 yr)				.28[a]
Kaufman et al. (1997)[l]	20		✓		8	✓	✓ (18 days)		.76	.81	
Cashel et al. (1998)	16			✓[m]	6	✓	✓	> .80[n]			
Cross-informant studies											
Orvaschel et al. (1982)	17		✓		2	✓		.64[o]			
Weissman et al. (1987)	38		✓		1	✓		.13[p]	.03		
Apter et al. (1989)[i]	40	✓	✓		6	✓		.19[i]	.42		.57[k]
Fendrich et al. (1991)	59	✓	✓		2	✓			.35		

Note. See Table 1.5 (p. 35) for a glossary of terms and abbreviations.

[a]Diagnosis of past episodes, with a retrospective account at follow-up.

[b]Intraclass coefficients (ICC) for 41 depressive, anxious, and psychotic symptoms.

[c]The r for summary scales.

[d]Participants from a study of family stress.

[e]Reported as the percentage of "exact agreement on scale ratings of symptom severity" (Hammen et al., 1987, p. 738).

[f]Based on K-SADS parent interview only.

[g]Given the very small number of fathers, this median is based on mothers.

[h]For child ratings alone, kappa = .79; parent ratings alone, kappa = .88.

[i]Hebrew translation.

[j]Based on 20 mood symptoms.

[k]ICCs for summary scales.

[l]K-SADS-PL version.

[m]Incarcerated delinquents receiving psychological services.

[n]Kappas > .80 were achieved for 80% of symptoms for child K-SADS.

[o]Based on 21 symptoms.

[p]Data were dichotomized and kappas used; for mother–father agreement, median kappa = .22.

used. K-SADS results were markedly variable. In three studies (see Table 6.1) that emphasized mood disorders, symptom consistency ranged from .13 to .64. Results for current diagnoses were also disappointing. As observed in child interviews generally, cross-informant consistency is very difficult to achieve even at moderate levels. In clinical practice, however, K-SADS inconsistencies are often resolved by sharing the discrepancies with the child being interviewed.

Validity

Research on the K-SADS has focused on its concurrent, convergent, and construct validity. Construct validity is examined via principal components analysis and Syndeham's criteria.

Concurrent Validity

Two studies have assessed the concurrent validity of the K-SADS based on other structured interviews. The two criterion measures were the CAS and the DISC; both are subsequently reviewed individually in this chapter.

Cohen, O'Conner, Lewis, Veliz, and Malachowski (1987) administered the DISC to 101 community children, ages 9 to 12, as part of an epidemiological study. K-SADS interviews occurred at an interval of 3–4 months after the DISC. In comparing DSM diagnostic criteria, termed "possible diagnosis," the kappas were low for the mother–child K-SADS, ranging from .08 to .30. Several problems constrained the interpretation of these findings. First, the DISC appeared to overdiagnose in these community samples (i.e., M of 1.41 *common* disorders per nonclinical participant). Second, the lack of observed association may have reflected clinical changes in the research population. As noted by Cohen et al., long intervals between tests, use of nonclinical populations, and mixing of lay and professional interviewers are likely to lead (individually and collectively) to poor levels of agreement.

Hodges, McKnew, Burbach, and Roebuck (1987) administered the K-SADS-E and the CAS to 29 children referred for outpatient services. Based on four diagnostic groupings (ADD, CD, anxiety and mood disorders), they found low-moderate kappas for child interviews alone (median = .44), with high-moderate coefficients for parent alone (median = .60). Diagnoses based on the combined parent–child K-SADS (median = .58) were comparable to the parent-only interview. Although based on a very small sample, the results suggest a moderate convergence of the two measures.

Several studies have examined the K-SADS in relationship to clinical diagnosis. For example, Carlson, Kashani, Thomas, Vaidya, and Daniel (1987) compared parent K-SADS and DICA administrations to clinical diagnoses. For six common disorders, the parent K-SADS evidenced moderate convergence (median kappa = .50; range from .16 to .69). Overall, the K-SADS performed slightly better than the DICA (median kappa = .40; range from .15 to .75). In light of the methodological constraint (no child-based interviews), the

K-SADS results appear generally positive. As a second example, Apter, Bleich, Plutchik, Mendelsohn, and Tyano (1988) examined the SADS summary scales in relationship to clinical diagnoses for 140 consecutive adolescent patients in a Tel-Aviv hospital. Comparisons across the three most common disorders (schizophrenia, major depression, and CD) revealed highly significant differences in the predicted directions for depression and schizophrenia. While lower on most scales, adolescents with CD evidenced a higher frequency of suicidal thoughts and behavior.

Convergent Validity

Studies have compared the K-SADS to several checklists and the Minnesota Multiphasic Personality Inventory—Adolescent (MMPI-A). Use of these studies as evidence of convergent validity is circumscribed because the K-SADS was sometimes used as the gold standard. Nonetheless, key findings are summarized as follows:

- Convergent data with the Child Behavior Checklist (CBCL; Achenbach & Edelbrock, 1983) offer general support for internalizing and externalizing disorders (Biederman et al., 1993; Carlson & Kelly, 1998; Kaufman et al., 1997).
- Grayson and Carlson (1991) compared the K-SADS disorders to the Stony Brook Child Psychiatric Checklist (SBC; Gadow & Sprafkin, 1987). As a screening measure, the SBC tended to overclassify over-anxious disorders and manic episodes. Despite this limitation, a moderate level of agreement was found (median kappa = .53).
- Cashel et al. (1998) examined MMPI-A correlates in relationship to K-SADS symptoms in a male delinquent sample. Most significant correlates were in the modest to low moderate range (.30 to .50) and appeared indicative of general impairment.

In summary, convergent validity studies provide general support for the K-SADS as a measure of broad diagnostic groups. However, these studies lack the necessary focus to evaluate the convergent validity of specific disorders.

Construct Validity

Ryan et al. (1987) evaluated the underlying dimensions of selected K-SADS symptoms in a clinical sample of 296 depressed children and adolescents. Utilizing principal components analysis, they found five factors that account for approximately 55% of the variance. With few exceptions, these factors were diagnostically logical, with components of depression, anxiety, and conduct disorder. Furthermore, the components were reported to be stable for both prepubertal youth and adolescents.

Construct validation of the K-SADS was addressed in relationship to

Syndeham's criteria. K-SADS research examined the clarity of diagnostic boundaries (i.e., inclusion and exclusion criteria) and longitudinal perspectives (i.e., outcome criteria). Carlson and Kelly (1998) investigated the diagnostic relevance of manic symptoms in hospitalized children. They found that manic symptoms were associated with other disorders (attention-deficit/hyperactivity disorder [ADHD], oppositional defiant disorder [ODD], and depression) but appeared to be distinguished by differences in cognitive abilities (e.g., digit span and coding) and interpersonal functioning (e.g., social problems and aggressiveness). Especially with young children, consideration of diagnostic boundaries appears to be a critical component of all child interviews.

K-SADS research has also addressed a critical element of construct validity via longitudinal perspectives of mental disorders; these studies include antecedents of first episodes and treatment outcome. Key findings are summarized as follows:

- Parental depression is linked with mood disorders in their children (Hammen et al., 1987; Orvaschel, 1990). One potential mediator for depression in offspring is cognitions about self-work and self-efficacy that are likely associated with the parent–child relationship (Hammen, 1988). Family history of mood disorders dramatically increases the likelihood that children will develop bipolar disorders at a prepubertal age (Geller, Fox, & Clark, 1994).
- A self-medication hypothesis has been proposed to explain subsequently high levels of substance abuse in adolescents with K-SADS anxiety disorders (Deas-Nesmith, Brady, & Campbell, 1998).
- Mattanah, Becker, Levy, Edell, and McGlashan (1995) evaluated the temporal stability of Axis I disorders in adolescents. After a 2-year follow-up, the large majority of adolescents with mood and externalizing disorders no longer warranted the diagnoses. Encouragingly, very few new cases of of externalizing disorders were observed.
- Mixed success (Ambrosini et al., 1999; Kye et al., 1996) has been had with pharmacological interventions for adolescent depression utilizing K-SADS mood symptoms.

In summary, construct validation of the K-SADS has focused almost exclusively on mood disorders. With this broad diagnostic category, meaningful dimensions, childhood antecedents, and treatment outcome provide useful data. More studies are needed to address construct validity in other diagnostic categories.

Clinical Applications

The K-SADS, like its adult counterpart, offers detailed clinical criteria for rating both the presence and severity of specific symptomatology. Clinical ratings are made separately for the parent and child for both the present episode and the previous week, and then combined into summary ratings. The complexity of the ratings is an advantage when carefully applied and, understandably, a disadvantage when faced with time constraints or less standardized administrations. A paramount question for each clinician is "Am I willing to administer the K-SADS, following its rigorous procedures?" If the answer is "no," then the K-SADS has the potential of becoming an elaborate pretense.

The K-SADS and its revisions offer clinicians a broad range of symptoms and clinical characteristics for mood and psychotic disorders that are likely to form a relatively complete diagnostic picture of these disorders. The most recent revisions, the K-SADS-III-R and K-SADS-IV, reflect the evolving DSM criteria; most of these clinical inquiries and concomitant ratings have a solid empirical foundation based on earlier versions. Therefore, clinicians are justified in using the K-SADS-III-R and K-SADS-IV except with those diagnoses in which substantive changes have occurred (e.g., CD). As noted in the introduction to the K-SADS, the K-SADS-PL is not currently recommended for clinical practice given the paucity of research on its validation and the fundamental changes in its organization and ratings.

The parallel coverage of the K-SADS and SADS allows for a systematic evaluation of symptoms from childhood to adulthood. Clinically, psychologists will need to choose which measure to employ with older adolescents. For example, Kutcher, Yanchyshyn, and Cohen (1985) found the adult SADS useful in the evaluation of adolescent depression with inpatients ranging in age from 13 to 18 (*M* age of 16.5). The advantage of the K-SADS-E and K-SADS-III-R is their coverage of childhood disorders. In contrast, the advantage of the SADS is its superior reliability and validity. One procedure is to screen older adolescent patients for possible childhood disorders. If none appear to be present, then the SADS might be employed.

The reliability estimates for child diagnostic interviews are generally lower than those for adults. The reason for this decline is not completely understood but probably reflects (1) routine use of multiple sources (parent and child), (2) the child's decreased ability for accurate and consistent self-reporting, and (3) less clearly defined symptoms in children and adolescents. Among child interviews, the K-SADS appears to be moderately reliable. Its particular strength is consistent and reproducible evaluation of symptoms and associated features. Like all child interviews, cross-informant consistency (parent and child) appears to be quite modest, with a tendency for children to underreport and parents to overreport symptoms.

The K-SADS studies provide moderate evidence of concurrent, convergent, and construct validity. Research spans both inpatient and outpatient setting, making the K-SADS useful in a range of professional settings. The strength of this research is mood disorders in children and adolescents.

A challenge for clinicians is the use of structured interviews with youth who have limited cognitive abilities. Preliminary data by Masi, Mucci, Favilla, and Poli (1991) suggest that the K-SADS might be successfully employed with adolescents who have limited intellectual abilities (*M* IQ = 61.08; *SD* =

4.08). The researchers found that these adolescents were able to report symptoms in response to K-SADS inquiries. Despite methodological limitations, the work is promising in that it provides a structured assessment for a traditionally underserved population.

In summary, the K-SADS is a clinically useful measure that is likely to be a strong candidate for child and adolescent diagnoses. The K-SADS has special merit in the examination of mood, schizophrenic, anxiety, and conduct disorders. The K-SADS should be strongly considered when a detailed examination of symptoms and associated symptoms is desired. For clinical settings that provide a family context for assessment and treatment, the parallel nature of the K-SADS and SADS is advantageous.

DIAGNOSTIC INTERVIEW SCHEDULE FOR CHILDREN (DISC)

Description

The original edition of the NIMH DISC was developed in 1979 as part of a feasibility study on child clinical interviews (National Institute of Mental Health, 1991). Box 6.2 provides a basic description and information on the

---

BOX 6.2. Highlights of the DISC

- *Description:* The DISC is a structured interview that is intended for use by both professionals and nonprofessionals. More than 30 DSM-III-R and DSM-IV diagnoses are covered by recent editions (DISC-2.1, DISC-2.3, and DISC-IV). Administrations typically involve both child (DISC-C) and parent (DISC-P) versions.

- *Administration time:* For use with patients, administration times are approximately 1½–2 hours each for the DISC-C and DISC-P.

- *Skills level:* Lay interviewers, typically at the BA level, require approximately 1 week of training followed by clinical supervision.

- *Distinctive features:* The DISC is the most extensively researched structured interview for children. It appears especially useful for addressing cross-cultural issues and epidemiological applications. The DISC provides extensive coverage of current diagnoses.

- *Cost:* Price list on 3/1/2001 for single copies = $50 + $10 shipping for each copy of the DISC-Y and DISC-P. Because the DISC is in the public domain, clinicians need only buy one copy of each version and reproduce their own copies as necessary.

- *Source:* DISC Development Group, by mail, 1051 Riverside Drive, Box 78, New York, NY 10032; by phone, (888) 814-3472; by fax, (914) 243-0492; or on the internet, *disc@worldnet.att.net.*

availability of the DISC. Three prominent researchers were brought together to develop a comprehensive child interview informed by their own research: Herjanic (DICA), Puig-Antich (K-SADS) and Conner (Conner's Rating Scales). These researchers attempted to assemble a comprehensive set of items addressing childhood psychopathology (Shaffer et al., 1993). Pertinent chronology of the DISC is summarized as follows:

1. DISC-1 represented revision and field-testing of the DISC by Costello and his colleagues (Costello, Edelbrock, & Costello, 1985; Costello et al., 1984) under the auspices of an NIMH contract. Corresponding to DSM-III diagnoses, DISC-1 addressed 205 standard questions and 852 optional probes (Shaffer et al., 1993).
2. DISC-R revised 83 unreliable items and was updated for DSM-III-R diagnoses (see Shaffer et al. 1988). DISC-R addressed 231 standard questions and 1,186 optional probes.
3. DISC-2.1 and DISC-2.3 represent further modifications, with the grouping of symptoms into six diagnostic modules and revisions of specific items. The DISC-2.3 was utilized in NIMH large-scale collaboration entitled "Methods for the Epidemiology of Child and Adolescent Mental Disorders" (MECA). It is published by NIMH (1991).
4. DISC-IV was developed in 1997 to evaluate current and lifetime childhood disorders for DSM-IV (Columbia DISC Development Group, 1999). It is composed of 358 standard questions and 1,341 optional probes.

An important feature of the DISC is the sustained effort to simplify the language and sentence structure in order to improve children's comprehension of questions. As reported by Edelbrock, Costello, Dulcan, Kalas, and Conover (1985), questions are composed of easily understood words and rarely exceed 10 words in length. In addition, complex inquiries are divided into simpler subquestions. To ensure the accuracy of responses, children are asked further questions to clarify their responses and may be asked to provide examples.

DISC studies suggest that circumscribed problems persist among children regarding the comprehensibility of specific inquiries. Key findings about comprehension are summarized as follows:

- Breslau (1987) found that many children and some parents are likely to misunderstand some questions regarding obsessions, compulsions, and certain psychotic symptoms. Care must be taken that children and informants understand the nature of the question; such understanding is often demonstrated through inquiries about characteristic examples.
- Fallon and Schwab-Stone (1994) evaluated the types of questions that typically cause problems for children. They found that certain types of questions markedly decrease reliability, including questions about (1)

frequency and duration or (2) comparisons of the child to other children.

- Breton et al. (1995), in a study of English-speaking children in Quebec, found that the length of questions had an inverse relationship with understanding: (1) approximately 80% accuracy for less than nine words, (2) approximately 63% accuracy for 10–19 words, (3) approximately 40% accuracy for 20 or more words.

The DISC and its revisions are composed of a structured interview in which both clinical inquiries and ratings of responses are highly standardized. Because of its epidemiological applications, the DISC is highly structured so as to enable nonprofessional interviewers to conduct interviews in a systematic and reliable manner. For the sake of simplicity, I limit the description to the two most recent editions, namely, DISC-2.3 and DISC-IV.

DISC-2.3 and DISC-IV are comprised of six modules: Anxiety Disorders; Miscellaneous Disorders (i.e., eating, elimination, and tic disorders); Mood Disorders, Schizophrenia and Other Disorders; Disruptive Behavior Disorders (e.g., ADHD, CD, and ODD); and Alcohol and Other Substance Abuse Disorders. Each module is organized by diagnosis and subdivided into components of the disorder. Besides the six modules, an introductory section is designed to survey sociodemographic information, history of health and mental health treatment, and a time line to establish important events in the previous 12 months. In addition to updating inquires to address DSM-IV, the DISC-IV provides a "whole-life" module for evaluating lifetime prevalences of mental disorders.

The DISC editions consist of two parallel versions designed for children (i.e., DISC-C) and parent informants (i.e., DISC-P). The primary difference between the two versions is the wording of the questions: "Do you . . ." in the child version versus "Does (he/she) . . ." in the parent version. For the DISC-R, interview times are approximately 1½ hours for children and 2½ hours for parents (Zahner, 1991). Efforts to shorten the DISC-IV were modestly successful (1 hour and 40 minutes for each). Still, many parents (41.9%) and the majority of children (55.4%) find the DISC-IV to be too lengthy (Fisher et al., 1997).

The scoring for the DISC is organized on a 3-point rating system: 0 for "no," 1 for "sometimes or somewhat," and 2 for "yes." According to Weinstein, Stone, Noam, Grimes, and Schwab-Stone (1989), ratings of 1 should be considered subclinical because their inclusion in diagnostic models leads to overdiagnosis. For evidence of psychotic symptoms, interviewers are required to provide detailed observations that may be rated by clinicians.

Reliability

The initial reliability studies of the DISC were conducted by Costello and his colleagues (Costello et al., 1985; Edelbrock et al., 1985). These studies do not address diagnostic validity per se. Rather, they evaluate either total symptom scores or symptom scores for specific disorders. Total scores provide little useful information because interviewers might be highly disparate in their individual ratings yet achieve similar totals. However, correlations for specific disorders provide dimensional data for these diagnoses. In this regard, Edelbrook et al. (1985) found a moderate level of agreement for the DISC-C (r = .68) and DISC-P (r = .78). The DISC-C was highly sensitive to age. Young children (ages 6–9) evidenced low consistency (r = .43) in comparison to older children (r = .60) and adolescents (r = .71).

The DISC has been subjected to large-scale investigations of it reliability since the original studies (see Table 6.2). The major emphasis of these investigations is the examination of test–retest reliability among outpatient and community settings. In general, the DISC evidences moderate test–retest reliability for current episodes. The key DISC findings are distilled from these studies and summarized as follows:

1. *Age.* Consistent with Edelbrook et al. (1985), younger children have substantial difficulty in responding to the DISC in a reliable manner (see Fallon & Schwab-Stone, 1994; Ribera et al., 1996). Reliability appears to be affected by a combination of age, intelligence, and impairment (Fallon & Schwab-Stone, 1994), and the complexity of questions (Breton et al., 1995). As a general benchmark, clinicians should be (a) generally concerned about DISC reliability with children ages 6 to 9 and (b) selectively concerned (e.g., impairment and intelligence) about DISC reliability with children ages 10 to 11.

2. *DISC-P versus DISC-C.* Partially due to age-related problems, parent versions (DISC-P) tend to have higher test–retest reliabilities than child versions (DISC-C). In practice, clinicians may wish to give greater weight to the DISC-P than DISC-C, especially when the parent informant appears to have detailed knowledge of his or her child's problems. This difference between DISC-P and DISC-C is greatly attenuated with adolescents.

3. *Diagnostic coverage.* A frequent problem for broad-based diagnostic interviews is that reliability studies often neglect less common diagnoses. The DISC is no exception. The majority of studies evaluate less than 10 of the more than 30 diagnoses. Clinicians should only consider the DISC to be reliable when applied to common disorders.

4. *Symptom reliability.* Several interrater reliability studies (Anderson, Williams, McGee, & Silva, 1987; Lahey et al., 1990) provide strong evidence of symptom reliability on the DISC.

5. *Dimensional diagnoses.* Symptom scores for specific diagnoses provide moderate to high correlations. The DISC symptom scores may be reliably used to evaluate changes in the severity of specific disorders.

6. *Spanish translation.* Several large-scale studies (Bird et al., 1987; Jensen, Roper, et al., 1995; Ribera et al., 1996) have established comparable reliability for the DISC Spanish translation with Puerto Rican samples. Reliability studies with other Hispanic groups have yet to be disseminated.

TABLE 6.2. Reliability Studies for the Diagnostic Interview Schedule for Children (DISC)

Study (year)	Ver	N	Setting			Dx	Raters		Reliability		Reliability estimates			
			In	Out	Com		Lay	Prof	Inter/Retest	(interval)	Sx	Cur-Dx	Life-Dx	Other
Costello et al. (1985)	C	316	✓	✓	✓	NA	✓	✓	✓	(1–2 wk)				.75[a]
	P	316	✓	✓	✓	NA	✓	✓	✓	(1–2 wk)				.84[a]
Edelbrock et al. (1985)	C	242	✓	✓	✓	12	✓		✓	(13 days)				.68[b]
	P	242	✓	✓	✓	12	✓		✓	(13 days)				.78[b]
Anderson et al. (1987)	C	60	✓			5	✓				≥.50	.70		
Bird et al. (1987)[c]	P[d]	91	✓	✓		13	✓		✓	(19 days)		.54		
Haley et al. (1988)	C	15	✓			1	✓		✓				.96[b]	
Lahey et al. (1990)	P	44	✓			5	✓		✓		.93			
Shaffer et al. (1993)	?	10	✓			5		✓			1.00[e]			
Schwab-Stone et al. (1993)	C	37	✓	✓		5	✓		✓	(1–3 wk)		.64		.66[f]
	P	37	✓	✓		5	✓		✓	(1–3 wk)		.82		.82[f]
Jensen, Roper, et al. (1995)[g]	C	97	✓	✓		5	✓		✓	(1–2 wk)		.46		
	P	97	✓	✓		5	✓		✓	(1–2 wk)		.69		
	C	278			✓	5	✓		✓	(2–4 wk)		.30		
	P	278			✓	5	✓		✓	(2–4 wk)		.57		
Ribera et al. (1996)[c]	C	78	✓	✓		11	✓	✓	✓	(<2 wk)		.50		
	P	78	✓	✓		11	✓	✓	✓	(<2 wk)		.56		
	C	248			✓	7	✓		✓	(<2 wk)		.37		
	P	248			✓	7	✓		✓	(<2 wk)		.60		

Study	Ver	N							
Schwab-Stone et al. (1995)[b]	C	247	✓[i]	✓	✓	8	✓	(1–15 days)	.31
	P	247	✓[i]	✓	✓	8	✓	(1–15 days)	.56
Breton et al. (1998)[j]	C	145	✓	✓		5	✓	(13 days)	.55
	P	260	✓			6	✓	(14 days)	.56
Fisher et al. (1997)	C	82		✓	✓	9	✓	(3–10 days)	.49
	P	84		✓	✓	9	✓	(3–10 days)	.58

Note. Ver = Version (C = child; P = parent). ? = information is not provided. See Table 1.5 (p. 35) for a glossary of terms and abbreviations.
[a]Correlation of total symptom scores for DISC.
[b]Correlations of total symptoms for specific disorders.
[c]Spanish version.
[d]Version not specified although the introduction reported more usefulness of the DISC-P because of comprehension problems with younger children.
[e]ICC.
[f]ICC for total symptoms for specific disorders.
[g]Multisite study that includes one Spanish-speaking (Puerto Rico) and two English-speaking (New York and Georgia) sites.
[h]Two samples are combined, one using lay–lay interviewers and the other lay–professional interviewers.
[i]Children were screened to ensure that slightly more than half (54.3%) were likely to qualify for at least one diagnosis.
[j]French version.

7. *Interviewer training.* The use of nonprofessional versus professional interviewers does not produce any consistent pattern. The current data support the use of nonprofessionals or paraprofessionals for conducting DISC interviews.

In summary, the DISC appears to have acceptable to excellent reliability depending on the version (DISC-C and DISC-P) and the population. Its diagnostic test–retest reliabilities tend to fall in the moderate range. Its strengths are symptom interrater reliabilities and dimensional test–retest ratings of specific disorders. In addition, current reliability data strongly support the Spanish translation with Puerto Rican samples.

Validity

The validation of the DISC has involved three major components: concurrent validity with traditional diagnosis, convergent validity with psychometric measures, and diagnostic validity via Syndeham's criteria. With respect to diagnostic validity, studies have investigated the discreteness of diagnostic boundaries (i.e., inclusion and exclusion criteria) and longitudinal dimensions of diagnoses (i.e., outcome criteria). Before addressing these major components, I briefly review the factor structure of the DISC.

The factor structure of the DISC was evaluated separately for 391 boys and 360 girls obtained from a community study by Williams, McGee, Anderson, and Silva (1989) via a higher-order factor analysis on the 13 DISC subscales. With a principal factor analysis rotated to an oblique solution, both boys and girls evidenced a similar factor of externalizing disorders comprised of inattention, impulsivity, hyperactivity, conduct, and oppositional features. Gender differences were observed for internalizing disorders. Boys had one internalizing dimension representing anxiety and depressive disorders. In contrast, girls had nonoverlapping dimensions: anxiety (separation anxiety, obsessive–compulsive, and phobia) disorders and depression (affective, suicidal, vegetative, and cognitive). The results provide support for an internalizing–externalizing dimension of child disorders and the conceptually logical division of anxiety and depression among girls.

Concurrent Validity

Cohen, O'Conner, et al. (1987; see also the K-SADS section) conducted the first diagnostic concordance study comparing the DISC with the K-SADS in a community sample. One methodological confound was the 3- to 4-month interval between the administration of the two structured interviews. The kappa coefficients were very modest (i.e., all < .40), which may reflect on (1) the low prevalence of disorders in a community sample and (2) the lengthy interval between administrations.

Weinstein et al. (1989) compared admission diagnoses with DISC diagnoses on a consecutive sample of 163 inpatient admissions. Characteristically, admission diagnoses tend to focus on the primary disorder (i.e., $M = 1.2$ disorders) in contrast to the DISC, with its multiple disorders (i.e., $M = 3.4$ disorders). As a result, diagnostic agreement between the two methods was very low (kappas < .20). Reassuringly, the DISC agreed with the majority of the admission diagnoses. As an important limitation, Weinstein et al. (1989) handicapped the study by use of admission diagnoses that did not have the benefit of inpatient assessments and observations. However, a further analysis (Aronen, Noam, & Weinstein, 1993) with discharge diagnoses failed to improve the level of agreement.

Several studies (e.g., Bird, Gould, & Staghezza, 1992; Lahey et al., 1990) have employed Spitzer's (1983) Longitudinal Expert Evaluation using All Data (LEAD) model for establishing childhood diagnoses. Bird et al. (1992) examined the Spanish translation of the DISC (see Bird, Canino, Rubio-Stipec, et al., 1987) and LEAD diagnoses on a community sample of 386 children. For five common diagnoses, the DISC-P yielded kappas in the low moderate range (median = .47). In comparison, the DISC-C produced only modest agreement (median = .35). In stark contrast to Bird et al., Lahey et al. (1990) compared the DISC to "best estimate" diagnoses that combined all available data. They found high agreement for three DSM-III-R disruptive disorders (kappas from .90 to .95) and two depressive disorders (.90 and .97) for outpatient samples. Beyond the obvious language dissimilarities, the studies differed strikingly in setting and prevalence of disorders. Importantly, both studies can be criticized for potential criterion contamination because DISC results were not independent of LEAD diagnoses.

Several research teams (Fisher et al., 1993; Pellegrino, Singh, & Carmanico, 1999; Piacentini et al., 1993; Schwab-Stone et al., 1995) have evaluated successive editions of the DISC. Key findings are summarized as follows:

- Piacentini et al. (1993) examined DISC-R diagnoses in comparison to informant-based clinical diagnoses that utilized the Clinical Assessment Form. For four diagnoses (ODD, ADHD, CD, and major depression), the median kappa was .44 (range from .32 to .46). Although the findings were relatively modest in absolute terms, the use of two separate sources of data (child vs. parent informant) militated against high levels of agreement.
- Fisher et al. (1993) tested the clinical usefulness of DISC-2.1 for the identification of rare disorders. Compared to clinical diagnoses, DISC-C or DISC-P alone had only modest sensitivity rates. When combined, the DISC-C + DISC-P yielded high sensitivity rates, ranging from 73% to 100%, with a median of 88%. The corresponding specificity rates were not reported.
- Pellegrino et al. (1999) compared DISC-2.1 and clinical diagnoses for inpatient and partially hospitalized youth. Interestingly, 26.0% of the sample

did not warrant a DISC diagnosis. Those warranting DISC diagnoses received 50.5% more DISC than clinical diagnoses. Not surprisingly, agreement of five specific disorders was negligible (median kappa = .09) and very modest for broad diagnostic groups (median kappa = .24).

• Schwab-Stone et al. (1995) compared eight DISC-2.3 diagnoses administered by nonprofessionals to clinician symptom ratings.[3] The DISC-C produced only modest agreement (median kappa = .33). In comparison, low-moderate levels of agreement were established for DISC-P (median kappa = .47) and DISC-P + DISC-C (median kappa = .49).

In summary, studies of concurrent validity yielded generally disappointing results. Even limiting the number of diagnoses rarely produced median kappas above .40. These studies represent the challenges of bootstrapping validity. Modest levels of agreement provide little evidence of concurrent validity.

Convergent Validity

Costello et al. (1985) performed the original validity study by contrasting DISC scales for 40 psychiatric and 40 pediatric referrals. Not surprisingly, significant differences were found for almost all the scales. Regarding convergent validity, total scores for the DISC-P were moderately correlated ($r = .71$), with the CBCL but not the DISC-C ($r = .14$ for the psychiatric sample). Overall, the study provides general evidence of convergent validity for the DISC-P as a measure of general impairment.

Considerable research has addressed the convergent validity of the DISC in relationship to the CBCL and the teacher's version of the CBCL, namely, the Teacher's Report Form (TRF). A summary of CBCL and TRF convergent studies is as follows:

- Edelbrock and Costello (1988, p. 223) found significant biserial correlations between CBCL scales and DISC diagnoses but did not report the magnitude of these correlations. Through an application of multiple regression to dichotomous variables, they reported a linear trend for the diagnoses of ADHD, CD, and depression with their respective CBCL scales.
- Weinstein et al. (1989) found significant differences on CBCL scales for youth with and without four specific DISC disorders. Although they found statistically significant differences in the expected direction, their interpretation is tempered by (1) clinically small differences (i.e., < 10 points), and (2) nonselective differences (i.e., except for CD, differences were general and not specific to any diagnosis).

---

[3]Although clinician-based DISC diagnoses are reported and have much higher levels, they are hopelessly confounded because the clinician administered both measures.

- Benjamin, Costello, and Warren (1990) evaluated 300 children enrolled in a health maintenance organization. They found significant differences in overall CBCL and TRF ratings for impaired (i.e., DISC-based anxiety and behavior disorders) and nonimpaired children. Their findings address only general impairment on the DISC.
- Jensen and Watanbe (1999) found a moderate convergence between DISC-P diagnoses and CBCL cut scores, with a sensitivity of .73 and specificity of .67.

In general, these studies provide strong convergent evidence for the DISC as a general measure of impairment. In contrast, they offer only modest evidence of convergent validity for specific disorders. Beyond the CBCL, convergent studies have focused on (1) general factors associated with psychopathology, and (2) depression and suicidal behavior.

Jensen et al. (1996) compared the number of DISC symptoms to indices associated with treatment needs, risk factors, and self-reported symptoms. In a large sample of military personnels' children with elevated CBCL scores, they found modest correlations (r's > .30 < .40) between total DISC symptoms and use of school services, family distress, and self-reported symptoms. Correlations also provided modest evidence for symptoms of specific disorders. For example, ADHD symptoms were modestly correlated ($r = .35$) with need for school services. One constraint of the magnitude of the correlations was the restricted range; only high CBCL scores were evaluated.

Two studies of convergent validity between DISC-based depression and specialized scales produced consistent results. In a nonreferred sample of adolescent mothers, Wilcox, Field, Prodromidis, and Scafidi (1998) found moderate correlations between DISC major depression and the BDI ($r = .53$) and the Center for Epidemiologic Studies—Depression scale (CES-D; Radloff, 1977; $r = .40$). Similar correlations were found for dysthymia (r's of .40 and .44, respectively). Among adolescent inpatients, King et al. (1997) found that DISC-C symptoms had moderate correlations of .59 with the Reynolds Adolescent Depression Scale (RADS; Reynolds, 1987) and .51 with the Children's Depression Rating Scale—Revised (CDRS-R; Poznanski et al., 1984). The DISC-P yielded low-moderate convergent correlations for females (.43 and .36, respectively) but not males (.12 and .22, respectively).

DISC correlates of suicidality were examined from several perspectives. King et al. (1997) found a linear trend between the Spectrum of Suicidal Behavior Scale (Pfeffer, 1986) and DISC symptoms reflecting suicidal thought and behavior. Gould et al. (1998) examined odds ratios (ORs) for suicidal ideation and attempts. While any DISC diagnoses increases the likelihood of ideation/attempts, mood disorders dramatically increased the likelihood of attempts (ORs from 14.5 to 15.9). In addition, substance abuse disorder markedly increased the likelihood of suicide attempts among boys (OR = 15.7) but not girls (OR = 3.3).

Construct Validity

Invoking Syndeham's criteria, a component of construct validity is the clear delineation of diagnostic boundaries, with evidence of effective inclusion and exclusion criteria. Anderson et al. (1987) examined diagnostic overlap on a New Zealand sample of 792 community youth. A reasonable discrimination was found for three diagnostic categories: (1) ADD, (2) anxiety disorders, and (3) combined CD and ODD. In contrast, depression/dysthymia appeared to be mostly subsumed within CD/ODD (78.6%), anxiety disorders (71.4%), and ADD (57.1%). In a Puerto Rican study, Bird et al. (1988) reviewed DISC diagnoses and found that 81.1% of 265 Puerto Rican children qualified for multiple diagnoses. In nearly one-half (46.1%) of the cases, diagnostic overlap crossed broad diagnostic categories (mood, anxiety, CD/ODD, and ADD). A troubling issue raised by Anderson et al. (1987) is whether depression constitutes a substratum of distress underlying most adolescent mental disorders.

Greenbaum, Prange, Friedman, and Silver (1991) examined diagnostic boundaries between substance abuse and other Axis I disorders in 547 emotionally disturbed adolescents. They reported that substance abuse disorders (primarily alcohol or marijuana) overlapped dramatically (> 80%) with depression and ADD, and moderately (> 60%) with CD. Although multiple Axis I disorders are common, this level of comorbidity is disconcerting.

A critical issue in the evaluation of troubled adolescents is the establishment of CD diagnoses. Research by Booth and Zhang (1996) on runaway adolescents has important implications for the diagnostic boundaries of CD. Irrespective of CD, more than one-half the sample had been arrested, dropped out of school, and had attempted suicide. Although aggressive behavior was more common among adolescents with CD, almost half (45.5%) of non-CD youth also had serious aggressive behavior. Most CD and non-CD youth came from maladjusted backgrounds. The important lesson from Booth and Zhang is that the clarity of diagnostic boundaries is likely to depend on samples and comparisons. Comparisons of CD youth to well-adjusted youth from stable environments are likely to produce marked differences. However, near-neighbor comparisons of different types of troubled youth from unstable environments are more clinically relevant for establishing diagnostic boundaries.

The longitudinal dimension of diagnostic validity is conceptualized in terms of (1) risk factors or precursors and (2) outcome variables, such as the course of the disorder and treatment outcome. A strength of the DISC is its substantial literature on predicting disorders and their outcomes.

Four large community studies have examined risk factors associated with DISC diagnoses. Key findings are summarized as follows:

- *Short-term.* Costello et al. (1988; see also Benjamin et al., 1990) assessed risk factors of childhood mental disorders in 300 children (ages

7–11) attending primary care pediatric clinics. With a 12-month follow-up, they found that (1) sociodemographic variables (gender, socioeconomic status, single-parent family) were linked with oppositional and conduct disorders, and (2) children's stress was associated with anxiety disorders.

- *Long-term.* Velez, Johnson, and Cohen (1989) conducted an elegant study of risk factors on 776 community children (*M* age = 5.7) after 8 and 10 years. Sociodemographic characteristics (particularly low income/parent education) represented a risk factor for externalizing disorders (ODD, CD, and ADD) and one internalizing disorder (separation anxiety).
  —Parental characteristics were logically related to risk factors (i.e., sociopathy with externalizing disorders; emotional problems with internalizing problems).
  —Childhood problems (academic failure, mental health intervention, and stressful life events) formed a general risk factor at the 10-year follow-up.
- *Retrospective.* Bird, Gould, Yager, Staghezza, and Canino (1989) examined risk factors linked to 386 Puerto Rican children with DISC diagnoses. Unlike prospective studies, Bird et al. evaluated children with a known outcome (i.e., mental disorders) and retrospectively assessed family history variables.
  —Socioeconomic status appeared to be a general factor associated with mental disorders.
  —Family dysfunction, stressful events, and parents' psychiatric history tended not to increase the likelihood of childhood diagnoses; the notable exception was depression.
- *Focused retrospective.* Flisher et al. (1997) explored the risk factors associated with retrospective accounts of physical abuse in children from New York and Puerto Rico. In examining ORs, high risks appeared to be associated with agoraphobia (6.7), GAD (4.6), and CD (4.3). The usefulness of the study is markedly constrained by its focus on physical abuse and inattention to other antecedents.

These large-scale community studies provide important insights into risk factors and antecedent conditions associated with specific disorders. Because the etiology of most specific disorders is not well understood, these general findings should be viewed as positive. Most encouraging are the differences between (1) externalizing disorders that are associated with disadvantaged and disrupted families and (2) internalizing disorders that are linked to stress and familial histories of mental illness. Because of the nonspecific nature of these risk factors, we cannot expect to identify precise precursors to particular mental disorders.

Studies of clinical populations have focused on predictors of specific disorders or environmental conditions. Key findings are summarized as follows:

- McCaskill, Toro, and Wolfe (1998) attempted to predict disruptive behavior and alcohol abuse/dependence with matched homeless and housed youth. Predictors of disruptive behavior included gender (male), maltreatment, low income, unsupportive family, and any episode of homelessness. Only two predictors were found for alcohol abuse/dependence: maltreatment and any episode of homelessness.
- Widom (1999) examined the role of childhood victimization in predicting adult PTSD. She found that 35.7% of those victimized had a lifetime episode of PTSD. However, childhood victimization did not predict PTSD when family breakup, substance abuse, and childhood behavioral problems were considered. However, childhood victimization does appear related to the number of PTSD symptoms experienced as an adult.
- Borst, Noam, and Bartok (1991) examined risk factors for suicide attempts for 219 adolescent inpatients. DISC diagnosis (especially combined mood disorder and CD), gender (female), and social conformity predicted suicide attempts.

DISC studies have also investigated intergenerational patterns of mental disorders. The following studies have attempted to predict childhood disorders based on parents' pathology:

- In a study of intergenerational disorders, Breslau, Davis, and Prabucki (1987) examined 331 mothers with the DIS, and one child per family with the DISC. They found that mothers' GAD did not increase the risk of anxiety or mood disorders in offspring. In contrast, depressed mothers were more likely to have overanxious disorder in younger (ages 8–17) and major depression in older (18–23) offspring.
- Rubio-Stipec, Bird, Canino, Bravo, and Alegria (1991) studied the effects of parental alcoholism on childhood adjustment. They found that children of alcoholics evidenced overall impairment; however, other Axis I disorders were more predictive of children's dysfunction.
- Lahey et al. (1990) conducted DISC interviews on 177 boys (ages 7–12) involved in outpatient treatment. They found that APD in biological fathers increased threefold (i.e., 35.5% vs. 11.1%) the probability of DSM-III-R CD. Moreover, a jail sentence served by any first- or second-degree biological relative doubled the likelihood (i.e., 43.3% vs. 20.0%) of CD.
- Lyon et al. (1995) examined genetic and environmental influences on CD and APD traits in a study of 3,226 pairs of male twins. CD traits were evenly divided: five traits related to genetic effects, and five to familial–environmental effects. Interestingly, APD appeared more related to genetic than familial–environmental effects.
- Prange et al. (1992) predicted three common DISC diagnoses (CD, al-

cohol/marijuana abuse, and depression) for 353 emotionally disturbed adolescents. They found that CD was related to parents' substance abuse and lack of family cohesiveness. Both substance abuse and depression were predicted by the lack of family cohesiveness.

Longitudinal dimensions of diagnostic validity have also been evaluated prospectively via treatment and treatment outcome. In this regard, Cohen, Kasen, Brook, and Struening (1991) sought to identify which youth would require subsequent treatment. From a community sample of 776 adolescents, disruptive disorders had a high probability of later treatment (ODD, OR = 4.84; CD, OR = 3.74); treatment was sought less often for internalizing disorders (major depression, OR = 2.02; overanxious disorder, OR = 1.11). In a more elegant study, Costello, Angold, and Keeler (1999) initially evaluated 300 children (ages 7–11) attending primary care clinic. In a 5- to 7-year follow-up, childhood behavioral disorders were clearly linked to adolescent behavioral disorders (males, OR = 38.4; females, OR = 8.1). For emotional disorders, the outcome was observed only for females (OR = 6.1). Combining across the two studies, externalizing/behavioral disorders appear to be more chronic and in need of treatment than internalizing/emotional disorders. Major gender differences clearly require further investigation.

The general course of child mental disorders based on DISC diagnoses have received relatively little attention. From a large sample of 13-year-old adolescents, McGee and Stanton (1990) selected five diagnostic groups ($N = 82$; ADD, CD, anxiety, depression, and mixed) and compared them to adolescents without these disorders ($N = 651$). In a 2-year follow-up, they found distinct patterns of disability associated with ADD (multiple deficits including communication and disruptive behavior) but not for other disorders. In addition, depression had the most ominous outcome, as measured by psychiatric hospitalizations.

Several investigations have focused on the course and outcome of disruptive disorders. Lahey et al. (1995) evaluated the diagnostic stability of CD in boys referred for disruptive disorders with four annual administrations of the DISC. Although a minority remained stable, most boys with CD evidenced a fluctuating course. The best predictors of positive outcome (i.e., reduced CD symptoms) was (1) at least average intelligence (≥ 100), and (2) no biological parents with APD. In a study of ODD, Speltz, McClellan, DeKlyen, and Jones (1999) conducted a 2-year follow-up on young boys (ages 4 to 5.5) with ODD (54.3%) and ODD + ADHD (45.7%) diagnoses. They found the following outcomes:

- 24.1% had no diagnoses.
- 26.6% had ODD, mostly from the ODD-only group.
- 26.6% had ODD + ADHD, mostly from the ODD + ADHD group.
- 16.5% had ADHD, mostly from the ODD + ADHD group.

Not included in these percentages were 2.5% of these young children (< 8 years) who already qualified for CD + ODD. In general, these data appear to support diagnostic stability for ODD and ODD + ADHD. In addition, they underscore the heterogeneity of outcomes possible among young children.

Wierson and Forehand (1995) conducted a follow-up (21 to 32 months) study of 75 juvenile detainees. Despite its modest sample, the study has important implications for the use of CD and other diagnoses as they relate to recidivism as an outcome. In the overall discriminant analysis, substance abuse diagnoses, but not CD, predicted recidivism. When divided by race, predictors for Anglo Americans were substance abuse disorders and CD; predictors for African Americans included no diagnoses, although ADHD evidence a nonsignificant trend ($p = .08$). As a stimulus for further research, CD cannot be equated with negative outcomes. Other diagnoses (e.g., substance abuse disorders and ADHD) mediated by moderator variables (e.g., ethnicity) are likely to play key roles in the outcome.

In summary, studies of diagnostic validity have addressed diagnostic boundaries of DISC disorders, risk factors, and diagnostic outcome. The majority of studies offer general evidence of the DISC's assessment of psychopathology but lack specific data on particular disorders. However, important findings relate to intergenerational patterns of childhood disorders and diagnostic stability, especially with externalizing disorders.

Generalizability

More than other child interviews, the DISC has paid close attention to factors that may influence its generalizability. These factors include ethnicity, gender, and language. Key findings are summarized as follows:

1. In a large epidemiological study (three states and Puerto Rico), Wu et al. (1999) examined sociodemographic differences associated with specific disorders. They found no differences due to age or family income. Predictably, females had a higher rate of depression. Hispanic children tended to have proportionately fewer disruptive disorders than other ethnic groups.

2. Beals et al. (1997) compared Native Americans from the Northern Plains to other epidemiological studies. Although overall 6-month prevalence of mental disorders appeared comparable, Native Americans tended to have fewer anxiety disorders and more externalizing disorders and substance abuse. Despite considerable exposure to trauma, the levels of PTSD appeared to remain low (Jones, Dauphinais, Sack, & Somervell, 1997). As expected, delinquent Native Americans had higher rates of substance abuse and CD than nondelinquent Native Americans (Duclos et al., 1998).

3. Several studies have examined the prevalence of mental disorders among disadvantaged youth. Buckner and Bassuk (1997) found high rates of anxiety symptoms and disruptive disorders among homeless youth and those

in low-income housing. An interesting gender difference was observed: High prevalence rates were observed for homeless boys and girls in low-income housing. Kupersmidt and Martin (1997) examined the prevalence of mental disorders in the children of predominantly Hispanic migrant and seasonal workers. Anxiety disorders, particularly simple phobias, were especially prevalent and observed in more than one-third of the sample.

4. Children of military families do not appear to have increased prevalences of mental disorders (Jensen, Watanabe, et al., 1995).

In addition to broad epidemiological research, studies have focused on ethnic and gender differences for specific diagnoses. Roberts, Chen, and Solovitz (1995) evaluated symptoms of major depression for adolescent outpatients. They found almost no differences between ethnic groups (Anglo American, African American, and Mexican American) or genders. Timmons-Mitchell et al. (1997) compared DISC diagnoses for male and female detainees and they found no differences for most Axis I disorders, including externalizing disorders. However, boys had much higher rates of substance abuse.

The DISC has been translated into eight languages and utilized in many different cultures. With respect of generalizability, Bird et al. (1988) evaluated prevalence rates with Puerto Rican children. They found relatively high rates of ODD and ADHD; although no ORs are reported, the other disorders appeared within the general parameters seen in U.S. studies. Verhulst, Ende, Ferdinand, and Kasius (1997) conducted a national study of childhood disorders in the Netherlands. They found very few gender differences; anxiety disorders accounted for the majority of the disorders.

Response Styles

Zahner (1991) conducted an important study on 138 preadolescents, 95 of whom were identified on the CBCL with elevated scores. She examined the quality of responses to the DISC-R based on interviewer ratings and found that 8.3% of children engaged in "yea-saying," while 10.1% responded with "nay-saying." In addition, 12.0% of the younger children (ages 6–8) tended to present themselves in an ideal light. Other response problems included attempts to please the interviewer (8.0%) and guarded responses (14.0%). She also pilot-tested a 10-item social desirability scale that appears to have promise with defensiveness and other response sets.

Adolescents' responses to the DISC are likely to be discrepant with those of their parents. Especially in the area of substance abuse, adolescents are likely to withhold information from their parents (Bidaut-Russell et al., 1995; Friedman, Glickman, & Morrissey, 1988). Clinicians should realize that the fear of punitive consequences may affect adolescents' reporting of substance abuse and delinquent behaviors to both parents and interviewers.

Clinical Applications

The DISC is a reliable diagnostic interview for children with extensive validity data drawn primarily from outpatient and community settings. It is certainly useful clinically in assessing risk factors, patterns of psychopathology, and overall impairment. The following paragraphs expand on its applications and limitations.

A strength of the DISC is the extensive research on its reliability with large outpatient and community samples. These studies suggest a moderate level of test–retest reliability. Clinicians should be cautious in trusting the reliability of younger children. The DISC appears to have two strengths with respect to reliability:

1. Symptoms appear to be adequately assessed for interrater reliability.
2. Dimensional ratings of DISC diagnoses demonstrate moderate to excellent reliabilities.

Validity studies clearly demonstrate the usefulness of the DISC as a measure of impairment and offer substantial findings on internalizing–externalizing disorders. This conceptualization of internalizing–externalizing disorders, which incorporates the more common childhood disorders, appears to have a well-defined factor structure (Williams et al., 1989) and to be significantly related to the emergence of mental disorders (see discussion of risk factors: Costello, 1989; Velez et al., 1989).

Concurrent validity studies have produced only modest results, with median kappas generally below .40. In most cases, the DISC is compared to clinical diagnoses (e.g., admission or chart diagnoses) that are likely to underdiagnose disorders. Still, these results are cause for concern because of low rates of concordance. Certainly, large-scale studies with other structured child interviews would be very helpful in establishing concurrent validity.

A major strength of the DISC is its usefulness in establishing risk factors for childhood disorders. Major studies have investigated both short- (Costello et al., 1988) and long-term (Velez et al., 1989) predictors. Research has also established the risk factors associated with trauma and adverse environmental conditions (e.g., homelessness). Likewise, studies have examined outcome criteria and the variables that predict both favorable and unfavorable outcomes.

Another strength of the DISC is its attention to generalizability. Studies systematically evaluate prevalence and comorbidity with different cultural groups. Especially well represented are Hispanic American and Native American youth. In addition, epidemiological research has explored the prevalence of mental disorders for disadvantaged populations (e.g., homeless and migrant families). For issues regarding different cultures, the DISC is likely to be the first choice among the child interviews.

Still another advantage of the DISC is its attention to response styles, which are often overlooked in both child and adult interviews. Two findings from the Zahner (1991) study are particularly relevant: (1) Substantial numbers of children distort their answers because they either adopt a response set (yea- and nay-saying) or exhibit defensiveness; and (2) a 10-item social desirability scale has promise in identifying these children. Other research has demonstrated the need to evaluate socially undesirable behaviors (e.g., use of drugs) carefully in adolescent populations.

The major drawback of the DISC is its rigid structure. Because of its intended use with paraprofessional populations, clinical inquiries and concomitant ratings are stringently controlled. Clinicians may feel constrained by the measure when they believe that the limited understanding negatively affects the accuracy of their ratings. Mental health professionals are then faced with the dilemma of breaking standardization or providing ratings of questionable accuracy.

CHILD ASSESSMENT SCHEDULE (CAS)

Description

Hodges, Kline, et al. (1982), in a collaborative arrangement between the University of Missouri and the NIMH, developed the CAS as a semistructured diagnostic interview for clinical use with children and adolescents ranging in age from 7 to 16 years. Box 6.3 provides a basic description and information

---

BOX 6.3. Highlights of the CAS

- *Description:* The CAS is designed to evaluate symptoms and psychological problems within the framework of school, friends, family, and activities. It is not intended as a formal diagnostic measure but is rather a clinical tool for gathering diagnostically relevant material.

- *Administration time:* Typically 45–75 minutes each for the C-CAS and the P-CAS.

- *Skills level:* The CAS requires a skilled clinician with experience in interviewing children. The CAS requires only minimal training for standardized administrations.

- *Distinctive features:* The CAS provides a problem-oriented interview for assessing potential difficulties and symptoms; this focus lends itself to the development of child- and family-based interventions.

- *Cost:* A nominal fee may be charged to cover copying expenses.

- *Source:* According to the most recent information, the author is Kay Hodges, PhD, Eastern Michigan University, Department of Psychology, Ypsilanti, MI 48197.

of the availability on the CAS. Its authors attempted to address what were considered substantial problems with earlier measures, namely, lengthy formats organized by symptom constellations that formed a barrier to rapport-building.

The CAS was first developed in 1978 and became available in 1981 (Hodges, Kline, Fitch, McKnew, & Cytryn, 1981). Hodges, Kline, et al. (1982) reported modeling the organization of the CAS after the Psychiatric Status Schedule (Spitzer, Endicott, Fleiss, & Cohen, 1970). The wording of the clinical inquiries corresponded to questions customarily employed by experienced investigators in interviewing children. In addition, Hodges, Kline, et al. constructed the clinical inquiries and ratings in order to match DSM-III and, subsequently, DSM-III-R diagnostic criteria.

The CAS, like most structured interviews for children, is composed of two parallel forms: one for children (i.e., C-CAS), and one for a parent serving as an informant (i.e., P-CAS). To improve user friendliness, the CAS is organized around 11 content areas, beginning with general topics (i.e., school, friends, activities, and family) and proceeding to more personal matters (i.e., fears, worries/anxieties, self-image, mood/behavior, physical complaints, acting out, and reality testing). Each form has slightly more than 250 clinical ratings that differ only slightly in structure (e.g., C-CAS, which often begins with the stem "Do you . . . ?" is altered in the P-CAS to "Does your child . . . ?"). An important feature of the CAS is that diagnostic criteria are embedded in topical questions so as to improve the flow of the interview.

The great majority of clinical inquiries are standard questions asked of each respondent. In addition, the CAS utilizes optional probes under two conditions: either an affirmative response that requires an additional follow-up or elective questions. In the latter case, interviewers may choose to probe further with elective questions designated by "If desired."

Responses to individual items are organized on a 3-point scale: 0 = "false or no," 1 = "an ambiguous response," and 2 = "true or yes." The CAS differs from other structured interviews in its use of the intermediate score (1) for responses that are not clearly present or absent. In contrast, most other structured interviews use the intermediate score as a positive endorsement either at a subclinical or clinical level. Given its explicitly equivocal nature, the score of 1 on the CAS appears less interpretable than more common alternatives.

CAS items are organized into content scales, symptom-pattern scales (originally termed "symptom complexes"), and total symptom scores. As described earlier, the 11 content scales address overall functioning and psychopathology. The C-CAS scales (see Hodges & Saunders, 1989) appeared to have a moderate level of internal consistency (median alpha of .68) when administered to 116 inpatient and outpatient children. However, two scales evidenced low levels of internal consistency (Activities at .09, Reality-Testing at .58). The P-CAS appeared to fare slightly less well (median alpha of .64), with three scales at low levels (Activities at .27, Reality-Testing at .47, and Fears at

.57). Attempts to reduce the number of variables to those with diagnostic significance appeared to have a negligible effect on alpha coefficients.

Reliability

Hodges and her colleagues (Hodges & Saunders, 1989; Hodges, Saunders, Kashani, Hamlett, & Thompson, 1990) investigated the internal consistency of the C-CAS and P-CAS. Via alpha coefficients,[4] Hodges and Saunders (1989) found relatively modest levels of internal consistency for C-CAS (median alpha = .71) and P-CAS (median alpha = .64) content scales. In contrast, alphas were moderately high for symptom patterns across both versions (median alphas of .80 for the C-CAS and .78 for the P-CAS). Two observations emerge from these studies:

- Several content scales (Activities and Reality Testing) have insufficient internal reliability.
- Unexpectedly, children's reports evidence comparable, if not greater, estimates of internal consistency than their parents' reports.[5]

The primary CAS reliability studies are summarized in Table 6.3. Because the CAS is not intended as a diagnostic measure, it focuses on dimensional ratings with content scales, symptom pattern scales, and total scores. Four key findings are enumerated:

1. The content and symptom-pattern scales evidence moderate to excellent interrater reliabilities (r's from .70 to .94). Clearly, the strength of the CAS is its dimensional ratings of these scales.
2. CAS ratings of individual symptoms/problems have a moderate level of interrater reliability. Although circumscribed, the CAS appears to have some value in reliably classifying a small number of diagnoses.
3. The CAS test–retest reliability has been neglected. While the sole study (Hodges, Cools, & McKnew, 1989) yielded promising results, the CAS should probably be avoided in cases where the stability of clinical findings is critical.
4. The CAS reliability has focused more on the C-CAS than the P-CAS.

On a practical level, CAS research (Hodges, Cools, et al., 1989; Hodges, Gordon, & Lennon, 1990; Merritt, Thompson, Keith, Johndrow, & Murphy, 1993; Thompson, Hodges, & Hamlett, 1990) has convincingly demonstrated that clinicians can be trained to achieve acceptable levels of reliability by the use of didactic materials, direct supervision, and the scoring of five practice

---

[4]With essentially categorical data (i.e., a rating of 1 reflects uncertainty), other estimates (e.g., Kuder–Richardson) may be more appropriate.

[5]This finding was supported by recent research on a Japanese translation (Sugawara et al., 1999).

TABLE 6.3. Reliability Studies for the Child Assessment Schedule (CAS)

Study (year)	N	Setting		Dx	Raters		Reliability	Reliability estimates	
		In/Out/Com			Lay/Prof		Inter/Retest (interval)	Sx/Content/Sx patterns	
Reliability studies									
Hodges, Kline, et al. (1982)	53	✓ ✓	✓	NA	✓	✓	✓	.60	.75[a] .70[a]
Hodges, McKnew, et al. (1982)	10	✓		NA		✓	✓		.94[a] .94[a]
Verhulst et al. (1987)	20	✓[b]		NA		✓	✓		.83[a]
Hodges, Cools, & McKnew (1989)	32	✓		6		✓	✓ (5 days)	.69[c]	.72[c] .64[d]
Vandvik (1990)[e]	30		✓[f]	NA		✓	✓		.72[g]
Hindley et al. (1994)[h]	12	✓[b]		NA		✓	✓		.63[g]
Sugawara et al. (1999)[i]	26	✓		4		✓	✓		.73[d]
Cross-informant studies									
Hodges, Gordon, et al. (1990)	48	✓		NA				✓ (12 days)	.35[a] .45[a]
Thompson et al. (1993)	49		✓	3[j]				✓ (0–6 wk)	.15[a] .07[a]

Note. See Table 1.5 (p. 35) for a glossary of terms and abbreviations.
[a]Correlations.
[b]School children rated with psychological problems.
[c]Phi coefficients.
[d]Diagnosis rather than symptom patterns.
[e]Norwegian translation.
[f]Medical inpatients.
[g]Kappa for total score.
[h]Study used American Sign Language.
[i]Japanese translation.
[j]Six disorders altogether but only three with sufficient representation.

cases. Typically, kappas ≥ .70 can be achieved with this level of training. The sustainability of this reliability in independent settings has been assumed but not formally tested.

Beyond reliability per se, two studies have investigated cross-informant consistency (see Table 6.3). Hodges, Gordon, et al. (1990) compared 48 inpatients at the time of admission to their mothers' P-CAS after a 12-day interval. Especially in light of the interval and intervening treatment, the results were generally positive, with median correlations of .35 for content and .45 for symptom-pattern scales. More recently, Thompson et al. (1993) evaluated cross-informant consistency in a nonreferred population from a general pediatric clinic. Their efforts (median r = .11) were stymied by very low endorsements rates; 85.7% of symptom-pattern scales averaged less than two symptoms across both C-CAS and P-CAS administrations.

In summary, CAS reliability emphasizes dimensional ratings of content and symptom-pattern scales. In contrast, relatively little attention is paid to diagnostic agreement, both the number of studies and the range of disorders. Therefore, clinicians may feel comfortable using the CAS to evaluate problems and symptom patterns rather than for diagnosis per se. The reproducibility of these scales over time (i.e., test–retest reliability) has only marginal evidence of effectiveness.

Validity

Hodges, Kline, et al. (1982) conducted the original validity study of the CAS, which combined known-groups design (i.e., comparisons of 18 inpatients, 32 outpatients, and 37 controls) with convergent measures. Of nine symptom scales, six met the predicted severity (inpatient > outpatient > controls). For the content scales, more variability was observed; however, the clinical groups had greater impairment that controls on all but two scales (i.e., Fears and Worries). Use of the CAS total score in a discriminant model predicted clinical status in 65.5% of the participants, a rate comparable to the CBCL. Subsequent research has investigated concurrent, convergent, and construct validity. These investigations are summarized in separate subsections.

Concurrent Validity

The deemphasis on diagnosis is reflected in the dearth of studies that compare the CAS to clinical diagnosis or other structured interviews. Described previously with the K-SADS, Hodges et al. (1987) conducted the first concurrent validity study comparing the CAS and the K-SADS. On a sample of 29 outpatient children and their mothers, both measures were administered in a counterbalanced order. Diagnoses were examined for four broad diagnostic categories: ADD, CD, and anxiety and mood disorders. Interestingly, when diagnosis was based on the child interview alone, nearly half the disorders were missed by both the CAS (48.8%) and the K-SADS (42.3%). When based on the parent interview alone or a consensus between parent and child interviews, the kappas were moderate (range of .51 to .75, median of .60).

Verhulst, Althaus, and Berden (1987) investigated the concurrent validity of the CAS in comparison to the Graham and Rutter (1968) parent interview on a sample of 116 Dutch children. Although not a perfect match, Verhulst et al. examined similar constellations of symptoms/problems. They found modest associations, expressed as median correlations, for content areas (.10), somatic concerns (.34), and observation judgments (.28). Overall, age played an important role with reliability: *M r*'s of .30 for 8-year-olds and .45 for 11-year-olds. As least with older children, the study demonstrated a moderate level of concordance.

Convergent Validity

Research on convergent validity has compared CAS results to various checklists and self-report measures. Key findings are summarized as follows:

- The CAS total score evidences moderate correlations with the CBCL and is a general indicator of psychological impairment among children with psychologogical problems (Hodges, Kline, et al., 1982; Verhulst et al., 1987). Some significant differences were observed between CAS symptom-pattern scales and CBCL scores on the Japanese translation (Sugawara et al., 1999).
- Consistent evidence of CAS convergent validity is found with depression. In particular, the CAS depression scale is moderately correlated with the Child Depression Inventory (CDI; see Hodges, Kline, et al., 1982) and the Beck Depression Inventory (BDI; Barrera & Garrison-Jones, 1988). Children classified as depressed on the CAS produce elevated scores on the CDI (Hodges, 1990) and a measure of hopelessness (Kashani, Reid, & Rosenberg, 1989).
- Several studies (Hodges, 1990; Hodges, Kline, et al., 1982) provide moderate evidence of convergent validity for CAS anxiety in comparison to the State–Trait Anxiety Inventory for Children (STAIC; Spielberger, 1973).

In summary, CAS convergent validity is more focused than that for other established child interviews. Results indicate that the CAS can be viewed as a general indicator of psychological impairment, with moderate support for its use with childhood depression and anxiety.

Construct Validity

In line with Syndeham's criteria, CAS research has examined longitudinal perspectives of depression and externalizing disorders. Although developmental trends are observed in diagnoses and symptoms (Kashani, Orvaschel, Rosenberg, & Reid, 1989), only longitudinal research can evaluate their diagnostic relevance. In addition, studies have addressed diverse mental health issues related to risk factors for depression, early pregnancies, and inability to cope following parental death.

Coie, Terry, Lenox, Lochman, and Hyman (1995) explored the relationships between childhood peer rejection and subsequent aggression and mental disorders. In a longitudinal study of African American youth, third-grade students rated their peers on social preference (low scores equated with rejection) and aggression. With follow-up data at the sixth, eighth, and 10th grades, C-CAS data revealed dissimilar gender patterns. Boys in the rejected–aggressive category had increased externalizing symptoms at an approximate rate of three symptoms every 2 years. In contrast, girls evidenced no significant differences based on rejection. Female aggression was associated with substantially more externalizing symptoms that remained stable during the follow-up period. The Coie et al. (1995) research is a superb model for predicting adolescent psychopathology on the basis of childhood interpersonal patterns.

Other predictive research has also yielded significant findings:

- Barrera and Garrison-Jones (1988) found significant but very modest relationships between social support and depression for adolescent inpatients. Family and parental support appeared to play a minor protective function, while peer support revealed a more complex relationship.
- West, Sandler, Pillow, Baca, and Gersten (1991) found that adjustment following parental death/bereavement was not related to previous symptoms. Instead, findings from structural equation modeling proposed that mediators (e.g., family support, lack of other negative family events, and stable positive family events) differentially predicted CAS depression, anxiety, and CD.
- Miller-Johnson et al. (1999), in a further study of Coie et al. (1995), found that aggression among African American girls in grades 3–5 predicted teenage births.

Clinical Applications

The CAS was specifically designed to assess key problems and symptoms in nonpsychotic DSM-III-R disorders in intellectually normal children. As such, the CAS has not been validated with psychotic or mentally retarded samples. The CAS differs fundamentally from other child interviews in its emphasis on problem areas and key symptoms rather than formal diagnosis. The CAS should not be faulted for its distinct focus. When clinicians are interested in differential diagnosis, the CAS is not the structured interview of choice. However, the CAS should be strongly considered when the focus is on clinical description and identification of salient problems with specific contexts (e.g., school, friends, or family). The format of the CAS lends itself to the development of detailed treatment plans and well-designed clinical interventions.

The CAS also lends itself to outpatient evaluations, particularly in clinics where common childhood disorders (CD, ADD, anxiety disorders) are prevalent. The CAS may be used in conjunction with standardized self-report measures for parents (CBCL) and teachers (TRF). The CAS, like other child-interview measures, should not be administered to the child alone. Research strongly suggests that child-only interviews substantially underreport psychopathology. When combined with the parent interview (see Hodges et al., 1987), the CAS may offer clinically useful information, often extending beyond DSM criteria (Greenhill & Malcolm, 2000).

An important feature of the CAS is its problem-oriented approach. Through its 11 content scales, clinicians can easily identify (1) troublesome problems and (2) discrepancies in child and parent perspectives. Within a treatment framework, both problems and discrepancies are important dimensions for clarification of treatment goals and improved communication. The CAS offers a systematic approach to common child and family problems that may assist in the treatment process via two types of data:

1. Convergent data provide a valuable foundation between the parent and child about areas of agreement. Treatment often builds from this foundation.
2. Discrepant data identify critical issues for subsequent treatment. An overriding issue for treatment is to understand and respect differing viewpoints, including parent and child perspectives.

Other focused applications of the CAS include populations that are hearing impaired or have chronic medical disorders. The CAS is the only child interview with established reliability using American sign language (Hindley, Hill, McGuigan, & Kitson, 1994; see Table 6.3). In addition, the CAS has been successfully employed in medical settings (Merritt et al., 1993) to evaluate chronic illness (Thompson et al., 1990).

For differential diagnosis, the CAS is circumscribed in its clinical usefulness. In addition to the already noted restriction with psychotic disorders, the reliability and concurrent validity of specific disorders have received only limited attention. In cases where diagnosis is paramount, clinicians may wish to consider other interview-based measures. The CAS is better utilized where clinical settings focus on dimensions of psychopathology rather than diagnosis, and where assessment becomes a problem-oriented basis for intervention.

DIAGNOSTIC INTERVIEW FOR CHILDREN
AND ADOLESCENTS (DICA)

Description

Herjanic et al. (1975; see also Herjanic & Campbell, 1977) were responsible for developing one of the very first structured interviews for children that was subsequently refined and named the Diagnostic Interview for Children and Adolescents (DICA). Initial studies of the DICA appeared in 1982 (Herjanic & Reich, 1982; Reich, Herjanic, Welner, & Gandhy, 1982), with the first published version available the following year (Herjanic & Reich, 1983a, 1983b).

The DICA, developed in line with the Renard Diagnostic Interview (RDI) and the DIS (Reich, 1992), was intended for use by lay interviewers with modest levels of training. Box 6.4 provides a basic description and information on the availability of the DICA. According to Hodges (1993), the DICA was first designed to assess childhood diagnoses in pediatric and psychiatric samples of children 6 to 17 years old. It has subsequently been employed in both clinical and epidemiological studies. Despite the intent that the DICA be administered by lay interviewers, the majority of investigations have utilized mental health professionals (Hodges, 1993).

Modification in accordance with DSM-III-R criteria resulted in the DICA—Revised (DICA-R). As described by Kaplan and Reich (1991), DICA-R questions were rephrased to achieve a much more conversational style and pretested for comprehension on children, adolescents, and their parents. In addition, questions were added to provide more comprehensive coverage of

---

BOX 6.4. Highlights of the DICA

- *Description:* The DICA is a structured diagnostic interview designed to cover lifetime diagnoses and render DSM diagnoses.

- *Administration time:* Highly variable, but averages 45 minutes each for the DICA-C and DICA-P.

- *Skills level:* The DICA was designed to be used by lay interviewers with training and experience in evaluating children.

- *Distinctive features:* The DICA can be used by trained paraprofessionals and yields useful diagnostic information. Validity data are strong in examining risk factors, especially in relationship to alcoholism and substance abuse.

- *Cost:* The cost of the DICA is $50, including child, adolescent, and adult versions, as well as a training manual scoring sheets, and tally sheets. For the computerized DICA-IV (*not* a structured interview), Multi-Health Systems charges $895 plus shipping.

- *Source:* For the DICA-R, contact Wendy Reich, PhD, by mail, 660 S. Euclid, Campus Box 8134, St. Louis, MO 63110; by phone, (314) 286-2263; by fax (314) 286-2265, by e-mail *Wendyr@twins.wustl.edu.* For the DICA-IV, contact Multi-Health Systems, or on the internet, *www.mhs.com*; by phone, (800) 456-3003; by fax, (888) 540-4484, or by mail, 908 Niagara Falls Boulevard, North Tonawanda, NY 14120-2060.

DSM-III-R criteria. Subsequent descriptions are limited to the most recent *interview* version of the DICA-R, namely, draft 7.3, which is available for children, adolescents, and parents (Reich, Shayka, & Taibleson, 1991a, 1991b, 1991c).

Clinicians should be aware that a DICA-IV has been published and is commercially available through Multi-Health Systems. While covering DSM-IV diagnoses, the DICA-IV represents a fundamental departure from earlier DICA versions (see Greenhill & Malcolm, 2000). It is a computer-administered questionnaire rather than a structured interview. Although the DICA-IV covers much of the same material, there is no trained interviewer to clarify responses or render clinical observations. Therefore, this chapter focuses on the most recent interview-based version, namely, the DICA-R.

The DICA is composed of three basic versions that are accompanied by an administration manual:

- The DICA-C, or Child Version, is administered to the youth being evaluated.
- The DICA-P, or Parent Version, is a corroborative interview completed by the parent or primary caretaker. A unique feature of the DICA-P is the option to evaluate as many as three children during a single administration.
- The DICA-A, or Adolescent Version, a slightly modified DICA-C, is intended for use with teenage youth.

The DICA is typically described as a *structured* interview since its questions and sequence of probing is clearly specified. Technically, the DICA is a *semistructured* interview, since clinicians are allowed on "rare" occasions to supplement the interview with their own unstructured questions (see Kaplan & Reich, 1991, p. 8).

The basic structure of the DICA is standard questions followed by optional probes. Standard questions are presented in bold print and should be asked verbatim. In cases where the answer is "yes" or even a tentative "no," the interviewer follows up with one or more probes. Probes are organized into three types: (1) question-specific probes, (2) standard probes, and (3) open-ended probes. Generally, standard and open-ended probes are only used when the interviewer remains unclear about the diagnostic criterion. The three types of probes are delineated as follows:

- Question-specific probes (presented in uppercase immediately following most standard questions) allow the interviewer to clarify or verify whether a particular diagnostic criterion is met.
- Standard probes (presented in lowercase at the beginning of some sections) assist primarily in establishing the magnitude of the problem. Examples of standard probes include "Does this happen a lot? Was this a big problem for you?"

- Open-ended probes, described in the test manual, are intended to elicit an example of the diagnostic criterion (e.g., "Can you give me an example of that?").

The DICA is scored on a 4-point scale organized primarily by the frequency of symptoms. The basic scoring is 1 for "no", 2 for "rarely," 3 for "sometimes or somewhat," and 5 for "yes." Additional scores include RF for refusing to answer a question and 9 for "don't know." Unless otherwise specified, symptoms are scored for lifetime occurrence.

The DICA provides comprehensive coverage through standard questions and probes. Approximately 900 items are presented in branching format, with screening questions for many sections (Sylvester, Hyde, & Reichler, 1987). As a result of this screening, the DICA-C is administered in approximately 40 minutes and the DICA-P in 45 minutes.

The DICA is organized into 15 major sections. The first two sections cover general and sociodemographic information. A total of 11 sections addresses mental disorders and symptomatology: behavior disorders (e.g., ADHD, CD, and substance abuse), mood disorders (e.g., symptoms of major depression and mania), dysthymic disorder, anxiety disorders, obsessive–compulsive disorder, PTSD, eating disorders, elimination disorders, gender identity, somatization, and psychotic symptoms. Other sections focus on menstruation, psychosocial stressors, and clinical observations. Parallel formats are found for the child, adolescent, and parent versions.

Care has been taken to make the DICA an understandable, positive experience for children and parents. Reich and Kaplan (1994) surveyed 50 parents and their children ($N = 72$). Nearly all the participants ($\geq 90\%$) reported the interview as a positive experience from which they learned more about themselves or their children. When children were asked about specific topics (e.g., school and family life), the majority reported that they "didn't mind" the questions.

The basic procedure is to administer the DICA-C and the DICA-P separately. As with all childhood interviews, the natural question is how interviewers should integrate the sometimes discrepant findings in achieving a diagnosis. Reich and Earls (1987) compared DICA data for 32 mother–child pairs to composite diagnoses that included additional interviews and data from teachers. They concluded that the children's report often had fewer reported symptoms but sufficient numbers to make most diagnoses. The children appeared much more accurate than parents and teachers in identifying symptoms associated with separation anxiety and overanxious disorders. Reliance on either source alone (DICA-C or DICA-P) would have resulted in missed diagnoses.

Reich and Earls (1990) tested the efficacy of telephone interviews in eliciting information on the DICA. Using matched samples (age, sex, alcohol status of parents), they compared elicited information on the DICA for 25 in-person and 25 telephone interviews. They found that in-person interviews resulted in slightly more symptoms being reported, although comparable numbers were found for "sensitive" questions (e.g., those related to drug use and sexual relations).

A self-administered, computerized version of the DICA was developed and pilot-tested for adolescents and parents (Stein, 1987). Preliminary data on 23 adolescents suggest that this format may have potential usefulness as an ancillary data source. However, supplementary findings of Stavrakaki, Williams, Walker, Rogers, and Kotsopoulos (1991) suggest that a computerized, self-administered DICA may be less effective than other self-report measures. Without any formal validation (comparability with in-person evaluations; reliability and validity studies), the computerized version should be used only for research purposes.

Reliability

The original studies of the DICA (Herjanic & Reich, 1982; Reich et al., 1982) focused on cross-informant consistency rather than reliability per se. As previously noted, cross-informant consistency involves an independent interview of the designated child, with a parallel interview by a closely-involved informant, almost always a parent. Sources of disagreement may include (1) different sources of data (e.g., self-disclosure vs. observation), (2) inconsistencies within the child's report (e.g., reporting different symptoms to parents and interviewer), and (3) unreliability of the structured interview. Because of these sources of variability, estimates of cross-informant consistency tend to be relatively low (e.g., kappas in the .30 range). Before examining cross-informant consistency, I review studies of DICA reliability.

DICA reliability studies have focused on test–retest reliabilities in two clinical samples and one large-scale community sample (see Table 6.4). The two clinical studies provide solid evidence of the DICA's test–retest reliability. For current diagnoses, Welner, Reich, Herjanic, Jung, and Amado (1987) achieved outstanding reliabilities on 27 consecutive inpatients, with kappas ranging from .76 to 1.00 (median = .87). In the second clinical study, Perez, Ascaso, Massons, and Chaparro (1998) utilized a Spanish adaptation of the DICA-R to test outpatient children and adolescents. They focused on individual symptoms and report averaged reliabilities for 12 diagnoses/syndromes. Although considerable variability was observed, the median kappas were in the moderate range for both children (.50) and adolescents (.51). For symptom reliability in a test–retest paradigm, these results are very positive.

Boyle et al. (1993; see also Boyle et al., 1997) conducted a large Canadian study of the DICA with schoolchildren. They oversampled students whose screening suggested the possibility of mental disorders. As a result, base rates were low, with three of the seven specific disorders resulting in very few cases (fewer than five cases per diagnosis). As a result, Boyle et al. (1993) reported data for broad diagnostic categories (e.g., externalizing and internalizing dis-

TABLE 6.4. Reliability Studies for the Diagnostic Interview for Children and Adolescents (DICA)

Study (year)	N	Setting In/Out/Com	Dx	Raters Lay/Prof	Reliability Inter/Retest (interval)	Reliability estimates Sx/Cur-Dx/Life-Dx/Other
Reliability studies						
Welner et al. (1987)	27[a]	✓	7	✓	✓ (1–7 days)	.87
Boyle et al. (1993)						
(ages 6–11)	114[a]	✓[b]	12	✓	✓ (10–20 days)	.20
(ages 12–16)	137[a]	✓[b]	12	✓	✓ (10–20 days)	.40
(ages 6–11)	114[c]	✓[b]	12	✓	✓ (10–20 days)	.44
(ages 12–16)	137[c]	✓[b]	12	✓	✓ (10–20 days)	.67
Perez et al. (1998)[d]						
(ages 6–12)	57[a]	✓	24	✓[e]	✓ (11 days)	.50
(ages 13–17)	52[a]	✓	24	✓[e]	✓ (11 days)	.51
Cross-informant studies						
Herjanic & Reich (1982)	307	✓	8	✓[f]	✓	.19
Reich et al. (1982)[g]	307	✓	8	✓[f]	✓	.36
Sylvester et al. (1987)	91	✓	6	✓[f]	✓	.24
	74	✓	6	✓[b]	✓	.54
Welner et al. (1987)	27	✓	7	✓[f] ✓	✓	.63
Earls, Reich, et al. (1988)	93	✓	5	✓[f]	✓	.35
Boyle et al. (1993)						
(ages 6–11)	114	✓[b]	12	✓[f] ✓	✓	.12
(ages 12–16)	137	✓[b]	12	✓[f] ✓	✓	.14

Note. See Table 1.5 (p. 35) for glossary of terms and abbreviations.
[a] DICA-C (version administered to the child).
[b] The community sample was screened to ensure that many participants had psychological problems.
[c] DICA-P (version administered to the parent).
[d] Spanish version.
[e] Interviewers are described as "trained"; their professional status is not reported.
[f] Parents served as the informants.
[g] Same data set as Herjanic and Reich (1982).
[h] Mother–father agreement on DICA-P.

orders). Not surprisingly, the kappa coefficients were generally modest in this community sample. Test–retest reliabilities for children ages 6 to 11 were negligible (median kappa = .20); however, the percentage of agreement remained high (median = 88%). Interestingly, limiting the reliability estimates to well-represented disorders did not improve the kappas. What accounts for differences between clinical and community samples? A possible explanation is greater involvement by clinical than community participants because of their (1) rapport with mental health professionals and (2) motivation for accurate diagnosis and effective treatment.

General conclusions from DICA test–retest reliability studies are as follows:

- The DICA had solid test–retest reliabilities for both current diagnoses and symptoms when employed in clinical samples.
- Data do not currently support the use of the DICA-C in community settings with children ages 6–11.

Several studies reported high interrater reliabilities but provide insufficient information to evaluate the quality of the data. For example, Bartlett, Schleifer, Johnson, and Keller (1991, p. 317) reported a kappa > .90 for DICA interviews with community adolescents, although the size of the sample and range of diagnoses (probably only depression) were not described. Similarly, Biederman, Rosenbaum, et al. (1990) reported an overall kappa of .88 but failed to specify sample size or diagnostic range. Finally, Ezpeleta et al. (1997) reported that clinicians were able to reach a high level of diagnostic reliability (kappas ≥ .80) after extensive training. No data were provided about the sample size, diagnoses in the reliability study, or specific kappa estimates.

Herjanic and Reich (1982) examined cross-informant consistency of 168 DICA ratings on 307 patients and their mothers. Only 15 symptoms evidenced good convergence (kappas ≥ .50), while an additional 30 symptoms had low to moderate convergence (kappas ≥ .30 < .50). Diagnostically, the convergence for current episodes was in the expected range (median kappa = .36; see Reich et al., 1982). In an additional study of cross-informant consistency with a clinical sample, Welner et al. (1987) reported very positive results, with moderate to high estimates (median kappa = .63).

Community studies of cross-informant consistency have modest results. Sylvester et al. (1987) found only modest convergence (median kappa = .24) in parent–child pairs. Interestingly, when parents were compared to each other, the level of agreement increased substantially (median kappa = .54). Earls, Reich, Jung, and Cloninger (1988) also found modest convergence (median kappa = .35). Finally, Boyle et al. (1993) produced the lowest convergence level, with basically negligible kappas (median of .12 for children and .14 for adolescents).

In summary, cross-informant consistency produced different levels of agreement between parents and children based on the setting. In clinical settings, the unweighted mean for kappa was .50. In community settings, the unweighted mean kappa was .24. The level of cross-informant consistency in clinical settings compared favorably to other Axis I child interviews. However, cross-informant consistency was very modest, with many symptoms evidencing only chance agreement.

Validity

Concurrent Validity

Two reviews by Hodges (1993) and Ezpeleta et al. (1997) summarized the concurrent validity studies for the DICA-C and DICA-P. Three studies (Carlson et al., 1987; Vitiello, Malone, Buschle, Delaney, & Behar, 1990; Welner et al., 1987) have evaluated the DICA-C with inpatient samples. For externalizing disorders, the convergence falls in the low-moderate range, with a median kappa of .43. Internalizing disorders addressed only a small number of mood and anxiety disorders; Ezpeleta et al. (1997) found kappas comparable to those for externalizing disorders, with a median of .48. In the Carlson et al. (1987) study, the DICA-P evidenced moderate kappas for both internalizing (median = .60) and externalizing (median = .43) disorders.

Ezpeleta et al. (1997) conducted their own concurrent validity study on 137 outpatients. They found modest levels of convergence for both children (DICA-C median = .27) and adolescents (DICA-A median = .31). In contrast, the parent version (DICA-P) evidenced low moderate convergence for both children (median = .49) and adolescents (median = .45).

In summary, these results indicate low-moderate concordance of the DICA-C and DICA-P. These results are consistent with concurrent validity studies with child interviews. A strength of the DICA interviews is that they have been tested in a variety of settings and yield generally positive results.

Convergent Validity

Research has compared DICA diagnoses to psychometric data from scales and inventories. For general diagnoses, the results vary markedly across studies. Brunshaw and Szatmari (1988) compared DICA diagnoses to the Survey Diagnostic Instrument (SDI; Boyle et al., 1987), which was derived from the CBCL. When parent SDIs were correlated with DICA and DICA-P, moderate kappas (.41 to .50) were generated for five common disorders in a sample of 100 children referred for outpatient treatment. Two studies with the Personality Inventory for Children (PIC; Lachar & Gdowski, 1979) yielded disparate results. Sylvester et al. (1987) examined the DICA–PIC relationship for children with mentally disordered parents. For four common disorders, kappa coefficients were modest (median = .26; range from .11 to .30). In a study of brain-injured children, Green, Foster, Morris, Muir, and Morris (1998) found moderate correlations between DICA and PIC cut scores (median r = .52) for four broad diagnostic categories.

Other convergent studies have targeted depression and ADHD, with the following key findings:

1. *Depression.* Evidence of convergent validity is provided by a range of specialized scales, including the Beck Depression Inventory (BDI; Beck et al., 1961; see Kashani, Strober, Rosenberg, & Reid, 1988; Marton, Churchard, Kutcher, & Korenblum, 1991), the Children's Depression Inventory (CDI; Kovacs, 1978; see Allen-Meares, 1991), and the Hamilton Depression Rating Scale (HDRS; Hamilton, 1960; see Bartlett et al., 1991).

2. *ADHD.* Consistent convergent data are also found for DICA ADHD diagnoses when compared to (a) specialized checklists with teachers (Biederman, Keenan, & Farone, 1990), Conners Teacher Rating Scale (CTRS; Conners, 1969; see Shapiro & Garfinkel, 1986) and (b) CBCL ratings and achievement tests (Livingston, Dykman, & Ackerman, 1990).

Construct Validity

As a component of construct validity, Syndeham criteria have been evoked to test whether the diagnostic constructs form discrete entities and follow predictable patterns. Regarding diagnostic overlap, Carlson, Loney, Salisbury, and Volpe (1998) found that young boys with manic symptoms appear to share many diagnostic characteristics of disruptive disorders. This finding raises questions about diagnostic boundaries for boys presenting with manic symptoms. One hypothesis is that irritability in children might lead to this diagnostic blurring. Alternatively, the distinctions between ADHD and mania may require further delineation.

DICA studies have focused on onset (particularly risk factors), course of the disorder, and familial/laboratory correlates. Of these studies, the majority have addressed risk factors for developing subsequent mental disorders. Major findings are summarized as follows:

1. Alcoholic parents dramatically increase the likelihood of DICA diagnoses in their children. In a 5-year follow-up study of 32 children with alcoholic parents and 22 children without alcoholic parents, Reich, Earls, and Powell (1988) found that behavior disorders increased exponentially with alcoholic parents (65.6% vs. 0.0%). More recently, Reich, Earls, Frankel, and Shayka (1993) found a linear relationship between parental alcoholism (0, 1, or 2 parents) and the likelihood of externalizing disorders and substance abuse in children.

2. Mood or anxiety disorders in parents may increase the general risk of

DICA disorders in their children. Sylvester et al. (1987) found parents with depression and panic disorder increase the likelihood of similar disorders in their children, although the data do not suggest any specific risk (e.g., parent-linked childhood depression).

3. Traumatic experiences during childhood increase the risk of mental disorders. Based on a natural disaster (i.e., a devastating flood), Earls, Smith, Reich, and Jung (1988) found that children's symptoms 1 year later did not appear to be associated with the intensity of their flood experiences. Instead, presence of preexisting disorders dramatically increased the likelihood of flood-related symptoms (i.e., prior diagnosis, 47.4% flood symptoms; no prior diagnosis, 0.0%). Famularo, Kinscherff, and Fenton (1992) found that serious maltreatment predicts extraordinarily higher risks (i.e., OR > 10) of ADHD, oppositional and defiant disorders, and PTSD based on both the DICA-C and DICA-P.

4. The basic temperament of behavioral inhibition (i.e., highly constricted behavior) increases the risk of mental disorders in children with mentally disordered parents. Biederman, Rosenbaum, et al. (1990) found much greater risks of DICA diagnoses (particularly anxiety disorders, ADD, and ODD) for inhibited children than either uninhibited children or controls with healthy parents.

Beyond risk factors, studies have examined biological correlates and treatment response of specific disorders. Gillis, Gilger, Pennington, and De-Fries (1992) evaluated the genetic etiology for DICA ADHD with 37 identical and 37 fraternal twin pairs. Concordance rates were significantly higher for identical (79%) than fraternal (32%) twins. These results are sustained when adjusted for age, intelligence, and reading level. For treatment response, Livingston, Dykman, and Ackerman (1992) evaluated children with ADHD with and without concomitant disorders. Children with ADHD and comorbid mood and oppositional/conduct disorders responded more effectively to higher dosages of psychostimulants.

Clinical Applications

The development of the DICA indicates careful crafting of questions and sequencing of sections to facilitate interviews of youth. Considerable care has been invested in increasing DICA acceptability among youth and their families. In addition, the DICA-A provides a slight rewording of some questions to make them more appropriate for this population. Finally, the DICA-P is easily adapted to family assessments, with the capacity to record symptoms on as many as three children simultaneously.

The DICA has fewer reliability studies than several other child interviews such as the K-SADS and the DISC. However, the test–retest reliabilities for current diagnoses compare favorably to other interviews when utilized with clinical populations. Much less is known about test–retest reliability on a symptom level. The sole study (Perez et al., 1998) produced very respectable results when applied to a Spanish version.

Like all child interviews, the cross-informant data indicate low to moderate convergence between child and parent versions of the DICA. Especially at a symptom level, reports are likely to be highly discrepant. In their original study of the DICA, Herjanic and Reich (1982) only managed to achieve a very modest median kappa of .19. In terms of professional practice, clinicians must take care to evaluate multiple sources of data with respect to key symptomatology. Even for diagnosis, no single data source is likely to cover child disorders adequately.

Concurrent validity studies generally produce moderate kappa coefficients for diagnoses. While higher levels would be preferred, diagnostic agreement between child interviews (structured and unstructured) tends to be in this range. Overall, the convergent validity studies produced positive results, with substantial research on depression and ADHD.

A distinguishing characteristic of the DICA is its emphasis on the child's or adolescent's confidentiality. In the introduction to the interview (Reich et al., 1991a, p. 2), the child is assured, "I won't tell anyone what you tell me— not even your parent(s), unless we find out that somebody might be getting hurt in some way." The likely trade-off is that (1) children, especially adolescents, are more likely to divulge personal problems and problematic behaviors, but (2) clinicians, particularly those employing family interventions, may be hampered in their treatment by an inability to address openly problems raised by the children/adolescents. In choosing the DICA, clinicians should be aware of both the positive and negative implications of confidentiality. For example, Famularo et al. (1987) employed the DICA in the evaluation of maltreated children. They found that the children reported nearly twice the frequency of PTSD as their abusive parents. We might safely assume that the assurance of confidentiality facilitated the children's self-disclosure.

The DICA, perhaps more than other measures, has been used with several specific populations:

- The DICA has been found to be especially useful in the study of children with alcoholic parents. Although these studies provide only a general understanding of risk factors associated with alcoholism and antisocial behavior, clinicians may feel comfortable in using the DICA in the assessment of these populations because of the availability of comparative data.
- The DICA has also been employed in delinquent samples. For example, Myers and his colleagues (Myers & Kemph, 1990; Myers, Burket, Lyles, Stone, & Kemph, 1990) have found the DICA useful in the assessment of juvenile delinquents, especially those with CD and substance abuse disorders. Myers et al. concluded that the DICA was helpful in eliciting clinical data from delinquents even when parent interviews were not possible.

CHILDREN'S INTERVIEW
FOR PSYCHIATRIC SYNDROMES (CHIPS)

Description

The Children's Interview for Psychiatric Syndromes (CHIPS; Weller, Weller, Fristad, & Rooney, 1999) is a semistructured diagnostic interview composed of 20 common disorders and 303 clinical inquiries. Box 6.5 provides a basic description and information on the availability of the CHIPS. Inquiries are designed to increase comprehension among children by utilizing brief questions written in simple language. Syndromes are organized by estimated prevalence, with the more common categories presented first. The CHIPS was intended to be used by trained nonprofessionals. Like most child interviews, it is composed of two parallel versions: CHIPS (child) and P-CHIPS (parent).

The CHIPS is distinguished from other child interviews in that its primary purpose is to screen for mental disorders. Therefore, it is intended to be time-efficient in (1) simply covering DSM-IV criteria and (2) eliminating disorders from consideration when cardinal questions are not endorsed. Unlike other child interviews, symptom endorsement is typically based on a single inquiry without supplementary questions. The explicit goal is the overidentifi-

---

BOX 6.5. Highlights of the CHIPS

- *Description:* The CHIPS is a structured interview designed to evaluate symptoms associated with 20 common DSM-IV disorders. It is intended as a screening measure for youth ages 6 to 18. As a screen, it is designed to overidentify potential symptoms and possible diagnoses.

- *Administration time:* Given its use of screening items, the CHIPS is relatively quick to administer. According to the test manual, average times correlate with impairment: 49 minutes for inpatients, 36 minutes for outpatients, and 21 minutes for community-based children.

- *Skills level:* The CHIPS is designed for use by trained lay interviewers under the supervision of a clinician.

- *Distinctive features:* Despite years in development, the CHIPS is a relatively new measure. It differs from the other major child interviews in that it is intended only to screen for disorders, not diagnose them. As such, the CHIPS evaluates symptoms categorically (present–absent).

- *Cost:* Price list on 3/1/2001 for CHIPS starter kit (CHIPS, P-CHIPS, scoring forms, and administration manual) = $123.

- *Source:* American Psychiatric Press, by mail, 1400 K Street, NW, Washington, DC 20005-2403; by phone, (800) 368-5777; by fax, (202) 789-2648; or on the internet, *www.appi.org.*

cation of symptoms for review and further evaluation by an experienced clinician.

Original work on the CHIPS began in the mid-1980s with an analysis of existing interviews. After a significant hiatus, five research studies were published in 1998 and summarized in the administration manual (Rooney, Fristad, Weller, & Weller, 1999). The basic focus of these studies was concurrent validity, with a comparison of diagnoses with the DICA.

The CHIPS is organized by syndromes, with affirmative answers typically associated with psychopathology. Most inquiries are standard questions asked verbatim. The scoring of the CHIPS is simpler than most child interviews. Items are scored dichotomously as present or absent.

Reliability

The reliability of the CHIPS is not adequately described. According to the CHIPS test manual, interviewers were trained on videotapes until they achieved an interrater reliability coefficient ≥ .90 (Rooney et al., 1999, p. 21). The following remain unspecified in the manual: the type of reliability coefficient, number of videotapes, included disorders, age of the participants, and version of the CHIPS (child or parent). After training, interviewers were observed on a single case, with random checks as "resources permitted" (p. 21). What was previously referred to as "an interrater reliability coefficient ≥ .90" is subsequently described as "this 90% cutoff rate." A vast difference can occur between a reliability coefficient and a percentage of agreement. Fristad et al. (1998b) specified that ICCs were used for interrater reliability and were presumably utilized on diagnostic agreement; however, details were not provided.

Validity

CHIP studies (see Rooney et al., 1999) have focused on its concurrent validity with the DICA (Herjanic & Reich, 1982) and clinical diagnoses. From the Rooney et al. research program, small samples were examined for their diagnostic agreement. Not surprisingly, very few diagnoses (six or fewer) had sufficient representation to calculate the standard kappas. As summarized in Table 6.5, two studies produced moderate to moderately high kappas (.53 and .68). The remaining two studies had modest (.34) to negligible (.18) kappas. For comparisons with other child interviews, clinicians should realize that the CHIPS limits its use of kappas to cases with at least 25% representation; this restriction optimizes CHIPS kappa coefficients.

For most diagnoses, researchers employed an infrequently used and potentially controversial statistic known as the "rare kappa" (Verducci, Mack, & Degroot, 1988). With standard kappas, uncommon disorders are held to a stringent standard that takes into account the very low base rates. In contrast, rare kappas are far less stringent and produce coefficients that generally exceed standard kappas (see Table 6.5). Considering the current standards for

TABLE 6.5. Concurrent Validity Studies for the Children's Interview for Psychiatric Syndromes (CHIPS) with the Diagnostic Interview for Children and Adolescents (DICA)

Study	Criterion	Sample	Dx	Kappa	Rare kappa[a]
Teare et al. (1998a)	DICA	42 inpatients	4	.34	.49
Teare et al. (1998b)	DICA	71 patients	5	.53	.58
Fristad, Cummins, et al. (1998a)	DICA	36 patients	4	.18	.45
Fristad, Cummins, et al. (1998b)	DICA	40 inpatients	6	.68	.64
Fristad, Teare, et al. (1998)	DICA	40 community	0	NA	.49
Teare et al. (1998b)	Clinical	26 patients	4	.11	.54
Fristad, Cummins, et al. (1998b)	Clinical	47 inpatients	4	.41	.48
Fristad, Cummins, et al. (1998a)	Clinical	21 patients	5	.49	.48
Fristad, Teare, et al. (1998)	Clinical	40 community	0	NA	.49

Note. For samples, patients = inpatients and outpatients; community = nonreferred community participants. Dx = number of disorders on which the standard kappas were calculated. Clinical = clinical diagnosis.
[a]Rare kappas (Verducci, Mack, & DeGroot, 1988) are not generally used with diagnostic interviews and represent a substantially less stringent measure of association.

evaluating diagnostic agreement, only standard kappas are recommended for clinical use.

The same studies also report concurrent validity research with clinical diagnoses (see Table 6.5). The interpretation of these results is constrained by even smaller samples than those used with the DICA. Of three clinical comparisons, two yielded low-moderate median kappas (.41 and .49). The third study (Teare, Fristad, Weller, Weller, & Salmon, 1998b) had two negative kappas (−.18 and −.01) and resulted in a negligible median kappa of .11.

In general, the studies evidence a low-moderate concordance between the CHIPS and two criterion measures: the DICA and clinical interviews. As previously noted, these results apply only to common disorders and are slightly attenuated by the elimination of any disorders that did not occur in at least 25% of the sample. However, for the purposes of a screening interview, these results appear acceptable.

Clinical Applications

Concurrent validity studies with the CHIPS suggest a low to moderate agreement rate with DICA-R. Larger studies with broad diagnostic coverage are indicated. However, the chief stumbling block in recommending the CHIPS for clinical practice is the lack of clear evidence concerning its reliability. The test manual provides insufficient empirical data to support CHIPS interrater reliability. Data are not forthcoming on its test–retest reliability. Until issues of reliability are resolved, the CHIPS cannot be endorsed for clinical practice.

OTHER DIAGNOSTIC INTERVIEWS

Interview Schedule for Children (ISC)

Kovacs (1983) developed the Interview Schedule for Children (ISC) as a semi-structured interview on which symptoms are rated on a 9-point scale. The ISC, designed to be used in conjunction with DSM-III, consists of parallel interviews first with a parent and then with the child. When discrepancies occur, parents' data are given greater weight than children's. Reliability data reported by Last, Strauss, and Francis (1987) suggest good-to-excellent diagnostic agreement (a median kappa of .81, range from .64 to 1.00) on 11 disorders.

Kovacs and her colleagues (Kovacs, Feinberg, Crouse-Novak, Paulauskas, & Finkelstein, 1984a; Kovacs et al., 1984b) conducted several longitudinal studies on childhood depression employing the ISC. Kovacs et al. (1984a) examined 65 outpatient children diagnosed with the ISC as depressed. In subsequent follow-up, major depression and adjustment disorder with a depressed mood evidenced greater recovery than "double depression" (i.e., major depression superimposed on dysthymia). Kovacs et al. (1984b), using the same sample, attempted to predict further episodes of depression. Subsequent follow-up, spanning upwards to 12 years, has demonstrated the outcome criteria for depression and dysthymia (Kovacs, Akiskal, Gatsonis, & Parrone, 1994).

Autism Diagnostic Interview (ADI)

Le Couteur et al. (1989) constructed the Autism Diagnostic Interview (ADI) to classify autism accurately by ICD-10 standards. The interview is intended for patients ages 5 to early adulthood in which a pervasive developmental disorder is suspected. The diagnostic questioning focuses principally on the parent's or caretaker's observations of the patient, with a concentration on three related areas: (1) reciprocal social interaction, (2) use of language, and (3) repetitive or stereotypical behaviors. Interrater reliability was on the basis of four experienced raters, with most weighted kappas for individual items exceeding .70. In addition, ICCs for the three areas, described earlier, were excellent, ranging from .94 to .97. Comparisons of 16 autistic and 16 mentally retarded patients indicated highly significant differences on symptomatic bases, leading to a perfect discrimination between the two groups. While in need of cross-validation, the results of this initial study appear highly promising. With the publication of DSM-IV, further refinements will be needed to differentiate autistic disorder from Rett's, Asperger's, and childhood disintegrative disorders.

Childhood Trauma Interview (CTI)

The Childhood Trauma Interview (CTI; Fink, Bernstein, Handelsman, Foote, & Lovejoy, 1995) is a brief semistructured interview for assessing interpersonal trauma (e.g., physical neglect, witnessing violence, and sexual abuse). Questions are asked directly to evaluate potential traumas with responses recorded on 7-point scales of severity and frequency. The interview has excellent interrater reliability (median r for items = .91) but its test–retest reliability has yet to be established. While the CTI evidences modest correlations with self-report data (Carrion & Steiner, 2000; Fink et al., 1995), external validity needs rigorous evaluation. In light of the controversies surrounding repressed memories, retrospective use of the CTI would demand extensive validation before application outside of research settings.

Home Environment Interview for Children (HEIC)

A structured interview designed to complement the DICA in assessing family/home conflicts and stresses, the Home Environment Interview for Children (HEIC; Reich & Earls, 1984), is available in parallel forms for parents and children. Content areas addressed by the HEIC include family and peer relationships as well as school adjustment. The HEIC may be particularly useful in assessing dysfunctional behaviors at home and school, and serves as a useful adjunct to diagnostic interviews (Reich & Earls, 1987). Unpublished data (cited in Reich et al., 1988) suggest good mother–child agreement and test–retest reliability.

Child and Adolescent Psychiatric Assessment Scale (CAPA)

The CAPA (Angold, Cox, Prendergast, Rutter, & Simonoff, 1987) was developed for use in the clinical assessment of children's disorders and level of impairment. CAPA interviews are administered by lay interviewers. Psychometric data are not yet available on the reliability and validity of this measure (see Hodges, 1993).

III

Differential Diagnosis for Axis II Disorders

7

Structured Interview for DSM-IV Personality Disorders (SIDP)

OVERVIEW

The original Structured Interview for DSM-III Personality Disorders (SIDP; Pfohl, Stangl, & Zimmerman, 1982) was subsequently revised to address DSM-III-R (SIDP-R; Pfohl, Blum, Zimmerman, & Stangl, 1989) and DSM-IV (Pfohl, Blum, & Zimmerman, 1995) Axis II disorders. The SIDP is a semi-structured interview organized into different facets of the patient's life; sections include Interests and Activities, Close Relationships, and Emotions. Sophisticated inquiries address Axis II criteria that are embedded in these facets.

SIDP-IV represents a major departure from the earlier SIDP versions. Because most of the validational research was conducted on these earlier versions, the major differences between the SIDP-R and SIDP-IV are outlined as follows:

1. *Inclusion criteria.* The SIDP-R utilizes anchored criteria, with detailed descriptions for each level of each criterion. In contrast, the SIDP-IV invokes the "50% rule" (i.e., the symptom is present more often than not). Unlike the SIDP-R, DSM-IV criteria are reproduced with corresponding SIDP-IV inquiries.
2. *Scoring gradations.* The SIDP-R has three gradations: 0 = not present, 1 = moderately present, and 2 = severely present. In contrast, the SIDP-IV has four gradations: 0 = present or rarely present, 1 = subthreshold (i.e., insufficient to rate as occurring), 2 = present, and 3 = strongly present.
3. *Organization.* The SIDP-R has 17 topical sections, while the SIDP-IV, with 10 topical sections, has a simpler organization.

4. *Optional diagnoses.* The SIDP-R has embedded inquiries about optional diagnoses among the standard diagnostic questions. In contrast, the SIDP-IV has placed these inquiries at the end of topical sections. SIDP-IV formatting allows clinicians to skip optional diagnoses, thereby reducing the administration time.

This chapter focuses on the SIDP-IV, although the SIDP-R remains available. Box 7.1 highlights the key features of the SIDP-IV. As an overview, subsequent paragraphs are devoted to its coverage, symptom ratings, and structure of clinical inquiries.

The SIDP-IV is composed of 160 clinical inquiries/ratings that entail the inclusion criteria for personality disorders. The items are organized into 10 topical sections that progress from relatively nonthreatening components, such as general interests and activities, to more potentially intrusive components that address disordered perceptions and thinking. The design of the SIDP-IV is intended to parallel a clinical interview in its progression through topical sections. The advantages of this organization are that (1) questions have a natural flow, and (2) patients may have greater difficulty in modifying their response styles because diagnostic criteria are not necessarily clustered together. The only disadvantage of this approach is that recoding patient responses based on DSM-IV criteria is a two-step process.

Consistent with the DSM model of personality disorders, SIDP-IV for-

---

BOX 7.1. Highlights of the SIDP-IV

- *Description:* Semistructured diagnostic interview that focuses on Axis II disorders.

- *Administration time:* The SIDP-IV requires 60–90 minutes for full administration. This time is shortened considerably by omitting optional diagnoses. For collateral interviews, an optional subset of approximately 50 clinical inquiries adds about 20 minutes.

- *Skills level:* Advanced, with clinical sophistication in interviewing and gradational ratings. Extensive training materials are available.

- *Distinctive features:* The SIDP-IV is unmatched in its natural flow of clinical inquiries that address Axis II criteria without transparent inquiries (i.e., questions that clearly signal the diagnostic criteria). The SIDP-IV is especially well suited for patients with both Axis I and Axis II disorders.

- *Cost:* Price list on 3/1/2001 for SIDP-IV booklets = $28.95 for a package of five.

- *Source:* American Psychiatric Press, by mail, 1400 K Street, NW, Washington, DC 20005-2403; by phone, (800) 368-5777; by fax, (202) 789-2648; or on the internet, *www.appi.org.*

mat emphasizes patients' characteristic functioning. Patients are asked to respond to questions about their general functioning based on "when you are your usual self" (Pfohl, Blum, et al., 1989, p. 4). With these directions, the authors hope to minimize any undue influence because of situational (e.g., a marital crisis) or psychopathological (e.g., a major depressive episode) factors. In cases where the patient reports significant personality changes, he or she is instructed to relate what has been typical for the greatest amount of time in the last 5 years.

Pfohl and his colleagues also recognized that Axis II patients are sometimes inaccurate in both their self-appraisals and self-reporting. To this end, the SIDP-IV provides the option for an "informant" interview with a family member or close friend. A subset of clinical inquiries (approximately one-third) form the basis for the informant interview; these questions are marked with asterisks. Unlike the SIDP-R version, permission is requested at the beginning of the interview. Even if the informant interview is not conducted, securing permission may reduce deliberate distortions.

Interviewers record the patient's and informant's responses to the SIDP-IV. Because many questions are open-ended, clinicians may find it necessary to follow the standard questions with optional probes that are provided for clarification. These probes are highlighted by conditional clauses presented in capital letters (e.g., "IF YES, . . ." and "IF IT HAS NOT HAPPENED . . ."). In addition, clinicians are also asked to make clinical observations regarding verbal and nonverbal behaviors; these observations are grouped near the midpoint in SIDP-IV administration. Finally, clinicians are asked to make judgments, often complex, regarding whether symptoms for certain personality disorders occurred exclusively during the course of specified Axis I disorders.

One valuable and possibly overlooked feature of the SIDP-IV is its clarity in the diagnosis of mixed personality disorder. In the DSM-IV, clinicians are given little guidance in how to diagnose mixed personality disorder. The disorder can be inappropriately applied to a range of characterological features with varying levels of dysfunction and distress. In this regard, the SIDP-IV imposes a rigorous and defensible standard. The mixed personality diagnosis is only invoked when the patient (1) does not meet criteria for any specific personality disorder, and (2) has one less than the necessary inclusion criteria for two or more personality disorders. The adoption of this standard may reduce the diagnostic slippage common with the diagnosis of mixed personality disorder.

The rationale and development of the SIDP are not described in detail. In the original study, Stangl, Pfohl, Zimmerman, Bowers, and Corenthal (1985) offered only a passing comment on the rationale for its development. They observed perennial problems in the assessment of personality disorders: (1) marked variations in traditional interviewing, (2) lack of differentiation between time-limited crises and stable personality characteristics, and (3) variable thresholds for meeting inclusion criteria. In light of these comments, the SIDP was developed to reduce substantially the considerable Axis II problems with information and criterion variances.

Stangl et al. (1985) reported that the development of the SIDP involved three major revisions over an 18-month period. Early versions of the SIDP were field-tested; "confusing" and "ineffective" questions were modified or replaced. The lack of any formal description of this refinement would suggest an intuitive, nonempirical approach. Similarly, no description is offered on the changes between SIDP and SIDP-R except to state that the SIDP-R is keyed to DSM-III-R. As noted, several important modifications were made with the SIDP-IV. For example, DSM-IV criteria were included with individual clinical inquiries. In this regard, Pfohl et al. (1995, p. i) observed that experienced SIDP interviewers "obtained the best results" when the specific DSM-IV criterion was immediately available. With the adoption of the 50% rule, the SIDP-IV introduced a "subthreshold" rating for traits that are often present but do not meet the 50% test.

VALIDATION

The SIDP and its subsequent revisions capitalized on the emergence of DSM-III Axis II diagnoses to provide the criteria and conceptual underpinnings for the systematic assessment of personality disorders. Therefore, a major emphasis in the early studies was to demonstrate the reliability of the SIDP; its validity was assumed because of the one-to-one correspondence of SIDP items and DSM criteria. Subsequent research has also addressed construct and predictive validity.

Diagnostic Reliability

Pfohl and his colleagues conducted the first reliability study of the SIDP (Stangl et al., 1985; Pfohl, Coryell, Zimmerman, & Stangl, 1986) and participated in several additional studies (Zimmerman & Coryell, 1990; Zimmerman, Coryell, Pfohl, Corenthal, & Stangl, 1986; see Table 7.1). In recent years, other researchers have closely examined the SIDP's diagnostic reliability.

As summarized in Table 7.1, reliability studies of the SIDP have focused almost entirely on clinical populations, most often patients with Axis I disorders. Studies of current diagnoses are relatively well balanced between inpatient and outpatient samples. As a benchmark, median reliabilities for SIDP diagnoses fall in the moderate to moderately high range (.66 to .80). Several exceptions are observed. First, a study by Brent, Zelenak, Busstein, and Brown (1990) evidenced substantially less agreement. However, this study utilized adolescents, a population for which the SIDP has not been validated. Second, two studies (Serper et al., 1993; Coccaro, Silverman, Klar, Horvath, & Siever, 1994) that were very focused in their Axis II coverage produced high reliabilities.

Research by Pilkonis et al. (1995) demonstrated that diagnostic disagreements were generally the result of marginal cases. They found that most dis-

TABLE 7.1. Reliability Studies for the Structured Interview for DSM Personality Disorders (SIDP)

Study (year)	N	Setting: In/Out/Com/Univ	Dx	Raters: Lay/Prof	Reliability: Inter/Retest	(interval)	Sx/Cur-Dx	Life-Dx	Other
Stangl et al. (1985)[a]	63	✓ ✓	5	✓ ✓	✓ ✓	(1 wk) ✓	.75		
Pfohl et al. (1986)[b]	46			✓	✓			.55	
Zimmerman, Rohl, et al. (1986)	23	✓ ✓	6	✓	✓		.66[c]		
Brent et al. (1990)[d]	21	✓ ✓	3	✓	✓		.53		
Hogg et al. (1990)	10	✓	10	✓	✓				.54[e]
Nazikian et al. (1990)	10	✓	10	✓	✓				.74[e]
Pica et al. (1990)	10	✓	10	✓	✓				.91[e]
Zimmerman & Coryell (1990)	104	✓	6	✓	✓		.80[f]		
Jackson, Grazis, et al. (1991)	27	✓	5	✓	✓		.67[g]		
Jackson, Whiteside, et al. (1991)	39	✓	7	✓	✓		.72		
Serper et al. (1993)[h]	45	✓	3	✓	✓		.81		
Coccaro et al. (1994)[i]	18	✓	1	✓[i]	✓		.81		
Trull & Larson (1994)	18	✓ ✓	11	✓	✓				.86[e]
Benstein et al. (1997)	62	✓ ✓	6	✓	✓		.70		
Oltmanns (1998)[k]	128	✓	4	✓	✓		.60	.53[l]	

Note. See Table 1.5 (p. 35) for a glossary of terms and abbreviations.

[a]The design combines three "research workers" with two clinicians; reliability estimates are combined for 43 interrater and 20 test–retest reliabilities.

[b]Reanalysis of Stangl et al. (1985)

[c]Median kappa is reported for SIDPs without informant interviews. When informant interviews were included, several diagnoses improved but the median kappa remained similar (.63).

[d]Sample composed of adolescents (below the age for SIDP); raters were described as "trained interviewers."

[e]Dimensional ratings of current diagnoses are reported as correlations.

[f]These kappas are based on personality disorders with two or more cases; for dimensional ratings, mean ICC = .91.

[g]For dimensional ratings of 11 personality disorders, median $r = .67$.

[h]The study was limited to schizotypal, borderline, and both diagnoses.

[i]One psychologist and four researchers (training unspecified) served as raters.

[j]Study was limited to borderline personality disorder.

[k]Unpublished data provided by Nancee Blum (personal communication, March 24, 2000).

[l]ICCs were used for categorical diagnoses. Use of dimensional diagnoses was far superior. For the 10 personality disorders, the median ICC was .78 for number of symptoms and .83 for symptom scores.

agreements occur when patients are within one symptom (more or less) of the minimum criteria for establishing an Axis II diagnosis. Integrating the Pilkonis et al. results with other reliability studies, the SIDP produces reliable diagnoses, especially when patients exceed the minimum diagnostic criteria by at least one symptom.

Reliability studies with modest samples have utilized dimensional diagnoses. Four such studies produced moderate to very high correlations (median r's from .54 to 91). These findings are useful when practitioners are describing the degree of personality traits rather than rendering a DSM diagnosis.

Like most Axis II interviews, the SIDP focuses on the interrater reliability of current personality diagnoses (categorical and dimensional). Relatively little attention is given to test–retest reliability. Although personality disorders are assumed to be chronic, test–retest reliability was only addressed in the original study (Stangl et al., 1985). Because interrater and test–retest data are amalgamated, specific reliability estimates are difficult to establish for the 20 patients in the test–retest condition.

Among Axis II interviews, the SIDP appears to be useful when clinicians are interested in measuring individual symptoms. Pfohl et al. (1986) were able to achieve a moderate reliability (median $r = .55$), with most items evidencing at least low-moderate agreement (> .40). Several personality disorders (dependent, avoidant, and borderline) evidenced high levels of agreement, with reliabilities for individual criteria at a uniformly satisfactory level (> .50). More recently, Svrakic, Whitehead, Przybeck, and Cloninger (1993) examined agreement on individual traits with 10 cases in an interrater reliability format. Although, they did not provide reliability coefficients Svrakic et al. achieved a very high concordance rate (95.4%).

Several studies (Berstein et al., 1997; Zimmerman, Coryell, et al., 1986) addressed the importance of collateral interviews in producing reliable diagnoses. Although Zimmerman et al. produced comparable median kappas with and without informant interviews, they found that informants were especially helpful in establishing dependent and histrionic personality disorders. Berstein et al. (1997) found that collateral interviews increase the frequency of Axis II diagnoses by more than 10% for paranoid, schizotypal, histrionic, and borderline personality disorders. Taken together, these data suggest that collateral SIDP interviews are likely to provide a more comprehensive coverage of Axis II disorders than patient interviews alone.

For the SIDP-IV, Oltmanns (1998; Nancee Blum, personal communication March 24, 2000) examined a large sample ($N = 128$) of Air Force recruits, two-thirds of whom were selected because of potential psychological problems. A major strength of the study was its examination of symptom reliability on a large sample with eight professional interviewers/raters. It produced very positive results for individual symptoms, with a median ICC of .60. A limitation of the study was the relative infrequency of categorical diagnoses (i.e., $N = 20$ for obsessive–compulsive personality disorder, and $N = 29$ for the other nine disorders combined). As a result, categorical diagnoses for four disorders with adequate representation ($n > 5$) were only moderate (median ICC = .53). However, the dimensional diagnoses were excellent for both number of symptoms (median ICC = .78) and the summing of symptoms (i.e., a total score, median ICC = .83). Overall, this study provides strong support for both individual symptoms and dimensional diagnoses.

In summary, the SIDP reliability estimates are generally comparable to other Axis II measures (see Chapter 9), although the Personality Disorder Examination (PDE) has superior reliability (see Chapter 8). Two major advantages of the SIDP include its focus on individual symptoms and use with Axis I patients. Clinicians are often interested in appraising key symptoms and evaluating changes in these symptoms. The SIDP provides moderate evidence of reliability for this purpose. In addition, clinical practice often addresses patients with both Axis I and Axis II disorders; SIDP reliability studies involve patients with a range of Axis I diagnoses.

A major limitation of the SIDP, common for Axis II disorders, is the lack of test–retest reliability studies. The stability of Axis II diagnoses was only addressed in an early study in which data were amalgamated with interrater reliability. Moreover, additional SIDP-IV studies with a focus on diagnostic reliability would be helpful.

Validity

Validational studies of the SIDP have approached this onerous task from several perspectives. As evidence of construct validity, studies have explored the discreteness of SIDP-diagnosed personality disorders (i.e., do inclusion–exclusion criteria distinguish specific disorders?) and their convergent validity via comparisons with self-report measures of personality disorders. In addition, investigations have addressed predictive validity of the SIDP, including (1) outcome criteria per se and (2) treatment outcome with Axis I–Axis II interactions.

Construct Validity

Diagnostic Boundaries and Clusters. Zimmerman and Coryell (1989) conducted an important SIDP investigation of diagnostic boundaries and overlap of personality disorders. In a nonreferred sample[1] of 797 community-based adults, they examined the comorbidity of Axis II disorders. They found that "pure" SIDP personality disorders ranged from 14.3% for paranoid to 71.4% for dependent and schizoid personality disorders (median = 47.9%).[2] Key findings from the study are summarized as follows:

---

[1]Most participants were recruited as first-degree relatives in a family proband study of psychiatric disorders. When administered the DIS as part of this study, substantial numbers evidenced a lifetime prevalence for mood, anxiety, and substance abuse disorders.

[2]An unexpected finding was that *none* of the 797 subjects warranted the diagnosis of narcissistic personality disorder.

- With reference to dimensional scores, schizoid and dependent personality disorders appeared uncorrelated (r's < .40) and independent of other disorders.
- Diagnostic overlap was observed with two pairs of disorders (i.e., paranoid and schizotypal; histrionic and borderline). With high correlations ($\geq$ .60), these pairs have limited discriminability. As might be expected, borderline personality disorder appeared to be moderately correlated (r's $\geq$ .50) with four other scales.
- The best way to understand the Zimmerman and Coryell (1989) results is to compare these SIDP findings with other research. Research on Axis II disorders has yielded pure personality disorders in as few as 1% of clinical cases (Blashfield, 1992). In contrast, the SIDP yielded pure diagnoses in roughly one-half of the cases. Except for the specific overlaps noted earlier, the SIDP scales have relatively discrete diagnostic boundaries.

Bell and Jackson (1992) explored the structure of SIDP diagnoses via hierarchical clustering. A three-cluster solution explained 69.1% of the variance, with 6 of the 11 DSM-III-R disorders loading on a single cluster. At best, these clusters provided mixed support for DSM-III-R conceptualization, ranging from moderate support (Cluster A) to modest support (Cluster B) and negligible support (Cluster C). One formidable challenge in the Bell and Jackson study was the presence of Axis I disorders that were likely to obscure the observed structure of Axis II disorders. From a psychoanalytic perspective, Torgersen and Alnaes (1989) attempted an entirely different cluster analysis based on the Basic Character Inventory (Torgersen, 1980) in relationship to SIDP diagnoses. They proposed that DSM-III-R personality disorders could be categorized by four decision points (reality contact, extraversion, oral focus, and obsessiveness). While theoretically interesting, the Torgersen and Alnaes study requires extensive validation before its clinical implications can be realized.

Trull (1992) approached the construct validity of the SIDP by examining its relationship to the five-factor model of personality (i.e., neuroticism, extraversion, openness to experience, agreeableness, and conscientiousness). He compared SIDP dimensional scores on 54 psychiatric outpatients with five-factor model as measured by NEO Personality Inventory (NEO-PI; Costa & McCrae, 1985). He found relationships that made conceptual sense and were consistent with other measures of personality disorders, namely, the MMPI personality disorder scales (Morey, Waugh, & Blashfield, 1985) and the Personality Diagnostic Questionnaire—Revised (PDQ-R; Hyler & Rieder, 1987).

Convergent Validity

Self-report measures (e.g., PDQ-R, Millon Clinical Multiaxial Inventory [MCMI], MMPI-2 personality disorder scales) do not provide DSM diagnoses. The reasons are abundantly clear; these measures assess neither chronicity nor impairment associated with specific personality traits. In addition, patients with personality disorders often have poor insight into their character pathology. Therefore, self-report measures are considered as evidence of convergent (i.e., related constructs) rather than concurrent validity (i.e., nearly identical constructs).

The majority of convergent validity studies have compared SIDP diagnosis to the PDQ, a self-administered questionnaire, and/or the Millon Clinical Multiaxial Inventory—II (MCMI-II; Millon, 1982), a multiscale inventory. Comparisons are most often made simply on the concordance of diagnoses across measures. Less frequently, investigators have examined dimensional scores across measures (see Table 7.2).

Table 7.2 summarizes the mean correlations of individual SIDP diagnoses by DSM clusters. Overall, the correlations are relatively modest in magnitude, with Clusters B and C (both r's = .34) performing slightly better than Cluster C (r = .32). Method variance appears to play an important role with these correlations. With .40 as a minimum for moderate correlations of individual scales, marked differences are observed between the MCMI and other measures:

- Zero of 12 correlations for the MCMI $\geq$ .40 (unweighted M = .28).
- Five of 9 correlations for the other measures $\geq$ .40 (unweighted M = .40).

Self-report measures are properly considered to be screening measures for Axis II diagnoses by measures, such as the SIDP. In the "Clinical Applications" section, the clinical usefulness of the PDQ-R and the MCMI as screens is briefly reviewed.

TABLE 7.2. Convergent Validity Studies of the Structured Interview for DSM Personality Disorders (SIDP) with Self-Report Measures for Personality Disorders

			Correlations for individual disorders		
Study (year)	Measure	N	Cluster A	Cluster B	Cluster C
Zimmerman & Coryell (1990)	PDQ	697	.34	.38	.37
Trull & Larson (1994)*	PDQ-R	57	.41	.43	.45
Trull & Larson (1994)*	MMPI-PD	57	.38	.40	.40
Hogg et al. (1990)	MCMI	37	.30	.29	.24
Nazikian et al. (1990)	MCMI	31	.21	.37	.34
Torgersen & Alnaes (1990)	MCMI	272	.33	.23	.22
Jackson, Grazis, et al. (1991)	MCMI	82	.25	.28	.33

Note. PDQ = Personality Diagnostic Questionnaire; PDQ-R = PDQ—Revised; MMPI-PD = Minnesota Multiphasic Personality Inventory—Personality Disorders; MCMI = Millon Clinical Multiaxial Inventory.

Concurrent Validity

Pilkonis and his colleagues (i.e., Pilkonis, Heape, Ruddy, & Serrao, 1991; Pilkonis et al., 1995) conducted several studies based on Spitzer's (1983) Longitudinal Expert Evaluation using All Data (LEAD) model for the SIDP and the PDE (see also Chapter 8, "Concurrent Validity" section). Experts with access to the Personality Assessment Form (PAF; Pilkonis & Frank, 1988; Shea, Glass, Pilkonis, Watkins, & Docherty, 1987), Axis I measures, clinical history, and the PDE rendered LEAD diagnoses. Because the PDE is not entirely independent of the external criterion (i.e., LEAD diagnoses), this design is constrained by criterion contamination. However, Pilkonis et al. (1995) allowed a direct comparison of the SIDP to the PDE under the same conditions. Median kappas between the SIDP and PDE fell in the low-moderate range for Clusters B (.40) and C (.49); insufficient numbers were available for Cluster A. These kappas were much higher than those reported for the PDE (.20 and .24).

Predictive Validity

Treatment Outcome with Axis I Patients. An important dimension of diagnostic validity is the longitudinal perspective, which is typically assessed in terms of either the course of the disorder or its response to treatment. More than other Axis II measures, the SIDP has paid close attention to treatment outcome. However, the studies have only addressed the issue indirectly by examining the effects of comorbidity (Axis I and Axis II interactions) on the treatment of Axis I disorders. Ideally, studies of specific personality disorders and tailored treatment programs would allow the investigation of theory-driven treatment outcomes. For example, we might speculate that persons with avoidant personality disorders might benefit more than individuals with other personality disorders from social skills training focused on their general deficits. In contrast, the existing studies, summarized below, simply evaluate their nonspecific effects on treatment.

The effects of SIDP-diagnosed personality disorders on the treatment of patients with mood and panic disorders are summarized in Table 7.3. Although Axis II disorders are generally considered a major impediment to treatment, SIDP studies provide a more comprehensive and less ominous picture of Axis I–Axis II interactions. The key findings are summarized as follows:

1. Most studies have found that the mere presence of an Axis II disorder does not reduce the effectiveness of treatment for depression. Instead, elevated dimensional scores that represent the total character pathology may reflect on poor treatment outcomes (Pfohl, Coryell, Zimmerman, & Stangl, 1987).

TABLE 7.3. Treatment Outcome Studies with the Structured Interview for DSM Personality Disorders (SIDP)

Pfohl et al. (1984)
- *Design.* Follow-up of 78 inpatients with major depression at time of discharge (approximately 4 weeks).

- *Key findings.* Depressed patients with personality disorders evidenced less improvement on the Hamilton Depression Rating Scale (HDRS) and the Global Assessment Scale (GAS) than those without Axis II disorders. Interestingly, the patients with personality disorder were more depressed at the beginning of the study and more likely to be suppressors on the dexamethasone suppression test (DST).

Zimmerman, Coryell, et al. (1986)
- *Design.* Six-month follow-up on 25 inpatients treated for major depression with electroconvulsive therapy (ECT).

- *Key findings.* Nonsignificant trend on the HDRS and the GAS toward a poorer outcome for patients with personality disorders.

Pfohl et al. (1987)
- *Design.* Six-month follow-up conducted on 65 inpatients with major depression; outcome measured on multiple indices, including (1) the HDRS and (2) absence of symptoms.

- *Key findings.* The presence of a personality disorder by itself did not appear to affect outcome on the HDRS. However, either the diagnosis of mixed personality disorder or the total number on personality disorder criteria (> 19) decreased the likelihood of a positive outcome. In general, patients with personality disorders evidenced poorer response to antidepressant medication (16% vs. 50%) but similar responses to ECT (see Pfohl et al., 1984).

Reich (1988)
- *Design.* Eight-week follow-up conducted on 52 panic patients receiving anxiolytic treatment.

- *Key findings.* Relatively few differences were found on (1) number of panic attacks and (2) HDRS ratings on depression between patients with or without personality disorders. Cluster B patients had more situational panic attacks than others.

Reich and Troughton (1988a)
- *Design.* Recovered panic ($n = 57$) and depressed ($n = 19$) patients were compared to controls without Axis I disorders ($n = 40$).

- *Key findings.* Recovered patients evidenced more personality disorders (particularly in Cluster C) than did controls.

Pfohl, Barrash, et al. (1989)
- *Design.* One-year follow-up on 42 hypertensive patients' compliance with medication.

- *Key findings.* No significant differences on the basis of personality disorders.

Reich (1990)
- *Design.* Panic patients ($n = 28$) who dropped out of "treatment" in a placebo condition were compared to those who completed at least 3 weeks.

- *Key findings.* A greater proportion of patients with personality disorders dropped out compared to those without personality disorders (41.7% vs. 12.5%).

(cont.)

TABLE 7.3 *(cont.)*

Baer et al. (1992)
- *Design*. Patients with obsessive–compulsive disorder were followed in a 10-week, double-masked, placebo-controlled study of clomipramine, with comparisons of treatment outcome between patients with (n = 33) and without (n = 22) personality disorders.
- *Key findings*. No differences were found between the presence of a single personality disorder and no personality disorder on the Yale–Brown Obsessive–Compulsive Scale (YBOC; Goodman et al., 1989). However, the presence of multiple Axis II disorders was related to more impairment at baseline and less improvement at follow-up.

Mellman et al. (1992)
- *Design*. Variable follow-up period (9–101 weeks) on 46 inpatients with panic and mood disorders.
- *Key findings*. No differences in outcome were found for either number of episodes or duration of hospitalization. Mood-disordered patients with personality disorders have a significantly earlier onset that those without personality disorders (M ages of 15.8 vs. 28.3 years).

Barrash et al. (1993)
- *Design*. A sample of 69 depressed inpatients from the Zimmerman, Coryell, et al. (1986) study were reassessed at a 4-year follow-up.
- *Key findings*. Eighteen patients with Cluster B personality disorders (mostly borderline in addition to other disorders) were compared to 16 patients without personality disorders. Only older patients with unstable features of Cluster B appeared to be affected negatively by depressive episodes and suicidal behavior.

Alnaes and Torgersen (1997)
- *Design*. A sample of 253 outpatients were reevaluated after a 6-year follow-up for relapses or new episodes of depression.
- *Key findings*. Cluster A disorders were infrequently associated with relapse (23.1%) or a new episode (5.9%) of major depression. With the exception of antisocial personality disorder, Cluster B disorders have a moderate risk of relapse (34.4%) or new episodes (31.3%). Finally, Cluster C disorders carried a moderate risk of relapse (36.4%) but lower risk of new episodes (21.6%).

2. Depressed patients with personality disorders from the "anxious" cluster may respond better to treatment (Reich & Troughton, 1988a) than other Axis II patients.
3. Older Cluster B (primarily borderline) patients may have many episodes of depression and frequent suicide attempts (both serious and manipulative). Importantly, ECT may be more effective than antidepressant medication for those with severe personality disorders (Pfohl et al., 1987).
4. Studies of patients with panic disorder found few differences between those with and without personality disorders.
5. The treatment outcome for 55 obsessive–compulsive (OCD) patients did not appear to be affected by a single Axis II disorder. Rather,

Baer, Jenike, Black, Treece, Rosenfeld, and Griest (1992) found that more than one personality disorder affected both baseline measure (i.e., more impairment) and treatment outcome (i.e., less improvement). Baer et al. speculated that severe OCD may be expressed as Axis II symptomatology. If this were true for other Axis I disorders, then the comorbidity of Axis I and multiple Axis II disorders might reflect generalized distress rather than multiaxial diagnoses.

6. Limited data (Pfohl, Barrash, True, & Alexander, 1989) suggest that Axis II disorders do not complicate treatment compliance for certain medical conditions.

These findings are logical and commonsensical. To consider all Axis II disorders as a single category would be to overlook their crucial differences. The presence of a single personality disorder, especially from the anxious cluster, is unlikely to affect treatment. In contrast, multiple Axis II disorders (especially with borderline personality disorder) are likely to complicate treatment compliance and outcome.

SIDP studies are instrumental in exposing the following myths or misassumptions about personality disorders and their treatment:

• Myth: Axis I and Axis II disorders are entirely separable. How else do we explain treating only Axis I disorders in patients with Axis I–Axis II interactions? Please note that the studies in Table 7.3 ignored the treatment of Axis II disorders. Thus, members of one group (Axis I only) received treatment for their mental disorders, while members of the other group (Axis I–Axis II) received treatment for only a component of their mental disorders. Should we be surprised that patients with untreated disorders (i.e., Axis II) did not show the same improvement?

• Myth: Axis II disorders will not respond to conventional treatments. How else do we explain that Axis II symptoms are evaluated only at the baseline and not at follow-up? The remarkable neglect of Axis II symptoms perpetuates the myth regarding the inalterability of personality disorders.

Regarding the second myth, Reich and Troughton (1988b) found that dysphoric mood, but not depression, was the strongest predictor of all three personality disorder clusters. This finding suggests the possibility that subclinical depression might form a substrate underlying all personality disorders. Would treatment of the subclinical depression improve patients' Axis II disorders?

Antecedents of Axis II Disorders. An important consideration in understanding the etiology of Axis II disorders is whether certain conditions predict an increased prevalence of specific personality disorders. Reich (1986) studied early childhood events in 82 outpatients who had both personality disorders and an Axis I diagnosis (typically depression or anxiety). He found that patients in Cluster B had a higher frequency of parental death or absence than those in Clusters A or C. The etiological significance of this finding is not understood, although, understandably, patients with APD frequently had an absent parent. Obviously, much more research is needed on the antecedent events for specific personality disorders.

Based on their own cluster analysis, Coryell and Zimmerman (1989) established Clusters 1, 2, and 3, for which they predicted familial patterns of Axis II disorders for patients with depression and schizophrenia. They did not find predicted results. For example, family members of patients with schizophrenia had slightly *lower* prevalence of Cluster 1 diagnoses. Interestingly, patients with major depression with mood-incongruent psychotic features (6.3%) were more likely to have family members with Cluster 1 disorders than other patients with depression (3.9%) or schizophrenia (3.1%). Also, Cluster 3 disorders, uncommon in family members of patients with schizophrenia (2.3%), were observed in family members of patients with depression (8.4%) or persons without mental disorders (7.0%).

CLINICAL APPLICATIONS

Practitioners and researchers must decide whether to use the SIDP-R or SIDP-IV with clinical populations. Because the versions differ substantially in clinical inquiries (questions and sequencing) and scoring, the SIDP-R and SIDP-IV cannot be considered equivalent measures. As a general parallel, comparisons of the SIDP and SIDP-R (Blashfield, Blum, & Pfohl, 1992) found moderately high correlations for symptoms (median $r = .74$) but disparities in diagnoses (median kappa $= .48$). The respective advantages of the SIDP-R and SIDP-IV are summarized as follows:

- The SIDP-R has more research on reliability and convergent validity than the SIDP-IV. Unlike the SIDP-IV and other Axis II interviews, the SIDP-R attempts to base its scoring on specific criteria.
- The SIDP-IV is completely compatible with DSM-IV diagnoses. In addition, its one major study of interrater reliability provided excellent data on both diagnoses and symptoms. Finally, the flow and organization of SIDP-IV clinical inquiries are generally superior to that of the SIDP-R.

The SIDP-R and SIDP-IV are clearly useful measures for the assessment of personality disorders (see Table 7.4). They are organized topically to address important facets of patients' day-to-day functioning as it relates to Axis II disorders. Both versions are distinguished from other Axis II measures by the quality of the clinical inquiries. With relatively little preparation, clinicians are able to evaluate Axis II disorders with queries that appear natural and nonthreatening.

TABLE 7.4. Advantages and Disadvantages of the Structured Interview for DSM Personality Disorders (SIDP)

Advantages

- *Good interrater reliability.* Particularly for dimensional scores, the SIDP has demonstrated excellent agreement. For diagnoses, the coefficients of agreement tend to be in the moderate range, although these estimates are negatively affected by small sample sizes and poor representation of specific personality disorders.
- *Clear boundaries for personality disorders.* The SIDP distinguishes itself from other Axis II measures in the discreteness of specific personality disorders, with as many as 50% of patients qualifying for a single or "pure" Axis II disorder.
- *Relationship to treatment.* The SIDP has investigated the role of Axis II disorders in the treatment of Axis I patients. Studies offer preliminary data on how treatment might be tailored to interventions for comorbidity.

Disadvantages

- *Little evidence of test–retest reliability.* Although small samples of patients were evaluated in a test–retest design (see Table 7.1), their amalgamation with interrater reliability participants prevents any accurate estimates.
- *Lack of cultural and cross-cultural studies.* Research of the SIDP, unlike the Personality Disorder Examination (PDE), has not focused on minority and cultural issues.

The topical organization of the SIDP-R and SIDP-IV is an important feature in maximizing patients' cooperation. The use of nonthreatening topics decreases the pathological focus often found with Axis II measures. In addition, SIDP-R and SIDP-IV items have relatively low transparency, which means that patients who want to distort the interview will have a comparatively more difficult time in deciding what character pathology is aligned with specific inquiries. Despite these advantages of the SIDP-R and SIDP-IV, recent research by Berstein et al. (1997) suggests that informant interviews may assist in identifying otherwise undisclosed personality disorders. Especially in cases where patients appear guarded or circumspect, collateral interviews may be very helpful in detecting Axis II disorders. Moreover, the SIDP-IV asks for patients' permission to contact a significant other prior to the SIDP-IV interview. This precaution alone may reduce blatant distortions.

The SIDP-R and SIDP-IV are highly recommended for patients with Axis I disorders. Both versions are intended to be used with patients manifesting a broad range of psychotic and mood disorders. Their results are clearly applicable to both inpatient and outpatient populations. A concomitant advantage of the SIDP-R and SIDP-IV is the concerted effort to understand the role of personality disorders in the treatment of Axis I disorders. The comorbidity of Axis I and Axis II disorders deserves our serious attention in addressing treatment compliance and treatment outcomes. The SIDP-R, more than any other Axis II measure, offers us this opportunity.

The real hallmark of the SIDP, and presumably the SIDP-R and SIDP-IV, is clear diagnostic boundaries that allow both clinicians and researchers to investigate single ("pure") personality disorders in a systematic and reliable manner. Lacking a gold standard, it is impossible to ascertain whether SIDP diagnoses represent "true" disorders. Despite this limitation on all Axis II interviews, versions of the SIDP offer a diagnostic clarity that is likely to improve clinical practice.

The SIDP also has several notable limitations in clinical practice (see Table 7.4). First, as noted previously, the test–retest reliability of the SIDP-R and SIDP-IV has been neglected. This oversight, easily remedied, curtails the current usefulness of the SIDP-R and SIDP-IV for evaluating treatment outcome on Axis II disorders.

A second limitation is the dearth of research addressing minority and cultural issues. Although there is no reason to believe that SIDP-R or SIDP-IV inquiries are biased for specific ethnic groups, this issue deserves rigorous evaluation. In terms of generalizability, SIDP diagnoses do not appear to be influenced by gender, age, or years of education (Pfohl, Stangl, & Zimmerman, 1984). Regarding specific personality disorders, some gender differences are observed (Jackson, Whiteside, et al., 1991). However, these differences appear to be consistent with the expected prevalence rates for particular disorders (e.g., APD is higher in males than females).

In summary, the SIDP-R and SIDP-IV are top contenders for the complicated task of assessing personality disorders. Both versions offer reliable diagnoses for patients with Axis I disorders. Extrapolating from early research, both the SIDP-R and SIDP-IV are likely to provide clear diagnostic boundaries with a high proportion of pure disorders. In addition, they offer preliminary data on treatment efficacy for patients with Axis I–Axis II interactions.

8

Personality Disorder Examination (PDE) and International Personality Disorder Examination (IPDE)

OVERVIEW

This chapter is devoted to the Personality Disorder Examination (PDE; Loranger, 1988; Loranger, Susman, Oldham, & Russakoff, 1987) which has been extensively researched during the last decade. In addition, the International Personality Disorder Examination (IPDE; Loranger, 1999a) was recently marketed for the assessment of Axis II disorders. The IPDE is composed of two separate modules:

- The IPDE DSM-IV module corresponds closely to the PDE in its clinical inquiries, organization of items, and ratings. A few differences are observed because of DSM revisions between the PDE (i.e., DSM-III-R criteria) and the IPDE DSM-IV.[1]
- The IPDE ICD-10 module is completely separate and entails the nine ICD personality disorders. In a number of instances, identical questions are used in ICD-10 and DSM-IV modules, although the rating criteria are generally different.

PERSONALITY DISORDER EXAMINATION (PDE)

Description

The PDE is an extensive, semistructured interview for the assessment of personality disorders. Box 8.1 summarizes its major features. The PDE is com-

---

[1]Although the items are established on DSM-IV, the IPDE validational studies were based on DSM-III-R.

BOX 8.1. Highlights of the PDE and IPDE

- *Description:* The PDE is organized by topics (e.g., work and interpersonal relationships) to evaluate Axis II disorders according to DSM-III-R criteria. IPDE is composed of two modules for DSM-IV and ICD-10. With parallel organization and some overlap in questions, the modules are designed to be administered separately.

- *Administration time:* The PDE often requires 60–90 minutes. The IPDE typically requires approximately 3 hours if both modules are administered.

- *Skills level:* Both the PDE and IPDE are intended for use by experienced psychiatrists, clinical psychologists, and other professionals with comparable training in the diagnosis of mental disorders. A moderate level of practice is required for both measures. However, clinicians administering the full IPDE have the additional responsibility to familiarize themselves with ICD-10 diagnoses.

- *Distinctive features:* As an Axis II interview, the PDE has strong reliability, especially with respect to dimensional ratings and diagnoses. The IPDE is distinguished from other Axis II measures by its emphasis on cultural issues.

- *Cost:* Price list on 3/1/2001 for IPDE DSM-IV Introductory Kit = $139.

- *Source:* The IPDE is commercially available through Psychological Assessment Resources (PAR), by phone, (800) 331-8378, by fax, (800) 727-9329; on the internet, *www.parinc.com*; or by mail, P.O. Box 998, Odessa, FL 33556. For the PDE, the simplest approach is simply to use the DSM-IV module of the IPDE.

---

posed of 126 criteria organized into six major categories to facilitate the interview flow: work, self, interpersonal relations, affect, reality testing, and impulse control. Because of the overlapping nature of this categorization, the organizing principle for ordering individual symptoms is the promotion of "user friendliness" through the logical sequencing of clinical inquiries. Each of the six major categories begins with open-ended inquiries for eliciting a general discussion of potential problems and issues. For example, the *work* category commences with inquiries such as, "How well do you function?" and "What annoyances or problems keep occurring?" Responses to these introductory questions provide points of comparison for the structured questions that follow.

The PDE is intended for use with patients who have concomitant Axis I disorders. Several important exceptions include (1) psychotic disorders, (2) severe depression, and (3) substantial cognitive impairment (e.g., mental retardation or dementia). Therefore, patients should be screened for certain Axis I disorders to assess the appropriateness of the PDE for the evaluation of Axis II disorders.

Structured questions are organized by DSM-III-R criteria. Typically, several clinical inquiries form the basis for making a decision regarding each criterion. Examples are often elicited for reported problems. Responses to the clinical inquiries are rated on a 3-point scale: 0 = behavior is absent or not clinically significant, 1 = behavior is present but of uncertain clinical significance, and 2 = behavior is present and clinically significant. The PDE provides extensive documentation (one-half page or longer) for scoring each DSM criterion. Importantly, criteria are not scored as present (either 1 or 2) unless supported by convincing examples. In this regard, the PDE imposes a more stringent standard than other Axis II interviews.

Because the PDE does not assume that all personality disorders begin in adolescence and follow a chronic pattern of maladjustment, it has several distinctive features regarding the onset and course of personality disorders. For example, clinicians must distinguish whether the age of onset was in early (< 25 years old) or late adulthood. In addition, the scoring of the PDE clearly recognizes that key symptoms may no longer be present; positive scores are not given if the symptom has not occurred in the last 12 months. When diagnostic criteria have been previously met, clinicians are allowed to diagnose *past* Axis II disorders. Both in terms of onset and possible remission, the PDE has considerable flexibility for describing the course of the disorder.

The PDE is designed for both categorical and dimensional scoring. The categorical scoring corresponds to the DSM inclusion criteria. A *definite* diagnosis is rendered when the minimum diagnostic criteria are met; a *probable* diagnosis is rendered when one criterion less than the minimum diagnostic criteria are met. Dimensional scoring involves the summing of individual ratings for each of the personality disorders.

Rationale and Development

The introduction of DSM-III had a profound effect on the diagnosis of mental disorders, especially personality disorders. This change was largely due to the multiaxial diagnoses and greater specification of Axis II disorders. In a study of 10,914 psychiatric inpatients, Loranger (1990) found a remarkable increase in the diagnosis of personality disorders, from 19.1% (DSM-II) to 49.2% (DSM-III). The increased attention to Axis II disorders spawned concerns about their diagnostic reliability and validity.

Loranger et al. (1987) developed the PDE to address several methodological problems with Axis II diagnoses. First and foremost, they recognized the limitations in diagnostic reliability for personality disorders, with most kappa coefficients not meeting the .70 benchmark of good agreement. Second, they believed that personality disorders represent a continuum of maladaptive traits best measured by a dimensional system. Third, Loranger et al. expressed concern over information variance and the lack of assessment techniques for standardizing the assessment process.

Loranger, Oldham, Russakoff, and Susman (1984) first attempted to modify existing measures in order to address the validity of Axis II diagnoses. Not satisfied with the results, they created the PDE to "systematically survey the phenomenology and life experiences relevant to the diagnosis of the personality disorders in DSM-III (Loranger et al., 1987, p. 3). They wrote as many PDE items as "deemed necessary" to establish reliability and validity. As observed by Green (1989), test materials do not reveal criteria imposed and procedures followed for test-item creation and revision.

The original form of the PDE was pilot-tested by pairs of clinicians on 25 patients with mental disorders. Although specific data are not reported, the primary goal was to improve the content, phrasing, and sequencing of clinical inquiries. Over a 5-year period, from 1983 to 1988, two preliminary drafts and a final version were created (Loranger, Hirschfeld, Sartorius, & Regier, 1991). The second draft of the PDE consisted of 249 questions and 79 clinician ratings of verbal and nonverbal behavior (Loranger, Susman, Oldham, & Russakoff, 1985). Modifications since the 1985 version have been essentially minor and incorporate changes found in DSM-III-R (Loranger, 1988). With the advent of DSM-IV, clinicians have the option of administering the IPDE DSM-IV module (see the description in the "IPDE" section).

Validation

Diagnostic Reliability

Reliability estimates with the PDE must take into account its dual scoring system, with kappa coefficients for categorical diagnoses and ICCs for dimensional diagnoses. Table 8.1 provides a distillation of the major reliability studies.

The predominant focus of the PDE is on diagnosis. Symptoms are only considered in aggregate for either (1) the number of symptoms associated with individual disorders or (2) the summing of symptom ratings for individual disorders. The only exception is Schmidt and Telch (1990), who examined the reliability of individual PDE symptoms on a small sample of women with bulimia. Therefore, this section is organized into categorical and dimensional diagnoses.

Categorical Diagnoses. PDE studies have extensively examined its interrater reliability for both inpatient and outpatient settings. For interrater reliability, kappa estimates range from moderate in two studies (i.e., .63 and .69) to exceptional in three studies (i.e., .80, .84, and .87). In addition, Raczek (1992) appeared to achieve excellent agreement on specific personality disorders (i.e., 92% agreement) but failed to report kappa coefficients. Importantly, the two studies with moderate reliability were artificially constrained by modest sample sizes ($N = 20$). In summary, PDE interrater reliability appears to be excellent despite low representation of certain personality disorders.

TABLE 8.1. Reliability Studies for the Personality Disorder Examination (PDE) and the International Personality Disorder Examination (IPDE)

Study (year)	N	Setting In/Out/Com/Univ	Dx	Raters Lay/Prof	Reliability Inter/Retest (interval)	Reliability estimates Sx/Cur-Dx	Life-Dx/Other
PDE studies							
Loranger et al. (1987)	60	✓	5	✓	✓	.80	.97[a]
Loranger (1988)	129	✓✓	NA	✓		.78	.96[a]
	82	✓✓	4	✓	✓ (1 to 26 wk)	.49	.71[a]
Standage & Ladha (1988)	20	✓	9	✓	✓	.63	.92[a]
Edell et al. (1990)	21	✓	NA	✓	✓		.89[b]
Schmidt & Telch (1990)	15	✓	NA	✓	✓	.93	
Loranger, Lenzenweger, et al. (1991)	84	✓	7	✓	✓	.87	
Riso et al. (1994)	20	✓	3	✓	✓	.69	.84[a]
	84	✓	5	✓	✓ (1 to 26 wk)	.57	
Pilkonis et al. (1995)	31	✓✓ ✓	NA	✓✓	✓		> .82[c]
Becker et al. (1999)	26	✓	> 4[d]	✓	✓	.84	
IPDE study							
Loranger et al. (1994)[e]							
DSM-III-R	143[f]	✓✓	4	✓✓	✓	.70	.89[a]
ICD-10	143[f]	✓✓	2	✓✓	✓	.74	.88[a]

Note. Full citations are included in the references. See Table 1.5 (p. 35) for a glossary of terms and abbreviations.
[a] Intraclass coefficients (ICCs) are reported on dimensional scores for Axis II disorders.
[b] Not all reliabilities are presented; however, 10 of the 12 kappas are greater than .89.
[c] The range of ICCs was from .82 to .92; the median was not reported.
[d] The number of Axis II disorders was not specified although kappas were reported for four disorders representing the lower and upper ranges.
[e] The same data are reported in the IPDE test manual (Loranger, 1999a).
[f] The IPDE—English version is much smaller and estimated at 29 cases.

223

Two studies by Loranger (1988; Loranger, Lenzenweger, et al., 1991) found moderate agreement (kappas of .49 and .57, respectively) for test–retest reliability of personality disorders. One methodological constraint on reliability estimates was the use of a highly variable interval in both studies (i.e., 1–26 weeks). Even with Axis II disorders, a 6-month interval is likely to introduce patient variance, thereby partially confounding the reliability estimates. In light of this constraint, these kappa coefficients might be viewed as the "lower bound" of PDE test–retest reliability. Overall, these test–retest estimates fall in the low-moderate range and are generally comparable with other Axis II interviews.

Dimensional Diagnoses. Dimensional diagnoses for the PDE have superb reliability. In examining interrater reliability studies (see Table 8.1), kappa coefficients for current diagnoses appear close to the .80 range.[2] For dimensional diagnosis, the ICCs are unparalleled. When clinicians are interested in levels or gradations of specific personality disorders, the PDE is clearly the instrument of choice. The interrater reliability of dimensional ratings represents the foremost strength of the PDE's psychometric development.

Dimensional ratings of test–retest reliability were reported by Loranger (1988). Based on a combined inpatient–outpatient sample, the PDE evidenced moderate reliability (median ICC = .71). As noted previously, this estimate is likely to be suppressed by a methodological design that allowed long intervals between administrations. Overall, this ICC is in the acceptable range for test–retest reliability.

Cross-Informant Consistency. Cross-informant consistency does not address reliability per se. Instead, it tests different sources of information for the same patients to evaluate the level of consistency. A high level of consistency would suggest that different sources are likely to provide similar perspectives. In contrast, a low level of consistency suggests divergent perspectives and argues for appraisals that include multiple data sources (e.g., both patient and informant PDE interviews). The two PDE studies of cross-informant consistency yielded disparate results.

Pilkonis et al. (1991) tested the interrater reliability of the PDE under several conditions: (1) at initial intake, (2) at 6-month follow-up, and (3) with use of informants. Very encouragingly, solid kappa coefficients were reported for both patient administrations (i.e., intake = .79; follow-up = .84) and use of informants (.76). The design for informants was unusual: whereas the same primary interviewers always interviewed the patient, the independent raters were often different. Even with two different sets of clinical information (patient + informant vs. informant only), the level of agreement was in the high-moderate range.

---

[2]Please note that two studies (Edell, Joy, & Yehuda, 1990; Pilkonis et al., 1995) did not report sufficient data to calculate a median kappa. Therefore, the reported kappas of .89 and .82, respectively, represent the lower ranges and not the medians.

In stark contrast, Riso, Klein, Anderson, Ouimette, and Lizardi (1994) examined patient–informant consistency for 105 outpatients. They found virtually no agreement for diagnosis (median kappa = –.01) and only a modest convergence for dimensional scores (median ICC = .39). The Riso et al. study differed from the Pilkonis et al. (1991) study in several significant ways. First, interviewers in the Riso et al. study were completely masked to patient interview data. In the Pilkonis et al. research, the primary interviewer, and occasionally the rater, knew the results of patients' PDEs. Second, the studies differed in terms of individuals used as informants. Specifically, the Riso study included a substantial proportion of friends (36.2%); Pilkonis use a stricter standard (i.e., *close* friends) and a smaller proportion (19.4%) of informants.

The divergence of cross-informant consistency between the two studies precludes any firm conclusions about the advisability of PDE informant interviews. Two issues should be considered: (1) the patient's willingness to disclose detailed information about personal problems and interpersonal difficulties, and (2) the closeness of the relationship between a potential informant and the patient. I suspect the type of relationship (e.g., spouse, sibling, or friend) is less important than the quality of the relationship and daily opportunities to observe the patient.

Validity

The PDE was developed with specific criteria that represent a one-to-one correspondence with DSM-III and, subsequently, DSM-III-R. Utilizing DSM versions as the official if not gold standard, the major Axis II interviews, including the PDE, provide substantial evidence of content validity. Beyond content validity, the PDE has been researched extensively with respect to concurrent and predictive validity. Regarding construct validity, research has addressed the discreteness of individual personality disorders and potential confounds between Axis I and Axis II diagnoses.

Concurrent Validity. PDE studies of concurrent validity focus primarily on the concordance between the PDE and SCID-II (see Chapter 9) DSM diagnoses. Because of their specific focus on categorical classification, we cannot examine dimensional ratings for individual personality disorders or the level of agreement of particular symptoms. As summarized in Table 8.2, four studies directly compared PDE and SCID-II results. Interestingly, three of the four studies (Hyler, Skodol, Oldham, Kellman, & Doidge, 1992; Hyler, Skodol, Oldham, Kellman, & Rosnick, 1990; Oldham et al., 1992) were conducted at the same site: a long-term psychodynamic inpatient service for the treatment of severe personality psychopathology.

The two major findings from the concurrent validity studies are summarized as follows:

TABLE 8.2. Concurrent Validity Studies of the Personality Disorder Examination (PDE) with Structured Axis II Interviews

Study (year)	Interview	N	Median kappas for individual disorders		
			Cluster A	Cluster B	Cluster C
Hyler et al. (1990)	SCID-II	87	.27	.55	.52
O'Boyle & Self (1990)	SCID-II	20[a]	.08	.83	.38
Oldham et al. (1992)	SCID-II	106	.23[b]	.59[c]	.44[d]
Hyler et al. (1992)	SCID-II	59	.55[e]	.35[f]	.37
Unweighted averages			.28	.58	.43

Note. SCID-II = Structured Clinical Interview for DSM-IV—Axis II Disorders.
[a]Initial assessment of inpatients
[b]Based on paranoid and schizoid personality disorder
[c]Based on antisocial and histrionic personality disorders
[d]Based on dependent and passive–aggressive personality disorders
[e]Based only on paranoid personality disorder
[f]Based on borderline, histrionic, and narcissistic personality disorders

1. Cluster A evidenced only modest concurrent validity, with kappas ranging from .08 to .55 ($M = .29$). The concordance between the two measures is not reflected in the kappa coefficients. For example, O'Boyle and Self (1990) reported the worst kappa (.08) but had an overall agreement rate of 88.3%.
2. Clusters B and C evidenced moderate concurrent validities, with mean kappas of .58 and .43, respectively. These levels of agreement are comparable to Axis I interviews.

As a general observation, the PDE appears to be more stringent than the SCID in establishing Axis II diagnoses. For example, Hyler et al. (1990) found that the PDE yielded on average 2.8 diagnoses ($SD = 3.7$) per patient versus 3.4 diagnoses ($SD = 3.8$) for the SCID-II. Likewise, Oldham et al. (1992) found that nearly twice (186.7%) as many patients on the PDE as on the SCID-II did not warrant any Axis II diagnosis. One hypothesis from these data is that PDE personality disorders are likely to be confirmed by the SCID-II.[3]

Pilkonis et al. (1991) evaluated the PDE with Spitzer's (1983) Longitudinal Expert Evaluation using All Data (LEAD) model for establishing personality disorders. Beyond the standard administration of the PDE, the investigators used informants' PDE data, the Personality Assessment Form (PAF; Pilkonis & Frank, 1988; Shea et al., 1987), the SCL-90 (Derogatis, 1977), the

---

[3]Given SCID-II's greater numbers, the inference is that more disagreements occur from nonconfirmed SCID-II than PDE diagnoses.

Beck Depression Scale (Beck et al., 1961) and the Hamilton Rating Scale for Depression (Hamilton, 1960). The PDE appeared slightly more stringent than either PAF or LEAD diagnoses; complete agreement across the three methods was achieved in 50% of the cases. Using the LEAD diagnosis as the gold standard, the PDE had a sensitivity of 71% and a specificity of 58%. Despite criterion contamination (i.e., PDE data were used in establishing LEAD diagnoses), the kappa coefficient was modest (.28) but appeared to be negatively affected by efforts to classify the residual category of "mixed personality disorders," which has no formal inclusion criteria.

Pilkonis et al. (1995) compared PDE data to LEAD diagnoses that were formulated by interviewers who had access to all the clinical data (i.e., history and interview data, Axis I measures, and the PDE). Despite criterion contamination, the results for 55 outpatients were modest. Median kappas between LEAD and PDE diagnoses were low for Clusters B (.20) and C (.24), with insufficient numbers to calculate Cluster A for specific disorders. An important finding was that changing the diagnostic criterion by one symptom had the potential of greatly improving classification rates. This finding is especially relevant in marginal cases that minimally meet or do not meet diagnosis (i.e., ± 1 symptom).

In summary, the emphasis on content validity (i.e., correspondence between Axis II interviews and DSM inclusion criteria) has detracted from rigorous examination of concurrent validity. The PDE and SCID-II have a total of four studies of concurrent validity. While limited, these studies surpassed efforts with the Structured Interview for DSM-III Personality Disorders (SIDP), which are restricted generally to convergent rather than concurrent validity. The studies find a moderate convergence between the two measures (unweighted grand mean kappa = .43), with higher agreement for Clusters B and C than for Cluster A.

Concurrent validity studies have mainly overlooked two key issues that would likely produce more positive results:

- Dimensional ratings of diagnoses are likely to produce superior results in measuring the concordance between Axis II measures.
- Exclusion of marginal cases (i.e., with one symptom of minimum criteria) is likely to improve classification. Based on the Pilkonis et al. (1995) study, it is likely that disagreements occur predominantly with marginal cases. Therefore, practitioners can have greater confidence in their diagnoses and lack of diagnoses in nonmarginal cases.

Convergent Validity. PDE studies of convergent validity assume a position of secondary importance given the previously reviewed studies of concurrent validity. Convergent validity addresses the relationship between similar clinical concepts. Because questionnaires and inventories do not measure DSM diagnoses, only evidence of convergent validity is possible. In general, moderate levels of agreement are expected.

Like the SIDP, the majority of studies address the relationship between the Personality Diagnostic Questionnaire—Revised (PDQ-R) and the PDE. As summarized in Table 8.3, a stable pattern between the PDQ-R and PDE emerges. The relationship is very modest for Cluster A ($M = .14$), modest for Cluster B ($M = .29$), and moderate for Cluster C ($M = .42$). As expected, these kappas are lower than studies of concurrent validity. It is interesting to note that the pattern of kappa coefficients parallels the concurrent validity studies, with concerns being raised about Cluster A diagnoses.

Several studies (e.g., Hart, Dutton, & Newlove, 1993; Soldz, Budman, Demby, & Merry, 1993a) have examined the PDE in relationship to the Millon Clinical Multiaxial Inventory—II (MCMI-II). Although the MCMI-II purports to assess Axis II disorders, the problems of employing the MCMI-II to evaluate DSM disorders are well-documented (Hart et al., 1993; Rogers, Salekin, & Sewell, 1999, 2000). Hart et al. (1993) examined the level of agreement between the PDE and the MCMI-II for categorical diagnoses with a sample of 34 wife assaulters. The agreement for the presence–absence of any personality disorder was below chance (kappa = $-.12$). Similarly, Soldz et al. (1993a) found that kappas ranged from $-.07$ to $.41$ for the five disorders with sufficient representation. The modest median kappa (.26) is further attenuated by the presence of two negative kappas. The lack of convergent evidence for categorical classification likely reflects the limits of the MCMI-II. When viewed simply from a dimensional perspective, Hart et al. found low-moderate correlations for Clusters A (median $r = .36$), and B (median $r = .37$). In contrast, Cluster C was highly variable (range from $-.15$ to $.46$) and yielded a negligible median correlation (.08). Soldz et al. (1993a) produced more positive results, with median correlations of .39 for Cluster A, .49 for Cluster B, and .40 for Cluster C.

In the final study of convergent validity, Barber and Morse (1994) utilized the PDE and SCID-II to validate the Wisconsin Personality Disorders Inventory (WISPI; Klein et al., 1993). The pattern of correlations for PDE di-

TABLE 8.3. Convergent Validity Studies of the Personality Disorder Examination (PDE)

Study (year)	Measure	N	Median kappas for individual disorders		
			Cluster A	Cluster B	Cluster C
Hyler et al. (1990)	PDQ-R	87	.12	.39	.45
Hyler et al. (1992)	PDQ-R	59	.18	.22[a]	.35
Hunt & Andrews (1992)	PDQ-R	40	.13	.26	.46
Barber & Morse (1994)	WISPI	52	.18[b]	.39[b]	.53[b]

Note. PDQ-R = Personality Diagnostic Questionnaire—Revised; WISPI = Wisconsin Personality Disorders Inventory.

[a]Based on three Cluster B disorders (not antisocial).

[b]Correlations with dimensional PDE diagnoses. Categorical diagnoses were not feasible because 8 of 11 PDE disorders were poorly represented (1 or fewer participants).

mensional diagnoses was consistent with other research (see Table 8.3). Cluster A evidenced a very modest median correlation (.18). Although this level of agreement may reflect problems with the WISPI, a corresponding analysis of the SCID-II and WISPI yielded very different results (median r = .43).

- As evidence of convergent validity, modest to low-moderate relationships were found for Clusters B and C diagnoses. This level of agreement falls in the expected range when employing similar but not identical clinical concepts.
- With the exception of the MCMI-II research, studies of convergent validity raise concerns about Cluster A disorders with very modest median coefficients (< .20). This concern is also observed with concurrent validity (see Table 8.2).

Construct Validity. Soldz, Budman, Demby, and Merry (1993b) examined whether the PDE measures personality disorder characteristics that are different from normal personality dimensions. After partialing out variables associated with the Big Five, they performed a factor analysis of the PDE on 102 outpatients referred for Axis II treatment. They found two factors: Factor 1 had high loadings ($\geq$ .60) on three of four Cluster B disorders, with moderate loadings ($\geq$ .35) on two Cluster C (dependent and passive–aggressive) disorders. Factor 2 was closely aligned with Cluster A, with the addition of avoidant personality disorder from Cluster C. Two implications of the study are that (1) PDE scales are clearly measuring clinical constructs beyond normal personality dimensions, and (2) these constructs appear aligned with Clusters A and B, and are conceptually meaningful.

Becker et al. (1999) evaluated the cohesiveness of individual personality disorders (internal consistency) and discriminant validity (diagnostic overlap) separately for adolescent and adult inpatients. Regarding internal consistency, alpha coefficients tended to be moderate to good for most disorders except for adolescent Cluster A disorders. In addition, scale intercorrelations were uniformly low (r's $\leq$ .21). Although Becker et al. expressed reservations about their findings, these results generally support the construct validity of the PDE.

Researchers have also grappled with the boundaries between Axis I and Axis II studies. Loranger, Lenzenweger, et al. (1991) evaluated whether Axis I disorders might distort perceptions of Axis II traits. With 71 inpatients and 13 outpatients, they tested the effects of treatment on PDE symptoms. Although symptoms were reduced at follow-up, the magnitude of these decreases was very modest (i.e., .39 fewer symptoms per Axis II diagnosis). Given these modest changes, it is not surprising that improvements in Axis I symptoms were not significantly correlated with changes in Axis II symptoms. These results are consistent with Gartner, Marcus, Halmi, and Loranger (1989) in suggesting that PDE results do not appear to be highly influenced with certain Axis I disorders (predominantly mood, anxiety, and eating disorders).

PDE studies have also examined the comorbidity of Axis I and Axis II disorders. This research has only indirect relevance to construct validity because multiaxial diagnoses allow for such comorbidity. However, high levels of comorbidity would raise questions about diagnostic boundaries. In general, PDE research has found only low to moderate comorbidity. For example, Mauri et al. (1992) examined Axis II disorders among a patient sample with generalized anxiety disorder (GAD), panic disorders, or depression. Patients with dependent, avoidant, and borderline disorders evidenced the most comorbidity but still at a low rate (15–20%). Marin, Kocsis, Frances, and Klerman (1993) failed to find even moderate levels of comorbidity among patients with depression superimposed on dysthymia (double depression). Only patients with double depression evidence moderate rates (29.2%) of avoidant personality disorder. Finally, Rees, Hardy, and Barkham (1997) evaluated Cluster C diagnoses in patients with mood and anxiety disorders. Single Axis I disorders had negligible comorbidity. In contrast, major depression + GAD evidence a moderate comorbidity with Cluster C (32.1%), especially avoidant personality disorder (15.5%). In summary, PDE studies do not report excessively high Axis I–Axis II comorbidity that would raise concerns about diagnostic boundaries.

Predictive Validity. PDE research has evaluated the course of personality disorders and treatment response for Axis I–Axis II interactions. Diagnostic validity is dependent on establishing clear diagnostic boundaries (discriminant validity) and predicting the course and outcome of specific disorders. Key findings that address personality disorders from a longitudinal perspective are summarized as follows:

- Antecedent conditions of personality disorders are rarely examined. In a retrospective study, Raczek (1992) compared outpatients with and without child abuse histories. Patients with reported child abuse qualified for more Cluster B disorders, particularly borderline and antisocial disorders. This line of research is promising in the advancement of our understanding of precursors to specific personality disorders.
- Prospective research on personality development (Korenblum, Marton, Golombek, & Stein, 1990) found that parent and teacher ratings of disturbed fifth graders appear to predict a greater likelihood of PDE personality disorders at age 18. While the age range is restricted, disturbed functioning in fifth grade nearly doubled the probability of a Cluster A diagnosis, borderline, or antisocial personality disorder.
- Although personality disorders are generally assumed to have a chronic course, the PDE takes into account the possibilities of late onset and remission. Several PDE studies yielded disparate results regarding temporal stability:
  —A small study ($N = 18$) by O'Boyle and Self (1990) found that most personality disorders (12 of 16, or 75.0%) were no longer diagnosed following 2 months of inpatient treatment for depression.

Even more surprising, 10 new PDE diagnoses were rendered following treatment.

—Loranger, Lenzenweger, et al. (1991) reevaluated PDE diagnoses after a variable interval (1 week to 6 months; the majority were ≤ 2 months) and found moderate stability (median kappa = .57) for five personality disorders. However, 15.5% of PDE diagnoses were no longer warranted at follow-up and 7.4% new diagnoses were rendered.

—On the DSM-IV component of the IPDE, Loranger et al. (1994) evaluated temporal stability after a 6-month interval, with moderate consistency for categorical diagnoses (median kappa = .48) and excellent consistency for dimensional ratings (median r = .83 when corrected for attenuation).

INTERNATIONAL PERSONALITY DISORDER EXAMINATION (IPDE)

Overview and Description

Under the aegis of the WHO, an International Personality Disorder Examination (IPDE; Loranger, Hirschfeld, et al., 1991) was developed. The format was modified to include both DSM-III-R and ICD-10 criteria for personality disorders. Some questions were reformulated to address ICD-10 disorders; the scoring manual also incorporated ICD-10 inclusion criteria so that both diagnostic systems could be implemented. The expanded IPDE requires approximately 3 hours to administer.

The English version of the IPDE has been translated into 10 languages: Dutch, French, German, Hindi, Italian, Japanese, Kannada, Norwegian, Swahili, and Tamil. In each case, the IPDE was translated into the language, with a back-translation by a psychiatrist or psychologist masked to the English version of the IPDE. Discrepancies in translations were reviewed by additional translators. The authors recognize that cultural issues may contaminate certain personality disorder characteristics. The IPDE was developed so that these cultural differences might be systematically assessed.

In addition to the IPDE, two screening measures are available. Lenzenweger, Loranger, Kofine, and Neff (1997) developed the IPDE—Screen (IPDE-S), which consists of a 250-item true–false inventory. They reported excellent internal consistency for the three Axis II clusters (alphas of .88, .93, and .88, respectively). Use of the cut scores identified all participants with personality disorders (sensitivity = 1.00) but with a poor positive predictive power (PPP) of .18. For each personality disorder correctly identified, slightly more than four false positives were generated. It is questionable whether the IPDE-S would be cost-effective in most clinical settings.

The IPDE—Screening Questionnaire (IPDE-SQ; Loranger, 1999b) is composed of two versions: (1) a 77-item true–false scale for DSM-IV disorders, and (2) a 59-item true–false scale for ICD-10 disorders. Endorsement of more than three symptoms for any individual disorder is considered "suggestive of the presence of the corresponding personality disorder" (Loranger, 1999a, p. 14). However, no empirical data are provided to justify this cut score. In the absence of utility estimates, the clinical use of the IPDE-SQ is not warranted.

Validation

Loranger, Hirschfeld, et al. (1991) and Loranger (1992) described the initial steps in the validation of the IPDE via a large-scale WHO study spanning 11 countries and 14 research sites. Loranger et al. (1994) summarized the results of this research collaboration. Issues of reliability and validity are addressed separately.

Reliability

Loranger et al. (1994) evaluated the interrater reliability of the IPDE with 143 patients from different sites and employed different translations (see Table 8.1). For purposes of dimensional diagnoses, the reliability estimates were exceptionally high. For the current 10 DSM personality disorders, the ICCs ranged from .85 to .94, with a median of .89. ICD personality disorders were comparable, with the range of ICCs from .86 to .93, and a median of .88. Data on categorical diagnoses are limited to four DSM-III-R and two ICD-10 disorders. They evidence moderate reliability for DSM-III-R (median kappa = .70) and ICD-10 (median kappa = .74) diagnoses.

The good news of the Loranger et al. (1994) study is that superb dimensional and acceptable categorical diagnoses were achieved in a rigorous study that spanned different cultures and translations. However, several important limitations must be noted:

- Reliability of individual IPDE symptoms was not assessed.
- Test–retest reliability of the IPDE remains unexamined.
- Categorical diagnoses were only evaluated for 4 of 11 DSM-III-R diagnoses.

On the final point, it is encouraging that a broad category (probable + definite IPDE diagnoses) yielded acceptable levels of agreement (median kappa = .75) for eight DSM-III-R personality disorders. Still, no data are available for schizotypal, narcissistic, and passive–aggressive personality disorder.

Lenzenweger et al. (1997) reported testing the interrater reliability of the IPDE with two clinical psychologists on a university sample. The sample size for the reliability estimates was not given. The reliability of dimensional diagnoses was very high, with a median ICC of .92. Insufficient diagnoses were available to evaluate categorical diagnoses.

An unexplored issue appears to be potential differences in interrater reliabilities for IPDE translations. It is quite possible that the IPDE is generally unreliable for specific diagnoses with particular translations. Unfortunately, the recent manual (Loranger, 1999a) does not address this critical issue.

Validity

Loranger et al. (1994) and Loranger (1999a) tackled only one circumscribed component of validity, namely, temporal stability. The average interval between administrations was 6 months, with 85% of intervals falling between 2 and 12 months. Categorical diagnoses evidenced low-moderate consistency (median kappa = .48) for five DSM-III-R disorders and high-moderate consistency (median kappa = .65) for two ICD-10 disorders. In contrast, dimensional ratings of disorders remained high for both DSM-III-R (median ICC =.79) and ICD-10 (median ICC = .77) disorders.

Loranger (1999a) described the lack of a gold standard as a major limitation to establishing diagnostic validity for the IPDE. He reported (p. 213; see also Loranger et al., 1994), "It was the opinion of most of the clinicians who participated in the field trial that the IPDE was a useful and essentially valid method of assessing personality disorders for research purposes." The absence of quantitative data and the focus on research rather than clinical practice are two areas of concern.

Verheul, Hartgers, Van den Brink, and Koeter (1998) studied the convergent validity of the IPDE Dutch translation in relationship to the PDQ-R. Not surprisingly, the PDQ-R identified many more personality disorders than the IPDE. As a result, the level of agreement was poor for personality disorders (median kappa = .15) and only marginally better for diagnostic clusters (median kappa = .29). These results may reflect the particular sample (treated alcoholics) or translation (Dutch).

Generalizability

Clinicians from research sites located in 11 different countries were surveyed regarding the cultural acceptability of the IPDE (Loranger et al., 1994). Surprisingly, only two items (monogamous relationships and harsh treatment of spouse/children) were viewed as culturally bound. However, the report would have benefited from quantitative data on the relative acceptability of different inclusion criteria. No published U.S. studies systematically address differences due to gender or ethnicity.

CLINICAL APPLICATIONS OF THE PDE AND IPDE

Use of the PDE

The PDE is distinguished from other Axis II interviews by its emphasis on dimensional ratings and diagnoses. In many clinical settings, practitioners are interested in the extent of Axis II pathology and its potential effect on treatment. The PDE is ideally suited for clinical settings where these considerations are consequential. In this regard, these measures have unmatched reliabilities for dimensional ratings, with median ICCs that generally cluster between .82 and .97.

DSM-IV diagnoses require a categorical classification of personality disorders. In this regard, the PDE evidences a moderate level of interrater reliability, with most median kappas at the .70 benchmark or higher. Because of modest reliability samples, more than half the studies (see Table 8.1) are focused on five or fewer personality disorders. This degree of focus naturally limits the generalizability of their findings for the 10 DSM-IV personality disorders. Overall, the PDE produces estimates of interrater reliability that are comparable to the SIDP and SCID-II. Like other Axis II interviews, test–retest reliabilities fall in the low-moderate range. These estimates may be slightly suppressed in cases where the interval is relatively long (i.e., $\geq$ 6 months); however, such cases appear to constitute a small percentage of the reliability cases.

The PDE has both strengths and weaknesses in its concurrent and convergent validity. A major strength is the availability of four concurrent studies to examine individual personality disorders. However, combined results from concurrent and convergent validity research raise concerns about Cluster A disorders. With the exception of Hyler et al. (1992), the level of agreement for Cluster A disorders remains modest (< .30; see Tables 8.2 and 8.3). In contrast to these marginal results, PDE disorders from Clusters B and C appear to have solid concurrent and convergent validity.

For the purpose of clinical applications, clinicians must observe the Axis I limitations on the PDE. The PDE is not intended for use with patients experiencing psychotic disorders, severe depression, or substantial cognitive impairment. On a practical basis, a thorough Axis I evaluation must precede the PDE interview to ensure that these important limitations are respected.

Use of the IPDE

For purposes of validity, the IPDE DSM-IV appears to be the stepchild of the PDE. Research has clearly demonstrated the IPDE DSM-IV's reliability for (1) dimensional ratings of all personality disorders and (2) categorical diagnoses of four DSM-III-R disorders. Beyond interrater reliability, the IPDE DSM-IV draws its validity from the PDE. Most IPDE DSM-IV questions correspond closely to the PDE in both wording and scoring criteria. Therefore, it would appear reasonable to assume that PDE validity studies are germane to the IPDE DSM-IV. In summary, the IPDE DSM-IV appears to have adequate reliability and validity for professional practice.

The IPDE ICD-10 represents a substantial departure from the PDE on both item and diagnostic levels. The inclusion criteria for the ICD-10 are substantively different from their DSM-IV counterparts. In addition, the ICD-10 includes disorders that differ fundamentally from DSM-IV (e.g., emotionally unstable personality disorder, impulsive type). Because of these differences, the IPDE ICD-10 does not derive its validity from the PDE. At present, clinicians are likely to consider the IPDE ICD-10 limited to research purposes only.

Use of the IPDE-S and IPDE-SQ as Screens

Self-administered screens provide a cost-effective means of evaluating only those patients likely to have Axis II diagnoses. Unfortunately, little research is available on the IPDE screens: (1) one study of the IPDE-S and (2) no published studies of the IPDE-SQ. Regarding the IPDE-S, the use of a nonclinical university sample markedly limited the number of Axis II diagnoses. Excluding the DSM-IV NOS (not otherwise specified) category, DSM-IV personality disorders are inadequately represented, with an average of 1.4 cases per diagnosis. In addition, its usefulness is further constrained by a very low PPP that produces a high number of false positives.

In summary, the IPDE screens should not be used for the following reasons:

- Validation of the IPDE-S has insufficient sampling of individual disorders. Therefore, the IPDE-S is not recommended for clinical practice.
- Validation of the IPDE-SQ has not been reported in the literature despite its commercial publication. Therefore, the IPDE-SQ is not recommended for clinical practice.

Advantages and Disadvantages of the PDE

The PDE is characterized by a topical format that allows clinicians to ask relatively nonthreatening and nonpejorative questions organized into six major categories. The PDE is also distinguished by its detailed scoring manual that provides specific criteria for each clinical rating. Beyond its ease of use, the PDE has several advantages, which are summarized in Table 8.4, including dimensional diagnoses with superb reliability and an international version, the IPDE. Based on IPDE reliability, reproducible findings are reported across diverse cultures and various translations.

The PDE also has several disadvantages (see Table 8.4). Because treatment of personality disorders often focuses on disabling symptoms, the PDE is limited in its applicability. Nearly all PDE research addresses dimensional and categorical perspectives of disorders rather than symptomatology.

The other two limitations of the PDE address constraints on its clinical applicability. The PDE is not intended for use with certain clinical populations. In addition, Cluster A diagnoses appear to have less validity than those of Clusters B and C. The use of Axis I interviews and effective screens (e.g., the PDQ-R) may assist in selecting those clinical cases for which the PDE will provide the most valid data.

TABLE 8.4. Advantages and Disadvantages of the Personality Disorder Examination (PDE) for the Assessment of Axis II Disorders

Advantages

- *Ease of use.* Clinical inquiries are conveniently organized into six major categories. A range of clinical inquiries is used, including open-ended questions, standard questions and optional probes.

- *Interrater reliability.* Studies have consistently shown superb interrater reliability for dimensional scores with acceptable levels for categorical diagnoses (see Table 8.1).

- *Dimensional diagnoses.* The PDE distinguishes itself by making available both dimensional ratings and DSM-III-R diagnoses.

- *International version.* The IPDE offers a direct opportunity for assessment and research with patients of different nationalities. Its international emphasis is likely to provide future crucial data regarding cultural influences on personality disorders. From a research perspective, the IPDE offers an unparalleled opportunity to compare DSM-IV and ICD-10 personality disorders.

- *Time perspectives.* Unlike other Axis II interviews, the PDE provides flexibility in classifying cases by onset and outcome.

Disadvantages

- *Symptom ratings.* The PDE focuses primarily on disorders rather than symptoms. Therefore, it has limited applicability in measuring changes in critical symptoms, which are often the focal point of therapy.

- *Cluster A.* Studies of concurrent and convergent validity raise concerns about PDE's validity with Cluster A disorders (see Tables 8.2 and 8.3).

- *Exclusionary diagnoses.* The PDE is constrained in clinical practice because it has not been validated for patients with psychotic disorders, severe depression, or cognitive impairment.

In summary, the PDE is an excellent Axis II interview that deserves consideration in a wide range of mental disorders. It provides unparalleled data on dimensional diagnoses and meets acceptable standards for DSM-III-R categorical diagnoses. Although not formally tested, the IPDE DSM-IV module should maintain these standards for reliability and validity.

9

Structured Clinical Interview for DSM-IV Personality Disorders (SCID-II) and Other Axis II Interviews

OVERVIEW

This composite chapter features the Structured Clinical Interview for DSM-IV Personality Disorders (SCID-II). During the last decade, the validity of the SCID-II has been greatly buttressed by international research on its reliability and validity. Besides the SCID-II, two additional Axis II interviews are considered: the Personality Disorder Interview—IV (PDI-IV) and the Standardized Assessment of Personality (SAP). Finally, two other less researched structured interviews are briefly summarized: the Diagnostic Interview for DSM Personality Disorders (DIPD) and the Personality Assessment Schedule (PAS).

STRUCTURED CLINICAL INTERVIEW FOR DSM-IV PERSONALITY DISORDERS (SCID-II)

Description and Rationale

As a complementary measure to the SCID, Spitzer et al. (1987c) constructed a semistructured Axis II interview called the SCID-II. The combined use of the SCID and SCID-II was designed to provide a comprehensive assessment of both Axis I and Axis II disorders. A slightly modified version of the SCID-II is commercially available (Spitzer, Williams, Gibbon, & First, 1990c); the most recent revisions (i.e., First et al., 1994; First, Gibbon, Spitzer, Williams, & Benjamin, 1997) incorporates minor changes in diagnostic criteria corresponding to the DSM-IV. As noted by First, Spitzer,

Gibbon, and Williams (1995a), a distinguishing characteristic of the SCID-II is its relative brevity of administration (30–45 minutes) in comparison to other Axis II measures. Box 9.1 provides a summary of the SCID-II and information for obtaining copies.

Like the SCID, the SCID-II is organized by diagnoses and has an identical 3-point rating system: 1 = absent or false, 2 = subthreshold, 3 = threshold or true. For each of the diagnostic criteria, the patient is typically asked one or two standard questions. If a patient responds affirmatively he or she is then asked to provide examples. As is the case with many structured interviews, all items are unidirectional, so that all endorsements are indicative of psychological impairment. The major advantage of the SCID-II is its user friendliness: Criteria are grouped by diagnosis and scored in the same direction. The SCID-II format has two major limitations: (1) Some patients may become reluctant to respond affirmatively given the inevitable requirement of providing examples; and (2) the transparency of the interview format lends itself to manipulation and distortion.

Spitzer et al. (1987a) also developed a self-report screen, originally called the SCID Personality Questionnaire that was later revised and renamed the SCID-II Questionnaire (SCID-II-Q; Spitzer, Williams, Gibbon, & First, 1990a). The SCID-II-Q is composed of one item per diagnostic criterion and

---

BOX 9.1. Highlights of the SCID-II

- *Description:* Semistructured Axis II interview that parallels DSM-IV personality disorders.

- *Administration time:* Averages 30–45 minutes; time can be reduced by using a self-administered screen, the SCID-II-Q.

- *Skills level:* Modest level of training required for mental health professionals.

- *Distinctive features:* The SCID-II is the simplest Axis II interview to administer and interpret. Its repetitive queries for examples can be burdensome for some patients.

- *Cost:* Price list on 3/1/2001 for SCID-II (user's guide and five questionnaires) = $54. The copyright statement for the 1990 version maintains that single copies can be made by "researchers and clinicians working in nonprofit and publicly owned settings" (Spitzer et al., 1990c, inside of front cover); this provision is not made for the First et al. (1997) version.

- *Source:* SCID-II, Version 1.0: HealthSource Bookstore, by phone, (800) 713-7122; on the internet, *www.healthsourcebooks.org;* or by mail, 1400 K Street, NW, Washington, DC 20005-2401. SCID-II, Version 2.0: Michael First, PhD, Biometrics Research, New York State Psychiatric Institute, 1051 Riverside Drive, New York, NY 10032.

parallels the SCID-II in its sequencing of criteria. The sole exception is the diagnosis antisocial personality disorder (APD), for which the SCID-II-Q provides questions with respect to conduct symptoms only, based on the apparent assumption that patients are more likely to acknowledge childhood than adult antisocial behavior. The answers for the SCID-II-Q are dichotomous ("no" or "yes") and are completed by the patient according to how he or she has "usually felt or behaved over the past several years."

Validation of the SCID-II

Reliability

Segal, Hersen, and Van Hasselt (1994) have provided an important summary of SCID-II reliability. The current review augments Segal et al., with systematic comparisons across settings and translations (see Table 9.1). As a caution, note that several studies include only data on the presence–absence of *any* personality disorder (e.g., O'Boyle & Self, 1990; Vaglum, Friis, Karterud, Mehlum, & Vaglum, 1993). Such studies are noninformative because they do not address reproducibility of specific diagnoses. More recently, large-scale U.S. and international research have produced respectable reliability data. Key findings about SCID-II reliability are summarized as follows:

- Regarding patients with anxiety disorders, the English SCID-II has been found in several studies (Brooks, Baltazar, McDowell, Munjack, & Bruns, 1991; Rennenberg, Chambless, Dowdall, Fauerbach, & Gracely, 1992) to have moderate interrater reliability, although several personality disorders, including APD, were not investigated.
- Regarding test–retest reliability, First et al. (1995b) examined 103 patients and 181 community participants that were retested over a short interval (1–14 days). Patients had a moderate test–retest reliability (median kappa = .62). Surprisingly, the community sample had comparable prevalence rates for Clusters A and C. However, the overall reliability estimates were relatively modest (median kappa = .49).
- Italian (Maffei et al., 1997) and Spanish (Gomez-Beneyto et al., 1994) SCID-II translations appeared to have excellent interrater reliability for current diagnosis.
- A Dutch SCID-II translation evidenced moderately high reliability for both symptoms and current diagnosis (Arntz et al., 1992; Dreessen & Arntz, 1998)

The Maffei et al. (1997) research is a large-scale, rigorously designed study that demonstrates SCID-II potential reliability. With eight clinicians paired randomly, Maffei et al. examined the interrater reliability on a large sample of inpatients and outpatients. Importantly, all Axis II disorders were

TABLE 9.1. Reliability Studies for the Structured Clinical Interview for DSM Personality Disorders (SCID-II)

Study (year)	N	Setting In/Out/Com/Univ	Dx	Raters Lay	Raters Prof	Reliability Inter/Retest (interval)	Reliability estimates Sx/Cur-Dx/Life-Dx/Other	
Malow et al. (1989)[a]	29	✓	2		✓	✓	.85	.88
Brooks et al. (1991)[b]	30	✓	8		✓	✓	.72	
Fogelson et al. (1991)	45	✓	5		✓	✓	.73	
Arntz et al. (1992)[d]	70	✓	8		✓	✓	.84[c]	.79
Rennenberg et al. (1992)[e]	32	✓	4	✓	✓	✓	.67	.53
Clarkin et al. (1993)	25	✓	1		✓	✓	.89[f]	
Gomez-Beneyto et al. (1994)[g]	60	✓	8		✓	✓	.80	.96
First et al. (1995b)	103	✓	9		✓	✓ (< 2 wk)	.62	
	181	✓	8		✓	✓ (< 2 wk)	.49	
Maffei et al. (1997)[h]	231	✓	10		✓	✓	.91[i]	
Dreessen & Arntz (1998)[j]	43	✓	6		✓	✓ (35 days)	.57[c]	.62[k]

Note. For reliability estimates, "Other" = Axis II clusters. See Table 1.5 (p. 35) for a glossary of terms and abbreviations.
[a]Borderline and APD diagnoses only.
[b]Axis I diagnoses limited to panic disorders with agoraphobia.
[c]Intraclass coefficients.
[d]Dutch translation; Axis I diagnoses were predominantly anxiety disorders.
[e]Axis I diagnoses limited to agoraphobia with and without panic attacks.
[f]Borderline personality disorder; range from .89 to .99.
[g]Spanish translation.
[h]Italian translation.
[i]Dimensional diagnoses, median kappa = .94.
[j]Dutch version (41 of 43 patients) with small numbers of other Axis I disorders.
[k]For dimensional diagnoses, median ICC = .62.

adequately represented (≥ 10 participants per diagnosis). This study of the SCID-II Italian version provides impressive reliabilities for nonpsychotic patients and compares favorably to other Axis II interviews.

The early U.S. studies of SCID-II reliability were relatively limited in their scope. However, First et al. (1995b) established respectable test–retest reliability for patient populations across inpatient and outpatient settings. Its two limitations were (1) its insufficient representation of schizoid and schizotypal personality disorders, and (2) a very low kappa (.24) for obsessive–compulsive personality disorder (OCPD) in both patient and community samples.

An interesting question is whether long-standing Axis II disorders can be reliably assessed after extended time periods. Weiss, Najavits, Muenz, and Hufford (1995) conducted a 12-month test–retest reliability study on 31 cocaine-dependent patients. The study found considerable instability in diagnoses; only 41 of 75 (54.7%) Axis II disorders found at baseline remained at follow-up. Moreover, 28 new personality disorders were diagnosed at follow-up. The modest level of agreement (median kappa = .47) may be accounted for by a combination of factors: (1) instability of Axis II disorders, (2) cocaine dependence obscuring personality disorders, and (3) limitations in the SCID-II. On the positive side, the Weiss et al. study suggests that some diagnostic stability in the low-moderate range is possible with several Axis II disorders.

An important consideration with Axis II disorders is cross-informant consistency. In this regard, Dreessen, Hildebrand, and Arntz (1998), using the Dutch SCID-II, compared 42 outpatient reports with collateral reports from close informants. In examining individual symptoms, the level of agreement was quite low (median ICC = .24). Several disorders (borderline, paranoid, and obsessive–compulsive) evidenced marginally higher levels of agreement. Interestingly, couples with very close relationships were substantially better informants. Specifically, low intimacy resulted in a median kappa of .20 for dimensional diagnoses; high intimacy had a much higher level of agreement (median kappa = .41). Two salient observations emerged: (1) The nature of the relationship was critical to the usefulness of collateral interviews; and (2) overall, patients reported many more symptoms than did collateral sources.

The SCID-II is not recommended for the assessment of key symptomatology. With the exception of the Dutch version, reliability research has largely overlooked the reproducibility of symptom ratings.

Validity

Validation research on the SCID-II is organized into three sections. The first two sections address criterion-related validity (i.e., concurrent and predictive validity); the final section summarizes construct validity. In addition, I briefly review the validity of the SCID-II-Q.

Concurrent Validity

As summarized in the previous chapter (see Table 8.2), four studies examined the concurrent validity of the SCID-II in relationship to the PDE. Briefly, the studies offered moderate support for specific disorders included in Clusters B and C. In contrast, specific disorders in Cluster A evidenced very modest agreement (i.e., kappas fewer than .30). Interestingly, the fact that the SCID-II resulted in many more Cluster A diagnoses than the PDE, militated against diagnostic agreement.

Predictive Validity

Personality disorders, by their nature, are predicted to have a chronic course beginning in early adulthood. Remissions without intensive treatment focused specifically on Axis II diagnoses are unexpected. Several studies of the SCID-II have examined the course and outcome of personality disorders:

- Contrary to predictions, O'Boyle and Self (1990) found diagnostic instability on the SCID-II in a small sample of depressed inpatients. They compared SCID-II results on 17 depressed patients before (T1) and after (T2) treatment that averaged 2 months' duration. SCID-II diagnoses (60.0%) at T1 were not observed at T2. Likewise, diagnoses at T2 (61.5%) were not observed at T1.
- In a chronic day treatment population, Vaglum et al. (1993) found a moderate decrease (17.8%) in personality disorders when reevaluated 2.8 years later. These results may be explained by treatment gains or method variance (i.e., clinical interviews vs. SCID-II).
- Childhood antisocial symptoms (Goodman, Hull, Clarkin, & Yeomans, 1999) appeared to be mildly predictive of Axis I and Axis II disorders. However, conclusions from this study are limited by its very focused sample comprised solely of female borderline inpatients.
- In chronic substance abusers, an important question is whether symptoms associated with Axis II disorders are attributable to substance abuse rather than personality. Weiss, Mirin, Griffin, Gunderson, and Hufford (1993) found that very few Axis II diagnostic criteria (7.5%) were met only during drug abuse episodes; this finding suggests that Axis II diagnoses are not likely to be confounded by chronic drug use. Surprisingly, substance abuse episodes may *reduce* Axis II diagnoses (23.4%), which suggests the intriguing possibility that substance abusers may be "medicating" Axis II pathology.

Across Axis II interviews, predictive validity studies generally demonstrate the expected chronicity of personality disorders. The two SCID-II studies produced mixed results, with marked variability in the O'Boyle and Self (1990) study and moderate stability in the Vaglum et al. (1993) study.

Construct Validity

Torgersen, Skre, Onstad, Edvardsen, and Kringlen (1993) conducted an elaborate first-order factor analysis, oblique rotation, on an early draft of the SCID-II with 445 participants from an ongoing twin–family study of patients. They factor-analyzed SCID-II, except for APD and CD symptoms, and established 12 factors. Factor scores were examined for each personality disorder. The results were strongly supportive of the current SCID-II typology, with fully two-thirds of the symptoms loading on the predicted personality disorder. Moreover, the majority of the remaining symptoms loaded on factor scores that were conceptually meaningful. While the stability of a 12-factor solution obviously needs confirmation, the Torgersen et al. (1993) study offers initial evidence for SCID-II construct validity.

Rennenberg et al. (1992) examined the convergent validity of the SCID-II with the MCMI-II. On a sample of 52 agoraphobic outpatients, they found relatively low correspondence between SCID-II diagnoses and MCMI-II elevations (i.e., > 74). For nine diagnoses, kappas ranged from .14 to .51, with a median of .25. Unfortunately, the authors did not report dimensional scores, which might have been more useful in comparing the two measures.

Research has examined the convergent validity of the SCID-II in relationship to multiscale inventories. In two studies of the SCID-II and the Millon Clinical Multiaxial Inventory (MCMI; Marlowe, Husband, Bonieskie, Kirby, & Platt, 1997; Renneberg et al., 1992). In both studies, the positive predictive power (PPP) was marginal; median values were .13 for Marlowe et al. and .21 for Renneberg et al. From a dimensional perspective, Marlowe et al. found modest correlations for convergent scales (median $r = .30$). While these results are disappointing, they likely reflect problems with the MCMI in establishing convergent and discriminant validity (Rogers et al., 1999). Beyond the MCMI, Barber and Morse (1994) explored the relationship of the SCID-II to the Wisconsin Personality Disorders Inventory (WISPI; Klein et al., 1993). Although correlations with SCID-II diagnoses were modest (median $r = .27$), dimensional scores produced moderate correlations (median $r = .46$). Taken together, these studies offer modest convergent validity for dimensional diagnoses on the SCID-II.

Validity of the SCID-II-Q

Modestin, Oberson, and Erni (1997) reported reliability data on the German translation of SCID-II-Q collected by Wittchen. For test–retest reliability (3-day interval), the kappas were strong (range from .70 to .85).

Several studies have evaluated the clinical utility of the SCID-II-Q in comparison to the SCID-II. Nussbaum and Rogers (1992), despite relatively low kappas (median = .31), found that slightly lower cut scores (i.e., one less than the minimum criterion) enable clinicians to screen for personality disorders effectively while maintaining high sensitivity and moderate specificity rates. Ekselius, Lindstrom, von Knorring, Bodlund, and Kullgren (1994) found moderately high dimensional ratings (median rho = .73) between the Swedish translations of the SCID-II-Q and the SCID-II. When cut scores were adjusted, the agreement on categorical diagnoses was moderate (median kappa = .56). With a German translation, Modestin, Erni, and Oberson (1998) compared the SCID-II-Q to the PDE with modest agreement for probable/definite diagnoses (median kappa = .38). Finally, Richman and Nelson-Gray (1994) examined patterns of SCID-II-Q diagnoses in a nonreferred university sample. Unexpectedly, large percentages were found for certain disorders (e.g., > 50% prevalence for paranoid personality disorder).

In summary, the SCID-II-Q may serve a useful function as a screen for personality disorders. Its level of agreement with categorical diagnoses clearly indicates that it cannot be substituted for clinical interviews. Moreover, data with nonreferred populations (Richman & Nelson-Gray, 1994) underscore its overinclusiveness, with improbably high prevalence rates.

Generalizability

Maier, Lichertermann, Klingler, Heun, and Hallmayer (1992) examined the generalizability of the SCID-II. In a large sample (N = 452) of normal controls, psychiatric inpatients, and first-degree relatives, they found relatively consistent prevalence rates for personality disorders across gender and age. One exception was older (≥ 40 years) males, who appeared to have a lower overall prevalence (6.7%) than their younger counterparts (13.5%). In contrast, females remained relatively stable for both older (9.2%) and younger (11.5%) groups.

Golomb, Fava, Abraham, and Rosenbaum (1995) found comparable prevalence rates between males and females for most SCID-II diagnoses in a sample of depressed outpatients. Unexpectedly, males scored significantly higher for both OCPD and narcissistic personality disorders. However, these results were consistent with PDQ-R research on a much larger sample.

Issues of ethnicity and culture have not been examined in any large-scale research on the SCID-II. Therefore, it is unknown whether the SCID-II has any systematic biases due to race or ethnic background.

Clinical Applications

The SCID-II is a user friendly structured interview for the assessment of personality disorders. Because of its parallel format with the SCID, the SCID-II can be employed selectively to examine specific personality disorders. Its organization and scoring simplify its application to individuals with personality disorders. Indeed, practitioners need relatively little training to apply the SCID-II to clinical populations.

In the past, the diagnostic reliability of the SCID-II has been a major stumbling block in recommendation for its clinical applications. However, recent studies have demonstrated adequate interrater reliability for most Axis II disorders. In addition, test–retest reliability studies have yielded moderate reliability coefficients for short intervals.

A major advantage of the SCID-II is the availability of the SCID-II-Q, which provides an item-by-item screening of Axis II criteria. By design, the SCID-II-Q is overly inclusive. Still, the combination of the SCID-II-Q, followed by the selective administration of specific SCID-II disorders, is likely to save time and provide reasonably reliable diagnoses. In light of research by Nussbaum and Rogers (1992), disorders should be evaluated if they either meet the minimum criteria or have one less than the necessary criteria. A limitation of the SCID-II-Q is that its questions are almost identical to SCID-II questions, which may make the SCID-II appear highly repetitive. An alternative screening measure is the Personality Diagnostic Questionnaire—Revised (PDQ-R), which has been tested with the SCID-II (Fossati et al., 1998; Hyler et al., 1990).

Specific applications of the SCID-II are based on (1) complications in the treatment of Axis I patients and (2) usefulness with forensic populations. The key findings are outlined below.

Studies suggest that co-occurring SCID-II personality disorders do not necessarily have a negative effect on Axis I treatment. Dreessen, Hoekstra, and Arntz (1997) found that Axis II disorders do not affect treatment compliance or outcome for OCD within a cognitive-behavioral paradigm. Sato et al. (1993) studied the effects of SCID-II diagnoses on patients taking antidepressant medication for major depression. Importantly, a single personality disorder did not necessarily affect treatment outcomes; the overall rates of remission were 72.7% for no Axis II diagnosis and 70.6% for a single Axis II diagnosis. Remission was much lower for (1) more than one Axis II diagnosis, especially from Cluster A, or (2) schizoid personality disorder. These studies dispute the commonly held notion that any Axis II diagnosis negatively affects treatment.

Use of the SCID-II with forensic populations has been closely examined. For example, Blackburn and Coid (1998, 1999) found violent offenders to be heterogenous in their Axis II presentation. Several clusters were unrelated to APD: borderline, compulsive + borderline, and schizoid disorders. Although highly correlated with APD ($r = .85$), psychopathy evidenced significant correlations ($p < .001$) with five additional personality disorders. In a related study, Stalenheim and von Knorring (1996) found that psychopaths had more SCID-II disorders, especially from Cluster B. Finally, research by Eppright, Kashani, Borison, and Reid (1993) suggests that youth with CD may also experience Axis II (borderline and paranoid) symptomatology. However, the SCID-II and other Axis II interviews have not been validated with adolescent populations.

In summary, the SCID-II is distinguished from the SIDP and PDE/IPDE by its twin attributes: user friendliness and transparency. Its ease of administration is characterized by (1) symptoms clustered by diagnosis, (2) questions incorporating DSM inclusion criteria, and (3) unidimensional scoring (i.e., affirmative responses always reflect psychopathology). As a result, the SCID-II is likely more transparent than other Axis II interviews.

The focus of the SCID-II is diagnostic reliability and validity. Especially with respect to the former, practitioners must make decisions regarding the relevance of prominent symptoms. When Axis II psychopathology becomes a focus in treatment, other Axis II interviews may be preferred because of their demonstrated symptom reliability. In cases where the focus is predominantly Axis I disorders, the SCID-II is likely to be a useful diagnostic measure for Axis II disorders.

PERSONALITY DISORDER INTERVIEW—IV (PDI-IV)

Description and Rationale

Widiger (1985) began the initial development of an Axis II interview that eventually evolved into the PDI-IV (see Box 9.2 for availability). In the original version, Widiger described the measure as the Personality Interview Questions (PIQ). One feature of the PIQ, unique among Axis II measures, was its use of nonprofessional interviewers. Curiously, the author (see Widiger & Frances, 1987, p. 53) assumed that "the use of lay interviewers minimizes the effect of clinical biases and expectations." This assumption does not appear to be tenable because the lay interviewers were trained by

---

BOX 9.2. Availability of Axis II Interviews

- The Diagnostic Interview for DSM-IV Personality Disorders (DIPD-IV) is available for $10 from Mary C. Zanarini, EdD, by mail, McLean Hospital, 115 Mill Street, Belmont, MA 02178; by phone, (617) 855-2660; or by fax, (617) 855-3550.

- The *Personality Assessment Schedule (PAS)* authored by Peter Tyrer, MD, is available by mail, Department of Public Mental Health, London, United Kingdom W2 1PD, by phone, 0207-886-1648; by fax, 0207-886-1995; or by e-mail, *p.tyrer@ic.ac.uk*.

- The Personality Disorder Interview—IV (PDI-IV) is commercially available as an introductory kit for $105 through Psychological Assessment Resources (PAR), by phone, (800) 331-8378; on the internet, *www.parinc.com*; or by mail, P.O. Box 998, Odessa, FL 33556.

- Standardized Assessment of Personality (SAP) is not published. The last correspondence address was John Pilgrim, MB, MRCPsych, by mail, Institute of Psychiatry, De Crespigny Park, Denmark Hill, London, United Kingdom SE5 8AF; by phone, 071-703-5411; or by fax, 071-277-0283.

mental health professionals and are therefore likely to have been inculcated with the same biases.

The PIQ was distinguished from other Axis II interviews in that symptoms and traits were rated on a 10-point scale of increasing severity. As reported by Trull, Widiger, and Frances (1987), the degree of severity was organized into the following format: 1 = absent, 2–4 = present but of a subclinical level; 5–9 = increasing severity in the clinical range. Initial data on 67 audiotaped interviews of nonpsychotic inpatients suggested that the PIQ was reliable, with a median kappa of .71 for diagnosis (Widiger, Frances, Warner, & Bluhm, 1986) and a median *r* of .80 for the number of symptoms per disorder (Widiger, Trull, Hurt, Clarkin, & Frances, 1987).

The PIQ-II (Widiger, 1987) was developed to incorporate changes made in the DSM-III-R. These modifications did not significantly affect its interrater reliability. For example, Widiger, Freiman, and Bailey (1990) assessed the reliability of the PIQ-II on two highly trained interviewers[1] for a sample of 47 inpatients that excluded diagnosis of mental retardation, and schizophrenic and organic disorders. Kappa coefficients for PIQ-II personality disorders ranged from .45 (schizotypal) to .92 (passive–aggressive), with a median of .73. In addition, the number of reported symptoms for each disorder was highly correlated across the two interviewers (*r*'s from .75 to .96; median *r* = .88).

The final revision consisted of two closely related stages. In anticipation of DSM-IV, the PIQ-III (Widiger, Corbitt, Ellis, & Thomas, 1992) was refined to address changes in diagnostic criteria. The structure of the PIQ-III was further modified, resulting in the current measure that has been renamed the Personality Disorder Interview—IV (PDI-IV; Widiger, Mangine, Corbitt, Ellis, & Thomas, 1995).

The PDI-IV, similar to other Axis II interviews, is scored on a 3-point scale: 0 = not present, 1 = meets DSM-IV criteria, and 2 = severe, exceeds DSM-IV criteria. The PDI-IV assesses each of the 94 diagnostic criteria for 10 established and 2 proposed personality disorders. It is organized into two formats: thematic and disorder. The thematic format addresses nine themes: attitudes toward self, attitudes toward others, security or comfort with others, friendships and relationships, conflicts and disagreements, work and leisure, social norms, mood, and appearance and perception. For the disorder format, the criteria are organized by specific personality disorders. Validation studies appear to be based on the thematic format.

DSM-IV criteria are evaluated with 317 standard questions that are utilized to establish particular diagnostic criteria. With the exception of observational items, each criterion is assessed by at least two and generally three or four standard questions. Because this is a semistructured interview, the interviewer is encouraged to ask unstructured questions to clarifying responses.

---

[1]Interviewers completed a 3-month training program with Widiger and continued discussions of problematic items throughout data collection.

Scoring issues and conventions are presented in separate chapters of the PDI-IV test manual devoted to each disorder.

The PDI-IV emphasizes the need for extensive questioning of the patient. Administration time is approximately 2 hours. Unlike the SIDP and the PDE, less attention is paid to collateral data. While acknowledging that corroboration may be helpful, no guidelines are presented on how patient and informant data should be integrated.

Reliability and Validity Studies

Widiger, as a chief architect of the DSM-IV personality disorders, devoted sustained attention to congruence between DSM-IV diagnostic criteria and the development of PDI-IV questions that closely reflect their meaning and intent. To a large extent, the validation of the PDI-IV has been a matter of face validity. The following important issues remain with respect to validity:

1. *Concurrent validity.* The results of the PDI-IV should substantially agree with clinical diagnosis and other Axis II structured interviews (especially the SIDP and PDE).
2. *Convergent validity.* The PDI-IV should evidence predicted associations in a theoretically coherent manner with measures of personality and psychopathology.
3. *Concordance between professional and lay interviewers.* Despite assumptions regarding possible clinical bias, mental health professionals are the mainstay for the diagnosis of mental disorders. If highly divergent findings occur between psychologists and college student interviewers, then the validity of the PDI-IV is brought into question.
4. *Generalizability across settings/training.* The PDI-IV should be tested across a variety of settings (inpatient, outpatient, and nonclinical). In addition, testing the usefulness of the PDI-IV with interviewers not extensively trained and supervised by its developer would be most helpful.

Important first steps have already occurred in the validation of the PDI-IV. I discuss this research with respect to PDI-IV reliability and validity. Additional studies are needed to address these four points.

The reliability of the PIQ-II was summarized in an earlier section on the development of the PDI-IV. With respect to interrater reliability, Widiger, Freiman, et al. (1990) found that the PIQ-II has satisfactory diagnostic reliability when employed by two highly trained doctoral students. Moreover, the use of dimensional scores appeared to yield very promising results.

Widiger et al. (1994) presented relatively little data on PDI-IV reliability. They reported data from an unspecified sample with excellent interrater reliability for personality disorders, with kappas ranging from .72 to .93 (median = .87). As yet, the test–retest reliability of the PDI-IV has not been investigated. Given the chronic nature of personality disorders, the test–retest reliability and temporal stability of PDI-IV personality disorders would appear to be critical components of its validity.

Several validity studies have been reported for the PIQ and the PIQ-II. For example, Trull et al. (1987) examined intercorrelations of symptoms for three PIQ disorders (avoidant, schizoid, and dependent) on 84 inpatients. Moderate correlations between avoidant and dependent symptoms raised questions regarding diagnostic boundaries and comorbidity. They also mentioned a moderate correlation ($r = .53$) between the MCMI avoidant scale and the number of PIQ avoidant symptoms.

Widiger et al. (1986) evaluated the PIQ-II criteria for borderline and schizotypal disorders in a sample of 84 inpatients, excluding those with diagnoses of schizophrenia, major mood disorders, and organic mental disorders. They found that borderline symptoms had moderate item-scale correlations (range from .15 to .46; median = .32) but schizotypal symptoms did not appear to correlate (range from –.21 to .35; median = .07). They expressed concern in the study about the substantial diagnostic overlap, with an average of 3.75 personality disorders per patient.

Widiger, Mangine, Corbitt, Ellis, and Thomas (1990) compared PIQ-II disorders to prototypical behaviors of 50 psychiatric inpatients for schizoid, histrionic, and compulsive personality disorders. They found that (1) three histrionic prototypical acts were significantly correlated with histrionic personality disorder, (2) none of the schizoid prototypic acts were significantly correlated with schizoid personality disorder, and (3) several other personality disorders were significantly correlated with these prototypical acts. Finally, researchers have found significant correlations between PIQ-II schizoid criteria and the Interpersonal Sensitivity scale of the SCL-90-R (Derogatis, 1977; median $r = .46$) and the Aloof–Introverted scale of the Interpersonal Adjective Scales (IAS; Wiggins & Broughton, 1985; median $r = .40$). Unfortunately, the authors do not present convergent and discriminant validity data for other PIQ-II personality disorders relative to the SCL-90-R and the IAS.

Bailey, West, Widiger, and Freiman (1993) addressed the convergent and discriminant validity of five schizotypia scales (Chapman & Chapman, 1987) with PIQ-II ratings. They found that these scales were moderately correlated (r's from .49 to .68, with a median of .56) with schizotypal criteria. In contrast, only a few of the other disorders (e.g., schizoid and avoidant) were correlated at all, and these associations were conceptually meaningful. The study provides useful convergent and discriminant validity for schizotypal personality disorder.

Kruedelbach, McCormick, Schulz, and Grueneich (1993) employed the PIQ-II in a study of borderline and nonborderline substance abusers seeking treatment from the VA. Using the NEO Personality Inventory (Costa & McCrae, 1985), they established significant differences between the two groups on anxiety, impulsivity, depression, and hostility. These data, as well as findings on research scales, demonstrated the convergent validity of the PIQ-II in its differentiation between borderlines and nonborderlines.

No validity studies have yet been reported on the PDI-IV. The critical issue is whether the PIQ-II studies should be employed in the validation of the PDI-IV. According to Widiger et al. (1995), DSM-IV and DSM-III-R criteria differ substantially with only 10.8% of the criteria remaining unchanged. Of the changed criteria, significant modifications were made in 52 criteria (55.9%) and an additional nine criteria (9.7%) were completely new. Since the PIQ-II is based on DSM-III-R and the PDI-IV on DSM-IV, generalizability across measures is seriously questioned. Although Widiger et al. (1994) reported a good correspondence (median kappa of .77) between PIQ-III and PDI-IV, they did not report any research comparing the PIQ-II and the PDI-IV.

In summary, the validity data on the PDI-IV and its predecessors are sparse. In the best available research devoted to the PIQ-II, a handful of studies has found convergent validity for borderline, schizotypal, schizoid, and histrionic personality disorders. Regrettably, other Axis II disorders have only been peripherally addressed. As previously noted, the comparability of the PIQ-II and the PDI-IV has yet to be established.

In reviewing the major facets of PDI-IV validity, considerable work remains to be completed. Although the interrater reliability appears to be satisfactory, only a very small number of interviewers were employed, who were extensively trained and personally supervised by the test's developer. Critical evidence of test–retest validity has yet to be accomplished. Moreover, the temporal stability of diagnoses has not been investigated.

A major shortcoming of the PDI-IV is that no studies have been reported on its concurrent validity with other established measures, such as the SIDP and the PDE. Additionally, matters of generalizability require careful attention. For example, does the PDI-IV yield comparable results when employed by clinicians and nonprofessionals? Furthermore, can the PDI-IV be used effectively in outpatient mental health settings, and at other health care facilities and community agencies? What happens when the PDI-IV is used with patients with schizophrenia and other psychotic disorders?

Clinical Applications

A primary strength of the PDI-IV is its value as a sourcebook on DSM-IV disorders (Kaye & Shea, 2000). The PDI-IV manual provides extensive and authoritative reviews of each of the personality disorders, with a thorough discussion of all Axis II diagnostic criteria. In addition, the PDI-IV provides a valuable template for evaluation of personality disorders and the provision of standard questions that closely reflect the diagnostic criteria.

The PDI-IV is not sufficiently validated for clinical practice. As noted in the previous sections, crucial questions remain with respect to its reliability and validity. Although intended for use by both professionals and nonprofessionals, existing reliability data on the PIQ-II and, presumably, the PDI-IV, were conducted exclusively with highly trained psychology staff. Therefore, the PDI-IV remains virtually untested with respect to its stated use by lay interviewers.

The first practical concern with the PDI-IV is the complexity of some of its inquiries, especially for APD, and the sophistication of its language. Its demands for concentration and complex understanding may undermine its usefulness among chronic mentally ill or intellectually limited patients. These matters are likely to be addressed in further refinements of the PDI-IV. A second practical concern is the sheer number of clinical inquiries. Given the competing demands on clinicians, a distillation of key questions followed by a greater number of optional probes may be an efficient alternative.

In conclusion, the PDI-IV has considerable promise as both a current resource and a future structured interview. Kaye and Shea (2000) report that continued work on its validation is likely to address many of these limitations in the coming years.

STANDARDIZED ASSESSMENT OF PERSONALITY (SAP)

Description and Rationale

The SAP was originally developed by Mann, Jenkins, Cutting, and Cowen (1981) as a brief measure of personality disorders that could be easily applied to large-scale studies (see Box 9.2 for availability). The three goals of the SAP consist of (1) evaluation of premorbid personality and its effects on the course and treatment of Axis I disorders, (2) standardization of personality assessment, and (3) development of a user-friendly measure that could be applied to clinical and nonclinical populations.

The SAP is distinguished from other Axis II interviews on several grounds. First and foremost, it does not rely upon accurate self-reporting by persons with personality disorders. Instead, the SAP depends entirely on close informants' interviews. In contradistinction to the SIDP and PDE, which both require and recommend a combination of patient–informant interviews, the SAP forgoes the patient interview altogether in favor of an informant's observations. Second, the SAP, developed in Great Britain, is based on ICD-9 and ICD-10 diagnostic standards. Compatible with ICD-10 criteria, the SAP covers eight diagnoses: paranoid, schizoid, dyssocial, impulsive, histrionic, anankastic (i.e., similar to OCD), anxious, and dependent disorders. In addition, Mann and Pilgrim (1992) reported that a DSM-III-R version has been prepared.[2]

A newly modified version of the SAP (SAD-ICD-10 Version or SAP/10; Mann & Pilgrim, 1992) is now available. The SAP/10 is utilized with an in-

---

[2]Only the ICD-10 version is described; no validity data are reported on the DSM-III-R version.

formant who has known the patient for at least 5 years. The informant is asked questions about periods of time when the patient was "illness-free." The unstructured portion of the interview requires that the informant provide a free-flowing description of the patient. Any relevant Axis II descriptors from a 72-item list are recorded. Following the unstructured portion of the interview, 10 general probes are asked verbatim. Again, any relevant descriptors are recorded.

The next step for the SAP/10 is a systematic review in a run-on-sentence format of all the criteria for any personality disorder for which any descriptors were endorsed. The number of criteria varies with the disorder (range from six to nine). For any personality disorder with three or more endorsed criteria, the clinician completes the final step, namely the assessment of impairment, which is evaluated on three separate indices: the patient's personal distress, occupational problems, and social problems.

The final classification for each disorder is a trichotomy. Patients with less than three endorsed criteria are classified as not having that trait accentuation or personality disorder. Patients with three or more endorsed criteria but no impairment are classified as having that trait accentuation. Patients with three or more endorsed criteria *and* significant impairment are classified as having that personality disorder.

The actual administration of the SAP/10 can be completed in 10 to 15 minutes (Pilgrim, Mellers, Boothby, & Mann, 1993). Because of its simplicity, the actual training for reliable use of the SAP/10 is relatively brief. According to Pilgrim and Mann (1990), sufficient training typically requires a single 2-hour session.

The rationale for the SAP/10 was the need for a brief but standardized structured interview that would circumvent problems with self-reports by individuals with personality disorders. Moreover, the SAP/10 was intended for use with inpatients as well as outpatients. Pilgrim and Mann (1990) expressed concern that customary evaluations of hospitalized patients (i.e., self-report and observation) might result in an overestimation of personality disorders because of patients' clinical presentation clouding the true diagnostic picture. Finally, the SAP/10 was developed to address the obvious need for a structured interview consistent with ICD-10 standards.

Reliability and Validity Studies

Mann, Jenkins, and Belsey (1981) examined the interrater reliability of the original SAP on a small sample ($N = 24$) of psychiatric inpatients. Employing pairs of psychiatrists, they established satisfactory reliability estimates, with weighted kappas from .60 to .85 (median = .64) for four personality disorders. Test–retest reliabilities after a 1-year interval ranged markedly, with reliability coefficients from .13 to .74, and a median of .42. McKeon, Roa, and Mann (1984) assessed the interrater and test–retest reliability (12-month intervals) for 25 OCD patients. Utilizing close relatives, clinicians evidenced a high level of agreement on three personality disorders, both on estimates of interrater (.88 to .93) and test–retest (.76 to .88) reliability.

Pilgrim et al. (1993) investigated the reliability of the SAP/10. For interrater reliability, they studied 16 elderly subjects suspected of dementia and 36 psychiatric patients. For the six disorders with sufficient representation (five or more), the kappa coefficients ranged from .60 to .82, with a median of .80. For test–retest reliability, they examined a consecutive sample of 77 inpatients. For the seven disorders with adequate representation, kappas ranged from .54 to .79, with a median of .69. In addition, they found that females and family members tended to be the most accurate in reporting personality disorders. In contrast, males and friends tended to give much more variable accounts of the same patient.

The diagnostic validity of the SAP/10, like that of many diagnostic interviews, is largely based on the face validity of its items and their correspondence to the ICD-10. Toward this end, Pilgrim and Mann (1990) assessed the prevalence rates of SAP personality disorders for 120 inpatients. Among individuals with personality disorders ($n = 43$), the SAP/10 produced relatively little diagnostic overlap, with subjects, on average, qualifying for 1.74 personality disorders. This number appears quite low for an Axis II structured interview, although direct comparisons cannot be made with measures based on DSM-III-R and DSM-IV criteria. Interestingly, significant gender differences were observed, with 50.0% of women and only 25.8% of men warranting diagnosis of a single personality disorder.

Mann et al. (1999) investigated the SAP's concurrent validity in relationship to the IPDE on outpatients from India. They found a low-moderate level of agreement (median kappa = .47) for seven ICD-10 personality disorders. While only moderate in magnitude, this level of agreement is typical for Axis II measures. Importantly, the SAP appeared to be effective (NPP = .97) in screening out patients with no personality disorders.

Initial validation of the SAP has focused on its relationship to overall functioning. For example, Mann, Jenkins, and Belsey (1981) followed 100 nonpsychotic outpatients for a 1-year period. Interestingly, they found that psychiatric morbidity was chiefly determined by estimates of psychological and social functioning. SAP personality dimensions appeared to play a peripheral role in predicting future mental disorders, although they proved significant in establishing future needs for psychotropic medication.

McKeon et al. (1984) examined 25 patients with OCD in a behavior treatment program. Surprisingly, those patients with premorbid personality disorders, as measured by the SAP, had fewer significant life events than their counterparts without personality disorders. This finding defies simple explanation. One possible explanation is that patients with personality disorders require fewer traumatic events before the onset of an additional disorder, in this case obsessive–compulsive neurosis. A second possibility is that obsessive–compulsive neurosis and the reported constellation of personality traits (obsessional, anxious, and self-conscious) are etiologically linked and unrelated to stressful events. A third explanation might be that the presence of these personality disorders insulates patients from substantial involvement in social and work spheres, thereby decreasing the likelihood of stressful events.

Validation of the SAP, as noted in the previous distillation of research findings, has focused largely on its reliability, with less attention to validity. The sole study by Mann et al. (1999) suggested a moderate level of concurrent validity. More research emphasizing concurrent and convergent validity studies of the SAP are strongly encouraged.

Clinical Applications

The SAP/10 clearly merits further attention because of its distinctive attributes. Focusing on critical descriptors, followed by standardized criteria and impairment probes, the SAP/10 provides a rapid and efficient method of assessing personality traits. For clinicians using DSM-IV criteria, the SAP/10 remains untested for diagnostic purposes. In light of Mann et al.'s (1999) findings, the SAP/10's potential as a screening measure deserves further consideration. More attention is needed regarding the comprehensiveness of the descriptor list and its refinement as an effective screen for personality disorders (Widiger & Frances, 1987).

Mental health professionals who work with patients with personality disorders may choose to use the SAP/DSM version as a secondary screen. In other words, a self-report screen such as the PDQ-R could easily be supplemented by the SAP/DSM version. In such cases, the SAP would provide valuable information about personality dimensions observed by others. In addition, it may provide information regarding treatment issues. For example, if a patient's spouse perceives overall problems in interpersonal functioning, these issues could potentially become a focus of individual and/or marital therapy.

The choice of an informant appears critical to the reliable use of the SAP/10. The ideal choice would be a close family member, preferably female. Use of nonfamily informants may lead to unacceptably inconsistent data. Of course, the use of multiple informants would appreciably improve the value of convergent data.

OTHER AXIS II INTERVIEWS

Personality Assessment Schedule (PAS)

Tyrer and Alexander (1979) developed one of the earliest semistructured interviews for the assessment of personality disorder, namely, the PAS (see Box 9.2 for availability). As noted by Widiger and Frances (1987), the PAS is comprised of 24 personality traits rated on a 9-point scale. Based on ICD classification, the PAS employs standard questions of the patient and an informant to assess the following personality disorders: explosive, asthenic, paranoid–

aggressive, histrionic, anankastic, and schizoid. Available studies suggest that the PAS may have adequate interrater reliability but only modest test–retest reliability (see Tyrer, Alexander, Cicchetti, Cohen, & Remington, 1979; Tyrer, Strauss, & Cicchetti, 1983). Kaplan and Kolvin (1994) found adequate interrater reliabilities (ICCs ≥ .60) for 16 of 23 traits on a modified 5-point scale. Interestingly, Brothwell, Casey, and Tyrer (1992) found spouses and siblings to be the most reliable, while friends and acquaintances were the least reliable.

Recent research has utilized the PAS to postulate a new diagnosis of hypochondriacal personality disorder (Tyrer, Fowler-Dixon, Ferguson, & Kelemen, 1990; Tyrer, Seivewright, & Seivewright, 1999). Additionally research has addressed the usefulness of the PAS in classifying personality clusters (Hassiotis, Tyrer, & Cicchetti, 1997) and evaluating chronic fatigue syndrome (Rangel, Garralda, Levin, & Roberts, 2000). No large-scale research has grappled with the PAS in terms of either concurrent or convergent validity.

Diagnostic Interview for DSM Personality Disorders (DIPD)

Zanarini, Frankenburg, Chauncey, and Gunderson (1987) constructed the DIPD in 1982 to assess DSM-III personality disorders systematically (see Box 9.2 for availability). The DIPD comprises 252 standard questions organized by each disorder and scored on a 3-point scale: 0 = absent or clinically insignificant, 1 = present and probably clinically significant, and 2 = present and definitely clinically significant. In addition, optional probes are provided for many questions and unstructured questions are encouraged in cases of ambiguity. Zanarini et al. (1987) provided the first study of its validity.

Reliability was assessed on nonpsychotic inpatients, employing three raters for both interrater ($n = 43$) and test–retest ($n = 54$) reliability. The resulting kappa coefficients were excellent for interrater reliability (> .85, median of .92) with the exception of paranoid personality disorder (kappa = .52). Moreover, the test–retest reliabilities tended to be relatively robust, with a range from .46 to .84 and a median of .68.

Comparatively little research has been conducted on the DIPD since its development. For example, Zanarini, Gunderson, Frankenburg, and Chauncey (1989) employed a revised version of the DIPD in research on borderlines (see Chapter 10) but offered little evidence of validity. Regrettably, the DIPD appears to be a reliable Axis II interview that has faltered not because of its psychometrics, which appear to be very encouraging, but because of a lack of sustained research effort. According to Kaye and Shea (2000), no DSM-IV studies have been published, although efforts are under way.

IV

Focused Structured Interviews

10

Diagnostic Interview
for Borderlines (DIB)

The connotations and denotations of the term "borderline" vary widely by clinical settings, diagnostic standards, and theoretical formulations. As observed by Stone (1985), six distinct usages can be found for the term "borderline" in current clinical practice: (1) psychic organization, (2) syndrome, (3) personality disorder, (4) dynamic constellation, (5) prognostic statement, and (6) descriptor for interjacent states of spectrum psychoses. From these multiple sources, two perspectives have emerged as the most influential, namely, those of Kernberg and Gunderson.[1]

Kernberg (1967) postulated that borderline organizations represent severe impairment of ego integration and disturbed interpersonal relationships. He delineated the relatively primitive use of defense mechanisms (e.g., denial, splitting, projective identification), impulsivity, and instability of identity. In contrast, Gunderson and Singer (1975) offered a syndromal approach characterized by lowered achievement, impulsivity, manipulative suicidal threats, mild or brief psychotic episodes, good socialization, and disturbed relationships. Perry and Klerman (1978) provided a penetrating analysis, of the two systems. They concluded that the two systems are highly divergent with respect to affect and cognitive processes, although they found some similarities in interview behavior (e.g., angry, manipulative, and devaluative) and thought content (e.g., depersonalization, derealization, and intolerance of anxiety). In addition, both systems describe (1) personal histories marked by unpredictable behavior, self-mutilation, and substance abuse, and (2) profound problems in establishing interpersonal relationships.

Spitzer, Endicott, and Gibbon (1979) attempted to amalgamate Kernberg and Gunderson systems by identifying schizotypal and unstable criteria with 808 borderline and 808 control patients. Of these, the eight unstable criteria became the basis for DSM-III borderline personality disorder (BPD; see Stone,

---

[1]Other influential models are by Knight (1953) and Grinker, Werble, and Drye (1968).

1985), with two criteria specifically from the Kernberg system (identity disturbance, and chronic feelings of emptiness and boredom), five from the Gunderson system (unstable and intense relationships, inappropriate and intense anger, physically damaging acts, affective instability, and intolerance of being alone), and one criterion shared by both (impulsivity). An ambitious study by Perry and Klerman (1980) compared 104 separate criteria identified in the literature as discriminating features of borderlines and provided empirical support for the DSM-III model.

This chapter is devoted to a review of the Diagnostic Interview for Borderlines (DIB; Gunderson, 1982). In understanding the DIB, clinicians should benefit from appreciating its place in the enduring controversies over "borderline" as both a personality organization and an Axis II disorder.

OVERVIEW

The DIB comprises 123 items for assessing clinical characteristics of borderlines in addition to symptoms chiefly associated with psychotic and affective syndromes. The time of administration across patients varies substantially from 50 to 90 minutes. Items are composed of (1) structured questions, (2) tables of information to be completed from multiple sources, and (3) clinical observations. These items/ratings are organized into 29 "statements" or criteria related specifically to borderlines. The 29 criteria are subsequently categorized into five "sections" or scales. Box 10.1 provides a summary of the DIB and DIB-R.

BOX 10.1. Highlights of the DIB and DIB-R

- *Description:* The DIB is a semistructured interview that addressed five broad areas of functioning related to BPD. The DIB-R is a substantial revision, with changes in inquiries, organization, and scoring.
- *Administration time:* 50–90 minutes.
- *Skills level:* The DIB and DIB-R require experienced clinicians for their administration; training for these measures is relatively modest.
- *Distinctive features:* The DIB and DIB-R provide a standardized method of assessing Gunderson's model of BPD. The DIB surpasses the DIB-R in terms of reliability and validity.
- *Cost:* Single copies (DIB and DIB-R), which can be reproduced, are available free of charge.
- *Source:* Mary C. Zanarini, EdD, by mail, McLean Hospital, 115 Mill Street, Belmont, MA 02178-9106; by phone, (617) 855-2293; or by fax, (617) 855-3522.

The DIB is a semistructured diagnostic interview. Standard questions are presented verbatim. These inquiries are followed by unstructured questions for the clarification of individual ratings (e.g., frequency, duration, and circumstances) for a particular patient. Clinical data from other sources are also integrated into specific ratings; however, no item is scored as "present" without some confirmation from the patient.

The purpose of the DIB (Kolb & Gunderson, 1980) is to assess comprehensively five general dimensions of borderline functioning:

1. The *social adaptation* dimension combines an instability at work/school with substantial and socially appropriate involvements with others.
2. The *impulse action patterns* dimension consists of potentially self-destructive behavior (e.g., suicide attempts, self-mutilation, and drug abuse) and behavior that does not conform to social norms (e.g., sexual deviance and antisocial actions).
3. The *affects* dimension incorporates negative affect (e.g., dysphoria, anhedonia, anger, and depression) with demandingness and an absence of flat or elevated mood.
4. The *psychosis* dimension refers to transient psychotic experiences (derealization, depersonalization, paranoid experiences) in the absence of prolonged psychotic symptoms such as hallucinations and delusions.
5. The *interpersonal relations* dimension is characterized by unstable and dependent roles, an active avoidance of isolation, and several facets of impaired functioning (e.g., devaluation, manipulation, and splitting).

In discriminating between borderline patients and those with other disorders, Gunderson and Kolb (1978) believed that these dimensions form important criteria. These dimensions are viewed as closely related to seven cardinal features: low achievement, impulsivity, manipulative suicide attempts, heightened affectivity, mild psychotic experiences, high socialization, and disturbed close relationships.

DIB scoring is a multistep process. Ratings of individual items use the following metric: 0 for "no," 1 for "probable," and 2 for "yes" or "definite." Two variations in the scoring (see Gunderson, Kolb, & Austin, 1981) include (1) negative weights for symptoms of schizophrenia and mood disorders, and (2) greater weights (maximum of 4) for two cardinal features: manipulative suicide attempts and dissociative experiences. Individual items are synthesized into a global rating for the presence–absence of the 29 criteria. Scores for the five sections are "scaled" so that each section is rated from 0 to 2. Based on the data of Kolb and Gunderson (1980), any scaled score of ≥ 7 is used to designate BPD.

Gunderson et al. (1981) reported that the DIB was developed over 4 years of pilot testing and item refinement. Its content and parameters were based on a comprehensive review of the borderline literature by Gunderson and Singer (1975) and two longitudinal studies (Carpenter & Gunderson, 1977; Gunderson, Carpenter, & Strauss, 1975). According to Hurt, Clarkin, Koenigsberg, Frances, and Nurnberg (1986), the first draft of the DIB was authored by Gunderson and Kolb in 1976. Preliminary evidence from training interviews (cited in Kolb & Gunderson, 1980) suggested adequate reliability for individual items (M ICC = .66) and descriptive statements (M ICC = .77).

Zanarini, Gunderson, Frankenburg, and Chauncey (1989) described the development of the Diagnostic Interview for Borderlines—Revised (DIB-R) undertaken in the fall of 1982. Further modifications in the DIB-R in 1992 resulted in the most recent version (Gunderson & Zanarini, 1992). The DIB-R requires that the clinician address 96 individual ratings, 22 ratings of statements, and 8 ratings of sections, for a total of 127 criteria.

The DIB-R differs substantially from the DIB in the following ways with respect to its inquiries, organization, and scoring:

- Section reorganizations include (1) the deletion of *social adaptation* and (2) incorporation of *psychosis* into a new section, *cognitions,* which also includes nonpsychotic but disturbed thinking.
- The time framework for applying these scores has been standardized in the DIB-R based on the preceding 24 months.
- The *interpersonal relations* dimension was recast, with statements addressing an intolerance of being alone; fears of abandonment, engulfment, and annihilation; counterdependency; and problems in psychiatric treatment (i.e., regression, object of countertransference, and a "special relationship" with the therapist).
- The scoring was altered: Two sections, *impulse action patterns* and *interpersonal relations*, were given greater weights (0–3). The total score was modified to ≥ 8 to designate BPD.

Because of these fundamental changes, the DIB and DIB-R should be considered separate measures. Given the appreciable differences in time framework, individual ratings, summary statements, composite ratings, and total cut score, attempts to generalize from the DIB to the DIB-R would be improper. Moreover, only one study (Marziali, Munroe-Blum, & Links, 1994) has addressed the equivalence of the DIB and DIB-R. With 41 outpatients, Marziali et al. found a 70.7% rate of agreement. In light of the differences between the DIB and DIB-R and the paucity of convergent data, we must assume that these are two different but related measures.

Clinicians have a natural tendency to use the most updated version of standardized measures. As observed by Kaye and Shea (2000), however, most of the research addresses the DIB and not the DIB-R. In many cases, clinicians are likely to prefer the DIB to the DIB-R.

The DIB and DIB-R have been adapted to child samples for research purposes and are used either in retrospective review (Guzder, Paris, Zelkowitz, &

Marchessault, 1996) or direct interviews (Guzder, Paris, Zelkowitz, & Feldman, 1999). Compared with other children, those with borderline pathology evidence greater abuse (physical and sexual), neglect, family instability (separations and divorces), and parental crime (Gudzer et al., 1996). Because they have not been rigorously evaluated, the children's versions are not recommended for clinical practice. With research applications, the establishment of interrater and test–retest reliability is essential.

VALIDATION

Reliability of the DIB

More than a dozen studies have addressed the reliability of the DIB. In stark contrast, no reliability studies were found that evaluate the DIB-R. The lack of established reliability for the DIB-R was recently confirmed: "The reliability of the DIB-R has not been reported" (Kaye & Shea, 2000, p. 728).

DIB reliability studies are balanced between inpatient and outpatient samples with nearly all the research conducted by mental health professionals (see Table 10.1). The primary focus is on interrater reliability of DIB sections and diagnoses. The key findings are summarized as follows:

- The DIB diagnosis evidences moderate to excellent interrater reliabilities, with kappas ranging from .63 to 1.00 and very high ICCs (.92 in both studies).
- Test–retest reliability for DIB diagnosis is in the moderately high range (ICCs of .71 and .78).
- Reliabilities of DIB sections were higher for the original study (Gunderson et al., 1981) than for subsequent studies. Still, the reliabilities of individual sections appear to be good for interrater (.65) and adequate for test–retest (.54 and .55) reliabilities.
- Reliabilities of the 29 statements and 123 items were investigated only by Gunderson et al. (1981). Their data provide promising results: (1) Median ICC = .82 for statements, and (2) the majority of items (63.4%) had correlations ≥ .60.

In summary, the interrater reliability of the DIB diagnosis has been extensively researched and has produced very favorable results. Although backed by less research, the test–retest reliability of the DIB is clearly acceptable. In addition, DIB sections have adequate interrater and test–retest reliabilities. At the statement and item levels, results are very promising but require further validation.

Research has also evaluated the homogeneity of DIB sections through the use of Kuder–Richardson (KR) coefficients. Hurt et al. (1986) found modest KR coefficients, with a range of .32 to .69 (median of .53). Both interitem (.04 to .36) and item-scale (.09 to .60) correlations evidenced marked vari-

TABLE 10.1. Reliability Studies for the Diagnostic Interview for Borderlines (DIB)

Study (year)	N	Setting In/Out/Com/Univ	Raters Lay/Prof	Reliability Inter/Retest	(interval)	Reliability estimates Stat/Section	Cur-Dx
Gunderson et al. (1981)	70	✓	✓	✓	.82[a]	.92[a]	.92[a]
Kroll, Pyle, et al. (1981)	30	✓	✓	✓		.74	
Cornell et al. (1983)	12	✓	✓	✓		.66[b]	.71[b]
	24	✓	✓		✓ (14 days)	.55[b]	.71[b]
Koenigsberg et al. (1983)	88	✓	✓ (Lay)	✓			≥.75
Frances et al. (1984)	76	✓		✓		.72	
Hurt et al. (1984)	40	✓	✓[c]	✓		.63	
McManus, Lerner, et al. (1984)	48	✓[d]	✓	✓		.72	
Links, Steiner, et al. (1985)	26	✓	✓		✓ (3 mo)	.54[b]	.78[b]
Hurt et al. (1986)	140[e]	✓	✓[c]	✓			≥.75
Kullgren (1987)	23	✓	✓	✓		.68[a]	.92[a]
Angus & Marziali (1988)	6	✓	✓	✓		1.00	
Links, Mitton, et al. (1990)	12	✓	✓	✓		1.00	
Kavoussi et al. (1990)	56	✓	✓	✓		.79	

Note. See Table 1.5 (p. 35) for a glossary of terms and abbreviations. It is important to observe that all reliability studies use the DIB and not the DIB-R. Stat = 29 statements; Cur-Dx = current diagnosis of BPD. Reliability estimates are kappa coefficients unless otherwise specified.
[a] Intraclass coefficients.
[b] Correlations.
[c] Raters are simply designated as interviewers trained by Gunderson and Kolb.
[d] Adolescents.
[e] An unspecified subset of the total sample (N = 140) was used.

ability. Of the five scales, social adaptation appears to have very poor homogeneity. In practical terms, these findings suggest that DIB sections are not likely to measure a single construct.

Validity of the DIB

Concurrent Validity

Approximately one dozen studies have investigated the concurrent validity of the DIB–DIB-R in comparison to DSM diagnoses. Most studies (11 of 13 samples) focused on the original DIB (see Table 10.2). Unfortunately, our conclusions are tempered by two methodological limitations: (1) The majority of studies simply report concordance rates that do not take into account

TABLE 10.2. Concurrent Validity of the Diagnostic Interview for Borderlines (DIB) and DIB—Revised (DIB-R)

Study	Version	Sample (BPD)	Measures	Kappa	Concordance
Kolb & Gunderson (1980)	DIB	70 inpatients (32)	Clinical	.52	.77
Kroll, Sines, et al. (1981)	DIB	117 inpatients (10)	Clinical		.33
Cornell et al. (1983)	DIB	24 inpatients (21)	Clinical		.92
Koenigsberg et al. (1983)	DIB	88 patients (40)	Clinical	.45	.58
McManus, Lerner, et al. (1984)[a]	DIB	48 inpatients (16)	Clinical		.75
Armelius et al. (1985)	DIB	16 inpatients (4)	Records	.64[b]	
Nelson et al. (1985)	DIB	51 inpatients (20)	Clinical		.78
Hurt et al. (1986)[c]	DIB	140 patients (33)	Clinical		.77
Angus & Marziali (1988)	DIB	22 outpatients (20)	PDE	.08	.35
Zanarini, Gunderson, & Frankenburg (1989)	DIB-R	237 patients (95)	Clinical		.80
Kavousssi et al. (1990)	DIB	56 outpatients (27)	SCID-II	.42	.64
Marziali et al. (1994)	DIB	171 outpatients (171)	Clinical		.77
	DIB-R	41 outpatients (41)	Clinical		.71

Note. BPD = number of participants with BPD; clinical = clinical diagnoses; patients = combined sample of inpatients and outpatients; PDE = Personality Disorder Examination; SCID-II = Structured Clinical Interview for DSM-IV—Axis II Disorders.
[a]Adolescent sample.
[b]Correlations of DIB ratings of hospital records with independent DIB interviews.
[c]Programmatic research apparently including data from earlier studies (Frances et al., 1984; Hurt et al., 1984).

base rates, and (2) three studies have very modest sample sizes (< 25). Nevertheless, two important observations emerge:

1. The five studies reporting kappas evidence a low-moderate agreement (median kappa = .45). This estimate is likely to be inflated given that the average base rate across these five studies (48.8%) is very high.
2. The overall concordance rate suggests approximately two-thirds agreement (unweighted M = .68) between the DIB–DIB-R and clinical diagnoses. The two studies using structured Axis II interviews produced lower concordances (i.e., .35 and .64).

Kaye and Shea (2000) cautions that the DIB[2] should not be used for rendering DSM-IV diagnoses because of differences in conceptualization. In light of its concurrent validity, I concur. The data in Table 10.2 suggest that the DIB is a construct closely related to the DSM BPD. However, the level of correspondence does not suggest that DIB classification could be substituted for DSM diagnoses.

Several studies (e.g., Bateman, 1989; Morika, Miyake, Minakawa, Ikuta, & Nishizono-Maher, 1993) that compare DIB classification with Present State Examination (PSE) diagnoses have produced disappointing results. However, interpretation of these negative findings must be tempered by the substantial differences in diagnostic systems and the lack of PSE syndromes that correspond to the cardinal features of BPD.

Discriminant Validity

In addition to studies of concurrent validity, researchers have investigated the extent to which DIB scores discriminate between diagnostic groups. By examining group differences, researchers have evaluated the discriminability of the DIB.[3] In the original study, Gunderson and Kolb (1978) sought to discriminate among 31 borderline, 22 schizophrenic, and 11 neurotically depressed inpatients. Although the results of a stepwise discriminant analysis were very promising, their interpretability is severely constrained by sample size. Since this first study, discriminant validity has been examined at three levels: 29 statements, five sections, and total scores.

Five studies systematically evaluated differences in DIB statements by diagnoses, with three studies focusing on Axis I comparisons (Hurt et al., 1986; McManus, Brickman, Alessi, & Grapentine, 1984; Soloff & Ulrich, 1981). Soloff and Ulrich (1981) compared 23 patients with BPD to 22 patients with schizophrenia and 20 patients with depression. They found sig-

---

[2]While directed at the DIB, Kaye and Shea (2000) concluded that the DIB-R lacks demonstrated reliability and has substantially less validation than the DIB.

[3]The capacity of cut scores to differentiate between criterion groups is often designated as "discriminant validity." This usage must be distinguished from the more common reference in construct validation to "convergent validity" and "discriminant validity."

nificant differences between borderlines and the other two diagnoses on many of the 29 statements. Unfortunately, the differences were highly variable by diagnostic group (i.e., schizophrenia vs. depression). Interestingly, the most pronounced differences were observed for statements in two sections: impulsive actions and interpersonal relations. In the second of the Axis I studies, McManus, Brickman, et al. (1984) used similar diagnostic groups but limited their sample to delinquent adolescents. They found relatively few differences between adolescents with BPD and those with (1) mood disorders (5 of 29 statements) and (2) schizophrenia (0 of 29 statements). In the third Axis I study, Hurt et al. (1986) found that 18 of 29 statements differentiated between BPD and schizophrenia. In summary, the McManus et al. (1984) study produced disparate results that may be explained by the questionable usefulness of the DIB with acting-out adolescents.

A different approach to discriminant validity is the use of near-neighbor comparisons by evaluating the discriminability of DIB statements between borderline and other personality disorders. For example, Barrash, Kroll, Carey, and Sines (1983) compared inpatients with BPD to those with other personality disorders. Limited by their methodology (i.e., 18 patients with BPD divided into two groups), they found differences on only 6 of the 29 statements. Likewise, Kullgren (1987) found relatively few differences (5 of 29) for DIB statements in comparison to other personality disorders. Interestingly, Kullgren's differences were exclusively in interpersonal relations. In contrast to Barrash et al. and Kullgren, Hurt et al. (1986) reported differences in 15 of 29 statements.

Discriminant validity has also been examined for section and total DIB scores. As summarized in Table 10.3, all sections except for social adaptation appear to have moderately good discriminant validity. In contrast, total DIB scores do not appear to have consistent discriminability. Of seven comparisons (see Table 10.3), only three are significant.

In summary, studies of DIB discriminant validity are mixed, with the most positive results for the DIB sections. An obvious challenge to discriminant validity is diagnostic overlap; Zanarini, Gunderson, and Frankenburg (1989) found that most patients with BPD also qualify for mood and substance abuse disorders. Not surprisingly, results for DIB statements appear greater for distant (e.g., schizophrenia) than for near-neighbor comparisons. What accounts for these mixed results? Research by Rippetoe, Alarcon, and Walter-Ryan (1986) provides important insights. They found that borderline symptoms appear to be moderated by comorbidity. For example, feelings of emptiness and boredom were much more frequent in patients with BPD plus depression (61.3%) than BPD alone (25.0%).[4] The formidable challenge to studies of discriminant validity is the substantial comorbidity of both Axis I

---

[4]Westen et al. (1992) also demonstrated qualitative differences in symptoms that may distinguish depression from BPD + depression.

TABLE 10.3. Significant Differences between BPD and Other Disorders on Diagnostic Interview for Borderlines (DIB) Section and Total Scores

Study	DIB sections						Total DIB
	Disorders	Social	Impulse	Affects	Psychosis	Interpersonal	
Soloff & Ulrich (1981)	MS	S	MS	S	MS	MS	*
Frances et al. (1984)	P		P	P	P	P	*
McManus, Brickman, et al. (1984)	MPS		P	MP	MP	P	*
Kroll, Sines, et al. (1981)[a]	MSP	*	*	*	*	*	MS
Koenigsberg et al. (1983)	PS	*	*	*	*	*	P
Bateman (1989)	NS	*	*	*	*	*	

Note. Disorders = diagnostic categories used for comparisons. For DIB sections, Social = social adaptation; Impulse = impulse action patterns; Interpersonal = interpersonal relations. Significant differences are denoted for specific diagnostic categories: M = mood disorders; N = neurotic disorders; P = other personality disorders; S = schizophrenia or other psychotic disorder. * = no comparisons are available.
[a]Statistics are not provided; both S and M have > 2.5 difference in total DIB score.

and Axis II disorders with BPD. In light of this comorbidity, the results (especially for the DIB sections) must be considered relatively robust.

Outcome Studies with the DIB

Consistent with the Syndeham criteria, DIB research has investigated the longitudinal perspectives of BPD, including studies of both antecedent conditions and outcome data. This research is organized into three categories: (1) antecedent conditions and risk factors, (2) course of BPD, and (3) treatment response and outcome.

Antecedent Conditions and Risk Factors. Research on the DIB has identified the following important risk factors and precursors of BPD:

1. Weiss et al. (1996) addressed an intergenerational hypothesis for BPD by comparing children of mothers with BPD to those with other disorders. Offspring of borderline mothers had an increased risk of not only borderline pathology (33.3% vs. 8.7%) but also disruptive behavior disorder (66.7% vs. 34.8%) and attention-deficit/hyperactivity disorder (ADHD; 42.8% vs. 13.0%). Based on this modest study, maternal BPD appears to be a general risk factor for child psychopathology not limited to BPD. Without long-term follow-up, the true nature of maternal and child BPD remains unknown.
2. Wood, Parmelee, and Arents (1992) explored symptoms that appear

best to predict childhood borderline syndrome, utilizing a retrospective DIB diagnosis. They found that the following symptoms occur frequently (≥ 75.0%): angry affect, unhappiness/anhedonia, depression, manipulation/devaluation, and suicidal thoughts/behavior. Interestingly, the three most prevalent symptoms addressed mood rather than behavior.

3. Predictors of borderline pathology in school-age children include physical and sexual abuse, neglect, parental separations and divorces, and parental criminality (Guzder et al., 1999).

4. Children with borderline pathology do not appear to differ in overall intellectual functioning from children with other disorders, although some deficits in executive functioning have been observed (Paris, Zelkowitz, Guzder, Joseph, & Feldman, 1999).

5. Adult inpatients with child sexual abuse histories evidence much higher DIB-R scores, especially on interpersonal relations, than their nonabused counterparts (Loebel, 1992).

In summary, DIB research has identified potential risk factors for borderline pathology that appear associated with unstable and conflictual families. Histories of abuse appear especially common. The relationship of adverse conditions and family pathology to BPD in offspring is complicated by the multiple comorbid diagnoses frequently observed in both children and adults with BPD.

Course of BPD. An important dimension of diagnostic validity is the establishment of a predictable course for BPD. Pope and his colleagues (Pope, Jonas, Hudson, Cohen, & Gunderson, 1983; Pope, Jonas, Hudson, Cohen, & Tohen, 1985) examined 33 patients with BPD (≥ 6 on the DIB) in a follow-up after an interval of 4 to 7 years. To complicate researchers' understanding of the course of BPD, most patients qualified for at least two additional diagnoses. Of clinical interest, the patients with BPD and a major mood disorder appeared to have marginally better outcomes (global rating of 1.86) than patients with BPD without the affective component (global rating of 1.27). Moreover, patients with BPD without mood disorders responded very poorly to medications. Overall, few patients with BPD were performing adequately in social relations and occupational functioning at follow-up. With respect to outcome criteria, the diagnosis of BPD remained stable for approximately two-thirds of the sample. In summary, the Pope et al. (1983, 1985) offer preliminary evidence of BPD as a chronic and debilitating disorder. Conclusions are hampered by the existence of multiple disorders and substantial changes in these disorders during the follow-up period.

Silk, Lohr, Ogata, and Westen (1990), in line with the Pope et al. (1985) study, followed up 9 borderline patients (interval from 1 to 3.5 years) with previous but not current depression. Patients improved significantly improvement on the DIB, particularly with respect to affect and psychosis, although most patients continued to meet the DSM-III BPD diagnosis. Without comparison groups of never-depressed and still-depressed borderlines, these results are difficult to interpret.

Programmatic research by Links and his colleagues (Links, Heselgrave, Mitton, Van Reekum, & Patrick, 1995; Links, Heselgrave, & Van Reekum, 1999; Links, Mitton, & Steiner, 1990) has investigated differences between chronic and remitted cases of BPD. At a 7-year follow-up, 52.6% were no longer diagnosed with BPD. Chronic cases were characterized by a high number of borderline symptoms at baseline and comorbidity for major depression and dysthymia. Impulsivity appeared to play a prominent role in maintaining chronicity (Links et al., 1999). Taken together, these studies suggest that problems with severity (high number of borderline symptoms) and comorbidity (depressive disorders) appear to play instrumental roles in influencing the course of BPD and potential its response to treatment.

In summary, BPD does not appear to be as chronic as once assumed. Either through treatment or the natural course of the disorder, substantial numbers of patients with BPD no longer warrant the diagnosis at follow-up. Drawing from the Links et al. studies, severity of BPD and comorbidity factors contribute to chronicity.

Treatment Response and Outcome. Outcome criteria for BPD have also been studied in relationship to treatment response. Kelly et al. (1992) found that our ability to study treatment response in patients with BPD is compromised by treatment refusal (25.4%) and treatment noncompliance (46.4%).[5] They found that premature terminations appear to be associated with greater impairment at baseline and less improvement during the initial 6 weeks of treatment. Those remaining in treatment demonstrated modest but significant gains. The study underscores both the challenges of successfully treating inpatients with BPD and treatment factors that may contribute to the chronicity of the disorder. Links, Steiner, Boiago, and Irwin (1990) also experienced high rates of noncompliance. Only 26 of 43 (60.5%) DIB borderline patients refused to participate in a drug treatment study, and 7 of the 17 (41.2%) did not complete the treatment protocol. Predictably, the marked instability of borderlines is reflected in problems with treatment compliance.

Zanarini, Frankenburg, and Gunderson (1988) evaluated treatment effectiveness for 50 outpatients with both DSM and DIB-R diagnoses of BPD. In response to various medications, approximately 50% of outpatients with BPD/APD evidenced some improvement, although marked improvement occurred in less than 15% of the cases. As acknowledged by the authors, the research was constrained by its methodological limitations.

---

[5]These percentages are not additive, because only a subsample of those agreeing to participate met all inclusion criteria.

Soloff, George, Cornelius, Nathan, and Schulz (1991) studied differences in pharmacological responses for BPD, schizotypal personality disorder (SPD), and combined BPD–SPD. The diagnosis of BPD was established with the DIB ($\geq$ 7). Of 85 consecutive admissions, 34 were diagnosed with BPD and 50 with BPD–SPD. Drug trials (i.e., haloperidol, amitriptyline, and placebo) lasted 5 weeks. As expected, BPD–SPD patients had a greater decrease in symptoms than patients with BPD when treated with haloperidol. However, the patients with BPD also evidenced considerable improvement. Interestingly, the clinical status of both groups significantly improved with antidepressant treatment.

Construct Validity

Barrash et al. (1983) examined DIB and DSM-III diagnosis of BPD via cluster analysis. Two clusters of BPD emerged. Cluster 1 borderlines (compared to Cluster 2 and nonborderline patients) exhibited social isolation, unstable work histories, less appropriate appearance, and less disturbed interpersonal relationships. In contrast, Cluster 2 borderlines were very social, intolerant of being alone, generally more impulsive, and involved in intense but unstable relationships. Both clusters were characterized by self-mutilation, manipulative suicidal gestures, splitting, and regression in treatment. Use of these clusters improved the identification of DSM-III-diagnosed borderlines.

Several studies (e.g., Derksen, 1990; Kullgren & Armelius, 1990) have examined the convergent validity of the DIB with the Structural Interview (SI) by Kernberg (1981). The term "structural" refers to personality structure (*not* a structured interview); the SI is a psychoanalytically oriented interview that evaluates identity diffusion and primitive defense mechanisms found in borderlines. Derksen (1990) administered the DIB and SI to 20 patients with eating disorders and 43 patients with Axis II disorders. The level of agreement between the two measures was only moderate (62.5%) and suggested that some persons may have borderline organization on SI without borderline behavior on the DIB. Kullgren and Armelius (1990) examined 44 psychiatric inpatients with the SI and DIB. They found that SI scores for the borderline organization were elevated (M= 5.7, SD = 1.9) but generally below the DIB cut score ($\geq$ 7) for borderlines. Both studies provide modest evidence of convergent validity across two distinct models of borderline pathology.

Swartz et al. (1990) developed from the DIS a borderline index consisting of 24 borderline symptoms (see Chapter 3). As a measure of concurrent validity this index was compared to the DIB. Using a cut score of $\geq$ 11, the two measures evidenced a high convergence (> 80%) and a moderate coefficient of agreement (kappa = .67) on 79 psychiatric patients. Similarly, D'Angelo (1991) found a high correlation (r = .82) between the DIB and the Borderline Syndrome Index.

Psychological Tests. Convergent validity for the DIB has also been examined with respect to traditional psychological tests. Key findings are summarized as follows:

1. Borderline patients appear to have markedly elevated clinical profiles on the MMPI. Hurt, Clarkin, Frances, Abrams, and Hunt (1985) found higher and clinically relevant elevations on Scales F, 6, 7, and 8 in comparison to non-BPD patients. Jonsdottir-Baldursson and Horvath (1987) found that BPD inpatients in treatment for alcoholism had similar MMPI elevations (Scales F, 2, 4, 7, and 8). Because these clinical elevations are common to other diagnoses, these studies offer only general evidence of impairment. Interestingly, practitioners should be cautious in interpreting Scale F because T scores ≥ 100 are not uncommon (Horvath & Jonsdottir-Baldursson, 1990).
2. Borderline inpatients tend to score higher than nonborderline inpatients on several SCL-90-R scales and the Global Severity Index (Edell et al., 1990). The usefulness of this finding is limited by the lack of clinical elevation in these scales, which remains generally low (i.e., less than 50 except for the Hostility scale, $M = 53.0$).
3. The DIB correlated moderately with the MCMI borderline scale ($r = .62$; Sansone & Fine, 1992), although the level of diagnostic agreement remained modest (55.6%; Sansone, Fine, Seuferer, & Bovenzi, 1989). The problem appears to be with the MCMI borderline scale, which is elevated with many personality disorders (Divac-Jovanovic, Svrakic, & Lecic-Tosevski, 1993). Given the fundamental differences between MCMI revisions, these findings cannot be extrapolated to the MCMI-II or the MCMI-III (see Rogers et al., 1999).
4. Initial data (Singer & Larson, 1981) suggested that a specialized Rorschach scoring system with 30 subscores on ego functioning may have promise in classifying patients with DIB-based BPD. However, without cross-validation, this specially constructed scoring system remains preliminary.

Not surprisingly, traditional psychological tests have little to offer in establishing the convergent validity of the DIB. As expected, patients with DIB tend to evidence more elevations than their non-DIB counterparts. Because these tests, with the exception of the MCMI, do not have specialized scales for BPD, the lack of definitive results is understandable.

Other Correlates. DIB studies have sought to link BPD classification to problematic behaviors (e.g., suicide attempts) and biological markers (e.g., EEG abnormalities). Not unexpectedly, these general efforts often have had only modest success. For example, Kullgren found that (1) patients with BPD were not overrepresented among completed suicides (Kullgren, Renberg, & Jacobsson, 1986), and (2) DIB scores did not differentiate between suicidal and nonsuicidal patients with BPD (Kullgren, 1988).

EEG and other biological markers have been explored in patients with BPD. Reynolds et al. (1985) found substantial differences in the sleep patterns of (1) patients with BPD and mood disturbance, and (2) controls. However, very few differences were noted between the BPD and depression-only groups. This lack of difference may be attributable to the depressive symptoms of the BPD group itself. Lahmeyer et al. (1988) found that patients with BPD slept more efficiently than patients with major depression, although the sleep architecture was very similar. Differences were observed in lithium transport, dexamethasone suppression, and mononamine oxidase activity, although these laboratory tests did not reveal consistent differences between BPD and major depression.

CLINICAL APPLICATIONS

The DIB and DIB-R are best conceptualized as two distinct, although related, measures of BPD. Fundamental differences in questions, time framework, and scoring argue against treating the DIB-R as simply an extension of the DIB (Kaye & Shea, 2000). Systematic studies of their comparability are clearly needed.

The great bulk of the research addresses the DIB, which is therefore likely to be the measure of choice in the clinical investigation of borderlines. In the absence of published data indicating its reliability, the DIB-R has very limited clinical applicability. Practitioners who wish to employ the DIB-R in their professional practices bear the rather onerous responsibility of establishing their own reliabilities in cooperation with their colleagues.

Simmering controversies over the nature and classification of BPD continue unabated. Whether the Gunderson and Singer (1975) model of borderlines is "correct" remains unresolved. For clinicians endorsing the Gunderson model, the DIB provides a format for conceptualizing patients' clinical characteristics vis-à-vis its five sections. Interpretations based on DIB sections appear warranted for the following reasons:

- A moderate level of reliability has been achieved consistently for the DIB sections.
- The DIB sections appear to have discriminant validity, especially with distant-neighbor comparisons. Given this validity and underlying theory, the DIB sections are likely to augment the conceptualization of BPD.

Interestingly, Gunderson (2000) has taken a much more conservative view of DIB sections. He has argued that they should *not* be used because "their reliability has not be demonstrated, and the developers did not intend for these scales to be interpreted" (p. 728). The first argument appears unduly negative; interrater reliability coefficients (see Table 10.1) appear more than adequate for three interrater reliability studies (i.e., median coefficients of .66, .68, and .92, respectively) and adequate for two test–retest reliability studies. The second argument about original intent is unpersuasive. The fundamental question is whether DIB validity supports these interpretations for the DIB sections.

The 29 statements are best viewed as explicit hypotheses. Although these statements may provide valuable suppositions about a patient's dynamics and functioning, their reliability and validity remain largely unknown. To avoid any misunderstandings, clinicians may wish to label specifically any of the 29 statements used in clinical reports as "hypotheses."

The DIB should not be employed as a substitute for BPD diagnoses. Very high scores on the DIB (≥ 8) are most often found with borderlines, although cases have been reported in which nonborderlines received a score of 10, the highest score (see McManus, Lerner, et al., 1984). Conversely, substantial numbers of BPD subjects score in the middle range (4–6) on the DIB. Despite moderate to high concordance rates between DIB and DSM, the DIB should not be used to establish DSM diagnoses. The reasons are twofold: First, coefficients that take into account base rates produce only moderate results (see Table 10.2); second, the two models are highly divergent in their conceptualization of BPD (see Gunderson, 2000). Although most DIB research was conducted before the publication of DSM-IV, the two substantive changes are likely to have little effect on the clinical usefulness of the DIB in relationship to the DSM. Indeed, one change in the DSM-IV inclusion criteria would appear to increase the correspondence between DSM-IV and DIB. Specifically, the DSM-IV addition of transient dissociative or paranoid symptoms is similar to the psychotic section on the DIB. The effect of the second change (i.e., the redefinition of identity disturbance) appears to be less clear in DSM-IV–DIB conceptualizations.

Borderline patients are often viewed as notoriously poor informants, with substantial numbers having a factitious component to their presentation (Pope et al., 1983). For example, Links, Steiner, and Mitton (1989) found that most patients (86.4%) with BPD had questionable psychotic symptoms. When limited to factitious symptoms, the percentage was substantially lower (13.2%). Beyond factitious symptoms per se, patients with BPD frequently engage in other forms of deception (Ford, King, & Hollender, 1988).

One potential problem with feigning and deception on the DIB is that its structure is relatively transparent. Transparency is observed in the face validity of its individual items, clustering of similar items, and unidimensional scoring (i.e., endorsements are almost invariably evidence of psychopathology). Intuitively, this transparency increases the likelihood that BPD and non-BPD patients can distort their clinical presentation without detection. In clinical practice, psychologists may wish to employ psychological tests in addition to structured interviews with borderline patients. For example, the Personality Assessment Inventory (PAI; Morey, 1991b) has both a borderline scale and well-established validity scales.

The DIB has been used successfully with adolescent and adult populations. One pilot study (Rosowsky & Gurian, 1991) with the DIB-R questioned its usefulness with geriatric populations. Based on clinical diagnoses, none of the 8 patients with BPD were identified. However, DSM-III-R diagnoses disagreed with clinicians' diagnoses in 75% of the cases. Given its minimal sample, poor concordance with DSM-II-R criteria, and use of the DIB-R, the relevance of this study to the DIB with geriatric patients remains obscure. Nevertheless, clinicians may wish to take special care in evaluating subthreshold geriatric patients.

The DIB has been successfully employed in a variety of mental health and medical practices. Among medical settings, the DIB has been utilized in primary health care facilities to evaluate medical conditions such as obesity (Sansone, Sansone, & Fine, 1992) and obstetric complications (Dahl & Bordahl, 1993). Clinicians may wish to consider selective application of the DIB in settings where borderline pathology is commonly observed.

The major advantages of the DIB are summarized as follows:

1. The DIB was carefully designed, based on the Gunderson and Singer (1975) model of BPD. This model has been tested and refined for more than two decades.
2. The DIB provides exhaustive coverage of symptoms associated with BPD. While rationally derived, its systematic review of BPD symptoms has substantial clinical value.
3. The DIB total score and sections have satisfactory to good reliability.

To provide a balanced review, the following major disadvantages of the DIB must also be delineated:

1. The DIB's exhaustive coverage is also a potential liability, since its 50- to 90-minute administration time may burden clinical resources. Other structured interviews, such as the PDE and SIDP, provide full coverage of Axis II interviews with approximately the same expenditure of time.
2. The DIB is not intended to yield DSM-IV diagnoses; clinicians must resist the temptation to substitute its classification for DSM-IV.
3. Relatively little is known about the usefulness of the DIB with different cultural populations. As an extrapolation from the DIB-R, research by Ikuta et al. (1994) provides a useful illustration. A Japanese translation provided small but significantly lower total scores, with differences on two of the four sections.

In summary, the DIB is likely to have specialized applications in settings where treatment and clinical interventions are consistent with the Gunderson and Singer model. The DIB provides the broadest coverage that is both more comprehensive and substantially divergent from the DSM-IV. In contrast to the DIB, the DIB-R is not recommended for clinical practice except in those rare circumstances in which practitioners are willing to establish their own reliability.

11

Structured Interview
of Reported Symptoms (SIRS)

Clinical assessment is highly dependent on patients' honesty and self-disclosure (Rogers, 1997; Rogers & Vitacco, in press). Among different response styles, malingering poses special challenges for mental health professionals, who must distinguish fabricated and grossly exaggerated symptomatology from genuine presentations. The assessment of malingering is not a simple dichotomy of feigning versus honest responding. A substantial but unknown percentage of malingerers also have genuine mental disorders.

One traditional perspective is that malingering has a very low base rate in most clinical settings; therefore, its assessment should occur on a very selective basis. Recent surveys (Rogers, Sewell, & Goldstein, 1994; Rogers, Salekin, Sewell, Goldstein, & Leonard, 1998) strongly rebut this perspective. Estimates from more than 500 forensic psychologists suggest that issues of malingering occur in approximately 7% of nonforensic cases. While these estimates are likely to be slightly inflated by the types of nonforensic cases referred to forensic specialists, these estimates remain substantial. Infrequency cannot be used as a justification for neglecting the assessment of malingering.

OVERVIEW

Description

The Structured Interview of Reported Symptoms (SIRS) was developed by Rogers and his colleagues (Rogers, 1992; Rogers, Bagby, & Dickens, 1992) to assess different response styles, particularly the feigning of mental disorders. Feigning is defined as the deliberate fabrication or gross exaggeration of

---

BOX 11.1. Highlights of the SIRS

- *Description:* The SIRS is a structured interview for the assessment of feigning and related response styles.
- *Administration time:* Typical administration time with impaired populations is 30–45 minutes.
- *Skills level:* SIRS administration requires clinicians with graduate training. High levels of reliability can be achieved with only moderate training.
- *Distinctive features:* The SIRS systematically evaluates eight detection strategies for feigning. Decision rules are implemented that greatly reduce the likelihood of false positives (< .03). Descriptive data are provided about defensive and random responding.
- *Cost:* As of 3/1/2001, the SIRS introductory kit (manual and 25 protocols) = $209.
- *Source:* The SIRS is commercially available through Psychological Assessment Resources (PAR), by phone, (800) 331-8378; by fax, (800) 727-9329; on the internet, *www.parinc.com*, or by mail, P.O. Box 998, Odessa, FL 33556.

---

psychological or physical symptoms. Unlike malingering, the term "feigning" does not specify the type of intentional motivation (Rogers & Vitacco, in press); it is the preferred term for psychological measures because a person's motivation cannot be inferred from his or her bogus performance.

The SIRS is composed of 172 items organized into eight primary and five supplementary scales. Box 11.1 provides information about the SIRS and its availability. Scales are designated as "primary" if their cut scores consistently differentiate feigners from clinical and community samples.[1] The eight primary scales are based on well-validated detection strategies:

- Three primary scales examine very unusual symptom presentation in terms of infrequency (i.e., rare symptoms [RS]), preposterous content (i.e., improbable and absurd symptoms [IA]), and atypical symptom pairs (i.e., symptom combinations [SC]).
- Four primary scales address the range and severity of symptom endorsements, including obvious symptoms of a major mental disorder (i.e., blatant symptoms [BL], symptoms more likely to be associated

---

[1]Statistically significant differences were also found for supplementary scales (see, e.g., Rogers, Gillis, Dickens, et al., 1991). However, the overlap of distributions militated against the effective use of cut scores.

with minor psychological problems (subtle symptoms [SU], indiscriminant endorsement of symptoms (i.e., selectivity of symptoms [SEL]), and overendorsement of symptoms with extreme or unbearable severity (i.e., severity of symptoms [SEV]).

• The remaining primary scale inspects differences between self-report and observation (i.e., reported vs. observed symptoms [RO]).

Some individuals who feign mental disorders focus mostly on the range and severity of symptoms (i.e., BL, SU, SEL, and SEV), while others manifest a less recognizable scattering of elevations. Persons who fabricate grossly psychotic presentations sometimes evidence marked elevations on the majority of primary scales.

The SIRS is a structured rather than a semistructured interview. In other words, the format disallows clinicians from asking their own unstructured questions during the formal administration of the SIRS. Once the SIRS is completed, clinicians are permitted to ask for an amplification of key questions. One valuable use of this postinquiry phase is to solicit examples. For instance, a clinician may desire examples of reported neologisms. The rationale for making the SIRS a structured interview is to minimize the possibility of interactional factors influencing either (1) the types of unstructured questions employed and (2) the nonstandardized interpretation of responses to these questions. In addition, a less structured format might occasionally allow a clinician to express implicitly or explicitly his or her perceptions of the patient's credibility, thereby negatively affecting rapport and possibly influencing subsequent responses to the SIRS.

SIRS items are scored on a 3-point scale: 0 = "no" or nondeviant responses, and 1 and 2 = increasing gradations of endorsement (Rogers, Bagby, et al., 1992). Different criteria are employed for scoring 1's and 2's based on the type of questions involved. For detailed inquiries, the scoring reflects severity: 1 = a "major problem," and 2 = an "unbearable problem." For general inquiries, the scoring reflects the level of certainty: 1 = a qualified endorsement, and 2 = an unconditional endorsement.

The chief purpose of the SIRS scales is the accurate classification of feigning and bona fide patients. Guidelines are offered for the further specification of feigning into malingering and factitious disorders.[2] In addition to DSM-IV (American Psychiatric Association, 1994) and the DSM-IV Text Revision (DSM-IV-TR; American Psychiatric Association, 2000) definitions of malingering, the SIRS manual offers an empirically derived model for the classification of malingering. Rogers (1990a, 1990b) proposed detection strategies for the overall classification of malingering that were cross-validated with both test and interview data. The SIRS integrated into these criteria in making classifications of malingering. Beyond malingering and facti-

---

[2]See Rogers, Bagby, and Rector (1989) for a discussion of diagnostic and conceptual problems inherent in factitious disorders with psychological symptoms.

tious disorders, the SIRS offers descriptive information on defensive and inconsistent responding.

Rationale

A structured interview was chosen over self-report inventories for several reasons (Rogers, Bagby, et al., 1992). First, in the absence of a gold standard, psychologists most often rely on clinical interviews in making their determinations of malingering and factitious disorders. The development of a structured interview would likely enhance this form of assessment. Moreover, research data (Tesser & Paulhus, 1983; Tetlock & Manstead, 1985) have clearly shown that persons may respond differently to self-report measures than to interview methods. To assume facilely that faked test results reflects a pervasive pattern of feigning is not empirically supported.

A second and closely related reason for developing a structured interview stems from the importance of the decisions related to response style and the concomitant need for a multimethod approach. Since determinations of feigning are likely to have far-reaching social consequences that often include the cessation of mental health services, clinicians should render their decisions on multiple sources, based on interview and psychometric data (Rogers, 1990a).

Development

Rogers (1984) conducted a comprehensive review of existing research and case studies on malingering, with the overriding goal of determining potential strategies for the identification of malingerers. This review yielded a total of 22 strategies, of which 15 were selected for further investigation with the SIRS. On a rational basis, a total of 330 items were generated preliminary to these 15 strategies. Items were refined and tested on several inpatient samples to examine their fluency and transparency (i.e., ease with which they were recognized as bogus symptoms; Rogers & Resnick, 1988).

SIRS items were refined by eight experts, who rendered independent judgments about their relevance to specific detection strategies for feigning. Combined with independent judgments by Rogers, only items with a minimum two-thirds concordance were included. In general, the concordance was very high for the selected items ($M = 88.2\%$). As a final refinement, scale homogeneity was enhanced by dropping three items that had very low item–scale correlations.

VALIDATION

Research on SIRS validation is summarized and described separately in three sections: reliability, validity, and generalizability.

Reliability

Research with 24 inpatients on an early version of the SIRS (Rogers, 1988, p. 265) suggested that good reliabilities (i.e., r's > .80) were achievable. In the final version of the SIRS, the major focus was on achieving superb interrater reliabilities for the SIRS scales for two reasons. First, response styles are seen as situational rather than invariant. Depending on individual circumstances and goals, patients may change their objectives from feigning to nonfeigning. Second, the SIRS is not intended for repeat administrations, especially with brief intervals. Knowledge and anticipation of SIRS items may influence responses. In a third consideration, the type of samples utilized for reliability, inpatient samples were considered the most stringent test because patients' level of impairment might affect the quality of their responses.

In the four reliability studies summarized in Table 11.1, interrater reliabilities were uniformly high for both professionals and paraprofessionals. Across these studies, the minimum reliability for any individual scale is .78. Median reliabilities range from .95 to 1.00. These estimates include both standardized administrations and a slightly modified version that assesses past episodes (Goodness, 1999).

Rogers, Bagby, et al. (1992) also evaluated the internal reliability of SIRS scales by computing alpha coefficients based on data from three separate studies. For the primary scales, alpha coefficients ranged from good to superb (i.e., .77 to .92; median = .87).[3] These alphas provided strong support of the internal reliability of SIRS primary scales. Although lower, SIRS supplementary scales evidenced satisfactory alphas (.66 to .82; median = .76).

Validity

Methodological Issues

Validation of response styles requires the use of specific research models. Rogers, Harrell, and Liff (1993) briefly defined the three most common research models:

1. *Simulation research* is an analogue design, with participants randomly assigned to honest and feigning conditions. In addition, a clinical comparison sample is typically employed for the crucial discrimination between genuinely disordered and feigned presentations. The simulation research capitalizes on internal validity but has serious limitations in generalizability.

2. *Known-groups comparison* uses independent classification by mental health professionals to categorize malingerers and genuine patients. The resulting comparisons capitalize on external validity in studying actual malin-

---

[3]Two primary scales (SEL and SEV) involve arithmetic summing for which measures of internal consistency are inappropriate.

TABLE 11.1. Reliability Studies of the Structured Interview of Reported Symptoms (SIRS)

Study (year)	N	Setting		Raters		Reliability	SIRS scales
		In/Out/Corr		Lay/Prof		Inter/Retest (interval)	Median (Range)
Rogers, Gillis, Dickens, et al. (1991)	27	✓		✓ ✓		✓	.96 (.89–1.00)
Rogers, Bagby, et al. (1992)	10	✓		✓		✓	1.00 (.92–1.00)
Linblad (1993)	6		✓	✓		✓	.95 (.87–.97)
Goodness (1999)[a]	10	✓		✓		✓	1.00 (1.00–1.00)
Rogers & Grandjean (2000)	14	✓[b]		✓ ✓			.99 (.78–1.00)

Note. See Table 1.5 (p. 35) for a glossary of terms and abbreviations.
[a]Modified SIRS was used for evaluating retrospective feigning; the content of the SIRS items was essentially identical.
[b]Offenders with mental disorders on a mental health unit of a metropolitan jail.

281

gerers in real-world settings. The chief constraint of a known-groups comparison is the establishment of its criterion groups (i.e., malingerers and genuine patients).

3. *Differential prevalence design* assumes different rates of malingering based on referral issues and settings. At best, this design provides only marginal evidence of validity. Even when differential rates are found in the predicted direction, researchers have no way of knowing (a) whether these prevalence rates are accurate, or more importantly, (b) whether deviant scores truly represent malingering.

Rogers, Bagby, et al. (1992) contended that no single model is sufficient for the validation of response styles. Instead, research must combine the respective strengths of two designs. Simulation research maximizes internal validity, whereas known-groups comparison maximizes external validity. A convergence of results across these designs is required to establish the validity of any measure for the assessment of malingering.

Simulation Research by the Original Investigators

Rogers and his colleagues conducted a series of four studies (Rogers, Gillis, & Bagby, 1990; Rogers, Gillis, Bagby, & Monteiro, 1991; Rogers, Gillis, Dickens, & Bagby, 1991; Rogers, Kropp, & Bagby, 1993) utilizing a simulation design. In each study, participants were given specific instructions to feign a mental illness and offered an incentive (financial or course credit) for providing a convincing performance.

The studies varied with respect to their settings and the use of experimental instructions. Rogers, Gillis, and Bagby (1990) and Rogers, Kropp, et al. (1993) employed correctional participants with prior experiences in psychological assessment and intervention to serve as simulators and controls. Rogers, Gillis, Bagby, et al. (1991) utilized college students, while Rogers, Gillis, Dickens, et al. (1991) used community participants. Experimental instructions set goals that ranged from avoiding placement in a more restrictive correctional institution to seeking voluntary hospitalization. In addition, two studies (Rogers, Gillis, Bagby, et al., 1991; Rogers, Kropp, et al., 1993) provided subgroups of simulators with coaching on the specific disorders being feigned or on detection strategies built into the SIRS.

The combined samples for the four simulation studies comprised 75 bona fide patients (35 outpatients and 40 inpatients), 170 simulators (70 from corrections, 40 from the community, and 60 from a university), and 97 controls (26 from corrections, 41 from the community, and 30 from a university). Rogers, Bagby, et al. (1992) combined these simulation studies and added 25 participants to the clinical group in order to increase the inpatient representation.

A primary focus of the SIRS was discriminant validity, addressing whether SIRS primary scales clearly differentiate between genuine and feigned protocols. For each study, the primary scales evidenced highly significant differences for simulators in comparison to clinical and nonclinical samples.[4] As reported by Rogers (1997), the effect sizes were very robust; the mean effect size (Cohen's *d*) was 1.74 between simulators and genuine patients. As expected, these effect sizes were even larger (*M*= 2.03) between simulators and controls. These differences appear to stand irrespective of the samples (clinical, community, college, or corrections), type of feigned disorder, and coaching.

A further test of discriminant validity by Rogers, Bagby, et al. (1992) involved a two-stage discriminant analysis to test overall differences in SIRS primary scales. To make the discriminant model more rigorous, they excluded nonclinical controls from the analysis. With both simulators and bona fide patients randomly divided into calibration and cross-validation samples, the discrimination function accurately classified 89.8% of the calibration and 88.3% of the cross-validation samples. From a methodological perspective, the next step was to examine whether the results of simulation research could be confirmed by known-groups comparison.

Known-Groups Comparison by the Original Investigators

Samples of actual malingerers are challenging to establish in the absence of a gold standard. Therefore, in their known-groups comparison, Rogers, Bagby, et al. (1992) designated the category of "suspected malingerers" to reflect a strong likelihood but not absolute certainty of malingering. Through systematic investigations of forensic inpatients, Rogers, Gillis, Dickens, et al. (1991) were able to identify 26 suspected malingerers that were independently classified by the assessment teams. Their primary SIRS scales were consistently elevated to levels comparable with simulators.

Rogers, Bagby, et al. (1992) combined the 26 suspected malingerers from the Rogers, Gillis, Dickens, et al. (1991) study and an additional 10 suspected malingerers to test for overall differences on the SIRS. In a comparison of SIRS scales, the average effect size was identical to simulators and patients, with a very robust mean Cohen's *d* of 1.74. In addition, the average Cohen's *d* was 2.19 between suspected malingerers and controls. Overall, these results demonstrated a strong correspondence between simulation research and known-groups comparison.

The discriminant validity of the known-groups comparison was also evaluated via discriminant analysis. The sample of suspected malingerers, which allowed only a single-stage analysis, yielded an overall classification rate of 94.3% that included 97.5% of the clinical groups and 84.6% of the suspected malingerers. Results of the discriminant analysis with suspected malingerers were generally comparable to the simulators when contrasted

---

[4]The sole exception was the SEL scale in the Rogers, Gillis, Dickens, et al. (1991) study.

with the same clinical samples. Moreover, the canonical correlations were virtually identical (i.e., .79 and .80) for the two discriminant functions.

Validation by Other Investigators

Connell (1991) tested the SIRS by comparing 60 offenders (30 simulators and 30 honest responders) and 30 psychotic inpatients with highly significant differences on the primary scales. He conducted a discriminant analysis on all three groups using the SIRS to differentiate (1) simulators from honest responders and (2) genuine patients from normal controls. Although the SIRS was not intended to differentiate patients and controls, the discriminant analysis still identified 23 of 30 simulators and 57 of 60 honest responders, for an overall classification rate of 88.9%.

Kropp (1992) addressed whether offenders with a high level of psychopathy as measured by the Psychopathy Checklist: Screening Version (PCL:SV; Hare, Cox, & Hart, 1989) would be more effective at feigning mental disorders than those with low PCL-SV scores. To this end, 100 male offenders were divided into 50 high- and 50 low-level psychopaths randomly assigned to honest and malingering conditions. Results indicated that high levels of psychopathy did not generally improve offenders' ability to feign. Highly significant differences were found in the predicted direction for all eight of the primary scales. Moreover, the SIRS appeared nonthreatening to simulators; approximately 90% of the feigning participants believed that they had successfully feigned mental illness.

Linblad (1993) conducted a within-subjects design on 66 participants recruited from correctional and forensic psychiatric settings. He compared three groups: (1) offenders without a mental health history, (2) forensic patients hospitalized with a primary diagnosis of major mental illness, and (3) forensic patients hospitalized with a primary diagnosis of personality disorder. The results indicated highly significant differences on the primary scales in the predicted direction, with an M effect size of 1.95. When the SIRS was combined with the MMPI-2, a very high rate of classification was achieved (95.5%). Experience as a psychiatric patient did not appear to improve simulators' ability to feign. As in the Kropp (1992) study, most simulators (77.6%) believed that they had successfully fooled both the SIRS and the MMPI-2.

Kurtz and Meyer (1994) tested the relative effectiveness of the the the SIRS, the MMPI-2, and the M test in discriminating between coached inmates feigning psychosis and psychotic patients. They found that the SIRS (88.9%) was significantly more effective than the MMPI-2 (81.3%) or the M test (< 75.0%). Indeed, data for the MMPI-2 were particularly worrisome: A majority of the patients tested under honest conditions were misclassified as malingerers. Combining the SIRS with either the MMPI-2 or the M test did not add to the incremental validity. The combined classification rates were nearly identical to the accuracy of the SIRS alone (i.e., 90.0% vs. 88.9%). These data suggest the superiority of the SIRS in the classification of malingerers in correctional settings.

Gothard (1993) performed an elaborate study of the SIRS with 60 offenders (30 simulators and 30 honest responders) compared to 48 patients referred for evaluation of competency to stand trial. She established highly significant differences between feigners and (1) patients incompetent to stand trial ($M d$ = 1.99), (2) patients competent to stand trial ($M d$ = 2.36), and (3) correctional controls ($M d$ = 2.99). In addition, 7 malingerers, independently identified and included as a known-groups comparison, yielded elevations similar to simulators. With the use of three or more scales in the probable feigning range (criterion established by Rogers, Bagby, et al., 1992), the overall classification rate was 97%. The convergence between simulators and malingerers was very encouraging in its combined simulation and known-groups design. Unlike earlier research, however, only a minority of patients (24%) believed they had successfully fooled the SIRS.

Convergent Validity

Research has examined the convergent validity of the SIRS by comparing its scales to other measures of feigning. The key findings of these studies are summarized as follows:

- A strong relationship was established (Rogers, Gillis, Dickens, et al., 1991) between the SIRS and MMPI fake-bad indicators, with nearly all correlations (97.5%) in the moderate to high range (i.e., r's $\geq$ .60).
- Marked elevations were found on SIRS scales for defendants suspected of feigning incompetence to stand trial (Michaela Heinze, personal communication, November 14, 2000); SIRS primary scales had moderately high correlations (median r = .66) with the MMPI-2 F scale.
- Adolescent comparisons of the MMPI-A to the SIRS primary scales yielded only modest correlations (Rogers, Hinds, & Sewell, 1996). Contrary to expectations, the correlations for honest responders were approximately double those for simulators (median r's of .40 and .19, respectively).
- Comparisons of the SIRS with the M test (Beaber, Marston, Michelli, & Mills, 1985), a screen for malingering, have yielded mixed results. Based on the original M test subscales, Rogers, Bagby, et al. (1992) found low to moderate correlations between SIRS primary scales and the two relevant subscales: Confusion, median r = .51; Malingering, median r = .26. Based on revised M test scales, Ustad (1996) reported moderate relationships ($M r$'s of .58 and .60).
- Correlations between the SIRS primary scales and the fake-bad scale (i.e., Negative Impression [NIM]) of the Personality Assessment Inventory (PAI; Morey, 1991b) produced moderate associations. Ustad,

Rogers, and Salekin (1996) found a moderate relationship ($M\ r = .58$) for inmates referred for psychological consultation. Wang et al. (1997) found a low-moderate relationship ($M\ r = .42$) for corrections-based inpatients.

In summary, studies of convergent validity have found moderate relationships in the predicted direction. While the principal focus of the SIRS validation is discriminant validity, this evidence of convergent validity should be viewed as ancillary but positive. The modest findings with adolescents are difficult to interpret in light of (1) the paucity of feigning research on the MMPI-A and (2) the lack of SIRS data with adolescents.

Construct Validity

Exploratory factor analyses have inspected the underlying dimensions of the SIRS separately for feigners (simulators and malingerers) and honest responders (patients, offenders, and community and university participants). For principal components analyses (PCAs) with varimax rotation, the following solutions were found:

- *Feigners.* Three factors were identified: feigning (49.5%), defensiveness (16.8%), and dishonesty/inconsistency (10.5%).
- *Honest responders.* Three factors were identified: nonbizarre faking (50.4%), bizarre faking (14.5%), and dishonesty/inconsistency (10.6%).

Gothard (1993) performed a combined PCA including both feigners and honest responders that resulted in one general dimension of faking (approximately 63% of the variance) and a second factor possibly associated with defensiveness (approximately 8%). Wynkoop, Frederick, and Hoy (2000) explored the underlying dimensions of the eight primary scales and the Cognitive Scale (i.e., word tasks involving opposites and rhyming). With a PCA, they found that the primary scales constituted the first dimension (61.5% of the variance) with high loadings (> .60) for each scale. These three studies suggest one general factor (accounting for 50–60% of the variance) for feigning, with positive loadings from all the primary scales. While confirmatory factor analyses (CFA) would be valuable, the existing data provide general support of the primary scales as forming one general dimension related to feigning.

Wynkoop et al. (2000) also investigated the internal reliability and correlates of the Cognitive Scale. With an inpatient forensic sample, the Cognitive Scale evidenced adequate internal reliability (alpha = .81) and was not significantly correlated with education ($r = .17$) and were relatively uncorrelated with primary scales (r's $\leq .35$). Wyncoop et al. suggested that errors on the Cognitive Scale might be indicative of feigned cognitive deficits. At present, the Cognitive Scale remains insufficiently validated for clinical use.

Generalizability

An important element of scale validation is the generalizability of results across sociodemographic backgrounds, the clinical status of patients, and the range of assessment settings. Rogers, Bagby, et al. (1992) examined the comparability of classification rules for 103 females and 299 males from the validation studies. Overall, the classification rates for nonclinical samples responding honestly remained similar. For the clinical samples, the SU scale appeared to classify more female (15.8%) than male patients in the probable feigning category. Combined across honest responders, the specificity for individual primary scales in the probable feigning range remained identical for both genders at 97.6%. The average sensitivity for individual primary scales was slightly higher for females (62.3%) than for males (56.3%).

Several studies have examined the generalizability of the SIRS with minorities. Connell (1991); who performed a multivariate analysis of variance (MANOVA) on 30 African American and 60 Anglo American participants, and found no significant differences due to race. Gothard (1993) reported a very high classification rate (97.4%) in a diverse sample that included 31 African Americans and 13 Hispanic Americans in her study of feigning and competency to stand trial. With an African American, Anglo American, and Hispanic American sample, Norris and May (1998) found no differences due to race on a self-report version of the SIRS. These results about the generalizability across several ethnic groups are very encouraging. However, the generalizability of the SIRS has not been investigated with other minority groups.

Rogers, Bagby, et al. (1992) investigated the comparative utility of the SIRS in correctional and noncorrectional settings. They found that the specificity rates remained similar (97.1% and 98.5%, respectively) for individual primary scales. The sensitivity of individual scales was slightly higher for correctional (60.1%) than noncorrectional (53.9%) participants.

The coaching of participants had no effect on specificity of individual primary but did cause a decrement, (from 65.2% to 49.1%) in the average sensitivity of individual scales (see Rogers, Bagby, et al., 1992). As a related issue, participants with knowledge of mental disorders gained through their own history did not appear to be more effective at feigning (see Linblad, 1993). Finally, persons with APD (Rogers, Gillis, & Bagby, 1990) and high levels of psychopathy (Kropp, 1992) do not have an increased likelihood of remaining undetected on the SIRS.

For the purposes of this chapter, unpublished pilot data on 9 forensic experts (psychologists and psychiatrists) who attempted to feign mental disorders on the SIRS were evaluated. In reviewing their protocols, 5 of the 9 experts were designated as malingering (*M* number of primary scales in the probable feigning range was 3.8) and an additional 3 were placed in the indeterminate range. Only 1 expert (11.1%) was miscategorized on the SIRS as an honest responder; however, he denied almost every symptom on the SIRS, including the DS and SU scales. Possible explanations are that either (1) he did not comply with the experimental condition, or (2) he feigned a very mild condition.[5] These preliminary data suggest that the majority of highly experienced forensic experts will be correctly identified as feigning, although some are likely to be placed in the indeterminate range.

Adolescents

The SIRS was designed (Rogers, Bagby, et al., 1992) for older adolescents ($\geq$ 18 years) and adults. Are SIRS results generalizable to younger adolescents? When adult cut scores were used with dually diagnosed adolescents in a corrections-based residential treatment program for substance abuse, the SIRS exhibited a superb NPP (1.00) and moderate PPP (.66). A slightly more liberal cutting score (i.e., two or more scales in the probable range) improved PPP (.79) at little cost to the NPP (.98). The study was limited by the absence of psychotic disorders among adolescents. While performing better than the MMPI-2, the SIRS should only be used for corroboration, not clinical classification.

Patients with Mental Retardation

Kurtz and Meyer (1994) found no differences based on IQ estimates in the ability of participants to feign mental disorders. However, the issue remains open as to whether the SIRS can be used with mentally retarded populations. Hayes, Hale, and Gouvier (1998) utilized a known-groups comparison to evaluate the SIRS with samples of forensic patients with mild retardation (*M* IQ's from 60.2 to 66.0). Using a discriminant analysis, they classified two groups of genuine patients (pretrial and adjudicated not guilty by reason of insanity) and malingerers. Despite the entry of three groups in the discriminant function, the overall classification rate was high. The PPP (feigning) was .89; the NPP (combined patient groups) was .97. However, two cautions must be observed: (1) Classification rates for the standard cut scores were not reported, and (2) the subject-to-variable ratio (i.e., 4.9:1) for the discriminant analysis was low. Pending further research, the SIRS should only be used for corroboration but not classification with persons with mild mental retardation. Cases with high Inconsistency of Symptoms (INC) scores should likely be excluded because of the heightened concern about impaired comprehension. Under no circumstances should the SIRS be used for persons with moderate or severe mental retardation.

---

[5]Interestingly, the one expert who was miscategorized as an honest responder endorsed relatively few symptoms (bogus or bona fide). His case represents the nettling dilemma for many malingerers: If very few symptoms are feigned, then the likelihood of detection decreases dramatically. By the same token, if very few symptoms are feigned, then the likelihood of achieving an external goal (e.g., compensation) also decreases dramatically.

CLINICAL APPLICATIONS

Many clinicians have discounted the importance of malingering and related response styles in their assessment and have facilely assumed that feigning is either very rare or easily detectable. As noted in the "Overview" section, malingering is not rare and occurs in a small but significant percentage of both forensic and nonforensic cases. In addition, the notion appears unfounded that malingering is likely to be so obvious that standardized methods are unnecessary. For example, malingering has gone undetected in disability cases simply because the feigning was not obvious to treating clinicians. Therefore, the question for clinicians is no longer *whether* to use standardized methods for assessing potential malingering. Rather, the question is *which* standardized methods should be used.

The assessment of feigning is a critical determination with far-reaching ramifications for patients in the provision of mental health services and other benefits. Given the importance and complexity of this decision, Rogers, Bagby, et al. (1992) advocate that any conclusions regarding feigning must be based on a multisource–multimethod approach. The SIRS may form an important component of this approach.

This section is organized into two components. I first evaluate the clinical usefulness of the SIRS. This component addresses SIRS strengths and limitations, and its comparative utility in relationship to self-report measures. Second, I review criticisms of the SIRS. Because I am also the author of the SIRS, I include published criticisms, so that readers may have multiple perspectives on the SIRS and its validation.

Clinical Usefulness

The SIRS has been established as a highly reliable measure that is cross-validated on diverse populations. Because of its extensive validation, the SIRS likely should be employed in clinical and forensic cases where the possibility exists that some or all of the patient's presentation is feigned. An explicit objective of the SIRS is to minimize the number of false positives because of the potentially devastating consequences of miscategorizing a genuine patient as a feigner. Toward achieving this objective, the SIRS institutes stringent criteria for determinations of feigning. Moreover, an "indeterminate" category was created to reduce errors in marginal cases.

The SIRS is intended for the evaluation of feigned symptomatology and mental disorders. It is not intended for use in cases of feigned cognitive deficits. Its only potential application in cases of feigned cognitive deficits is the evaluation of psychological symptoms that reportedly accompany the precipitating event (e.g., a head injury). In this case, clinicians evaluate the legitimacy of the psychological sequelae but not the cognitive deficits per se.

Typically, the SIRS can be administered to a wide range of patients, including those with active psychotic symptoms. Naturally, care must be taken to avoid interviewing patients who are untestable. Fortunately, most of such patients are hospitalized and may be observed extensively to evaluate whether grossly disorganized speech or bizarre and highly regressed behavior (e.g., smearing and eating feces) are feigned or bona fide. Once patients are stabilized, the SIRS has an advantage over paper-and-pencil methods because the clinician presents the questions and records the responses, thus minimizing administration problems. As a guideline for untestable patients, psychologists are asked to discontinue testing if more than 15 minutes are spent on the first set of detailed inquiries. In such cases, for whatever reason, the administration is obviously bogged down and unlikely follow the standardized procedure.

Use of the SIRS is consistent with DSM definitions of malingering. Successive DSM editions (DSM-III: American Psychiatric Association, 1980; DSM-III-R: American Psychiatric Association, 1987; DSM-IV: American Psychiatric Association, 1994; DSM-IV-TR: American Psychiatric Association, 2000) have offered virtually identical definitions of malingering. Therefore, SIRS cases of suspected malingering in the early 1990s were equally applicable to DSM-IV and DSM-IV-TR. The DSM category of malingering does not offer formal inclusion and exclusion criteria; instead, four potential risk factors are enumerated (for a discussion, see Rogers & Vitacco, in press). These risk factors have also remained consistent from DSM-III to DSM-IV-TR.

Malingering versus Factitious Disorders

Both malingering and factitious disorders are defined by the intentional production or feigning of psychological or physical symptoms. The key difference is motivation. Patients with factitious disorders are assumed to be motivated by the desire to assume a "sick" role, whereas malingerers are apparently motivated by other, external incentives. As observed by Rogers, Bagby, and Rector (1989), a clinician's attempts to establish motivation are thwarted by the patient's obvious distortions and the competing theories for his or her feigning. More explicitly, if we cannot trust the patient's self-reporting, how can we rely on his or her account of motives? Conversely, should we assume willy-nilly the patient's motivation from the context of the evaluation? Following this logic, a *per saltum* inference that all patients in personal injury cases are motivated to feign by financial incentives is logically and empirically insupportable.

Preliminary SIRS data by Rogers, Bagby, and Vincent (1994) suggested substantial overlap between the malingerers and patients with factitious disorders with psychological symptoms (FDPS). They found (see also Rogers, Bagby, et al., 1992, p. 26), however, that some malingerers had marked elevations on primary scales that were not generally observed in factitious patients. For example, 50% of malingerers had *BL* scores > 13 as compared to 12.5% of FDPS patients. Moreover, malingerers tended to be less consistent in their presentations, with 48.5% scoring > 6 on the INC scale in contrast to FDPS patients (10.0%). However, the real diagnostic task is to attempt to establish the patient's past and current relationships with doctors and health care systems. If the patient's admiration and dependency on health care professionals can be firmly established, at least one important component of factitious disorders can be determined. The clinician is then left to consider the role played by secondary gain and external benefits (e.g., disability insurance or removal of household responsibilities while hospitalized). If any other external goals are identified, then the classification of malingering is rendered.

The presence of malingering does not preclude treatment (Rogers, 1997), but may complicate clinicians' ability to assess accurately current diagnosis and treatment effectiveness. Whether the exaggeration of psychological problems represents a "cry for help" (i.e., strong motivation) or a breakdown/manipulation of the therapeutic relationship (i.e., low motivation) has not been explicated and likely varies from case to case. Unpublished data on the SIRS (Rogers, Bagby, & Prendergast, 1993) would suggest that a significant minority of chronic schizophrenic patients tend to be unreliable in their presentation and may dissimulate some of their symptoms. In spite of this, these patients continue to be involved in treatment. Within a treatment context, a frank but nonconfrontational discussion of SIRS results is recommended, with a sincere attempt to include the feigning patient in treatment decisions.

Strengths of the SIRS

The major advantages of the SIRS include its rigorous validation, classification rates, and information about styles of feigning. Its four key strengths are summarized as follows:

1. *Interrater reliability.* Because of standardization, the SIRS is a highly reliable structured interview that produces virtually the same results when administered by mental health professionals with sufficient training.
2. *Validation with simulation and known-groups.* As noted in the "Overview," validation of feigning measures relies on the respective strengths of simulation design (internal validity) and known-groups comparison (external validity). The SIRS is distinguished by its painstaking validation that integrates both research models.
3. *Stable cut scores.* The SIRS cut scores are both stable and effective in classifying persons who feign disorders.
4. *Specific information about feigning.* An important feature of the SIRS, beyond the classification of feigning and honest responding, is its attention to the description of response styles. For example, treating psychologists may choose different interventions with patients who simply exaggerate the severity of their symptoms, as opposed to others who fabricate preposterous or incongruous symptoms.

In addition to these advantages, the SIRS has attended to issues that could possibly affect its generalizability, including gender, ethnicity, and referral (forensic vs. nonforensic) issues. In summary, the SIRS is a highly reliable structured interview with cross-validated primary scales utilizing both simulation research and known-groups comparison. Importantly, SIRS scales and classification have been effectively tested by outside investigators.

Limitations of the SIRS

The SIRS has not been validated for the assessment of feigned cognitive deficits. While reported psychological sequelae of a traumatic injury can be reviewed, feigning of these symptoms does not address feigning of cognitive impairment. For example, a patient may malinger psychological symptoms following a head injury but still experience genuine cognitive decline. Please also note that the Hayes et al. (1998) study, while addressing patients with mental retardation, evaluated the malingering of symptoms and mental disorders, and not feigned cognitive deficits.

The SIRS is not intended for repeat evaluations at brief intervals. Although Norris and May (1998) found close agreement after a 2-day interval between the standard SIRS and a self-report version,[6] the SIRS has not been validated for repeat administrations within a short time period. I am aware of several cases in which the results of a feigned SIRS protocol appeared to be shared with the patient. Not surprisingly, results of the second administration evidenced marked changes in responses and a consequent change in SIRS classification. While research data suggest that the SIRS is largely resistant to general coaching, specific feedback about failed performances is likely to confound subsequent results. This concern is substantially lessened by extended intervals (e.g., > 6 months) addressing different episodes or presenting problems.

Comparative Utility of the SIRS and MMPI-2

Clinicians are frequently concerned with the relative usefulness of different scales and indicators of feigning. In my workshops, a common question is "Why not simply use the MMPI-2 with its fake-bad indicators?" This section outlines the comparative validity and utility of the SIRS in comparison to the MMPI-2. To facilitate the comparisons, the following key questions are raised and addressed:

1. *Are results tested on suspected malingerers?* SIRS studies with known-group comparisons (Rogers, Bagby, et al., 1992; Gothard, 1993; Hayes et al., 1998) have yielded strong and consistent results that cross-validate findings from simulation research. In contrast, the MMPI-2 has a dearth of research

---

[6]The self-report version is likely to confound the usefulness of the standard SIRS; therefore, it is not available for clinical use.

on suspected malingerers. The available study (Lees-Haley, English, & Glenn, 1991) produced different results from MMPI-2 simulation research.

2. *Are the same cut scores validated across different studies?* SIRS studies rely on the same cut scores for purposes of standardization and replication. In direct contrast, the MMPI-2 has been plagued with problems in establishing stable cut scores. In a meta-analytic study of the MMPI-2, Rogers, Sewell, and Salekin (1994) found a lack of consistent cut scores for the classification of feigning. As a specific example, the reported cutting scores for *F* ranged widely from > 8 to > 30. With the SIRS, stable cut scores greatly facilitate clinical interpretation.

3. *Are conclusions about feigning confounded by other alternatives?* The SIRS is designed and validated for discrimination between feigned and nonfeigned presentations. In contrast, MMPI-2 fake-bad indicators are confounded by lack of reading comprehension, compromised attention, and severe mental disorders. The SIRS has eliminated literacy problems and reduced the demands for concentration (e.g., response to direct inquiries with clarification available). Clearly, MMPI-2 problems with confounds are not trivial. As an illustration of this point, Kurtz and Meyer (1994) found that MMPI-2 validity indicators had an unacceptably high false-positive rate of 60.0%.

4. *Are the conclusions valid with minority populations?* While more studies of the SIRS are needed, available research about the applicability of the SIRS with African American and Hispanic American samples is very encouraging. Feigning on the MMPI-2 remains untested regarding its usefulness with minority populations. This oversight is of special concern given observed ethnic differences on validity scales (see, e.g., Greene, 2000).

In summary, the SIRS and the MMPI-2 should not be considered comparable in either their validation or clinical usefulness. Clinically, the use of far-ranging cut scores and inattention to minority issues limits the conclusions drawn from the MMPI-2. With these limitations in mind, the SIRS and MMPI-2 are frequently used together for the assessment of feigning. Convergent data between the two measures help to satisfy the requirement that determinations of feigning are multimethod. In cases where defensiveness appears to a be a key issue, the MMPI-2 provides substantial information, especially when specialized indicators such as Wiggins social desirability (Wsd) or positive malingering (Mp; see Baer, Wetter, & Berry, 1992; Rogers & Shuman, 2000) are used.

An important distinction must be made between convergence of methods and incremental validity. With the joint use of the SIRS and the MMPI-2, clinicians have additional data from two sources to support their conclusions. However, this convergence should not be equated with incremental validity (i.e., greater accuracy in classifying criterion groups). Kurtz and Meyer (1994) found that the SIRS alone was comparable to the SIRS plus the MMPI-2 in classifying participants as feigning and nonfeigning. With the advent of specialized MMPI-2 scales (see Rogers, Sewell, & Salekin, 1994), further research on this issue would be helpful (see, e.g., Rogers, Hinds, & Sewell, 1996). At present, clinicians should not assume that multiple measures of feigning add incremental validity.

Criticisms of the SIRS

The SIRS has generally received very positive reviews and commentaries (e.g., Melton, Petrila, Poythress, & Slobogin, 1997; Phillips & Fallon, 2000). However, the purpose of this section is to identify criticisms leveled at the SIRS, so that readers will have the benefit of others' perspectives. Toward this end, criticisms with brief commentaries are summarized as follows:

• *The SIRS is susceptible to acquiescent responding and suggestibility.* Pollock (1996) utilized several scales to evaluate the SIRS in terms of research scales addressing suggestibility, compliance, and acquiescence, and concluded that the SIRS is susceptible to these influences. Three issues should be considered:

1. These research scales have not been validated on samples with mental disorders; therefore, the meaning of these scales with clinical samples remains unknown.
2. These research scales have not been used in malingering studies; it is likely that malingerers would attempt to appear impaired on these scales as well (e.g., easily influenced and willing to contradict themselves).
3. The strength of any interpretation is constrained by the magnitude of the correlations, which are relatively modest (M r's = .36 for total suggestibility and .36 for acquiescence).

• *The SIRS lacks cut scores for malingering.* With reference to malingering, Meyer and Deitsch (1996, p. 422) concluded that the SIRS is of "questionable usefulness since even its author has consistently declined to offer cut-off point decision rules." Two issues must be considered:

1. The SIRS offers consistent cut scores for feigned and nonfeigned responses; this information is clearly useful to clinicians.
2. The SIRS does not, and should not, offer cut scores for malingering. The complex determination of motivation (see "Overview") is beyond the scope of any quantified measure. Clinicians must search for direct (e.g., statements to others) and indirect (past relationship with health care staff) information in distinguishing malingering from factitious disorders.

• *Knowledge of the referral question may vitiate SIRS effectiveness.* Edwards, Stearns, Yarvis, Swanson, and Mirassou (1997) reported the case of a male malingerer who modified his results after learning that the test "assessed malingering." Two issues should be considered:

1. The SIRS is a measure of response styles rather than malingering. Many clinicians use it to (a) establish nonfeigned (i.e., "honest") responding or (b) describe inconsistent responding. It should not be misportrayed as a measure to "catch you malingering."
2. Close review of the cited case revealed that the SIRS was a repeat administration, with some information about the SIRS being shared after the first administration. Repetitive administrations, especially with feedback, are likely to be confounded.

12

Focused Forensic Interviews

Forensic assessments have burgeoned with broad applications and increased sophistication during the last two decades (Heilbrun, Rogers, & Otto, 2000). Among the developments, several focused interviews have been constructed and validated. Foremost among these interviews is the Psychopathy Checklist (PCL; Hare, 1980) and its more recent versions for adults (PCL-R and PCL:SV) and adolescents (PCL:YV), featured in this chapter's first major section (see Box 12.1).

With research spanning the last two decades, focused forensic interviews have emphasized competency to stand trial. The second major section of this chapter provides an integrated review of four competency interviews (see Box 12.2). The first three interviews are available for clinical practice: the Georgia Court Competency Test (GCCT; Wildman et al., 1979), the Fitness Interview Test (FIT; Roesch, Webster, & Eaves, 1984), and the MacArthur Competency Assessment Tool—Criminal Adjudication (MacCAT-CA; Poythress et al., 1999). The fourth interview is available to forensic clinicians for research collaboration: the Evaluation of Competency to Stand Trial—Revised (ECST-R; Rogers & Tillbrook, 1995).

PSYCHOPATHY CHECKLIST (PCL)

Overview of Psychopathy and APD

The related constructs of antisocial personality disorder (APD) and psychopathy have crucial ramifications for how psychologists evaluate and treat individuals in conflict with the law. As noted by Rogers and Dion (1991), mental health professionals remain undecided as to how to distinguish between antisocial "behavior" (i.e., a choice of actions) and antisocial "personality" (i.e., a mental disorder embedded in childhood antecedents and characterological

---

BOX 12.1. Highlights of the PCL-R and PCL:SV

- *Description:* Both the PCL-R and PCL:SV are semistructured interviews that evaluate psychopathy and its two components: core personality features and antisocial behavior. The PCL-R has a much stronger emphasis on criminal activity.

- *Administration time:* PCL-R = 1½ to 2 hours for the interview plus 1 hour for record review; PCL:SV = 1 to 1½ hours for the interview plus 1 hour for record review.

- *Skills level:* Both measures require doctoral-level trained clinicians with specialized training in forensic practice. A moderate level of training is required to attain proficiency with the PCL-R and PCL:SV.

- *Distinctive features:* Both interviews have exceptional reliabilities for dimensional ratings of psychopathy. The lack of direct correspondence from clinical inquiries to criteria (1) complicates the scoring and (2) reduces the potential transparency of these inquiries.

- *Cost:* The basic PCL-R package (i.e., the PCL-R manual, rating booklet, 25 score sheets, and 25 interview guides) = $215. The basic PCL:SV package (i.e., the PCL:SV manual, 25 score sheets, and 25 interview guides) = $120.

- *Source:* Multi-Health Systems, on the internet, *www.mhs.com;* by phone, (800) 456-3003; by fax, (888) 540-4484; or by mail, 908 Niagara Falls Boulevard, North Tonawanda, NY 14120-2060.

---

deficits). This indecision about what constitutes APD is clearly chronicled in successive versions of the DSM. In the DSM-II, the emphasis was placed on characterological dimensions that reflected "grossly selfish, callous, irresponsible, impulsive, and unable to learn from experience and punishment" (American Psychiatric Association, 1968, p. 43), with no specification of criminal actions. In the DSM-III (American Psychiatric Association, 1980), the focus centered on dysfunctional behavior that indicates a lack of socialization and achievement both as a child and adult and a pervasive willingness to violate the rights of others. In the DSM-III-R (American Psychiatric Association, 1987), attention was refocused on violent criminal acts, particularly those that emerge prior to adulthood. In the development of the DSM-IV (American Psychiatric Association, 1994), three divergent models (DSM-III-R, ICD-10, and psychopathic personality disorder) were vigorously debated (Hare, Hart, & Harpur, 1991) before settling on a similar though simplified version of the DSM-III-R.[1] As simply a text revision, the DSM-IV-TR (American Psychiatric Association, 2000) did not alter the APD criteria.

---

[1]Although field trials were supposed to play a major role in establishing the optimal criteria for APD (Widiger, Frances, Pincus, Davis, & First, 1991), political and nonempirical considerations appear to have won out (see Hare & Hart, 1995; Widiger & Corbitt, 1993).

Psychologists are confronted with a bewildering array of symptoms associated with the diagnosis of APD. As outlined in Chapter 1, Rogers and his colleagues (Rogers, Dion, & Lynett, 1992; Rogers, Duncan, & Sewell, 1994; Rogers, Salekin, Sewell, & Cruise, 2000) established broad dimensions of APD through prototypical analysis. In the Rogers et al. (1994) study, four distinct factors emerged: (1) *unstable self-image, unstable relationships, and irresponsibility,* (2) *manipulation and lack of guilt,* (3) *aggressive behavior,* and (4) *nonviolent delinquency.* While relying on the DSM-IV APD diagnosis, clinicians may find these dimensions helpful in the conceptualization of what constitutes APD.

Hare (1980, 1985a) initiated his efforts to assess psychopathy as a construct relatively independent of the DSM versions. The concept of psychopathy (Hart, Hare, & Harpur, 1992) is seen as more encompassing than recent versions of APD because of its inclusion of affective and interpersonal dimensions. According to Hare and Hart (1993), psychopathy is defined as "a cluster of personality traits and socially deviant behaviors: a glib and superficial charm; egocentricity; selfishness; lack of empathy, guilt, and remorse; deceitfulness and manipulativeness; lack of enduring attachments to people, principles, or goals; impulsive and irresponsible behavior; and a tendency to violate explicit social norms" (p. 104). Hare's work resulted in the development of the PCL.

Description of the PCL Measures

The PCL is a semistructured interview designed specifically for the assessment of psychopathy with underlying dimensions of core personality traits (i.e., F_1) and antisocial behavior (F_2). It is presently available in four closely related versions:

- The Psychopathy Checklist (PCL) is the original measure with 22 criteria; ratings are based on an extensive interview and record review.
- The Psychopathy Checklist—Revised (PCL-R) is composed of 20 criteria; modifications (see Rogers, Salekin, Hill, et al., 2000) included changes in (1) criteria (two criteria dropped and 11 modified), (2) descriptions of criteria, and (3) rating system.
- The Psychopathy Checklist: Screening Version (PCL:SV[2]) composed of 12 criteria, was developed for use in noncorrectional populations.
- The Psychopathy Checklist: Youth Version (PCL:YV) parallels the PCL-R with 20 corresponding criteria; inquiries and criteria were modified for adolescent populations.

This review focuses primarily on the PCL-R because of its extensive validation and commercial availability. The PCL:SV is also featured because of

---

[2]The PCL:SV was originally described as the PCL: Clinical Version, or PCL:CV.

its validation and applicability to clinical populations. In contrast, the PCL and PCL:YV are deemphasized. Despite its high correlations with the PCL-R, the PCL appears to be slightly outdated and no longer the focus of programmatic research. Unlike the PCL, the PCL:YV is a newly developed measure with relatively little empirical research.

PCL-R Description

The PCL-R is composed of a 16-page Interview and Information Schedule and a 2-page answer sheet. The Interview and Information Schedule is organized into 10 sections: School Adjustment, Work History, Career Goals, Finances, Health, Family Life, Sex/Relationships, Drug Use, Childhood/Adolescent Antisocial Behavior, and Adult Antisocial Behavior. Unlike most semistructured interviews, these sections and their concomitant questions are not explicitly linked to specific ratings. Instead, clinicians are required to integrate data from multiple responses and collateral information to address specific PCL-R criteria.

The PCL-R Interview and Information Schedule is organized into (1) standard questions, which are enumerated and asked of all respondents, and (2) optional probes, which are bracketed and asked when more detailed information is required. In addition, several branching questions are asked depending on responses to earlier questions. Although the Interview and Information Schedule provides very limited space for recording responses, all ratings are made on a separate answer sheet. Some clinicians may wish to save considerable expense by recording patients' responses elsewhere and reusing the Interview and Information Schedule.

Responses to the Interview and Information Schedule are scored on an answer sheet that includes a list of the criteria the possible ratings. The 20 criteria are rated on a 3-point scale: 0 = no, 1 = maybe/in some respects, and 2 = yes. Unfortunately, the actual descriptions of the criteria are not included on the answer sheet. Rather, clinicians must consult a third source, the PCL-R Rating Booklet, in order to make the necessary ratings.[3] In addition to rating the PCL-R, the answer sheet provides tables for prorating scores when individual ratings are omitted as well as percentile ranks for use with male inmates and forensic patients.

Most PCL-R criteria (17 of 20) are assigned to one of two underlying dimensions. The PCL-R test manual (Hare, 1991) does not provide any extensive description on how practitioners should make differential use of factor scores in their clinical use of the PCL-R. According to Hart et al. (1992), high scores on F_1 should be interpreted as reflecting interpersonal and affective characteristics of psychopathy that are linked to narcissistic and exploitative dimensions. In contrast, high scores on F_2, indicative of criminal and impulsive behaviors, are associated with APD diagnosis.

---

[3]An unexplored issue is the number of administrative and interpretative errors that occur from this unnecessarily complicated organization.

The PCL-R also yields an overall or global score that is intended as "a dimensional score that represents the extent to which a given individual is judged to match the 'prototypical psychopath'" (Hare, 1991, p. 17). In addition, a cut score of ≥ 30 is provided, which has a sensitivity of .72 and specificity of .93 when employed with white male inmates (Hare, 1985a).

Hare (1991) warned against problems in cut scores based on the standard error of measurement (SE_M). The SE_M for the PCL-R total score was 3.25. If a liberal standard (1 SE_M) were employed, then a cut score of ≥ 33 should be used. If a conservative standard (2 SE_M) were employed, then a cut score of ≥ 37 should be used. Similar adjustments should be made for determination of nonpsychopathic individuals. If a conservative standard (based on 2 SE_M) were fully implemented, then the cut scores would be (1) 0–23 = nonpsychopathic; (2) 24–36 = indeterminate; and (3) 37–40 = psychopathic. Of course, a significant problem with this categorization is that most psychopaths would be missed.

PCL:SV Description

The PCL:SV shares many common characteristics with the PCL-R. The purpose of this brief section to highlight the following three major differences:

1. The PCL:SV has fewer questions about criminality.
2. The PCL:SV has less emphasis on various forms of antisocial and dyssocial behavior (e.g., early behavior problems, promiscuous sexual behavior, many marital relationships, and revocation of early release).
3. The PCL:SV has normative data for use with general patients without legal involvement.

The PCL:SV was originally conceptualized as a "stand-alone" measure for the assessment of psychopathy in clinical and nonclinical populations. Hart et al. (1997) were cautious in their publication of the PCL:SV, indicating that it should simply be used as a "screening measure" with results confirmed by the PCL-R. This recommendation is problematical for several reasons:

- The overlap of clinical inquiries is very substantial. Over one-half of PCL:SV inquiries are identical or closely related to PCL-R inquiries. Given this similarity, the difference appears to be in focus between criminal (PCL-R) and noncriminal (PCL:SV) content.
- The PCL:SV corresponds closely to the PCL-R (i.e., $r = .80$ for total score; Hart et al., 1997); its items closely parallel the PCL-R, with six of eight criteria (75.0%) for F_1 and six of nine criteria (66.7%) for F_2. Importantly, no incremental validity is reported for the PCL-R over the PCL:SV. Furthermore, the likelihood of incremental validity is negligible given these exceptional similarities.

- Recent research (see Validity) has addressed most concerns about the reliability and validity of the PCL:SV.

In summary, the role of the PCL:SV as simply a screen for the PCL-R is strongly questioned. The two interviews appear both empirically and conceptually to be measuring the same construct. Therefore, clinicians should select the PCL-R and PCL:SV as "stand-alone" interviews based on the referral question and populations. The PCL-R is preferred for risk assessments in correctional populations. The PCL:SV is preferred for the evaluation of non-forensic patients. Both the PCL-R and PCL:SV appear comparable for addressing clinical issues with forensic patients.

PCL:YV Description

The PCL:YV closely parallels the PCL-R in criteria and ratings. The interview format is expanded to 99 standard questions with subcomponents and optional probes. Unlike the PCL-R, some subcriteria are explicitly categorized (i.e., "yes" or "no") or quantified (e.g., frequency of suspensions). In addition, the scoring manual offers some specific guidelines on how data are to be integrated into ratings of the criteria.

Rationale and Development

Hare and Cox (1978) originally devised a series of 16 ratings apparently derived from Cleckley's (1976) conceptualization of psychopathy. These global ratings were organized on a 7-point Likert scale and required interviewers to be highly versed in Cleckley's theory and sophisticated in interviewing inmates and integrating relevant data. This approach evidenced considerable promise as a reliable assessment method. For example, Hare (1985a) established high interrater reliability (.90) on 229 inmates.

Several problems were observed with this "global-ratings" approach. First, as previously noted, interviewers were required to have sophisticated training. Second, the rating items themselves varied in the accessibility of required information and the range of resulting scores. Third, the global-ratings approach provided only partial standardization of criterion variance and offered little assistance with information variance. For these reasons, Hare (1980) decided to develop a more criterion-based checklist approach.

The first step in the development of the PCL was the generation of characteristics that would likely differentiate between psychopathic and nonpsychopathic inmates (Hart et al., 1992). Based on literature reviews and practical experience with criminals, a list of over 100 characteristics was constructed. Although specific details are not available, Hart et al. (1992) described the general process of item selection and refinement. Items were selected that appeared to discriminate between psychopaths and nonpsychopaths, and met the following conditions: (1) nonoverlapping, (2) sufficiently correlated with global ratings, (3) not extreme in base rates, and (4) generally reliable. According to Hare (1985b), a series of analyses was carried out to refine these items and create the PCL.

The original PCL was composed of 22 items that reflect interpersonal, affective, and behavioral indicators of psychopathy. As previously noted, the PCL was further refined as the PCL-R. Hare (1991, p. 1) described the PCL-R as intended to assess "a widely understood clinical conception of psychopathy, perhaps most clearly exemplified by Cleckley's (1976) *The Mask of Insanity*." Although originally based on Cleckley's conceptualization, the resulting PCL actually deviated significantly from its own theoretical underpinnings. Table 12.1 summarizes the differences between Cleckley's (1976) formulation and Hare's interpretations and refinements on the PCL and PCL-R. Of the 16 Cleckley criteria, only four characteristics (untruthfulness, remorse, affect, and planning) are closely paralleled by the PCL–PCL-R. Three other characteristics (charm, sex, and egocentricity) share key elements.[4] The remaining nine characteristics are not represented on the PCL–PCL-R.

Hare (1991) reported other theoretical contributions to the PCL–PCL-R, including the work by McCord and McCord (1964), Craft (1965), Karpman (1961), and Buss (1966). These studies focus on affective, impulsive, dishonest, and antisocial aspects of psychopathy. Hare also presented evidence that the PCL criteria were similar to those employed clinically by Canadian psychiatrists (e.g., Gray & Hutchinson, 1964) and British physicians (e.g., Davies & Feldman, 1981).[5]

Hare (1985b) described the modifications made in the PCL to create the revised 20-item version, the PCL-R. One PCL item (alcohol/drug) was dropped because of difficulty in scoring, and a second item (previous diagnosis as psychopath) was deleted because of its redundancy with the PCL itself. The PCL-R manual (Hare, 1985b) provided detailed descriptions of each PCL-R item and its scoring. The more recent PCL-R manual (Hare, 1991) corresponds closely to the 1985 manual in its description of 11 items. However, the remaining nine items evidence small but observable changes in the wording and resulting criteria. Given the fact that these descriptions constitute the actual scoring criteria, the lack of data on the comparability of these two versions is a rather serious oversight. In other words, do validity data on the 1985 version generalize to the 1991 version?

Reliability of Recent PCL Measures

This section provides a composite review of reliability of the PCL-R, the PCL:SV, and the PCL:YV. Table 12.2 allows practitioners to make direct comparisons across these closely related interviews. In contrast, the validity section addresses each PCL version separately and focuses primarily on the PCL-R and the PCL:SV.

---

[4]Please note, however, that egocentricity was eliminated in the PCL-R version.

[5]Following Hare's (1991, p. 41) own description, however, the PCL-R appears to be consistent with only five characteristics from the Canadian study and six from the British study.

TABLE 12.1. Similarities and Differences between Cleckley's Formulation of Psychopathy and Hare's PCL/PCL-R

Similar constructs for Cleckley, PCL, and PCL-R

Source	Item descriptor
Cleckley	Superficial charm and good intelligence
PCL	Glibness/superficial charm
PCL-R	Glibness/superficial charm
Cleckley	Untruthfulness and insincerity
PCL	Pathological lying and deception
PCL-R	Pathological lying
Cleckley	Lack of remorse or shame
PCL	Lack of remorse or guilt
PCL-R	Lack of remorse or guilt
Cleckley	General poverty of major affective reactions
PCL	Lack of affect and emotional depth
PCL-R	Shallow affect
Cleckley	Sex life impersonal, trivial and poorly integrated
PCL	Promiscuous sexual relations
PCL-R	Promiscuous sexual behavior
Cleckley	Failure to follow any life plan
PCL	Lack of realistic, long-term plans
PCL-R	Lack of realistic, long-term plans
Cleckley	Pathological egocentricity and incapacity for love
PCL	Egocentricity/grandiose sense of self-worth
PCL-R	Grandiose sense of self-worth

Dissimilar constructs—Cleckley

Absence of delusions/irrational thinking
Absence of nervousness and psychoneurotic manifestations
Unreliability
Inadequately motivated antisocial behavior
Poor judgment/failure to learn by experience
Specific loss of insight
Unresponsiveness in general interpersonal relations
Fantastic and uninviting behavior with drink and sometimes without
Suicide rarely carried out

Dissimilar constructs—Hare

Previous diagnosis of psychopath[a]
Proneness to boredom/low frustration tolerance[b]
Conning/lack of sincerity[b]
Callous/lack of empathy
Parasitic lifestyle
Early behavior problems[b]
Short tempered/poor behavioral controls[b]
Impulsivity
Irresponsible as a parent[b]

(cont.)

TABLE 12.1 *(cont.)*

Dissimilar constructs—Hare *(cont.)*

Frequent marital problems[b]
Juvenile delinquency
Poor probation or parole risk[b]
Failure to accept responsibility for own actions
Many types of offense[b]
Drug or alcohol abuse not direct cause of antisocial behavior[a]

Note. Cleckley's (1976) criteria; PCL = Psychopathy Checklist; PCL-R = Psychopathy Checklist—Revised
[a]Deleted in the PCL-R revision.
[b]Modified in PCL-R.

PCL-R

Hare (1991) summarized the interrater reliability regarding the total PCL-R scores for four inmate and two forensic-psychiatric samples. The ICCs for total scores were relatively high across four inmate samples (range from .78 to .89, with a median of .84). Moreover, the sole forensic study appears to have excellent interrater reliability, with an ICC of .91 for the total score. In addition, the PCL-R demonstrated excellent interrater reliability on both symptom (median ICC = .59) and factor (median ICC = .80) levels.

Approximately one dozen studies have investigated the PCL-R's interrater and test–retest reliability following its publication (Hare, 1991). Table 12.2 summarizes these studies plus reliability data on the PCL:SV and PCL:YV. Key findings on the reliability of the PCL-R are highlighted as follows:

- For dimensional ratings of psychopathy, the interrater reliability for total scores produced superb results for PCL-R interviews. Clinicians can clearly use the PCL-R as a highly reliable interview for evaluating the overall level of psychopathy.
- For categorical ratings of psychopathy, surprisingly few studies reported classification rates for psychopaths versus nonpsychopaths. Three of eight studies produced good reliabilities: (1) Darke, Kaye, Finlay-Jones, and Hall (1998) found perfect interrater agreement, (2) Alterman, Cacciola, and Rutherford (1993) found moderately high test–retest reliability, and (3) Brandt, Kennedy, Patrick, and Curtin (1997) had a moderate reliability in classifying delinquents with low, medium, and high psychopathy. Other studies generally producing reliabilities in the low-moderate range are slightly disappointing in light of the dichotomous classification.[6]
- For dimensional ratings of PCL-R factors, a moderate level of interrater and test–retest reliability was observed.

[6]The kappa becomes a more stringent test as the number of disorders/classifications increases. These kappas are only disappointing because of the simplicity in classification, namely, the presence or absence of psychopathy.

TABLE 12.2. Reliability Studies of the PCL-R, PCL:SV, and PCL:YV

Study (year)	Version	N	Setting In/Out/Com/Con				Raters Lay/Prof		Reliability Inter/Retest (interval)	Reliability estimates Sx/Factor/Total/Classify			
Cacciola et al. (1990)	PCL-R	10	✓[a]				✓	✓	✓ (1 mo)			.94[b]	
Hare (1991)[c]	PCL-R	1,632	✓	✓			?	✓	✓	.59[b]	.80	.84	.54[c]
Kropp (1992)	PCL:SV	15	✓					✓	✓	>.38[b]		.96	
Alterman et al. (1993)	PCL-R	88	✓[a]				✓	✓	✓ (1 mo)	.78		.80	.76[d]
Serin (1993)	PCL-R	120			✓	✓	?	?	✓				.45[e]
	PCL-R (F)	35			✓	✓	?	?	✓			.85[b]	
Gacono & Hutton (1994)	PCL-R	146	✓					✓	✓			.98	
Hart, Forth, & Hare (1995)	PCL:SV	295	✓	✓	✓		?	?	✓	.60[b]	.81	.82	.51
Miller, Goddings, et al. (1994)	PCL-R	32	✓	✓			?	?	✓			.96[b]	
Cornell et al. (1996)	PCL-R (F)	26[f]			✓		✓		✓	.77	.83		
Forth et al. (1996)	PCL:SV	150	✓				?	?	✓			.88	
Brandt et al. (1997)	PCL-R (F)	130[f]	✓				✓		✓			.87	.71[g]
Darke et al. (1998)	PCL-R	50	✓[a]				?		✓	.51[b]		.94[b]	1.00
Grann et al. (1998)[i]	PCL-R (F)	40	✓				✓		✓	.31[b]	.79	.88	.58
Heilbrun et al. (1998)	PCL-R	232	✓				?		✓		.86	.92	.63[i]
Newman & Schmitt (1998)	PCL-R (F)	80				✓						.77	

(cont.)

TABLE 12.2 (cont.)

Study (year)	Version	N	Setting In/Out/Com/Con	Raters Lay/Prof	Reliability Inter/Retest (interval)	Reliability estimates Sx	Factor	Total	Classify
Rutherford et al. (1998)	PCL-R	10[k]	✓	? ?	✓	.78		.88	
Rutherford et al. (1999)	PCL-R	225	✓[a]	? ?	✓ (2 yr)	.32	.55	.63	.58[d]
Loving & Russell (2000)	PCL:YV	66[l]	✓	✓	✓			.94[b]	
McDermott et al. (2000)	PCL-R	20	✓[a]	✓ ✓	✓			> .80	
Cruise (2000)	PCL:YV	10	✓	✓	✓			.98	
Molto et al. (2000)[m]	PCL-R	49	✓	✓	✓			> .87[b,n]	> .50[n]

Note. See Table 1.5 (p. 35) for a glossary of terms and abbreviations. PCL-R = Psychopathy Checklist—Revised; PCL.SV = Psychopathy Checklist: Screening Version; PCL.YV = Psychopathy Checklist: Youth Version; (F) = file information only; ? = information not provided; Total = PCL total score; Classify = classification of psychopathy. Unless otherwise specified, ICCs are used as reliability coefficients except for Classify (i.e., kappas).

[a] Methadone patients.
[b] Correlation.
[c] Eleven male samples, mostly inmates and forensic inpatients; the kappa for classification is derived from a further analysis by Hart, Forth, and Hare (1991).
[d] Used ≥ 25 for psychopathy rather than the standard cut score ≥ 30.
[e] Simply percentage of agreement on psychopathy (25 of 56 cases) between file and file plus interview; Serin (1993) reported an out-of-range kappa (2.75).
[f] Adolescents in a residential treatment program for severe delinquency.
[g] Classified as low (< 22), medium (22–27), and high (> 27).
[h] kappas.
[i] Swedish translation.
[j] Used ≥ 33 for psychopathy rather than the standard cut score ≥ 30.
[k] Hare's training videotapes.
[l] Exact number not given; "most" of 66 participants were involved.
[m] Spanish translation.
[n] No measures of central tendency are reported on three small samples.

- For categorical and dimensional ratings of PCL-R criteria, the results were mixed. Hare (1991) and Darke et al. (1998) produced very respectable reliability estimates. Two other studies produced modest results, although these findings may be explainable by their methodology: Grann, Langstrom, Tengstrom, and Stalenheim (1998) used file information only (i.e., no PCL-R interview) with a Swedish translation, while Rutherford, Cacciola, Alterman, McKay, and Cook (1999) examined test–retest reliability after a 2-year interval. In light of these limitations, a reasonable conclusion is that PCL-R criteria have moderate reliability when used in the standardized format (interview plus file information) for the current time.

Four reliability studies have attempted to substitute the review of file information for the standardized administration (PCL-R interview plus file review). In general, these studies have produced moderately high interrater reliabilities for total scores. However, these reliability estimates are typically lower than standard administrations. More critical than whether two raters can agree about file information is whether file reviews used in research approximate standard administrations in clinical practice. In this regard, Serin (1993) found only a moderate relationship between file reviews and standard administrations for 120 cases. In addition, six items on the PCL-R could not be routinely rated on file information alone. The obvious conclusion is that clinicians should not rely on file reviews for PCL-R criteria and classifications.

Psychopathy is conceptualized as a personality constellation that remains stable throughout most of adulthood, with possibly some attenuation in later years (Harpur & Hare, 1994). The stability (i.e., test–retest reliability and temporal stability) of the PCL-R has generally been assumed rather than rigorously tested. For test–retest reliability, the most startling discovery was the use of overly focused samples. In particular, each of the three test–retest studies relied exclusively on methadone patients. Data are not available on PCL-R test–retest reliability with forensic-psychiatric or general offender populations.

Rutherford et al. (1999) rigorously evaluated the test–retest reliability of the PCL-R after a 2-year interval. This extended interval is only justifiable because psychopathy is believed to be a very stable personality construct. Interestingly, the overall trend was for PCL-R scores to increase slightly during a 2-year period. While total scores evidenced a moderate relationship for men and women, important gender differences were observed: (1) ratings on F_1 were *less* reliable for men (.43) than for women (.63), and (2) ratings on F_2 were *more* reliable for men (.60) than for women (.50). Classification of psychopathy was worrisome. Because very few participants met the standard cut score for psychopathy (≥ 30), the researchers lowered the cut score to ≥ 25.[7] Potentially inflated reliability estimates remained in the low-moderate range

---

[7]Two points should be observed. First, this expediency does not appear to be empirically justified. Second, ICC estimates are likely to be inflated by artificially raising the prevalence rates.

for 200 men (.48) and the high-moderate range for 25 women (.67). Especially with men, clinicians cannot assume, "Once a psychopath, always a psychopath."

PCL:SV

Hart et al. (1997) conducted the primary PCL:SV reliability study, which combined 295 participants from seven diverse samples. Although some variability was observed within and between samples, the PCL:SV demonstrated a moderate level of reliability for individual criteria. Its correlations for criteria (median r = .60) are comparable to the PCL-R. Kropp (1992) also appeared to have moderate Kropp's correlations for PCL:SV criteria. While not reporting central tendencies, correlations for individual criteria ranged from .39 to .98. Regarding the reliability of the two factors, the PCL:SV appears highly reliable, with median ICCs of .80 (F_1) and .81 (F_2).

Like the PCL-R, the PCL:SV evidences high reliabilities for total scores. Across three studies, the PCL:SV total scores ranged from .84 to .96. For dimensional ratings of psychopathy, the PCL:SV produced superb ratings. Like the PCL-R, less attention was paid to the classification of psychopathy. Hart et al. (1997) obtained a pooled kappa of .51 across four samples. Agreement about classification fell in the low-moderate range.

The PCL:SV has neglected test–retest reliabilities. Hart et al. (1997) provided estimates of test–retest reliability based on extrapolations from the PCL-R. However, the reproducibility of PCL:SV ratings and classification needs to be evaluated across time within a test–retest paradigm.

PCL:YV

Reliability studies for the PCL:YV are likely to be forthcoming in the next several years as this measure is published and widely disseminated. At present, two studies have evaluated its interrater reliability for total scores. They found very promising results with correlations > .90.

Validity of Recent PCL Measures

PCL-R

Concurrent Validity. Hare (1991) reported two studies of the PCL-R that compare its scores to the previously described global ratings of psychopathy. Both studies evidenced strong correlations with the PCL-R total (i.e., .87 and .90) and factor (range from .70 to .87; median = .79) scores. Despite its divergence from Cleckley's conceptualization, the PCL-R appears to be closely related to notions of psychopathy found in clinical practice.

Predictive Validity. The PCL-R has been extensively researched, especially the extent to which its scores predict violent and antisocial behavior.

Two meta-analyses (Hemphill, Hare, & Wong, 1998; Salekin, Rogers, & Sewell, 1996) have evaluated the PCL-R in relationship to violent behavior. Salekin et al. (1996) summarized five PCL-R studies, with Cohen's d's ranging from .42 to 1.18 (median = .70). While not especially strong, Salekin et al. demonstrated a low to moderate effect size for violence. More recently, Hemphill et al. (1998) evaluated six studies of the PCL-R and violence, with correlations as a measure of effect sizes. They found very modest correlations ranging from .06 to .34 (median = .26) that accounted for a very small proportion of the variance (i.e., generally less than .10). Despite these disappointing results, high PCL-R scores were obtained with during a 12-month follow-up period. In comparing high and low PCL-R scores, with midrange scores removed, Hemphill et al. found a relative risk of 2.26 (OR = 3.82) for violent recidivism. Importantly, low and middle PCL-R scores had nearly identical recidivism rates (20.2% and 21.4%, respectively).

Meta-analyses have also addressed general recidivism. Salekin et al. (1996) found relatively modest effect sizes in three studies (.56, .58, and .71). Similarly, Hemphill et al. (1998) reported modest correlations (range from .10 to .39; median = .27). With predominantly federal inmates, they found a relative risk of 1.87 (OR = 5.31) for high versus low PCL-R scores. Interpretation of this relative risk is constrained by the sampling's high prevalence rates (i.e., low = 39.7%, middle = 54.9%, and high = 74.1%).

Three general studies of the PCL-R were not included in these meta-analyses. Cornell et al. (1996) examined differences based on instrumental (i.e., goal-oriented) and hostile aggression among a male inmate population. Inmates with instrumental violence had higher PCL-R scores than those with either hostile aggression or nonviolent offenses. However, the actual differences in PCL-R total scores appeared relatively small. Salekin, Rogers, Ustad, and Sewell (1998), studying female detainees in a large metropolitan jail, found only a modest relationship ($r = .20$) between PCL-R scores and subsequent recidivism. Among convicted sex offenders, Birt, Porter, and Woodworth (2000) found that the classification of psychopathy significantly increased the likelihood of recidivism for both sexual and nonsexual crimes.

An important consideration is whether the predictive validity of the PCL-R can be demonstrated among offenders with Axis I disorders. Simply put, do disorders such as schizophrenia affect PCL-R predictive validity? Rice and Harris (1995) found that among patients with schizophrenia recidivism was low whether patients were classified as psychopathic (.23) or nonpsychopathic (.15). In contrast, other psychopaths (.57) compared to nonpsychopaths (.27) evidenced increased prevalence recidivism. Tengstrom, Grann, Langstrom, and Kullgren (2000) produced very different results with patients with psychotic disorders: .48 for psychopaths and .14 for nonpsychopaths. Whether Axis I disorders are an important moderator variable in the PCL-R prediction of recidivism remains an unresolved issue.

Predictive validity has also been examined with respect to treatability. In particular, psychopaths have often been viewed as less treatable than other offenders, although the empirical literature is far from conclusive (Wong &

Elek, 1989). Ogloff, Wong, and Greenwood (1990) studied the treatability using their own idiosyncratic classification: psychopaths (PCL-R > 26), nonpsychopaths (PCL-R < 18), and mixed psychopaths (PCL-R = 18–26). In a predictive study, they found that psychopathic inmates were less motivated and showed less improvement than either of the other two groups. Interestingly, the nonpsychopathic and mixed groups had comparable scores on all indices. As an unexpected complication, Barbaree (1999) studied effects of treatment on sex offenders classified as psychopaths and nonpsychopaths. Surprisingly, he found that "successfully treated" psychopaths had a higher recidivism rate than "unsuccessfully treated" psychopaths. One interpretation of this study is that psychopaths were able to deceive clinicians about their treatment progress. Several observations are salient about psychopathy and treatment:

- Psychopathy is likely to complicate treatment and treatment outcome.
- More predictive studies are needed on how psychopathy affects treatment. Recent reviews of treatment for psychopathy (see Millon, Simonsen, Birket-Smith, & Davis, 1998) describe interventions but do not test their efficacy directly.

Construct Validity. Two important facets of PCL-R construct validity have been closely evaluated. Researchers have explored and evaluated the PCL-R's underlying dimensions via factor analysis. In line with Syndeham's criteria, the diagnostic boundaries for the psychopathy construct have also been investigated.

The establishment of PCL-R underlying dimensions appears central to its construct validation. If its factor structure is either unstable or poorly formed, then the ability to utilize these factors in clinical practice is severely compromised. Hare (1991) performed an analysis of congruence coefficients for four separate factor analyses rotated to oblique solutions. Of the 17 items loaded on the two factors, 10 items were replicated across the four studies. Of the remaining seven items, five were consistent across three of the four studies. Although a confirmatory factor analysis (CFA) would be preferable, the congruence coefficients proved general support for a stable, two-factor solution.

Hare (1991) described the two factors: F_1 is characterized as "selfish, callous, and remorseless use of others" (p. 38); F_2 is depicted as "chronically unstable and antisocial lifestyle; social deviance" (p. 38). Rogers and Bagby (1994) have taken issue with these descriptions. They contended that F_1 has the highest loadings on two interpersonal components of psychopathy overlooked by Hare (1991): glibness/superficial charm (.86) and grandiose sense of self-worth (.76). They also noted that Hare's F_2 misses important problems in the self-modulation of behavior, as observed in impulsivity (.66), poor behavioral controls (.44), and need for stimulation (.56).

Brandt et al. (1997) attempted to replicate the Hare (1991) factor structure on adolescent offenders and yielded a comparative fit index of .83. They described this as a "moderate fit" (p. 432), although the typical benchmark for fit indices is $\geq$ .90 (Bentler, 1995). With reported congruence coefficients, agreement appeared stronger for F_1 (.91) than F_2 (.84). Unfortunately, specific information is lacking about which criteria were replicated for each factor.

Cooke and Michie (1997) evaluated PCL-R data on 2,067 participants with an item response theory (IRT). Despite finding support for both dimensions, they concluded that F_1 criteria were more prototypical than F_2 criteria. While acknowledging Hare's (1991) argument for two subordinate factors, they determined that F_1 represents the core of psychopathy and should be given greater weight than F_2.

Two recent CFA studies have questioned the appropriateness of Hare's two-factor model for both offender and substance abuse populations. McDermott et al. (2000) evaluated the PCL-R on 956 prisoners and patients with substance dependence. They concluded that Hare's two-factor model was neither generalizable nor stable in these samples. Darke et al. (1998) reached a similar conclusion about Hare's two-factor model for community and prison-based patients on methadone maintenance. They concluded that this model was a poor fit for the data. They performed an exploratory principal components analysis (PCA) suggesting the possibility of a five-factor model. In light of these recent studies, a reanalysis of Hare's (1991) results would be helpful using rigorous CFA methodology.

Bodholdt, Richards, and Gacono (2000), in their analysis of the study by Cooke and Michie (1997), indicated that a three-factor solution optimizes the discriminability on the PCL-R. The three factors were composed of affective (most discriminating), interpersonal, and lifestyle. The three-factor alternative requires further examination with CFA methods.

In line with Syndeham's criteria, an important consideration is whether PCL-R psychopathy represents a distinct clinical construct, distinguishable from other syndromes and disorders. Blackburn and Coid (1998) evaluated the overlap between psychopathy and SCID-II personality disorders among violent offenders. Among psychopaths, four Axis II disorders (paranoid, narcissistic, antisocial, and borderline) were very prevalent (65–95%; M = 74.8%). In contrast, nonpsychopaths from the same sites had low to moderate prevalence rates (22–54%; M = 34.8%). Further work is needed to test whether PCL-R psychopathy is potentially confounded by other character pathology, especially among offenders with significant mental health histories.

Convergent Validity. PCL-R studies have evaluated both core personality features (F_1) and antisocial behavior (F_2) in relationship to convergent measures. Key findings for the two factors are outlined as follows:

- F_1 is associated in personality-based psychopathic characteristics as measured by the newly developed Interpersonal Measure of Psychopathy (IM-P). As strong evidence of convergent validity, Kosson, Steuerwald, Forth, and Kirkhart (1997) found much higher correlations for F_1 (r_{pbi} of .33 and .62) than F_2 (r_{pbi} of .15 and .31).

- F_2 evidences positive correlations with specific scales designed to evaluate antisocial tendencies and aggression. Specifically, F_2 is correlated moderately with the MCMI-II Antisocial scale (Hart, Forth, & Hare, 1991), moderately with the MMPI-2 Pd scale (Molto, Poy, & Torrubia, 2000), and modestly with the MMPI-A Pd scale (Sullivan & Gretton, 1996). For measures of aggression and anger, correlates are modest for the MCMI-II—Aggression scale (Hart et al., 1991), the MMPI-2—Anger scale (Molto et al., 2000), the MMPI—A Anger scale (Sullivan & Gretton, 1996), and the Multidimensional Personality Questionnaire Aggression scale (Lavoro, Geddings, & Patrick, 1994).
- Moderate correlations are generally found between the PCL-R and APD symptoms in offender populations (Hare, 1991; Hart et al., 1991; Toupin, Mercier, Dery, Cote, & Hodgins, 1995).
- For adolescent offenders, moderate correlations were found between PCL-R and conduct symptom constellations, especially aggression and deceit/theft (Rogers, Johansen, Chang, & Salekin, 1997).
- Low-moderate correlations were found between the PCL-R and Millon Adolescent Clinical Inventory (MACI) Unruly and Delinquent Predisposition scales (Murrie & Cornell, 2000).

In general, PCL-R studies provide moderate evidence of convergent validity, with correlates of F_1 and F_2 consistent with a priori expectations. Higher correlations are typically not expected because specific scales of multiscale inventories often have only modest evidence of external validity.

Generalizability. Original PCL-R studies (Hare, 1991) conducted predominantly on Canadian offenders greatly overrepresented males and Caucasians. Therefore, the validity of the PCL-R with diverse populations must be considered. Recent PCL-R research on gender and ethnicity is reviewed.

A higher prevalence of psychopathy is expected for men than women in light of extensive epidemiological research on the APD diagnosis. Prevalence is not the issue in evaluating the generalizability of the PCL-R. Rather, issues of predictive (e.g., recidivism) and construct (e.g., underlying dimensions) validity must be addressed. Very little is known about female psychopaths:

- Female substance abusers ($r = .66$) evidence marginally higher correlations between PCL-R and APD symptoms than their male counterparts ($r = .41$; Rutherford, Alterman, Cacciola, & McKay, 1998).
- The PCL-R scores of female offenders were not significantly correlat-

ed ($r = .20$) with recidivism in a 14-month follow-up on jail detainees (Salekin et al., 1998).

- The PCL-R factor structure appears substantially different for women than men (Salekin, Rogers, & Sewell, 1997). For instance, only four of the nine F_2 criteria were replicated for female offenders. Likewise, Jackson, Rogers, Neumann, and Lambert (2001) could not replicate the two-factor model with CFA. Instead, the data suggested a three-factor solution similar to Cooke and Michie's (in press).

Psychopathy research must grapple with differences due to ethnicity. The seminal study by Kosson, Smith, and Newman (1990) utilized the original PCL in comparisons of African American and Anglo American male inmates. Regarding reliability, small but not statistically significant differences were observed for ethnicity: African American (.78) and Anglo American (.85; $z = 1.91$). For validity, low congruence was found between ethnic groups on F_1. In addition, differences in violent and nonviolent offenses were evaluated. For both ethnic groups, psychopaths committed more offenses than nonpsychopaths. However, one cause of concern was the comparable level of offenses between Anglo American *psychopaths* and African American *nonpsychopaths*.

Several PCL-R studies have addressed components of ethnicity, although many aspects remain unexplored. Based on an elaborate IRT analysis of the PCL-R, Cooke and Michie (1997) found that the lack of racial differences in item functioning likely reflected a lack of difference between African American and Anglo American offenders. This argument would be more compelling if comparative data were provided. In predicting adolescent psychopathy on the PCL-R, Rogers et al. (1997) found ethnicity to be an important variable, with a decreased likelihood for Anglo Americans.

Is psychopathy, as measured by the PCL-R, generalizable to cultures outside of North America? Cooke (1998) found that a cut score of ≥ 25 resulted in only 8% of Scottish prisoners being classified as psychopaths compared to 29% in North American samples using the standard cut score (i.e., ≥ 30). Similarly, Anderson, Sestoft, Lillebaek, Mortensen, and Kramp (1999) evaluated the applicability of the PCL-R to Danish criminals. Using standard cut scores, only 6.2% of this inmate population would be classified as psychopaths; a much lower cut score (≥ 24) still produced a low prevalence rate (12.4%). The results of these studies raise important questions about the generalizability of psychopathy to countries outside North America.

PCL:SV

Concurrent Validity. Hart et al. (1997) summarized the comparisons of PCL:SV and PCL-R on five samples. Overall, the weighted M correlations were high (i.e., .80), with more agreement on F_2 (.81) than F_1 (.68). Problems in achieving agreement were observed with the inpatient New York sample, with only moderate correlations for the total (.55) and factor (.52) scores. Explanations for this disparity may include (1) the type of clinical sample (i.e., inpatients), (2) the level of training (i.e., four other samples were collected by the Hare group), and (3) the content of interviews (i.e., differences in criminal content between the PCL-R and PCL:SV).

Hart et al. (1997) also compared the PCL:SV to Hare's Self-Report Psychopathy scale (SRP; Hare, 1985b). Four samples revealed a moderate correlation for total scores (median $r = .64$), with slightly higher scores on F_2 (median $r = .57$) than F_1 (median $r = .47$). Although characterized as a measure of psychopathy, the SRP's validity has not been rigorously tested. Therefore, these moderate results should be viewed as generally positive.

Predictive Validity. Like the PCL-R, validation of the PCL:SV includes major studies of predictive validity, with salient findings summarized as follows:

- The PCL:SV can be used to evaluate future violence and management problems among male patients in a maximum security hospital (Hill, Rogers, & Bickford, 1996).
- Adolescent psychopaths have more violent and nonviolent institutional infractions while in a maximum security juvenile setting. However, the PCL:SV scores are significantly correlated with number of infractions for only African Americans, not Anglo Americans or Hispanic Americans (Hicks, Rogers, & Cashel, 2000).
- Nonforensic patients are rarely classified as psychopaths based on PCL:SV total scores. However, elevated PCL:SV scores produced an OR of 9.9 for violent offenses (Douglas, Ogloff, & Nicholls, 1997).
- As predicted, offenders using goal-oriented violence (i.e., instrumental aggression) had much higher PCL:SV scores than those using emotionally based violence (i.e., reactive aggression; Cornell et al., 1996). Salient criteria included (1) lack of remorse, (2) lack of empathy, and (3) manipulativeness.

In summary, predictive studies have found that high PCL:SV scores are predictive of antisocial and socially disruptive behavior. Overall, the use of dimensional scores appears promising with elevated scores indicative of increased risk. Current data provide mixed support for the use of cut scores.

Construct Validity. Rogers, Salekin, Sewell, et al. (2000) investigated the PCL:SV factor structure on two adult samples. Unlike earlier factor analyses, they conducted a first-order principal axis factoring using the 58 subcriteria as items. Results supported a two-factor solution; most subcriteria had unique and substantial loadings on the predicted factor. As further evidence of construct validity, the relationship between criteria and subcriteria was explored. Treating the criteria as individual scales, the subcriteria yielded moderate to excellent alphas ($\geq$ .75) on 10 of the 12 criteria. As initial evidence of convergent–discriminant validity, item–scale correlations for each criterion (M = .63) substantially exceeded correlations with other criteria (M = .23).

Cooke, Michie, Hart, and Hare (1999) utilized IRT to perform a corresponding analysis of the PCL:SV. They found that 8 of the 12 PCL:SV criteria had strong parallels on the PCL-R. The remaining four items were equal or superior to the PCL-R in terms of their discrimination. They found that PCL:SV items constituted a good predictor along the entire continuum of PCL-R scores. Cooke et al. (1999) concluded that the PCL:SV was a good, shortened version of the PCL-R.

Convergent Validity. Hart et al. (1997) summarized the PCL:SV's convergent validity for several samples with the California Psychological Inventory (CPI) and the MCMI-II. Results were in the predicted modest to moderate range. The PCL:SV evidences moderate convergent validity in relationship to APD symptoms (Forth, Hart, & Hare, 1990; Hart et al., 1997).

Adolescent studies provided mixed support for the PCL:SV. Moderate correlations were observed between the PCL:SV and conduct symptoms (Vitacco, Rogers, Neumann, Durant, & Collins, 2000). However, a similar relationship was not observed between the PCL:SV and the MMPI-A Pd scale. Hicks et al. (2000) reported a negligible correlation (r = .06); this finding may be partly explained by the general elevations on this scale for delinquents in a maximum security placement.

Generalizability. Hart et al. (1997) correlated total PCL:SV scores with race (Caucasian vs. non-Caucasian), which yielded negligible correlations (range from .00 to −.26; median = −.08). While useful, these data do not address whether similar scores should be interpreted differently based on ethnicity. As previously noted, Hicks et al. (2000) found that the PCL:SV was more correlated with violent and nonviolent crimes for African Americans than Anglo Americans and Hispanic Americans. A supplementary analysis of Vitacco et al. (2000) revealed similar ethnic differences when the PCL:SV was compared to conduct problems: .66 for African Americans, .53 for Anglo Americans, and .40 for Hispanic Americans. As expected, women tended to score lower than men on the PCL:SV (Hart et al., 1997). Whether this finding reflects problems with generalizability remains to be investigated.

PCL:YV

The test manual for the PCL:YV is forthcoming and should thoroughly address its validation (Forth, Kosson, & Hare, in press). Forth and Mailloux (2000) indicated higher interrater reliabilities for total PCL:YV scores. Cruise (2000) evaluated the construct validity of the PCL:YV via a multitrait–multimethod approach. While not supporting the two individual factors, this study found general support for the PCL:YV. Dodds (2000) found that the PCL:YV did not add incremental validity to the prediction of violent crimes after the prior contacts with the criminal justice system were considered. However, several unpublished studies (see Forth & Mailloux, 2000) have found the PCL:YV moderately useful in predicting recidivism.

Clinical Applications

Two versions of the PCL are not recommended for clinical practice. The original PCL has been largely superseded by the PCL-R. Despite extensive research, the original PCL has been eclipsed by the breadth and sophistication of recent PCL-R studies. Ethical standards (American Psychological Association, 1992) disallow the use of outmoded measures. Antipodally, the PCL:YV continues in its early stages of development. The publication of its test manual, anticipated this year, will likely prompt a critical reevaluation of its clinical status.

Because of its implications for clinical practice with the PCL-R and the PCL:SV, one PCL:YV study is worthy of a brief description. Rogers, Vitacco, et al. (2001) tested whether uncoached adolescents could substantially modify their PCL:YV total and factor scores. They found marked differences occurred for response styles of social desirability and social nonconformity. These data suggest that clinicians must be concerned about response styles, especially social desirability, in conducting PCL-R or PCL:SV evaluations.

PCL-R

The PCL-R is a highly reliable semistructured interview, especially for dimensional ratings of psychopathy. For the classification of evaluatees (i.e., psychopaths vs. nonpsychopaths), reports vary across studies but generally fall in the moderate range. The constraints of moderate reliability coupled with a large SE_M are addressed in the next paragraph. PCL-R factors, especially dimensional ratings, have moderate reliability. Finally, individual criteria of psychopathy are likely to have moderate reliability if clinicians are well trained and follow standardized procedures (i.e., PCL-R interview and file review).

Clinicians often neglect to consider SE_M when making classifications of psychopathy. The designation of psychopathy typically carries very negative consequences for the evaluatee with exceptionally little hope for treatment or remediation. Especially in light of the moderate reliability for psychopathy classification, clinicians should add 1 SE_M to the cut score. Based on standard cut scores, the following guidelines are proposed:

1. PCL-R scores $\geq$ 33 are needed for the classification of psychopathy.
2. PCL-R scores from 27 to 32 are described as "indeterminate."

These guidelines represent a practical compromise. A lax standard ($\geq$ 30) would ignore entirely the variability in scores and moderate classificatory reliability. A stringent standard (≥ 37) would insist on 2 SE_M's to achieve a 95% confidence level; however, this cut score greatly restrict the usefulness of the PCL-R. Therefore, the cut score ≥ 33 balances the twin needs for rigor and clinical applicability.

Clinicians should be especially wary of attempts to make overly refined classification. For example, Gacono and Hutton (1994) suggested that total scores of 28–29 be labeled as "high moderate," 30–32 as "low severe," and ≥ 33 as "severe." Three compelling reasons argue against overly refined classification. First, such classifications lack empirical justification. Second, problems with SE_M render such narrow ranges infeasible. Third, referral sources are unlikely to appreciate these subtle distinctions and may treat the "high moderate" category in a similar fashion as the "severe" category.

The bulk of PCL-R research has addressed its usefulness in the context of risk assessment. In most cases, risks are defined in terms of violent behavior, recidivism, or management problems within an institutional setting. When should clinicians offer PCL-R conclusions about risk assessment? The answer is very complex. Two important facets are addressed in the subsequent paragraphs: placement and background.

Placement. Clinicians must consider the evaluatee's current placement; the majority of studies only consider those (1) convicted and incarcerated or (2) involuntarily hospitalized in maximum security forensic hospitals. With these populations, the PCL-R can be especially useful. An important issue is whether the PCL-R should be used at the "front end" (e.g., pretrial evaluations) when most of the validation has occurred at the "back end" (e.g., after conviction and incarceration). PCL-R results are likely to be different if both "successes" (e.g., acquittals, dropped charges, and probated sentences) and obvious failures (e.g., imprisonments) are included. As a rough analogy, studying the effectiveness of birth control methods in a maternity unit might bias the outcome. Clinicians will need to decide whether available research justifies the use of the PCL-R on offenders who are not convicted or adjudicated. Clinicians who find sufficient data may wish to offer an explicit caution about the certitude of PCL-R findings.

Background. Clinicians must also take into account a host of sociodemographic variables in using the PCL-R for risk assessment: gender, ethnicity, age group (i.e., adolescents, adults, and older adults), and culture. PCL-R results do not carry the same risk for men and women; available data suggest that women are likely to have a much lower risk, although more research with diverse populations is needed. Regarding ethnicity, PCL-R factors are different for Anglo Americans and African Americans; however, high total PCL-R scores appear to be associated with greater risk with both ethnic groups. The usefulness of the PCL-R with Hispanic Americans and other ethnic groups remains virtually untested. PCL-R studies clearly show differences between adolescents and adults, while its use with older adults has not been fully explored. Finally, PCL-R risk assessment should be confined to North

America; clearly, European studies have produced dissimilar results that are likely to have a marked effect on risk assessments.

The question remains, "When should clinicians offer PCL-R conclusions about risk assessment?" In North America, a virtual consensus for using the PCL-R is likely to be achieved for the following five criteria: (1) forensic assessments conducted at (2) the postconviction (i.e., "back-end") phase with (3) adult, (4) male, (5) Anglo Americans. Each exception to the criteria adds uncertainty. While many clinicians may feel comfortable making one exception, more than one exception has a multiplying effect on uncertainty. For a fuller treatment of risk assessment and its inherent complexities, see Rogers (2000) for a review of risk factors, protective factors, moderator effects, and mediating effects.

Some clinicians appear one-sided in rendering risk assessment. Especially in forensic reports, elevated PCL-R scores are routinely addressed. However, *low* PCL-R scores are equally important. In reviewing utility estimates, clinicians are likely to be more effective at "ruling-out" future recidivism than determining who is likely to reoffend. Informed by these five criteria, low scores should be given equal if not greater weight as high scores.

A concern about the PCL-R, especially in forensic evaluations, is whether its top-down approach to ratings lends itself to halo effects and potential bias. Clinicians are asked to make global ratings of the 20 PCL-R criteria that incorporate multiple subcriteria and attempt to integrate responses, interview behavior, and file information. The sheer complexity of these ratings make them vulnerable to the halo effect. In a separate but related issue, Hare (1998a) expressed concerns about potential bias influencing PCL-R scores in forensic cases. An additional bias likely occurs when conflicts in scoring are not resolved. In unresolved scoring, clinicians are instructed to apply the more psychopathic rating (Hare, 1991, p. 6).

The empirical data on the PCL-R are very limited with respect to treatability. Ogloff et al. (1990) indicated that psychopaths are less likely to continue in treatment. Barbaree (1999) suggested that psychopaths with sex offenses are likely to recidivate, despite being designated by clinicians as "successfully treated." Psychopathy clearly complicates treatment but should not be viewed as an insurmountable barrier to treatment. In both studies, researchers appeared to apply standard treatment to psychopaths and nonpsychopaths. Clearly, treatment must focus on psychopathy if it is likely to be successful.

The PCL-R is likely to be useful with nonforensic populations for improving clinical understanding and subsequent interventions. Outside of offender populations, the treatment implications of psychopathy are unknown. Clinicians are cautioned against using the forensic data to limit treatment access. Instead, PCL-R factors and criteria may inform practitioners about issues that must be addressed in either (1) the context of other treatment goals or (2) the focus of treatment itself.

Should psychopathy as measured by the PCL-R be considered a chronic and invariant syndrome? Surprisingly little information is available to address this key issue. Based on Rutherford et al. (1999), we know that chronic substance abusers are likely to manifest a moderate level of agreement across a 2-year period, although the agreement level in only fair for men (ICC = .48) even when potentially inflated by using a low cut score ($\geq$ 25). An additional concern is the number of new cases (e.g., more than 7.5% of men) during this 2-year period. Given the age of the male sample (i.e., approximately 40), new cases of psychopathy are unexpected. Given (1) the equivocal findings of Rutherford et al. (1999) and (2) the dearth of research on other forensic and nonforensic populations, clinicians likely should refrain from making any long-term (e.g., > 1 year) conclusions and recommendations based on the PCL-R. Without demonstrable proof of its long-term stability, judgments based on PCL-R classifications may not remain accurate for extended periods. Obviously, clinicians can have greater confidence in extreme scores (e.g., $\geq$ 37), which are less likely to be affected by minor variations in total PCL-R scores.

PCL:SV

Hart et al. (1997) and Bodholdt et al. (2000) maintain that the PCL:SV should only be used a screen for psychopathy. If the PCL:SV is elevated, then the complete PCL-R is administered. A troubling oversight is that not a scintilla of research evidence is presented for the incremental validity of this cumbersome procedure. The procedure is described as "cumbersome" because more than half the PCL-R inquiries parallel those asked on the PCL:SV. Moreover, PCL:SV ratings match PCL-R factors in 70.6% of the criteria. The onus falls squarely on Hart et al. to demonstrate how this highly redundant procedure improves either collection of relevant information or accuracy of consequent ratings. Indeed, the opposite appears to have occurred. Both Hart and Hare, coauthors of the Cooke et al. (1999, p. 11) analysis of the PCL:SV, concluded, "The PCL:SV total scores were so strongly and linearly related to the PCL-R total scores that the scales can be considered metrically equivalent measures of the same psychological construct." In case of any lingering doubts, Cooke et al. (p. 3) affirmed, "The PCL:SV is an effective short form of the PCL-R."

The PCL:SV test manual proposed a cut score of $\geq$ 18 for psychopathy classification. The Cooke et al. (1999) study indicated that a cut score of $\geq$ 20 would be the equivalent of the PCL-R $\geq$ 30 cut score. Using the PCL:YV cut score of $\geq$ 20 is warranted for two reasons: (1) It establishes equivalence with the PCL-R and (2) takes into account the SE_M, which ranges from 1.34 to 1.94. The two following guidelines are proposed:

1. PCL:SV scores of $\geq$ 20 are needed for the classification of psychopathy.
2. PCL-R scores from 16 to 19 are described as "indeterminate."

Should clinicians use the PCL:SV or the PCL-R for risk assessments in correctional settings? With incarcerated populations, the PCL-R is the obvious choice based on its being more extensively researched. To avoid the redundancy and unnecessary time expenditure of the PCL:SV, practitioners may wish to use the SRP (Hare, 1985a) to screen out patients who evidence no psychopathy.

For other evaluations, the PCL:SV may serve as a useful measure of psychopathy, with helpful data regarding the two underlying dimensions of psychopathy. Use of the 1985 PCL:SV score sheet, which includes both criteria and subcriteria, is likely to provide accurate ratings with demonstrable psychometric qualities. Several advantages accrue from the expanded score sheet (see Rogers, Salekin, Hill, et al., 2000):

- The "top-down" PCL:SV and PCL-R ratings require clinicians to amalgamate information about multiple subcriteria from several sources into a single rating. By systematically rating each subcriterion, the obvious vulnerability of the PCL:SV to halo effects is likely to be greatly reduced.
- Alpha coefficients and interitem correlations are available to demonstrate how these subcriteria constitute a homogenous scale.
- Most subcriteria directly contribute to clinicians' understanding of the two underlying dimensions of psychopathy.

The PCL:SV is recommended in clinical and forensic practice for the assessment of psychopathy and its components. With the exception of risk assessment with incarcerated offenders, studies have demonstrated that the PCL:SV has more than adequate validity. Given its compact focus and deemphasis of criminality, the PCL:SV is likely to be best suited for nonforensic applications. In many clinical settings, psychopathy is a valuable dimensional construct with direct relevance for the effective treatment and safe management of patients.

In these cases, the PCL:SV is preferred to the PCL-R for two reasons:

1. The PCL:SV is simpler to administer and avoids marginally relevant inquires about crimes and adjustment to correctional settings.
2. The PCL:SV's expanded answer sheet systematically collects additional data that bolster the basis of criteria ratings and likely reduce halo effects.

COMPETENCY INTERVIEWS

Several structured interviews have been developed to address the psycholegal abilities required for competency to stand trial. Unlike most interviews, competency interviews face the formidable challenge of operationalizing components of a specific legal standard, namely, the *Dusky* standard (i.e., *Dusky v. United States*, 1960). Prior to reviewing the competency interviews, I present a nontechnical summary of the *Dusky* standard.

The *Dusky* standard is embodied within a single sentence issued by the U.S. Supreme Court: "The test must be whether he has sufficient present ability to consult with his lawyer with a reasonable degree of rational understanding—and whether he has a rational as well as factual understanding of the proceedings against him" (*Dusky v. United States*, 1960, p. 789). Except for a minor elaboration in *Drope v. Missouri* (1975), the substantive criteria of *Dusky* have remained unchanged for last four decades (Cruise & Rogers, 1998). How is *Dusky* conceptualized as basic components (i.e., "prongs")? The three basic options (Rogers & Grandjean, 2000) are outlined as follows:

1. Three prongs are used by most clinicians: (a) factual understanding of the proceedings (e.g., knowing the role of the judge), (b) rational understanding (e.g., comprehending the potential risks of being found guilty), and (c) rational capacity to consult with counsel (e.g., sufficient trust in one's attorney).
2. Two prongs, based on the syntax of *Dusky*, are favored by many legal scholars: (a) factual and rational understanding, and (b) rational capacity to consult with counsel.
3. Two prongs, based on the level of rational abilities, have also been proposed: (a) factual understanding and (b) rational understanding and rational capacity to consult with counsel.

Competency interviews have favored the first option and attempt to evaluate three related constructs of the *Dusky* standard. Importantly, the mixed success of these measures may be due to several nonexclusive possibilities. First, the three-prong model may not accurately reflect the *Dusky* standard. Second, the *Dusky* standard may not reflect an empirically demonstrable partitioning of human capacities. Third, the competency measures may have limited usefulness in measuring components of *Dusky*, irrespective of their organization.

Clinicians are likely to select one of the four competency interviews as a primary measure for their forensic practices. To facilitate comparisons, Box 12.2 provides an integrated overview of these competency interviews. In addition, a single clinical applications section addresses their strengths and limitations.

Practitioners should be aware that a fifth competency interview, the Interdisciplinary Fitness Interview (IFI; Golding, Roesch, & Schreiber, 1984), is not covered by this section. Despite promising data on the original study, no further research has been generated in the last 15 years. In summary, the IFI should not be used in forensic practice, although some practitioners may have a heuristic interest in its structure (see Melton et al., 1997).

BOX 12.2. Comparative Summary of the GCCT, FIT, MacCAT-CA, and the ECST-R

- *Descriptions:*
  - The GCCT is a 22-item, semistructured interview for evaluating competency to stand trial; a 1992 revision includes an additional eight-item screen for possible feigning.
  - The FIT is a 28-item, semistructured interview for assessing the Canadian competency standard.
  - The MacCAT-CA is a structured interview using two formats: (1) 16 questions addressing a hypothetical assault case and (2) 6 inquiries involving a comparative analysis of the defendant's case to other cases.
  - The ECST-R is a semistructured interview with 30 questions devoted to components of competency and a separate 28-item screen for feigning.

- *Administration times:*
  - GCCT: 10–20 minutes.
  - FIT: 15–30 minutes.
  - MacCAT-CA: 25–55 minutes.
  - ECST-R: 30–45 minutes.

- *Skills levels:*
  - GCCT: mental health professionals with forensic training and experience
  - FIT: health care professionals (e.g., nurses and social workers) with modest training.
  - MacCAT-CA: mental health professionals with forensic training and experience.
  - ECST-R: mental health professionals with forensic training and experience.

- *Distinctive features:*
  - GCCT: Its visual display is useful with very impaired clients. The GCCT is weak on the prong "consult with counsel"; the 1992 revision is useful as a brief screen for feigning.
  - FIT: A Canadian version of the CAI with additional items to address psychological impairment.
  - MacCAT-CA: Good reliability for individual items. Its limitations include reliance on a hypothetical case and no indices for feigning.
  - ECST-R: The longest competency interview, with detailed questions for "rational understanding" and "consult with counsel." The ECST-R includes a formal scale for the evaluation of feigning; it is currently available for only circumscribed clinical applications.

(cont.)

BOX 12.2 *(cont.)*

- *Costs:*
  - GCCT: no charge.
  - FIT: nominal charge for manual but not for the FIT itself.
  - MacCAT-CA: $75 for professional manual and 10 interview booklets.
  - ECST-R: no charge.

- *Sources:*
  - GCCT: No central source is available. The GCCT basic 21 items are reproduced in Nicholson, Briggs, and Robertson (1988). The 1992 addition of the AP scale is reproduced in Gothard, Rogers, and Sewell (1995).
  - FIT: Available from Program in Law and Forensic Psychology, Simon Fraser University, Burnaby, British Columbia V5A 1S6, Canada.
  - MacCAT-CA: Commercially available through Psychological Assessment Resources (PAR), by phone, (800) 331-8378; by fax, (800) 727-9329; on the internet, *www.parinc.com;* or by mail, P.O. Box 998, Odessa, FL 33556.
  - ECST-R: Available for a limited time to qualified forensic psychologists and psychiatrists who formally agree to share their ECST-R data with its developer. Contact Richard Rogers, PhD, ABPP, by mail, Department of Psychology, University of North Texas, Box 311280, Denton, TX 76203-1280, or by e-mail, *rogersr@unt.edu.*

Georgia Court Competency Test (GCCT)

Overview

The GCCT (Wildman et al., 1978) was originally a 17-item, semistructured interview for assessing knowledge of the courtroom proceedings, awareness of the charge and its severity, and ability to assist counsel. Robert Wildman (personal communication, Robert A. Nicholson, May 22, 1991) developed the GCCT as a brief screen to reduce the number of time-intensive competency evaluations. Nicholson, Briggs, and Robertson (1988) slightly expanded the original version to 21 items with (1) two questions addressing courtroom activities and (2) two questions about the attorney's name and the defendant's ability to contact him or her. Gothard, Rogers, and Sewell (1995) added the Atypical Presentation Scale (APS) as a simple screen for feigning.

The first portion of the GCCT assesses the defendant's orientation to the courtroom; he or she is asked to identify the typical location of persons in court (e.g., witness, judge, and jury). The second portion asks the defendant to describe the role and duties of key persons (e.g., prosecutor and defense counsel). The third portion asks questions about the defense attorney and current charges. Its final question asks for an account of the events prior to the defendant's arrest. The fourth and final portion asks questions about unusual symptoms; these address predominantly psychotic symptoms (e.g., ideas of reference, illogical thinking, and atypical delusions).

Validation

Reliability. Wildman et al. (1979) conducted the original study of GCCT reliability and found its test–retest reliability to be moderately high (r = .79; see Table 12.3). Since then, several investigations have evaluated both its interrater and test–retest reliability with uniformly positive results. As a composite summary of published and unpublished data, Nicholson (1992) concluded that the GCCT had excellent interrater reliability with coefficients > .90. Nicholson (1992) also reported test–retest reliability data (n = 25) with high agreement (r = .84). When reliabilities were computed on scales corresponding to factual and rational understanding, the correlations remained moderate (M r = .74). Two key findings about the GCCT reliability are summarized as follows:

1. As an overall measure, the GCCT has excellent internal consistency and interrater and test–retest reliability.
2. The interrater reliability of scales representing two *Dusky* prongs is moderate. With reference to internal consistency, however, Rogers and Grandjean (2000) found disappointing alphas for "factual understanding" (.65), "rational understanding" (.45), and especially for "consult with counsel" (.41).

Validity. Nicholson and Kugler (1991) evaluated the concurrent validity of the GCCT by combining studies (total N = 527) and comparing their results to competency status.[8] They found low-moderate correlation (r = −.42). While less than expected, the magnitude of this relationship is similar to results found with other competency measures.

Convergent validity studies have yielded mixed results in comparison to other competency measures. Nicholson, Robertson, Johnson, and Jensen (1988) found a moderately high correlation (r = .76) between the GCCT and the Competency Screening Test (CST; Lipsitt, Lelos, & McGarry, 1971). In contrast, Ustad, Rogers, Sewell, and Guarnaccia (1996) found a low-moderate association (r = .47).

GCCT research has sought to establish construct validity by evaluating its underlying dimensions. Bagby, Nicholson, Rogers, and Nussbaum (1992) conducted principal axis factoring on two competency samples (i.e., Nicholson, Briggs, et al., 1988, and the current study). Using congruence analysis,

---

[8]Competency status was determined by forensic experts; it does not represent legal outcome.

TABLE 12.3. Reliability Studies of Competency Interviews

Study (year)	Interview	N	Setting In	Out	Con	Raters Lay	Prof	Reliability Inter/Retest	(interval)	Reliability estimates Criteria/Scales	Total
Wildman et al. (1980)	GCCT	160	✓				✓	✓	✓ (several days)		.79[a]
Roesch et al. (1984)	FIT	8[b]	✓	✓		✓	✓	✓		.64[c]	
	FIT	270		✓	✓	✓[d]		✓		.75[a]	.53[e]
Nicholson et al. (1988)	GCCT	35	✓				✓	✓			.94[c,f]
McDonald et al. (1991)	FIT	29	✓				✓	✓			.79[c]
Tillbrook (1997)	ECST	25			✓[g]			✓			.75[b]
Poythress et al. (1999)	MacCAT-CA	47			✓	✓[i]		✓		.75[c,f]	.85[c,f]
Rogers & Grandjean (2000)	GCCT	14			✓		✓	✓		.95[i]	.82
	MacCAT-CA	14			✓		✓	✓		.97	.99
	ECST-R	14			✓		✓	✓		.99	1.00
Tillbrook (2000)	MacCAT-CA	33			✓		✓	✓			.76[k]
	ECST-R	33			✓		✓	✓			.82[l]

Note. See Table 1.5 (p. 35) for a glossary of terms and abbreviations. GCCT = Georgia Court Competency Test; FIT = Fitness Interview Test; ECST = Evaluation of Competency to Stand Trial; MacCAT-CA = MacArthur Competency Assessment Tool—Criminal Adjudication; ECST-R = ECST—Revised.
[a]Correlation.
[b]Videotapes.
[c]Intraclass coefficient.
[d]Criminology students without clinical training.
[e]Kappa for agreement on three categories: competent, questionably competent, and incompetent; kappa excluding questionable case = .98.
[f]Interscorer reliability.
[g]Outpatient competency referrals interview at the county jail.
[h]Phi coefficient; 89.3% agreement.
[i]Simply described as research assistants.
[j]Based on factual and rational understanding prongs.
[k]Phi coefficient; 85.5% agreement.
[l]Phi coefficient; 88.4% agreement.

the factor solutions appeared reasonably comparable with mean diagonal co-efficients of .92. The three factors were general legal knowledge, courtroom layout, and specific legal knowledge. While not matching the *Dusky* prongs, the first two factors appeared to be related to "factual understanding," while the third factor combined elements of "rational understanding" and "consult with counsel."

Several more recent studies have failed to confirm the GCCT's factor structure, such as the Ustad et al. (1996) study of 111 defendants adjudged legally incompetent. Perhaps because of the skewed sample (i.e., only incompetent patients), two confirmatory factor analyses yielded poor goodness-of-fit Indices (.78). A subsequent principal axis factoring indicated a two-factor solution (i.e., legal knowledge and courtroom layout) accounting for 36.0% the variance. Because of this disparate finding, Rogers, Ustad, Sewell, and Reinhart (1996) conducted a CFA on 125 pretrial mentally disordered offenders. They failed to confirm either the Bagby et al. or Ustad et al. solutions. A less stringent congruence analysis suggested a "fair" correspondence between the Rogers et al. (1996) and Ustad et al. (1996) results. Key conclusions are summarized as follows:

- The congruence analysis indicated a "fair" to "good" correspondence for three factors on the GCCT with defendants evaluated for competency to stand trial.
- Attempts to replicate this factor solution on either incompetent defendants or pretrial offenders with mental disorders proved unsuccessful.
- Both three- and two-factor solutions did not appear to match the *Dusky* prongs.

Rogers and Grandjean (2000) examined the construct validity of the GCCT in a multitrait–multimethod matrix. The three *Dusky* prongs were evaluated by rationally selected GCCT items that were compared to corresponding scales on the MacCAT-CA and ECST-R. Not unexpectedly, the three items pertaining to the attorney were not homogenous. Two items (name and method of contacting) involved simple recall, while only the third item addressed "consult with counsel." For the remaining two prongs, convergent validity was established for factual but not rational understanding.

The 1992 GCCT revision incorporated an Atypical Presentation (AP) scale to serve as a basic screen for potential feigning. Given the transparent nature of competency measures, feigning incompetency would appear to be a relatively straightforward task. Gothard et al. (1995) confirmed this hypothesis; jail detainees in the general population were able to achieve severely impaired scores ($M = 37.47$) without any coaching or assistance. Gothard and her colleagues found that the AP scale appeared very promising. A cut score of ≥ 6 had good sensitivity (.89) and specificity (.82). Rogers and Grandjean (2000) tested this cut score in a known-groups design comparing suspected malingerers and genuine patients. They found that the AP scale had only modest sensitivity (.33) but moderately high specificity (.89). Combining the two studies, the specificity of the GCCT AP scale suggests that it has clinical applicability in eliminating cases that are likely to be genuine from a full evaluation of feigning.

In summary, the GCCT provides a highly reliable screen of competency to stand trial. When compared with clinical determination of competency, the GCCT demonstrated a moderate relationship. Because the GCCT is the first competency interview, concurrent validity is largely a bootstrapping operation, building on unstandardized methods. As such, high correlations are not expected. In relationship to the *Dusky* standard, the GCCT does not appear to have clear parallels except for "factual understanding." In addition, the GCCT AP scale appears to have some value in identifying defendants who are unlikely to be feigning.

Fitness Interview Test (FIT)

Overview

Roesch, Webster, et al. (1984; Roesch, Zapf, Eaves, & Webster, 1998) altered the Competency to Stand Trial Assessment Instrument (CAI; Laboratory of Community Psychiatry, 1973) with three major modifications. First, the CAI was changed from a rating scale with suggested questions into a structured interview. Second, its terminology was adapted to a Canadian law. While the CAI ratings were developed for the *Dusky* standard, the FIT was intended to measure the Canadian standard. Third, the FIT added items to address psychopathology that might impair competency.

The FIT is composed of 28 items rated on 38 criteria; ratings of incapacity are rendered on a 5-point scale from "none" to "total." For most items, very brief questions are provided. For example, the seriousness of the charges is appraised by the following question: "If found guilty, what might happen?" Questions on psychopathology focus predominantly on cognitive impairment (concentration, abstraction, memory deficits, mental retardation, and amnesia for the offense). The FIT also covers psychotic (hallucinations, delusions, and formal thought disorder) and other (disorientation, mood disturbance, and impaired judgment) symptoms.

Validation

Reliability. Roesch, Webster, et al. (1984; see also Roesch, Jackson, et al., 1984) conducted the original FIT reliability study using eight videotapes rated by psychiatrists, social workers, psychiatric nurses, and lawyers/law students. As observed in Table 12.3, reliability of the individual criteria was moderately high (median ICC = .64). Minor variations were observed across professions from psychiatrists (median ICC = .61) to lawyers (median ICC = .67). A limitation of these videotaped interviews is that roughly one-third

(34.2%) of the FIT items could not be scored by at least 20% of the raters. Because the FIT interviews were conducted by psychiatrists, these data do not address the feasibility of using other health care professionals or attorneys.

Two studies evaluated the FIT's interrater reliability with actual competency referrals. Roesch, Webster, et al. (1984) used two nonprofessionals (i.e., criminology students) in a large sample of outpatient evaluations. Results for individual criteria were in the high-moderate range (median = .75). However, their overall classification was disappointing, with a kappa of .53. As expected, the greatest level of disagreement occurred with the marginal cases; the concordance was only 35.1% on questionably competent cases. On 29 competency referrals, McDonald, Nussbaum, and Bagby (1991) evaluated interrater reliability on pooled FIT criteria and achieved a moderate ICC of .73. Regarding agreement in classification, a high percentage (89.7%) was found, although no kappa was reported.

Validity. Roesch, Webster, et al. (1984) compared FIT results with independent evaluations by experienced forensic psychiatrists. Utilizing the three categories (competent, questionably competent, and incompetent), the level of agreement was relatively modest, with kappas of .46 and .47. Obviously, these kappas improve when difficult-to-rate (i.e., questionably competent) cases are removed; however, these estimates should not be considered.[9]

McDonald et al. (1991) attempted to evaluate the discriminant validity of the FIT by comparing FIT scores to overall classification. Although significant differences were found between competent, questionably competent, and incompetent groups, the authors readily acknowledged the serious problem with criterion contamination. Simply put, the criteria and classifications, derived from the same source, were obviously not independent.

Roesch, Webster, et al. (1984) investigated the underlying dimensions of the FIT via a factor analysis rotated to a varimax solution. On a subset of 24 items, they reported a two-factor solution addressing factual understanding and legal process/psychopathology. At best, this solution appears marginal; 9 of the 14 criteria on F_2 had substantial cross-loadings (> .50) with F_1. With congruence analysis, Bagby et al. (1992) attempted to replicate this factor structure. This attempt, with 72.7% of the items cross-loading, appears to suggest that the FIT is unidimensional.

Whittemore, Ogloff, and Roesch (1997) evaluated a revised version of the FIT (Roesch, Webster, & Eaves, 1994) and found that it was moderately useful as a screen. However, the FIT produced somewhat different results than measures estimating both competency to confess and competency to plead guilty.

---

[9]If participants had been forced to choose between competent and incompetent decisions, these reliability estimates would be relevant. However, the simple removal of problematic cases artificially inflates the level of agreement and renders invalid the results. Reliability must be demonstrated for all cases, not simply clear-cut cases.

In summary, the FIT is a reliable measure of specific criteria related to competency to stand trial. Agreement about classification is complicated by the introduction of an intermediate category (i.e., questionably competent). Predictably, marginal cases cause the highest levels of disagreement. Validity data suggest that the underlying dimensions of the FIT are not well understood. In addition, its relationship to competency status appears to be relatively modest, indicating that the FIT is best used as a screen.

MacArthur Competency Assessment Tool— Criminal Adjudication (MacCAT-CA)

Overview

The MacCAT-CA was derived from a lengthy research measure, MacArthur Structured Assessment of the Competencies of Criminal Defendants (MacSAC-CD; Hoge, Bonnie, et al., 1997). The MacSAC-CD was heavily influenced by Bonnie's (1992) formulation of competency, which extended beyond *Dusky* (see Cruise & Rogers, 1998) to include a contextualized concept of decisional competence. Decisional competence extends beyond the *Dusky* criteria to address such capacities as (1) expressing a preference, (2) understanding the choices, (3) reasoning, and (4) understanding implications of decisions relative to one's own case. Hoge, Bonnie, et al. (1997) postulated two underlying dimensions (adjudicative and decisional competencies) but did not formally test them. To address this oversight, Cruise and Rogers (1998) performed a principal axis factoring on the Hoge, Bonnie, et al. (1997) data but was unable to establish two factors. Instead, the MacSAC-CD appeared to be clearly unidimensional.

The MacCAT-CA was distilled from the MacSAC-CD as a clinical measure of competency to stand trial. It is composed of 22 items rated on a 3-point scale: 0 = no credit; 1 = partial credit; 2 = full credit. Sixteen items relate to a hypothetical case of aggravated assault alleged to have occurred in a pool hall altercation between two adult males. In the remaining six items, the defendant is asked to make comparative judgments about his or her own case and to explain his or her reasoning.

The MacCAT-CA was designed to assess three discrete competencies (see Otto et al., 1998, p. 436): "*understanding* (the ability to understand general information related to the law and adjudicative proceedings), *reasoning* (the ability to discern the potential legal relevance of information and capacity to reason about specific choices that confront a defendant in the course of adjudication), and *appreciation* (rational awareness of the meaning and consequences of the proceedings in one's own case)." How do these match with *Dusky*? Poythress et al. (1999, p. 20) posited that: (1) "understanding" corresponds with *Dusky*'s "factual understanding," (2) "reasoning," with *Dusky*'s "consult with counsel," and (3) "appreciation," with *Dusky*'s "rational understanding." Clinicians must take care to understand these complex formulations. The three key *Dusky* elements are outlined as follows:

1. *Dusky* requires that the defendant have a *factual* understanding of the proceedings *against him or her*. MacCAT-CA neglects this requirement by asking about a hypothetical case that is likely to be dissimilar to the defendant's particular circumstances.

2. *Dusky* also requires that the defendant have a *rational* understanding of the proceedings *against him or her*. MacCAT-CA focuses on the defendant's perceptions of fairness and equality regarding his or her own trial. Impairment is measured by (a) failure to give reasons or (b) implausible reasons based on delusions or impaired reality testing. Although not comprehensive, the MacCAT-CA appears to match *Dusky*'s rational understanding.

3. *Dusky* requires that the defendant be able consult with *his or her lawyer* with a reasonable degree of rational understanding. The MacCAT-CA disregards the requirement that these capacities relate to the defendant's own attorney. In addition, the ability to consult with counsel includes rational communication and mutual understanding; the MacCAT-CA reduces this complex construct to simple disclosures of hypothetical information.

Validation

Reliability. Otto et al. (1998) summarized the first MacCAT-CA reliability study. Based on 47 cases, excellent interscorer reliabilities were established for both individual criteria (median ICC = .75) and scales (range from .75 to .90; median = .85). With this paradigm, scored protocols are independently rated by research assistants. This procedure is likely to result in inflated estimates because some items are conditional. Depending on initial ratings, other inquiries are made. Therefore, research assistants cannot be truly independent. To illustrate this point, the median ICC for conditional items = .88, while the median ICC for other items = .71.

The interrater reliability of the MacCAT-CA has not been formally tested by its authors. However, Rogers and Grandjean (2000) found superb reliabilities for the three MacCAT-CA scales (median r = .97) for a small sample of offenders with mental disorders. In classifying competency to stand trial, Tillbrook (2000) found moderately high agreement when comparing forensic examiners. These results are very promising. As a caution, conditional responses compose 36.4% of the MacCAT-CA and may inflate interrater reliabilities for individual criteria and the "factual understanding" prong. Test–retest reliability with a brief interval (e.g., 1–2 days) would be the best method for assessing independent reliability.

Otto et al. (1998) investigated MacCAT-CA concurrent validity for hospitalized patients previously adjudicated as incompetent. Clinician ratings on a 6-point scale were compared to MacCAT-CA scores on three scales. The results were in the low-moderate range (r's from .36 to .49; median = .42). The interpretation of these results is constrained by the knowledge of the legal outcome; clinicians and, presumably, research assistants were aware of patients legally adjudicated as incompetent. With adolescents, Hughes, Denney, and Cannedy (2000) found moderate correlations (.71 to .75) between Mac-CAT-CA scales and the Competence Assessment for Standing Trial for Defendants with Mental Retardation (CAST-MR; Everington, 1990).

No factor-analytic studies are reported that investigate the three Mac-CAT-CA scales postulated to measure "three discrete competence-related abilities" (Otto et al., 1998, p. 436). The test manual (Poythress et al., 1999) even omitted the intercorrelations of the three scales. When applied to adolescents, the three MacCAT-CA scales appear to be highly intercorrelated (r's of .64, .69, and .79, respectively; see Hughes et al., 2000). With adults, Rogers and Grandjean (2000) found slightly lower intercorrelations ($M\ r = .57$). Plainly, these three scales need to be tested to determine whether they represent three discrete abilities.

Rogers, Grandjean, Tillbrook, Vitacco, and Sewell (2001) recently conducted a principal axis factoring of the MacCAT-CA, integrating samples from Alabama, Florida, and Texas. A two-factor solution appeared optimal F_1 combined factual understanding and consult with counsel, and F_2 was composed primarily of rational understanding. This solution appears somewhat inconsistent with typical formulations of *Dusky*. Moreover, this solution is potentially confounded by the type of MacCAT-CA inquiries: nearly all the hypothetical items loaded on F_1, and all the case-specific items loaded on F_2.

Rogers and Grandjean (2000) evaluated the construct validity of the MacCAT-CA in relationship to GCCT and ECST-R. The high heterotrait–monomethod correlations militated against positive findings. They found that the intercorrelations of MacCAT-CA scales (i.e., heterotrait–monomethod correlations; $M\ r = .45$) exceeded the convergent validity for each of the three prongs (i.e., .38, .32, and .04, respectively). Unexpectedly, a strong association ($r = .69$) was found between "factual understanding" and "consult with counsel."

Convergent validity was examined by Poythress et al. (1999) in relation to the Brief Psychiatric Rating Scale (BPRS) and the MMPI-2. Most correlations were modest (< .35) but in the predicted direction.[10] The primary exception was BPRS psychoticism which evidenced moderate correlations with reasoning (.48) and appreciation (.52) scales. Rogers and Grandjean (2000) found modest correlations between MacCAT-CA and SADS-C psychotic symptoms (.22) and global assessment (.22).

In summary, the MacCAT-CA corresponds to one prong of *Dusky* (rational understanding) but differs from the remaining two ("factional understanding" and "consult with counsel"). Reliability data are very positive for inter-

---

[10]These correlations are actually negative, because high scores refer to more impairment on the BPRS and less impairment on the MacCAT-CA.

scorer and interrater reliability, but research has yet to be conducted on truly independent estimates (i.e., test–retest reliability) with appropriate populations (i.e., actual referrals for competency evaluations). Studies provide moderate evidence of concurrent validity and modest evidence of convergent validity. Critical questions about construct validity still need to be investigated.

Evaluation of Competency to Stand Trial—Revised (ECST-R)

Overview

Rogers (1995) developed the ECST as a semistructured competency interview. The goals of the ECST were threefold: (1) a standardized measure to address satisfactorily the more complex *Dusky* prongs (i.e., "rational understanding" and "consult with counsel"); (2) a well-validated screen for feigned incompetence; and (3) a competency measure with more depth than existing screens. To ensure that the ECST was conceptually similar to the *Dusky* prongs, five national experts rated the prototypicality of potential competency items. For those items selected, the prototypical ratings were high; M ratings on a 7-point scale were 5.70 for "factual understanding," 6.36 for "rational understanding," and 6.15 for "consult with counsel." Three scales were developed on the basis on the prototypical analysis corresponding to the *Dusky* prongs. In addition, the AP scale was devised to assess psychotic and nonpsychotic feigning. The ECST was revised in 1998, with minor clarifications of items and ratings; this modified version is the ECST-R (Rogers & Tillbrook, 1998).

The primary objective of the ECST-R is to collect standardized data that are germane to the *Dusky* standard. The ESCT-R is intended to assemble systematic descriptions of the defendant and to render severity ratings. Both descriptions and ratings are considered essential to competency determinations. Four scales are summarized as follows:

1. *Consult with Counsel* (CC). This scale covers the nature of the client–attorney relationship, each person's expectations, areas of agreement, areas of disagreement, the resolution of disagreements, and any special methods of communication.
2. *Factual Understanding* (FU). This scale covers courtroom proceedings. Incorrect responses are addressed by prompts and education.
3. *Rational Understanding* (RU). This scale covers decisions about testifying, plea bargaining, and communication with the prosecutor. It asks for the defendant's appraisal of the best, worst, and most likely outcome of the trial. Finally, the RU inquires about unusual experiences or atypical behaviors in the courtroom.
4. *Atypical Presentation* (AP). Atypical questions with psychotic and nonpsychotic content are interleaved with realistic questions. For all questions answered affirmatively, the defendant is queried about

severity: "Has this made it difficult for you to go to court and try to help yourself?"

Validation

Reliability. Tillbrook (1997, 2000) compared the interrater reliability on two samples of 25 and 33 competency referrals. He found a moderately high level of agreement, with median phi coefficients of .75 and .82 for the final classification. These coefficients were associated with relatively high percentages of agreement (i.e., 89.3% and 88.4%). More recently, Rogers and Grandjean (2000) examined internal consistency and interrater reliability for the three competency scales. They established moderate to high alphas for the scales: .72 for CC, .86 for RU, and .90 for RU. For interrater reliability, they found extremely high levels of agreement (median r = .99; range from .97 to 1.00). For scales and overall classification, the ECST-R appears to have very good reliability.

Validity. Tillbrook (1997) compared ECST conclusions to forensic experts' opinions and legal outcomes. Phi coefficients averaged .75 for forensic experts and .66 for legal outcome. Diagnoses were dichotomized (psychosis–mental retardation vs. other disorders) and found to be significantly associated with ECST competency (r_{pb} = .66). More recently, Tillbrook (1999) found a moderate correlation (M r = .65) between the ECST-R and expert opinions by forensic examiners on a larger sample (N = .70) of defendants. This relationship is comparable to the MacCAT-CA and forensic examiners (M r = .58) for the same defendants. Finally, ECST-R ratings do not appear to be influenced by sociodemographic variables.

Rogers and Grandjean (2000) examined ECST-R construct validity via a multitrait–multimethod study. As evidence of low heterotrait–monomethod coefficients, they found low intercorrelations among the three *Dusky* scales (M r = .10). However, the convergent correlations for factual and rational understanding were below .30 threshold (M r = .25), indicating very modest relationship with corresponding scales on the GCCT and MacCAT-CA. No relationship was found for CC between the MacCAT-CA and the ECST-R (r = −.07). Content analysis of the two scales offers some clues to their dissimilarities. The MacCAT-CA utilizes a hypothetical case to assess what information would be more relevant to disclose and how the defendant might decide between several alternatives. In stark contrast, the ECST-R addresses the defendants' actual attorney and his or her expectations, perceptions, and methods of communication.

Rogers, Grandjean, et al. (2001) recently conducted a principal axis factoring of the ECST-R for forensic samples from Alabama, Florida, and Texas. A two-factor solution separated factual and rational abilities required by the *Dusky* prongs. The first dimension was aligned with factual understanding (FU scale). The second dimension combined rational understanding of the proceedings (RU scale) and rational ability to consult with counsel (CC scale). Two dimensions of cognitive complexity (factual recall vs. rational abilities) form the conceptual basis for the ECST-R assessment of *Dusky*.

Rogers and Grandjean (2000) evaluated ECST-R potential usefulness as a screen for feigned incompetence. They found that the AP psychotic subscale was effective at distinguishing feigned from genuine presentations. More specifically, this subscale had a sensitivity of .67 and a specificity of .86. It also evidenced a moderate PPP (.56) and an excellent NPP (.92). With additional validation, the AP psychotic subscale may be effective at identifying genuine patients for whom feigning is very unlikely.

In summary, the ECST-R has carefully operationalized the *Dusky* prongs for competency to stand trial. The *Dusky* scales have good internal consistency and low interscale correlations. Reliability data suggest excellent interrater reliability for the scales, with moderately high agreement on classification. Available validity data found a moderate relationship between expert opinion and legal outcome.

The ECST-R is not sufficiently validated to be considered a formal structured interview. However, it may be useful as a systematic guide for standardizing clinical inquires and resulting descriptions. It provides (1) a useful template for the *Dusky* prongs, which is not available with competency interviews, and (2) a moderately effective screen for distinguishing genuine cases from those suspected of feigning. Forensic psychologists, psychiatrists, and other qualified examiners may contact me about data-sharing arrangements. For experts with sufficient training and experience, the ECST-R is made available for no charge in exchange for ECST-R data (see Box 12.2).

Clinical Applications of Competency Interviews

No competency interview emerges as a rigorously tested operationalization of the *Dusky* standard. Moreover, a survey (Borum & Grisso, 1995) on forensic practices suggest that neither competency interviews nor scales are commonly used in competency evaluations. While this survey does not take into account recent developments in competency interviews, it does appear to signal a skepticism toward the use of simple, first-generation measures to capture the potential complexities of competency assessments. Whether employing traditional methods or competency interviews, the critical issue is whether the psycholegal abilities implicit in the *Dusky* standard are adequately addressed. As cogently observed by Skeem, Golding, Cohn, and Berge (1998), competency evaluations often deemphasize the more complex decisional abilities that are necessary to satisfy *Dusky*'s "rational understanding" prong.

What are the key issues to consider in selecting competency interviews? These issues are presented as a series of four inquiries:

1. Is the competency interview intended simply for screening or for a comprehensive evaluation?

2. What elements of the *Dusky* standard are adequately covered?
3. Does it screen for feigned incompetence?
4. Has its reliability and validity been demonstrated on actual competency referrals?

Competency interviews are examined individually in light of these inquiries. These brief reviews should assist clinicians in deciding how to choose competency interviews in their forensic practices.

GCCT

The GCCT was intended as a brief screen for defendants' competency to stand trial. As such, the critical issue is whether impaired performance on the GCCT accurately identifies defendants when competency issues should be addressed. In this regard, the GCCT appears to be a satisfactory screen (Nicholson & Kugler, 1991; Rogers & Mitchell, 1991). As a screen, the GCCT does not need to address the individual *Dusky* prongs.

• *Strengths.* The GCCT has been extensively validated on actual competency referrals and includes two valuable screens: (1) competency to stand trial and (2) feigned incompetence. Recent data suggest that the AP scale has moderate specificity but lacks sensitivity.
• *Limitations.* The GCCT has no major limitations when used as a screen for competency. Attempts to use the GCCT for comprehensive determinations must be avoided because (1) the GCCT does not address *Dusky* prongs and (2) it emphasizes simple recall rather than more complex rational abilities. The AP scale should not be used to indicate likely feigning; scores above the cut score simply indicate a need for a fuller evaluation.

FIT

The FIT differs from other competency interviews in that its intent is to evaluate competency to stand trial in light of the Canadian Criminal Code. No published analyses were found that evaluated components of the FIT in relationship to the Canadian standard, although a recent revision (Roesch et al., 1994) is said to parallel the Canadian Criminal Code (see Whittemore et al., 1997). Needless to say, the FIT has not been validated against the *Dusky* prongs.

• *Strengths.* The FIT has a moderate reliability for dimensional ratings of competency and has been tested with actual competency cases from several leading forensic facilities.
• *Limitations.* The use of an intermediary category (i.e., questionably competent) has led to problems in reliable classification. In addition, the FIT does not address more complex rational abilities or feigned incompetence.

MacCAT-CA

The MacCAT-CA differs from other competency interviews in its reliance on a hypothetical assault case. Defendants are asked to remember details about this case while answering sequential questions involving rational abilities. One concern is that some defendants may have difficulty in answering hypothetical questions but still be competent in terms of their own case. Clinicians wishing to use the MacCAT-CA will need to supplement this competency interview with inquires to address the *Dusky* prong, "consult with counsel."

- *Strengths.* The MacCAT-CA is outstanding in its coverage of rational abilities under the *Dusky* prong. While presented hypothetically, factual abilities are also adequately covered.
- *Limitations.* The MacCAT-CA has several psychometric limitations, such as no data on actual competency referrals and modest data on interrater reliability. Other limitations include (1) a lack of congruence with the *Dusky* standard, especially with respect to "consult with counsel," and (2) no data on feigned incompetence.

ECST-R

The ECST-R currently lacks sufficient validation to be recommended as a formal interview for competency evaluations. Rather, it is available as an interview guide to provide standardization and structure to these assessments. As an interview guide, the ECST-R does not produce formal "test results," although available data are very promising with regard to its reliability and construct validity.

- *Strengths.* As an interview guide, the ECST-R has formally addressed the three prongs of the *Dusky* standard, with questions, probes, and ratings for each prong. It is distinguished from other competency interviews by its focus on the complex issues surrounding "consult with counsel." It also addresses more complex rational thinking and feigned incompetence.
- *Limitations.* As an interview guide, the ECST-R has no major limitations. Attempts to use the ECST-R as a formal competency interview are impermissible because further validation is required to establish its reliability and validity.

In conclusion, forensic clinicians are likely to use different competency measures for different purposes. The GCCT appears to be moderately effective as a very brief screen that is often completed in less than 15 minutes. As such, the GCCT is likely to be useful in high-volume court referrals to screen patients for possible incompetency. In these cases, practitioners are likely to use not only the quantitative cut score (< 70) but also their clinical observations in determining which defendants receive a complete evaluation of their competency to stand trial. The MacCAT-CA would appear to be highly useful in cases where defendants appear to (1) meet rudimentary requirements of competency but (2) lack more complex decisional abilities. Its focus on reasoning is likely to be especially valuable to these cases. The ECST-R is likely to be useful as structured format to provide questions and ratings about potentially complex issues found with "consult with counsel" and "rational understanding" prongs. In addition, the ECST-R can be used to screen out defendants who are unlikely to be feigning incompetency.

13

Other Structured Interviews for Specific Disorders

Structured interviews that have been developed to address many specific disorders and syndromes (Wiens, 1990) vary considerably in terms of validation and clinical applicability. As a result, this chapter is organized into three broad categories:

1. Several structured interviews with extensive research and broad applicability are featured. Featured interviews include (a) the Anxiety Disorders Interview Schedule for DSM-IV (ADIS-IV; Brown, DiNardo, & Barlow, 1995), (b) the Addiction Severity Index (ASI; McLellan, Luborsky, Woody, & O'Brien, 1980; McLellan et al., 1992), (c) the Clinician-Administered PTSD Scale for DSM-IV (CAPS; Blake et al., 1998), and (d) the Eating Disorder Examination (EDE; Fairburn & Cooper, 1994). Each featured interview follows the standard outline: (a) description, (b) reliability and validity, and (c) clinical applications.

2. Brief descriptions are provided for several additional interviews that have more circumscribed clinical applications: the Structured Clinical Interview for DSM-IV Dissociative Disorders (SCID-D; Steinberg, 1994), the Interview for the Retrospective Assessment of the Onset of Schizophrenia (IRAOS; Hafner et al., 1992), and the Comprehensive Drinker Profile (CDP; Marlatt & Miller, 1984).

3. Concise synopses are presented for a broad array of other focused interviews.

FEATURED FOCUSED INTERVIEWS

Anxiety Disorders Interview Schedule (ADIS)

Description

The ADIS, developed by DiNardo and his colleagues (DiNardo, O'Brien, Barlow, Waddell, & Blanchard, 1982) after the emergence of DSM-III, had the following objectives: to provide differential diagnosis of anxiety disorders, to rule out other disorders (e.g., psychotic, substance abuse, and mood disorders), and to supply additional clinical data regarding anxiety (see DiNardo, O'Brien, Barlow, Waddell, & Blanchard, 1983). The ADIS was derived in part from other diagnostic interviews (i.e., the SADS and the PSE).

The ADIS, a semistructured interview, is organized by diagnosis (i.e., GAD, PTSD, acute stress disorder, panic disorder, agoraphobia, specific and social phobias, and OCD), with sections for other diagnoses, including mood disorders, hypochondriasis, somatization, substance abuse, and psychosis. Unlike most structured interviews, the ratings of responses vary widely across the ADIS. Many symptoms are rated on a nominal (yes or no) scale. In addition, 9-point scales are used to determined intensity of specific symptoms in terms either of severity or frequency.

The ADIS has also been modified for use with children. Silverman and Albano (1996) adapted the ADIS-IV-C so that the language and ratings would be appropriate for children. For example, children are asked whether a particular problem "messes things up for you." In addition, symptoms often address school-related behaviors (e.g., asking a teacher for help and taking tests). Symptoms are rated on a 5-point scale that reflects the degree of children's fear, avoidance or distress. An optional "feelings thermometer" is available for the visual depiction of intensity ratings.

See Box 13.1 for an overview and availability information for the ADIS and ADIS-IV-C.

Reliability and Validity

ADIS reliability studies have focused on current diagnoses. As summarized in Table 13.1, kappa coefficients are in the moderate to moderately high range for both interrater and test–retest reliabilities. In the most ambitious study, DiNardo et al. (1993) evaluated the test–retest reliability of the ADIS-R on a large sample ($N = 267$) with varying intervals (0–44 days). For principal diagnoses, the kappas were generally in the moderate range (median = .65). These estimates compare favorably to general Axis I interviews for anxiety disorders within a test–retest paradigm. Low to mediocre estimates for mood disorders are partially attributed to their low base rates in a sample predominated by anxiety disorders.

The question arises whether the ADIS is actually more reliable than gen-

---

BOX 13.1. Highlights of the ADIS-IV and the ADIS-IV-C (Child)

- *Description:* The ADIS-IV, an extensive, semistructured interview for the evaluation of anxiety disorders, also provides coverage of mood and psychotic disorders.

- *Administration time:* For patients with anxiety disorders, the ADIS-IV may require 2 hours to complete the detailed ratings of symptoms and situations. Like most child interviews, the ADIS-IV-C is composed of child and parent interviews that require approximately 1 hour each.

- *Skills level:* The ADIS-IV may be administered by professionals or trained paraprofessionals. When paraprofessionals are used, clinicians directly review the protocols, decide whether additional data are needed, and render diagnoses. The ADIS-IV-C is intended to be administered by clinicians with a moderate level of training.

- *Distinctive features:* The ADIS-IV provides a template for treatment planning by examining symptoms based on common circumstances. Symptoms are rated by their frequency and the degree of distress/impairment they cause. The ADIS-IV-C includes the optional use of a "feeling thermometer" that provides a visual, 5-point scale of impairment.

- *Cost:* As of 3/1/2001, the price for the ADIS = $18; 10 interview booklets = $48. The price for ADIS-IV-C manual = 18; 10 interview booklets (child) = $64; 10 interview booklets (parent) = $72.

- *Sources:* Contact the Psychological Corporation, on the internet, *www.psychcorp.com;* by phone, (800) 211-8378; or by mail, 535 Academic Court, San Antonio, TX 78204-2498.

---

eral Axis I interviews for the diagnosis of anxiety disorders. The answer is far from clear. Studies such as that of DiNardo et al. (1993) have very positive results for several anxiety disorders. However, these studies have a major advantage over Axis I interviews utilized with more heterogenous populations, producing low base rates of anxiety disorders. The most prudent course is to consider the ADIS a reliable measure of anxiety disorders, without making comparative judgments about its possible superiority.

The chief shortcoming of the ADIS is the lack of reliability data on symptoms and intensity ratings. Burns, Formea, Keortge, and Sternberger (1995) provided only preliminary data on the presence–absence of specific symptoms. Based on 8 community participants, they produced very high kappas. Because detailed ratings of frequency and severity are hallmarks of the ADIS, this general neglect of such ratings limits the research and clinical applications of the ADIS. A second limitation is the reliance on earlier versions (i.e., ADIS and ADIS-R) for reliability studies.

TABLE 13.1. Reliability Studies for the Anxiety Disorders Interview Schedule (ADIS) and ADIS—Child Version (ADIS-C)

Study (year)		N	Setting In/Out/Com/Univ	Dx	Raters Lay/Prof	Reliability Inter/Retest (interval)	Reliability estimates Sx/Cur-Dx/Life-Dx/Other
Adult studies							
DiNardo et al. (1983)		60	✓	6		✓ (< 3 wk)	.68
DiNardo & Barlow[a]		125	✓	5		✓ (NA)	.86
Paradis et al. (1992)		93[b]	✓	6	✓	✓[c]	.82
DiNardo et al. (1993)		267	✓	9	✓	✓ (< 45 days)	.65
Abel & Borkovec (1995)		40	✓	1[d]	✓	✓	.95[e]
Burns et al. (1995)		8	✓	2	✓	✓	.96 1.00
Child studies							
Silverman & Nelles (1988)	(C)	51	✓	4	✓	✓	.69[f] .98[g]
	(P)	51	✓	4	✓	✓	.61 .99[g]
Silverman & Eisen (1992)	(C)	50	✓	4	✓	✓ (10–14 days)	.79 .61[g]
	(P)	50	✓	4	✓	✓ (10–14 days)	.64 .46[g]
Rapee et al. (1994)	(C)	131	✓	4	✓		.79
	(P)	131	✓	4	✓		.81
Silverman & Rabian[h]	(C)	66	✓	4	✓	✓ (10–14 days)	.46[i]
	(P)	66	✓	4	✓	✓ (10–14 days)	.67[i]

Note. See Table 1.5 (p. 35) for a glossary of terms and abbreviations. For child studies, (C) = child's report; (P) = parent's report.

[a] Unpublished study cited in Sanderson, DiNardo, Rapee, and Barlow (1990).
[b] Sample mostly limited to African Americans (91.5%).
[c] Reliability derived from patient responses, technically, interscorer reliability.
[d] Generalized anxiety disorder.
[e] Only percentage of agreement (kappa not reported).
[f] Kappa evidence a marked split (i.e., .35, .38, 1.00, and 1.00).
[g] Correlations of symptom scales.
[h] Further analysis of data in Silverman and Eisen (1992).
[i] Only for select symptoms of separation anxiety disorder, avoidant disorder, and overanxious disorder.

The reliability of the ADIS-IV-C has also been investigated in child and adolescent outpatients. Silverman and her colleagues (see Table 13.1) found a moderate level of interrater and test–retest reliability for a subset of anxiety disorders. ADIS-IV-C child interviews produced more reliable diagnoses than did parent informants. However, parents appeared more reliable in the description of symptoms (median kappa = .64) than their children (median kappa = .46). Interestingly, age did not appear to be a major factor influencing the reliability of children's self-reporting.

Rapee, Barrett, Dadds, and Evans (1994) addressed cross-informant consistency in the form of parent–child agreement. Like most child interviews, the convergence was very modest, with a median kappa of .24 for young children (< 10 years) and .34 for older children. These findings are somewhat lower than expected in light of the circumscribed range (i.e., four disorders).

Like many DSM-based interviews, diagnostic validity appears to be assumed rather than rigorously tested. No large scale studies were found that compared ADIS disorders to independent classifications based on clinician diagnoses or other structured interviews. The available studies have produced somewhat mixed results:

- Blanchard, Gerardi, Kolb, and Barlow (1986) examined the concurrent validity of the ADIS for PTSD. Perhaps influenced by demand characteristics, a high level of agreement (93.0%; kappa = .86) was found for 43 male Vietnam combat veterans when compared to clinical diagnoses.
- Paradis, Friedman, Lazar, Grubea, and Kesselman (1992) compared ADIS-R panic disorders to intake diagnoses. Although 24.7% of patients warranted ADIS-R panic disorders, none were diagnosed by clinical staff. The researchers used these negative findings to advocate the use of the ADIS for an apparently neglected diagnosis in minority populations.
- DiNardo et al. (1983) attempted to establish convergent validity with clinicians' ratings on the Hamilton Anxiety (r = .56) and Depression (r = .77) scales. Because the clinicians were not masked to the Hamilton scales, the study is limited by criterion contamination.
- Concordance rates between the ADIS-IV and self-report measures have yielded positive results for the general categories of anxiety disorder (Sinoff, Ore, Zlotogorsky, & Tamir, 1999) and GAD (Roemer, Borkovec, Posa, & Borkovec, 1995).

In line with the Syndeham criteria, ADIS research has also investigated diagnostic boundaries (inclusion and exclusion criteria) and longitudinal dimensions of anxiety disorders (outcome criteria). Several studies have examined the diagnostic boundaries of GAD. For example, Barlow, Blanchard, Vermilyea, Vermilyea, and DiNardo (1986) found that symptom clusters for GAD were endorsed at comparable rates by patients with other anxiety disorders. This finding led them to speculate that GAD should be considered a residual category. Brown, Marten, and Barlow (1995) also found substantial symptom overlap; they proposed increasing the minimum inclusion criteria to four, in order to differentiate more clearly GAD from other anxiety disorders. Not surprisingly, GAD anxiety symptoms are not very common in healthy controls (Abel & Borkovec, 1995). However, this comparison constitutes a nonrigorous test of diagnostic boundaries.

Problems with diagnostic overlap are not restricted to GAD. Barlow, Di-Nardo, Vermilyea, Vermilyea, and Blanchard (1986) found that most referrals to an anxiety disorder clinic qualified for several disorders, including phobias and depression. Likewise, Sanderson, DiNardo, Rapee, and Barlow (1990) found that approximately 70% of anxious patients qualified for more than one anxiety diagnosis, while 33% had a concomitant mood disorder. Other Axis I and II disorders were not sufficiently evaluated to know how much additional overlap occurs. These studies call into question the inclusion and exclusion criteria for DSM–ADIS disorders. Alternatively, these studies from specialized anxiety clinics may reflect more demanding and complicated cases, and have limited generalizability to other samples and settings.

In line with Syndeham's criteria, several studies have used the ADIS-R to evaluate treatment outcome. Brown, Anthony, and Barlow (1995) examined patients with panic disorder, including their response to treatment and functioning at follow-up. They found that comorbidity did not necessarily affect outcome; patients with panic disorders and social phobia evidenced greater symptom improvement that those with only panic disorders. Immediate reductions in comorbidity were not sustained during a 24-month follow-up. In a second study, Tsao, Lewin, and Craske (1998) found that treatment for panic disorders had positive effects on comorbid anxiety disorders. However, comorbidity constituted a nonsignificant trend toward less improvement. Combining results of both studies, panic disorders do not appear to be treatment-specific; at least short-term improvement is found for the broad category of anxiety disorders.

In summary, the ADIS appears to assume that the DSM-III-R and DSM-IV are gold standards of diagnosis. Unfortunately, little attention has been paid to concurrent validity via structured interviews and clinical diagnosis. Moderate evidence of convergent validity is reported. Although problems with diagnostic overlap are observed, they likely represent constraints in DSM-IV anxiety disorders rather than limitations in the ADIS-R and ADIS-IV.

In contrast to the ADIS, the ADIS-IV-C has not been subjected to extensive validation. Messer and Beidel (1994) found that children with anxiety disorders scored higher on trait anxiety and lower on perceived self-confidence than children with test anxiety only or no disorders. While useful in examining the overall category of anxiety disorders, the study has little bearing on specific diagnoses. Additionally, levels of psychosocial maturity appear to differentiate among children with separation anxiety versus overanxious disorders (Westenberg, Siebelink, Warmenhoven, & Treffers, 1999). Miller and

Kamboukos (2000) reported that no published studies are available on ADIS-IV-C validity.

Clinical Applications

The ADIS-IV provides exhaustive coverage of anxiety symptoms. For example, symptoms of agoraphobia are specified for 20 situations (e.g., driving, bridges, and movie theaters). Likewise, social phobias are systematically reviewed for 12 situations (e.g., eating in public, dating, and using public restrooms). Ideally, the ADIS-IV provides a template for treatment by identifying key symptoms and specific circumstances. A treatment program can be generated in cooperation with patients to address individual symptoms in particular situations. To assess progress in treatment, ADIS-IV criteria include ratings of intensity (i.e., the severity and frequency). Improvements are easily quantified for patients and provide additional motivation for further progress.

Because of its treatment focus, the ADIS-IV has paid less attention than other well-established interviews to the reliability of individual symptoms and intensity ratings. From a treatment point of view, emphasis has been placed on patients' perspectives rather than necessarily the veridicality and reproducibility of symptoms. Therefore, the ADIS-IV deemphasizes reliability and cross-informant consistency. In light of this information, when should clinicians utilize the ADIS-IV? The answer depends of the purpose of the assessment:

- *Treatment.* The ADIS-IV is strongly recommended for cases in which the focus is the treatment, especially from cognitive-behavioral and behavioral paradigms. The specification of symptoms, situations, and severity provides a comprehensive assessment of treatment needs.
- *Current diagnosis.* The ADIS-IV is recommended in cases in which the focus is on the diagnostic reliability of the current episode.
- *Symptomatology.* The ADIS-IV is not recommended in cases in which the reliability of key symptoms is central to the assessment.

The ADIS-IV-C is a promising, semistructured interview for childhood anxiety disorders. In the absence of programmatic research on its concurrent, convergent, and construct validity, its current clinical applications are limited. It not recommended as the primary measure for establishing childhood anxiety disorders and screening for mood and psychotic disorders. However, the ADIS-IV-C is likely to be a useful adjunct for case conceptualization and treatment planning (Miller & Kamboukos, 2000).

Clinician-Administered PTSD Scale for DSM-IV (CAPS)

Description

The Clinician-Administered PTSD Scale for DSM-IV (CAPS) was first developed by Blake et al. (1990) and subsequently modified to address DSM-IV symptoms and associated features (Blake et al., 1998). The CAPS is a structured interview designed to evaluate DSM-IV PTSD inclusion criteria in detail. Each inclusion criterion is rated on frequency and intensity (i.e., degree of distress and impairment); descriptive information is also sought for salient examples and constraints on the accuracy of self-reporting (i.e., "questionable validity"). The time framework allows clinicians to evaluate both current (i.e., past week and past month) and lifetime episodes. Although first developed to address combat-related PTSD, the CAPS is now used for a broad range of traumas (Shear et al., 2000).

See Box 13.2 for highlights and availability information for the CAPS.

Reliability and Validity

A small group of reliability studies have yielded consistently high interrater reliability estimates for current diagnosis and overall ratings of symptom intensity and frequency (see Table 13.2). The level of diagnostic agreement is generally excellent. However, the design was straightforward, with the diagnostic task of differentiating between PTSD and non-PTSD participants. A more rigorous research design would compare PTSD to a range of diagnoses, including near-neighbor comparisons (e.g., social phobia and panic disorder).

The diagnosis of PTSD is distinguished from most DSM-IV diagnoses in its three clusters of symptoms (i.e., intrusive, avoidant, and arousal). Several studies have examined the reliability of these symptom clusters (Table 13.2)

BOX 13.2. Highlights of the CAPS

- *Description:* The CAPS is a structured interview for the assessment of PTSD, with dimensional ratings of frequency and severity.
- *Administration time:* 45 to 60 minutes.
- *Skills level:* The CAPS can be administered by either professionals or paraprofessionals with substantial interviewing experience and a moderate level of training.
- *Distinctive features:* PTSD symptoms and concomitant impairment are rated for three periods: past week, past month, and lifetime. The CAPS can be administered for the targeted event plus two other traumatic events.
- *Cost:* The CAPS is in the public domain; contact Terence M. Keane to inquire about any nominal charges.
- *Source:* Contact Terence M. Keane, PhD, by e-mail, *Terry.Keane@med. va.gov;* by phone, (617) 232-9500, ext. 4143; or by mail, National Center for PTSD (116B2), VA Boston Healthcare System, 150 South Huntington Avenue, Boston, MA 012130.

TABLE 13.2. Reliability Studies for the Clinician-Administered PTSD Scale (CAPS)

Study (year)	N	Setting In/Out/Com/Univ	Dx	Raters Lay/Prof	Reliability Inter/Retest (interval)	Reliability estimates Sx/Cur-Dx/Life-Dx/Other	
Blake et al. (1990)	7	✓[a] ✓[a]	1	✓	✓	1.00	>.92[b]
Neal et al. (1994)[c]	43	✓	1	✓	✓	.90	
Malekzai et al. (1996)[d]	30	✓	1	✓	✓		.98[e]
Fleming & Difede (1999)	7	✓[f]	1	✓	✓	.90	.99[g]
Weathers et al. (1999)[h]	84	✓[a] ✓[a]	1	✓	✓ (2–3 days)	.76	.85[i]

Note. See Table 1.5 (p. 35) for a glossary of terms and abbreviations.

[a]Status (inpatient or outpatient) is unreported

[b]Correlations for three subscales; *r*'s > .98 for intensity ratings; *r*'s > .91 for frequency.

[c]The CAPS compared to a computerized CAPS.

[d]Translated in Afghan languages of Pushto and Farsi and administered to Afghan refugees living in the United States.

[e]ICC for symptom intensity and symptom frequency ratings.

[f]Hospitalized burn patients.

[g]Intensity of symptom ratings; .98 for symptom frequency ratings.

[h]These data from two samples are reported previously (e.g., Blake et al., 1995) and incorporated from earlier studies (e.g., Weathers et al., 1992).

[i]Agreement of the three PTSD symptom clusters.

and produced excellent results. The findings of Weathers, Ruscio, and Keane (1999; see also Blake et al., 1995) revealed a high level of agreement (.77 to .96) for these clusters when examined in a test–retest design. While not reported on an individual-symptom level, the current research provides strong support for the reliability of symptom clusters.

The CAPS has excellent interrater reliability in establishing dimensional ratings of overall symptom intensity and frequency. Three studies yielded superb estimates. Because only global estimates are provided, it is difficult to know how much variation occurs at the cluster and symptom levels. Nonetheless, such high estimates suggest very little variation, especially at the cluster level.

Validation of the CAPS has been evaluated through concurrent, convergent, and construct validities. Two major studies (Hyer et al., 1996; Weathers et al., 1999) have compared large samples of combat veterans to SCID diagnoses. Hyer et al. (1996) validated older veterans against a computerized SCID; they found a concordance rate of 92.8%, with a resulting kappa of .75. Weathers et al. (1999) combined samples from earlier studies of Vietnam veterans referred to the National Center for PTSD. They investigated different decision rules for classifying SCID-based PTSD. In general, empirically derived rules calibrated to SCID symptoms yielded a moderate kappa (.75), while those based on overall severity were slightly lower (kappas from .65 to .74). In summary, these studies provide solid evidence of concurrent validity for combat-related PTSD.

For convergent validity, the CAPS typically is compared to self-report PTSD scales, such as the Mississippi Scale for Combat-Related Posttraumatic Stress Disorder (Mississippi Scale; Keane et al., 1988), PTSD Checklist (Weathers, Litz, Herman, Huska, & Keane, 1993), and Impact of Event Scale (IES; Horowitz, Wilner, & Alvarez, 1979). With these specific scales, correlations are typically in the moderate range for veterans and nonveterans (e.g., Blake et al., 1990, 1995; Blanchard, Jones-Alexander, Buckley, & Forneris, 1996; Shear et al., 2000). Other studies have found that higher CAPS scores result in significant differences for self-report scales. For example, Weathers et al. (1999) found that more stringent CAPS criteria were reflected in significantly higher scores on the Mississippi Scale and the PTSD Checklist. For burn patients, Fleming and Difede (1999) found that changes in symptom severity resulted in corresponding changes on the IES and measures of anxiety and depression. Blanchard et al. (1995) found a nonsignificant trend toward greater impairment as CAPS rules were made more stringent. In summary, studies provide consistently strong evidence supporting CAPS convergent validity.

King, Leskin, King, and Weathers (1998) examined the construct validity of the CAPS via confirmatory factor analyses (CFAs) of its symptom clusters. Combining results across earlier studies, a large sample ($N = 524$) of data from male veterans was assembled for several CFAs. The best solution was a four-factor, first-order solution. This solution corresponded to DSM-IV symptom clusters with one modification: Avoidant symptoms were divided into "effortful avoidance" and "emotional numbing." This disaggregation of avoidant symptoms into two factors has strong support theoretically and empirically. In summary, the King et al. study provides strong support for the CAPS–DSM-IV conceptualization of PTSD.

In line with Syndeham's criteria, the longitudinal perspectives of PTSD have been addressed via research on the emergence of PTSD and treatment outcome studies. Salient findings are summarized as follows:

- CAPS results 1 month following a trauma were the best predictor of later PTSD (Shalev, Freedman, Peri, Brandes, & Sahar, 1997). The CAPS outperformed the Mississippi Scale, the IES, and several additional self-report scales.
- CAPS intensity and frequency ratings appeared effective, as measured by other scales, in documenting changes in PTSD symptoms as a result of behavioral treatments.
- CAPS scores and subscale scores appear useful in documenting changes in PTSD as a result of medication trials. Studies have included an anticonvulsant (i.e., divalproex; Clark, Canive, Calais, Qualls, & Tuason, 1999) and a range of antidepressants: nefazodone (Davis, Nugent, Murray, Kramer, & Petty, 2000), bupropion (Canive, Clark, Calais, Qualls, & Tuason, 1997), fluoxetine (van der Kolk et al., 1994), and brofaromine (Baker et al., 1995)

In summary, the CAPS studies provide strong evidence of concurrent and convergent validity. The research on construct validity, including both symptom clusters and outcome data, is very positive for a focused interview. The only major drawback is the lack of research on noncombat-related PTSD cases. While studies have included different traumas (e.g., motor vehicle accidents and severe burns), concurrent and construct validity research with a range of traumas would be very helpful.

Clinical Applications

The CAPS is the measure of choice for the systematic evaluation of male veterans suspected of PTSD. It provides an extensive assessment of diagnosis, symptom clusters, and severity ratings. Data are also available on its usefulness in treatment planning and outcome with this population. The CAPS should be a standard component of PTSD evaluations for male veterans.

Less data are available on the CAPS with other populations, namely, women and civilians. Therefore, the CAPS is likely to have only circumscribed applications with these populations. A primary application is the detailing of symptom clusters and individual symptoms as part of an individualized treatment plan. The provision of dual ratings of severity (intensity and frequency) affords standardized comparisons for the evaluation of treatment progress. Despite limited data on validity, this dual structure is likely to be useful in the development and implementation of treatment programs.

In summary, (1) CAPS is recommended for diagnosis and treatment of PTSD among male veterans, and (2) the CAPS is recommended for treatment of PTSD in other populations. In these cases, diagnosis can be established with an Axis I interview, while the CAPS provides critical data about treatment needs.

Addiction Severity Index (ASI)

Description

McLellan et al. (1980) created the ASI, semistructured interview for assessing the level of substance abuse and its negative consequences in different facets of patients' functioning: family/social, legal, medical, psychological, and employment/support. Unlike most structured interviews, the ASI is relatively unrestricted in its use, permitting both paraprofessionals and nonprofessionals (e.g., receptionists) to administer it with appropriate training (Rounsaville & Poling, 2000). See Box 13.3 for an overview of the ASI and information on its availability.

The fifth edition of the ASI attempts to quantify information for two time parameters: last 30 days and lifetime. Additionally, patients are asked to make severity ratings on a 5-point scale about their own perceptions of prob-

---

BOX 13.3. Highlights of the ASI

- *Description:* The ASI is a semistructured interview for assessing functional domains often impacted by substance abuse (e.g., employment, family and social status, and psychiatric status).

- *Administration time:* Initial evaluations require from 45 minutes to 1 hour and 15 minutes.

- *Skills level:* With relatively modest training, the ASI can be administered by professionals, paraprofessionals, or nonprofessionals.

- *Distinctive features:* The ASI is intended to aid in the development of a comprehensive treatment plan; brief follow-up versions are available to measure treatment progress.

- *Cost:* The ASI is in the public domain and available at no cost; training and reference materials are available at nominal charges.

- *Source:* DeltaMetrics, by mail, One Commerce Square, 2005 Market Street, 11th Floor, Philadelphia, PA 19103, or by phone, (800) 238-2433. The National Institute on Drug Abuse (NIDA) has training materials and videotapes available via National Technical Information Service, (703) 487-4650, Order Number: AVA19615VNB2KVS.

lems in different facets of their lives. For most sections, patients rate their de-gree of distress and motivation for treatment. Finally, interviewers identify potential distortions that either result from a lack of understanding or inten-tional misrepresentation.

Reliability and Validity

Reliability studies of the ASI are summarized in Table 13.3, with the primary emphasis placed on content scales and severity ratings. Key findings on the ASI reliability are as follows:

- Uniformly high reliabilities are reported for the severity ratings.
- Problem scales addressing facets of substance abuse produce generally high reliabilities.
- Individual symptoms and features have been investigated in only one study that produced moderate to moderately high ICCs.

In summary, the ASI is a reliable measure for assessing different facets of substance abuse and providing severity ratings. Less attention has been paid to the stability of these ratings across time. However, the two studies of test–retest reliability have produced very positive findings.

Validity

McClellan et al. (1980) performed the original validity study on a large sam-ple of male VA patients with substance abuse. As evidence of convergent va-lidity, they compared six problem scales with independent criteria. The results were very robust with a median r of .62 ; scales ranged from the lowest for family/social (M r = .48) to legal (M r = .67). To assess differences in treat-ment needs, McClellan et al. compared VA patients with alcoholism versus drug abuse and found modest differences in medical problems (higher in alco-holism) and legal problems (higher in drug abuse).

McClellan, Luborsky, Cacciola, and Griffith (1985) conducted the sec-ond major study of ASI validity with 181 male and female substance abusers. They compared ASI scores to a battery of psychological tests and external measures. Key findings for construct validity are outlined as follows:

- For patients with alcohol abuse, convergent correlations were in the low-moderate range (median r for severity ratings = .42; median r for problem scales = .47); most discriminant correlations were below .30.
- For patients with drug abuse, convergent correlations were generally modest (median r for severity ratings = .36; median r for problem scales = .38); most discriminant correlations were below .25.

Given the complexity of this multitrait–multimethod approach, the con-vergent validities fall in the expected range. Importantly, the convergent cor-

TABLE 13.3. Reliability Studies of the Addiction Severity Index (ASI)

Study (year)	N	Setting In/Out/Com/Univ	Dx	Raters Lay/Prof	Reliability Inter/Retest (interval)	Reliability estimates Sx/Scales/Severity
McLellan et al. (1980)	25	✓	2	✓	✓	.90[a] .89[a]
McLellan et al. (1985)	30	✓ ✓	NA	✓ ✓	✓	.89[a,c] > .93[a]
	40[b]	✓ ✓	NA	✓ ✓	(3 days)	> .91[a]
Hodgins & Guebaly (1992)	15	✓	6[d]	✓ ✓	✓	.85[e] .80[e]
Cacciola et al. (1997)	5[f]	✓	NA	✓ ✓	✓	.59[e]
Cacciola et al. (1999)	108	✓		✓	✓ (1–3 mo)	.52[g]

Note. See Table 1.5 (p. 35) for a glossary of terms and abbreviations.
[a]Spearman–Brown reliability coefficients.
[b]Same interviewers were used for both administrations in 15 of the 40 cases.
[c]Correlations were lower (.74 to .91) but no average was reported.
[d]Common diagnoses for entire sample.
[e]Intraclass coefficients (ICCs).
[f]Videotapes of simulated patients.
[g]Based on 53 family history, family/social lifetime, and psychiatric lifetime items; the median ICC for 40 variables is .67.

relations generally exceed the discriminant correlations, providing general evidence of construct validity. Of the seven scales, the family/social scale appeared the weakest, with convergent correlations less than .30 for both samples.

Subsequent studies have examined the utility of the ASI with clinical populations. McClellan et al. (1992) provided normative data on the use of the ASI with abusers of alcohol, opiates, cocaine, and polysubstances. Hodgins and El-Guebaly (1992) studied the usefulness of the ASI in evaluating patients with comorbid conditions that included substance abuse and an additional Axis I disorder (e.g., mood disorder or schizophrenia). Independent variables significantly predicted ASI problem scales.

Clinical Applications

The ASI is intended as an efficient, semistructured interview for assessing treatment needs in self-referred substance-abusing populations. It provides a highly reliable measure for assessing seven problem scales that are likely to be affected in patients with substance abuse histories. Although recent concerns have been raised about the reliability of severity ratings (Butler et al., 1998), proper training should adequately address this issue.

In patients who voluntarily seek substance abuse treatment, the ASI is an effective and efficient interview for identifying level of impairment and treatment needs. While primarily validated on male VA patients, studies have extended its usefulness to women and non-VA populations. In addition to assessing treatment needs, the ASI has proven valuable as a measure of treatment progress when readministered periodically.

The major limitation of the ASI involves attempts to extend its usefulness to patients coerced into treatment via either social or legal sanctions. As observed by Rounsaville and Poling (2000), the ASI's high face validity allows patients to manipulate their presentations and, consequently, their ASI scores. Although interviewers are asked to evaluate every patient's forthrightness on each problem scale, this judgment is largely dependent on the skill of the interviewer and his or her knowledge of the patient. The apparent susceptability of the ASI to faking is a general problem for all substance abuse measures (Rogers & Kelly, 1997).

Eating Disorder Examination (EDE)

Description

Cooper and Fairburn (1987) developed the EDE, as a semistructured interview for the assessment of psychopathology associated with eating disorders. Among the 62 ratings are items that address behavioral (e.g., diet, self-induced vomiting, and exercise) and attitudinal (preoccupation with food, fear of fatness, guilt about eating) dimensions of eating. With few exceptions, individual items are measured on a 7-point scale of increasing severity. The most recent version (Fairburn & Cooper, 1993) has four subscales: restraint, eating concern, weight concern, and shape concern. Box 13.4 provides an overview of the EDE and information on its availability.

The EDE questions were selected for their ability to differentiate among four criterion groups: (1) patients with anorexia nervosa, (2) patients with bulimia nervosa, (3) age-matched controls with current concerns about weight and shape, and (4) age-matched controls without such concerns. Because of patients' problems with accuracy in long-term recall, the EDE is intended to assess only current (i.e., the last 4 weeks) characteristics of eating disorders.

Reliability and Validity

Cooper and Fairburn (1987) reported very high interrater reliability for individual EDE items with a small sample of three raters and 12 participants. With correlations for dimensional ratings, the agreement was superb, with 95.2% of EDE items having *r*'s > .90. Subsequent research (see Table 13.4) has been very limited. Rosen et al. (1990) found excellent interrater reliability for the EDE scales. The only study to evaluate test–retest reliability was by

---

BOX 13.4. Highlights of the EDE

- *Description:* The EDE is a semistructured interview for the evaluation of psychopathology associated with eating disorders. It is designed to assess both DSM-IV criteria and the severity of eating disorder pathology.

- *Administration time:* 30–60 minutes.

- *Skills level:* The EDE requires extensive training for interviewers experienced in the assessment of eating disorders.

- *Distinctive features:* The EDE provides a conceptual model for evaluating four facets of eating disorders: (1) restraint, (2) eating concerns, (3) weight concerns, and (4) shape concerns. It also addresses behavioral dimensions, including overeating and methods of weight control.

- *Cost:* The EDE, with scoring instructions, is available in Fairburn and Cooper (1993), a chapter in the book *Binge Eating: Nature, Assessment, and Treatment* (Fairburn & Wilson, 1993). Single copies of the EDE are also available free from the first author.

- *Source:* The book is available from the Guilford Press, on the internet, *www.guilford.com;* by phone, (800) 365-7006; or by fax, (212) 966-6708. Copies of the EDE are available from Christopher G. Fairburn, DM, FRC Psych, Department of Psychiatry, Warneford Hospital, Oxford OX3 7JX, United Kingdom.

TABLE 13.4. Reliability Studies for the Eating Disorder Examination (EDE) and Eating Disorder Examination—Self Report Questionnaire (EDE-Q)

Study (year)	Measure	N	Setting In/Out/Com/Univ	Dx	Raters Lay/Prof	Reliability Inter/Retest (interval)	Reliability estimates Sx/Scales
Cooper & Fairburn (1987)	EDE	12	✓	2	✓[a]	✓	> .90[b]
Rosen et al. (1990)	EDE	20	✓	2	✓[a]	✓	.95
Luce & Crowther (1999)	EDE-Q	139	✓	NA		✓ (2 wk)	.90

Note. See Table 1.5 (p. 35) for a glossary of terms and abbreviations.
[a]Simply referred to as "trained interviewers."
[b]Correlations.

Luce and Crowther (1999), based on the questionnaire version (EDE-Q); they found excellent reliability for the EDE scales (median r = .90; range from .81 to .94). Overall, the following two conclusions can be drawn about the EDE reliability:

1. The EDE scales and symptoms appear very promising based on initial studies.
2. The absence of large-scale reliability data suggests that the EDE should only be used as an ancillary measure for the assessment of eating disorders.

Pike, Wolk, Gluck, and Walsh (2000, p. 670) provide an excellent summary of past research on the EDE subscales and their discriminant validity. Combined studies evaluate differences among patients with bulimia nervosa (n = 218) and anorexia nervosa (n = 97), participants concerned with weight (n = 114), and psychologically healthy controls (n = 379). Although effect sizes were not reported, the EDE subscales clearly differentiate among criterion groups:

- Healthy controls average well below 1.00 across scales.
- Participants concerned with weight generally averaged < 2.00 across scales; only a small sample of restrained eaters exceeded this benchmark.
- Patients with anorexia nervosa scored highest on restraint (M = 3.49), with patients with bulimia scoring the lowest (M = 1.74), and the other three scales generally scoring in the range of 2.00 to 3.00.
- Patients with bulimia nervosa tended to have the highest scores, with most subscales elevated above 3.00 except for eating concern (i.e., mostly in the range of 2.00–3.00).

In summary, these subscales appear to have moderate discriminant validity in distinguishing among criterion groups (see also Cooper, Cooper, & Fairburn, 1989). This discriminant validity has also been extended to binge-eating disorders (Wilfley, Schwartz, Spurrell, & Fairburn, 2000).

Validation studies have also investigated EDE convergent validity in relationship to eating behavior and other eating-related scales. Rosen, Vara, Wendt, and Leitenberg (1990) found predicted relations for eating records and caloric intake, although the magnitude was often modest (r's < .40). However, EDE scales associated with weight and shape concerns were highly correlated (r's > .75) with the Body Shape Questionnaire (Cooper, Taylor, Cooper, & Fairburn, 1987). Fitcher et al. (1991) compared the EDE scores with the Stuctured Interview for Anorexia and Bulimia Nervosa (SIAB; see "Synopsis of Focused Interviews") with positive but modest correlations.

Several studies have also investigated the usefulness of the EDE in research on longitudinal studies of treatment outcome. Employing pre- and postmeasures, Smith, Marcus, and Kaye (1992) found the EDE useful in recording changes as a result of cognitive-behavioral treatment. In contrast, Wilson and Eldredge (1991) divided patients with eating disorders in terms of poor and good outcomes as a result of 20 sessions of cognitive-behavioral treatment. Improvement was not documented by the EDE. One potential confound in the study was that patients' initial psychopathology appeared to influence the efficacy of treatment.

Studies have also sought to use EDE results in predicting the course of eating disorders. In a large-scale study of female twins, Wade et al. (1999) established both genetic and environmental influences on the prevalence of eating disorders. Morgan, Lacey, and Sedgwick (1999) studied the effects of pregnancy on the course of bulimia nervosa. They found that most participants improved during the pregnancy. Following delivery, the outcomes diverged: 34% were no longer bulimic but 57% relapsed into more severe symptoms than those experienced before the pregnancy. Finally Turner, Batik, Palmer, Forbes, and McDermott (2000) found the EDE to be valuable in predicting future laxative use among patients with anorexia nervosa.

Clinical Applications

Validity data consistently demonstrate highly significant differences between patients with and without eating disorders. Less pronounced differences are found between specific diagnoses that may reflect either (1) limitations in the differential diagnosis of DSM eating disorders or (2) constraints in the EDE's diagnostic validity. A major limitation of the EDE is its reliability data; while very positive, larger studies are needed to confirm the current findings.

The EDE provides both categorical and dimensional data on eating disorders. Pike et al. (2000) reported that sufficient information is covered for the diagnosis of anorexia nervosa, anorexia bulimia, and eating disorder NOS. However, the EDE's validation emphasizes its dimensional ratings rather than differential diagnoses of DSM-IV eating disorders. Therefore, clinicians are likely to choose the EDE because of its focus on important psychological dimensions of eating disorders. In particular, the EDE assists mental health professionals in examining how critical issues (e.g., restraint, weight, and shape) affect patients' perceptions and treatment needs.

The EDE is clinically useful in planning treatment interventions for patients with eating disorders. Researchers have used the EDE with some success to document treatment progress. From this perspective, the EDE may prove beneficial in providing patients with systematic feedback about their accomplishments in treatment. Such feedback may stimulate additional motivation and further progress.

Several alternative forms of the EDE are available. The EDE-Q is a self-report version intended as a screen for the EDE. Wilson, Nonas, and Rosenblum (1993) cited unpublished data supporting its use. In addition, Pike et al.

(2000) described the Children EDE (ChEDE), which simplifies the language of the EDE to faciliate comprehension.

In summary, the EDE appears to be clinically appropriate for the assessment of eating disorders. Establishment of DSM-IV eating disorders would require independent evaluation. Patients with eating disorders should also be evaluated for comorbidity, since other disorders (see Wilson & Eldredge, 1991) may negatively affect treatment. Overall, the EDE would appear to be a top candidate as a focused interview for the dimensional assessment of eating disorders.

OTHER FOCUSED INTERVIEWS OF CLINICAL INTEREST

Structured interviews within this section are briefly summarized. These interviews either have circumscribed clinical applications (SCID-D and IRAOS) or limited availability (CDP). Information on accessing these measures is summarized in Box 13.5.

Structured Clinical Interview for DSM-IV Dissociative Disorders (SCID-D)

The SCID-D (Steinberg, 1994) is a semistructured interview for the evaluation of dissociative disorders and symptomatology. The SCID-D is composed of 276 questions organized into eight sections: psychiatric history, amnesia, depersonalization, derealization, identity confusion, identity alteration, associated features of identity disturbance, and follow-up. Questions are organized into standard questions, branching questions, and optional probes.

Highlights on reliability of the SCID-D are as follows:

- Interrater reliability appears excellent (kappas > .80) for two disorders: dissociative identity disorder (kappa of .90) and dissociative disorder NOS, with good agreement for five core symptoms (median kappa = .78) on 48 outpatients of whom approximately one-half had dissociative disorders (Steinberg, Rounsaville, & Cicchetti, 1990). Steinberg et al. found that the SCID-D yielded excellent reliability for the two disorders that were adequately represented (kappa of .82). Agreement of symptom scales was generally good (weighted kappas ranged from .59 to .88, with a median of .78).
- Test–retest reliability appears to be excellent for the five core symptoms and the presence–absence of a dissociative disorder (Steinberg, 1994, see also Putnam, Noll, & Steinberg, 2000). Unfortunately, because these estimates are not published, independent examination of the reliability coefficients is impossible.
- A Dutch translation appears to show promise for its interrater reliability. Boon and Draijer (1991) achieved nearly perfect agreement on di-

BOX 13.5. Resources for Focused Interviews

- *Structured Clinical Interview for DSM-IV Dissociative Disorders (SCID-D)* is available from American Psychiatric Press through HealthSource Bookstore, by phone, 800 713-7122; on the internet, *www.healthsource-books.org;* or by mail, 1400 K Street, NW, Washington, DC 20005-2401.

- *Interview for the Retrospective Assessment of the Onset of Schizophrenia (IRAOS)* is authored by Heinz Hafner, Head, Central Institute of Mental Health, P.O. Box 122120, D-6800, Mannheim 1, Germany.

- *Comprehensive Drinker Profile (CDP)* is no longer published by Psychological Assessment Resources. Contact its first author, William R. Miller, PhD, Department of Psychology, University of Mexico, Albuquerque, NM, 87131-1161, by phone, (505) 277-2805, by e-mail, *WRMiller@unm.edu.*

- *Structured Interview for the Five-Factor Model of Personality (SIFFM)* is available through Psychological Assessment Resources (PAR), by phone, (800) 331-8378; on the internet, *www.parinc.com;* or by mail, P.O. Box 998, Odessa, FL 33556.

- Acute Stress Disorder Inventory (ASDI) is available on the internet, *www.psy.unsw.edu.au/~richardb/asdi/,* or by contacting the author, Richard Bryant, by e-mail, *r.bryant@unsw.edu.au,* or by mail, School of Psychology, University of New South Wales, 2052, Australia.

- *Clinical Eating Disorders Rating Instrument (CEDRI)* is authored by Robert Palmer, MB, Academic Department, Psychiatric Unit, Leicester General Hospital, Gwendolen Road, Leicester LE5 4PW, United Kingdom.

- *Interview for the Diagnosis of Eating Disorders—IV (IDED-IV)* is available from Vesna Kutlesic, University of New Mexico Health Sciences Center, Children's Psychiatric Hospital, 1001 Yale Boulevard, NE, Albuquerque, NM 87131.

- *Structured Interview for Anorexia and Bulimia Nervosa (SIAB)* is authored by Manfred M. Fichter, MD, Medical Director, Nevernklinik der Universität München, Psychiatrische Klinik, Nussbaumstrasse 7, 800 Munich 2, Germany.

- *Dissociative Disorders Interview Schedule (DDIS)* is available as an appendix of C. A. Ross (1997). The DDIS is also available at no cost from Colin A. Ross, MD, 1701 Gateway, Suite 349, Richardson, TX 75080.

- *Structured Clinical Interview for the Mood Spectrum (SCI-MOODS)* is authored by Giovanni B. Cassano and his colleagues. Contact Dr. Cassano by mail, Department of Psychiatry, Neurobiology, Pharmacology, and Biotechnology, University of Pisa, Via Roma 67, 56100 Pisa, Italy; by phone, +39-50-385419; or by fax +39-50-21581.

- *Primary Care Evaluation of Mental Disorders (PRIME-MD)* is reproduced in Spitzer et al. (1994). It is also available from Robert L. Spitzer, MD, Biometric Research Department, Unit 60, New York State Psychiatric Institute, 1051 Riverside Drive, New York, NY 10032.

(cont.)

BOX 13.5 *(cont.)*

- *Structured and Scaled Interview to Assess Maladjustment (SSIAM)* is authored by Barry J. Gurland and colleagues. According to 1972 articles, Dr. Gurland was at the Biometric Research Department, New York State Psychiatric Institute, 1051 Riverside Drive, New York, NY 10032.

- *Biographical Personality Interview (BPI)* is authored by Detlev von Zerssen, Ottostrasse 11, D-82319 Starnberg, Germany; academic address: Max Planck Institute of Psychiatry, Clinical Institute, Kraepelinstrasse 2, D-80804, Munich, Germany; or by fax, +49-8151-4116.

- *Gender Role Assessment Schedule—Child (GRAS-C).* Its first author, Dr. Heino F. L. Meyer-Bahlburg, PhD, is a research scientist at New York State Psychiatric Institute, 1051 Riverside Drive, New York, NY 10032.

- *Derogatis Interview for Sexual Functioning (DISF)* is available from Clinical Psychometric Research, Inc., by mail, 100 West Pennsylvania Avenue, Suite 302, Towson, MD 21204; by phone, (410) 321-6165; or by fax, (410) 321-6341.

---

agnosis (97.7%) but did not report any reliability estimates. Goff, Olin, Jenike, Baer, and Buttolph (1992), with a very modest sample of 16 patients, found a range of kappas (.66, .73, and 1.00) for three disorders. Reliability for the five core symptoms was more impressive (.85 to .96, with a median of .92).

- Other U.S. studies have been sparse. Bremmer, Steinberg, Southwick, Johnson, and Charney (1993) evaluated only total SCID-D scores and found nearly perfect agreement (ICC = .95).

In summary, the SCID-D appears to have good to excellent reliability for its five core symptoms. Additionally, it appears reliable for diagnosis, although the adequacy of the sampling for certain dissociative disorders is a cause for concern. Finally, the reliability of individual items remains unknown.

Validity studies have focused on discriminant validity, namely, whether SCID-D core symptoms differ between patients with and without dissociative disorders. Steinberg et al. (1990) found consistent differences between 18 patients (M = 3.46) with and 23 patients (M = 2.02) without dissociative disorders. While limited by criterion contamination, Boon and Draijer (1991) found highly significant differences in the expected direction for core SCID-D symptoms. Interestingly, Bremner et al. (1993) examined veterans with PTSD and found their core symptoms (M = 3.40) comparable to those of dissociative disorders. While patients with PTSD may have dissociative symptoms, the overall similarity in SCID-D symptoms raises questions about discriminant validity.

The SCID-D is a useful, semistructured interview for addressing core symptoms of dissociative disorders. Clearly, its reliability and validity have focused primarily on the five core symptoms and concomitant diagnoses. Practitioners faced with extensive SCID-D interviews (1–3 hours for dissociative disorders) will likely question the exhaustive coverage, with its paucity of validation. This issue is especially salient for diagnostic cases. For treatment, SCID-D coverage is likely to make sense in planning treatment interventions for patients already diagnosed with dissociative disorders. In this regard, Steinberg (1996b; Steinberg & Hall, 1997) provides specific guidelines for how SCID-D data can assist in treatment planning.

The SCID-D has been advocated for both forensic and adolescent populations. With respect to the former, Steinberg, Bancroft, and Buchanan (1993) discussed the forensic applications of the SCID-D in evaluating dissociative disorders, especially in criminal cases. Clearly, the SCID-D standardizes the assessment and facilitates the comparison of self- and informant reports in forensic evaluations. However, forensic clinicians are likely to be concerned about the dearth of validity data on individual SCID-D items. The recommendation that the SCID-D be used clinically with children and adolescents appears premature. In advocating SCID-D use, Steinberg (1996a) cites only four case studies with adolescents.

Interview for the Retrospective Assessment of the Onset of Schizophrenia (IRAOS)

The IRAOS (Hafner et al., 1992) is a semistructured interview that retrospectively evaluates the onset of 66 specific symptoms and signs. Each symptom/sign is rated on three criteria: presence during the course of the disorder, onset, and manifestation (e.g., continuous or reoccurring). Mental health professionals typically administer the IRAOS to patients in remission. Corroborative interviews with close informants are frequently used.

Highlights of IRAOS reliability are summarized as follows:

- Hafner et al. (1992) reported excellent interrater reliability (.73 to .97) for various aspects of symptomatology.
- Cross-informant agreement addressed the presence of specific symptoms during the early course of the disorder. The data (Hambrecht, Hafner, & Loffler, 1994) evidenced a moderate percentage of agreement (median = 67.9%) but only modest kappas (median = .27).
- Cross-informant agreement also addressed the onset of specific symptoms; the relationship between reports was impressive (median r = .49) given the retrospective requirements.
- Test–retest reliability on a small sample indicated a moderate level of reliability even after an extended interval (M = 10.4 months). Maurer and Hafner (1995) found a median kappa of .39, with a moderately high percentage of agreement (74.3% had ≥ 60.0% concordance).

The primary emphasis of IRAOS validation is the establishment of relia-bility and consistency across sources (patient and informant). Although the kappa coefficients are generally in the low to moderate range, these should be viewed positively given the demands on patients to recall accurately symp-toms that occurred years before and often during an actively psychotic episode. Especially with the age of onset, subsets of individual symptoms evi-dence moderate to exceptionally high cross-informant consistency: 20 symp-toms with r's $\geq$ .70, and 13 symptoms with r's $\geq$ .80.

Current investigations have focused primarily on early symptoms of pa-tients with schizophrenia. In order to establish the longitudinal dimensions of specific disorders, comparisons with other diagnoses would be extremely helpful. As reported by Hambrecht et al. (1994), the earliest symptoms of pa-tients with subsequent psychotic episodes were very general, covering (1) de-pression, anxiety, worry, self-confidence, and lack of energy, as well as (2) suspicion, persecutory delusions, and delusions of reference. Diagnostic com-parisons would allow clinicians to know which symptoms are likely predic-tive of specific disorders. In a variation of this idea, Hambrecht and Hafner (1996) investigated the role of substance abuse in relationship to the onset of schizophrenia. Alcohol and drug abuse were associated with earlier onset for first negative and first positive symptoms. For drug abusers, the difference was most pronounced for positive symptoms, averaging more than 5 years. In addition, specific psychotic symptoms were associated with substance abuse. For example, patients with alcohol abuse are more likely than others to evi-dence auditory hallucinations and expansive mood.

The IRAOS has also been used to predict the course of schizophrenic dis-orders. Eggers and Bunk (1997) used the IRAOS to examine patients' early symptoms of childhood schizophrenia and their relationship to further episodes over a span of four decades. Earlier onset, but not the number of positive or negative symptoms, predicted unremitted cases.

Clinically, the IRAOS has limited applications. Clinicians are rarely called upon to establish the earliest signs and symptoms of a particular disor-der. Without any differentiating patterns between specific disorders, knowl-edge of early symptoms is unlikely to be predictive of the first psychotic episode or the course of a schizophrenic disorder. Instead, the great strength of the IRAOS is its contribution to clinical research. The IRAOS has the po-tential to assist in (1) establishing the diagnostic boundaries of near-neighbor disorders, (2) demonstrating the prodromal courses of specific disorders, and (3) determining possible treatment interventions prior to the first full episode.

Comprehensive Drinker Profile (CDP)

The CDP (Marlatt & Miller, 1984) is a structured interview to assess alco-holism and potential for alcoholic treatment. In addition, Miller and Marlatt (1987) devised several related measures: an abbreviated version (Brief Drinker Profile), a treatment outcome version (Follow-up Drinker Profile), and a corroborative version (Collateral Interview Form). The CDP is organized into three sections: demographic information (e.g., family and employment history), drinking history (e.g., alcohol consumption, alcohol-related life problems, other substance abuse, and related medical history), and motivational information (e.g., reasons for drinking, and motivation for treatment). Most inquiries require nominal ratings (presence or absence). One notable exception is the computation of alcohol consumption, which is calculated in Standard Ethanol Content (SEC) units across days and episodes. From these data, estimates of blood alcohol concentrations (BACs) are derived. Embedded in the alcohol-related problems are two scales: the Michigan Alcoholism Screening Test (MAST; Selzer, 1971) and 12-item Ph score for physical dependence.

Highlights on reliability of the CDP are as follows:

- Moderate agreement exists between patients and informants on alcohol consumption.[1] Self-referred alcoholics had low-moderate levels of agreement at intake (median $r = .44$; Miller, Crawford, & Taylor, 1979). These levels improved at the completion of treatment (median $r = .53$) and at a 3-month follow-up (median $r = .72$). Other studies (Brown & Miller, 1993; Miller, Benefield, & Tonigan, 1992) have produced generally positive results with cross-informant consistency.
- Interrater reliability on 26 CDP interviews for 22 indices was evidenced excellent agreement (r's from .86 to 1.00; Miller, Leckman, Delaney, & Tinkcom, 1992).

In summary, the data are very encouraging for cross-informant consistency on the level of alcohol consumption. Interestingly, patients were as likely to underestimate as overestimate alcohol use. For interrater reliability, dimensional ratings were highly reliable. Additional studies focused on both interrater and test–retest reliability would be very helpful. Overall, these results are limited in their generalizability because of the emphasis on self-referred patients who abuse alcohol.

Test manuals for the CDP (Miller & Marlatt, 1984, 1987) do not directly address validity. From one perspective, the convergence of self-report and informant data could be perceived as convergent validity, particularly with respect to alcohol consumption and peak BAC. With reference to predictive validity, CDP scores predicted treatment success. A substantial body of treatment literature (e.g., Bien, Miller, & Boroughs, 1993; Harris & Miller, 1990; Miller, 1978; Miller & Dougher, 1989; Miller, Gribskow, & Mortell, 1981; Miller, Sovereign, & Krege, 1988; Miller & Taylor, 1980; Miller, Taylor, & West, 1980) suggests that high SEC and BAC scores at intake, despite treatment improvement, are likely to predict relapses. In addition, Miller, Hedrick, and Taylor (1983) found that improvements in alcohol-related problems were associated with concomitant decreases in alcohol use.

---

[1]The one sample that included court-referred alcoholics (37.0%) had substantially lower correlations.

Research has also demonstrated that alcoholics' beliefs about drinking (e.g., Miller, Benefield, et al., 1992) and treatment goals (Graber & Miller, 1988), as measured by the CDP, produced expected differences in treatment outcome. Miller, Leckman, et al. (1992) predicted long-term outcomes through the integration of four earlier studies. In a discriminant analysis, they found that data from the CDP at intake predicted long-term outcomes. Surprisingly, MAST scores at intake did not predict outcome.

Clinically, the CDP appears to be particularly effective as an adjunct to treatment with self-referred alcoholics. A substantial literature describes its efficacy, especially as treatment continues, in accurately assessing alcohol use (SEC and BAC) and alcohol-related problems. Moreover, the CDP appears, at least in general terms, to document overall improvement and decreased likelihood of relapse.

The focus of the CDP in documenting alcohol use by time of the day, day of the week, and type of alcohol is likely to assist problem drinkers in not glossing over the amount of alcohol they consume. Without such structure, patients with alcohol abuse are likely to overlook/disregard important elements of their drinking patterns. Of course, alcoholics may still choose to minimize their consumption. As a protection against minimization, clinicians may elect to conduct routine, corroborative interviews.

SYNOPSIS OF OTHER FOCUSED INTERVIEWS

In the last several decades, we have seen the proliferation of focused interviews with limited clinical applications. This section identifies promising measures that often require further testing and validation prior to their adoption in clinical practice. For availability of these focused interviews, see Box 13.5.

Specific Disorders and Syndromes

Acute Stress Disorder Inventory (ASDI)

The ASDI (Bryant, Harvey, Dang, & Sackville, 1998) is composed of 19 items related to DSM-IV criteria for acute stress disorder. Items are rated dichotomously as absent or present. ASDI test–retest reliability (2- to 7-day intervals) yielded high correlations for cluster scores (median $r = .86$); diagnostic agreement appeared moderately high at 80.8%; however, no kappa was reported. For validation, five experts rated content validity high on relevance and clarity. In addition, Bryant et al. investigated concurrent validity based on independent clinical interviews; they found moderate agreement for the diagnosis (kappa = .75) and the clusters (median kappa = .65). As noted by the authors, the ASDI is in its early stages of scale validation.

Clinical Eating Disorders Rating Instrument (CEDRI)

The CEDRI (Palmer, Christie, Cordle, Davis, & Kedrick, 1987) is a semi-structured interview composed of 31 ratings, of which 22 items cover symptomatology associated with eating disorders. The CEDRI was tested on two small reliability studies (N's = 10 and 11 female participants, respectively). For the 22 items that specifically address eating disorder symptomatology, the median Kendall's coefficient was .88, indicating an excellent agreement on individual symptoms. Large-scale research on the CEDRI is needed prior to its adoption in clinical practice.

Interview for the Diagnosis of Eating Disorders—IV (IDED-IV)

The IDED-IV (Kutlesic, Williamson, Gleaves, Barbin, & Murphy-Eberenz, 1998) contains both a semistructured (e.g., history of eating and other mental disorders) and a structured (i.e., systematic ratings of DSM-IV criteria) interview. Interviewers rate the severity or frequency of specific symptoms on a 5-point scale. Through a series of four related studies, Kutlesic et al. (1998) evaluated the reliability and validity of the IDED-IV. Interrater reliability for three eating disorders and two controls (obese and normal weight) was excellent for both diagnoses (median kappa = .88) and individual symptoms (median kappa = .78). Content validity was established through ratings by 10 experts on eating disorders. Convergent validity was explored via relationships with self-report measures of eating disorders; most measures evidenced moderate correlations with the three IDED-IV subscales. In summary, the IDED-IV demonstrates superb reliability and satisfactory convergent validity. Research is needed on its concurrent validity. Presently, the IDED-IV could be used in clinical practice to evaluate individual symptoms and their changes as a result of treatment interventions.

Structured Interview for Anorexia and Bulimia Nervosa (SIAB)

The SIAB (Fitcher et al., 1991) was constructed to assess a broader range of individual and family psychopathology than is found on most eating disorder measures. Compatible with both the DSM-III-R and the ICD-10, the SIAB is organized into two components: the SIAB-P for psychopathology (62 items) and the SIAB-FAM for family interaction and pathology (25 items). Items are scored on a 5-point scale and interpreted in relationship to diagnosis and factor scores. For reliability, high levels of Kendall's coefficient of concordance were reported for composite scales using six videotapes and six lay interviewers. For construct validity, a principal components analysis (PCA) yielded a six-factor solution: body image (12% of the variance), social integration (12%), depression (11%), anxiety/compulsion (7%), bulimic behavior (6%), and laxative abuse (5%). Unfortunately, the stability of this solution has not been evaluated. For convergent validity, comparisons with the EDE were in the predicted direction but modest in magnitude (i.e., < .40). Additional research is needed on the construct, convergent, and concurrent validity of the SIAB. At present, it is not recommended for clinical practice.

Structured Interview of Sleep Disorders (SIS-D)

The SIS-D (Schramm et al., 1993) was developed for the standardized assessment of sleep–wake disorders in accordance with DSM-III-R. The SIS-D is composed of (1) a semistructured component for assessing physical health, substance abuse, medications, and mental health, and (2) a structured component for assessing sleep disorders. With an initial validation study of 68 patients from sleep laboratories and an inpatient psychiatric unit, two interviewers were able to achieve good test–retest reliability at 1- to 3-day intervals (kappas from .49 to .91; median = .79). Initial data on 30 patients suggests that the diagnosis was confirmed by sleep laboratory findings in 90% of the cases. The SIS-D shows considerable promise as a potential measure for the evaluation of sleep disorders.

Dissociative Disorders Interview Schedule (DDIS)

The DDIS (Ross, 1997; Ross et al.,1989) is a fully structured interview for the evaluation of dissociative disorders and other diagnoses of interest (e.g., somatization, borderline personality disorder, and major depression). Its initial validation was based on relatively small numbers (e.g., 20 patients with dissociative identity disorder [DID]). According to Ross (1991; see also Putnam, Noll, & Steinberg, 2000), the DDIS has a moderate interrater reliability for DID (kappa = .68). For concurrent validity with clinical diagnosis, the DDIS had produced superb agreement for DID, with kappas of .95 and .96 in two studies (see Ross, 1997). One main limitation of the DDIS is the lack of programmatic research on its interrater and test–retest reliability (Putnam et al., 2000). A second limitation is that concurrent validity has focused predominantly on DID and not on all dissociative disorders. For clinical practice, mental health professionals would need to establish their own interrater reliability. A further consideration is the DDIS's extensive coverage of childhood physical and sexual abuse, which appears to be associated with dissociative symptoms (Anderson, Yasenik, & Ross, 1993). Given the enduring controversies over repressed and recovered memories, clinicians are likely to be divided over the merits of extensive queries on this potentially explosive issue.

Structured Clinical Interview for the Mood Spectrum (SCI-MOODS)

The SCI-MOODS (Cassano et al., 1999) was developed to detect bipolar symptoms and characteristics extending beyond DSM criteria. The SCI-MOODS focuses on subthreshold criteria related to physical experiences, energy levels, mood phenomenology, and cognitive changes. Because Cassano et al. did not provide empirical data on the SCI-MOODS's reliability and validity, it consequently cannot be recommended for clinical practice.

Substance Use Disorders Diagnostic Schedule (SUDDS)

The SUDDS (Kruedelbach et al., 1993) assesses the 23 DSM-III-R substance abuse and dependence disorders. It is a 99-item, structured interview for assessing all major symptoms related to either current or lifetime substance abuse, including onset, duration, and effects on functioning. Kruedelbach et al. evaluated the SUDDS with borderline and nonborderline patients evaluated at a VA substance abuse treatment center. They found that patterns of polysubstance abuse (three or more drugs) were more common among borderline than nonborderline patients. More systematic research is needed to demonstrate the SUDDS clinical utility and ability to establish substance abuse disorders.

Nonsyndromal Focused Interviews

Structured Interview for the Five-Factor Model of Personality (SIFFM)

The SIFFM (Trull & Widiger, 1997) was developed to evaluate the five-factor model (FFM) with more emphasis on maladaptive components of personality. The SIFFM evidenced outstanding interrater reliability for both the five domains (mean ICC = .96) and 30 facets (mean ICC = .92). Comparable estimates were found with both college and clinic samples. Test–retest reliabilities (2-week intervals) were also excellent (r's > .80) for domains. For construct validity (see Trull et al., 1998), a FFM accounted for 89% of the variance and corresponded closely to factor structure of the NEO Personality Inventory—Revised (NEO-PI-R; Costa & McCrae, 1992). The SIFFM also has good convergent validity when compared to other measures of personality and personality disorders. It has clearly demonstrated the requisite reliability and validity to be adopted for clinical practice. The challenge for practitioners is deciding how the SIFFM contributes to specific evaluations. In cases where DSM-IV personality disorders do not appear relevant, the SIFFM offers a valuable alternative in conceptualizing maladaptive personality patterns. These personality patterns are likely to be germane to the assessment of functioning (e.g., a poor match between personality style and work environment) and complications of treatment (e.g., low scores on agreeableness).

Primary Care Evaluation of Mental Disorders (PRIME-MD)

The PRIME-MD (Spitzer et al., 1994) is intended as a rapid screen (< 10 minutes) for common Axis I disorders. Its 25 questions tap symptoms associated with depression, anxiety, alcohol abuse, and eating disorders. When compared with clinical interviews by mental health professionals, a low-moderate agreement was achieved (kappas from .15 to .73; median = .55). As a screening measure, PRIME-MD specificities were very high (> .90) for specific disorders, suggesting that medical patients without these disorders could be successfully screened out. Its sensitivity was much more variable (range from .22 to .83; median = .57), indicating that many disorders might be missed by this brief screen. A serious oversight is its lack of any formal testing of interrater or test–retest reliability. Although Skodol and Border (2000, p. 67) have suggested that a comparison of similar measures might be substituted for reliability, this approach addresses concurrent validity, not reliability. Without systematic research on reliability, the PRIME-MD cannot be recommended for medical or clinical practice.

Structured and Scaled Interview to Assess Maladjustment (SSIAM)

The SSIAM (Gurland, Yorkston, Stone, Frank, & Fleiss, 1972) was developed as an overall measure of impaired functioning. It measures the effects of mental disorders on five general dimensions: work, social, family, marriage, and sex. The SSIAM consists of 45 items that evaluate behavior, friction, and distress for each of the five dimensions. An exploratory factor analysis yielded six factors: social isolation, work inadequacy, friction with the family, dependence on the family, sexual dissatisfaction, and friction outside the family. Gurland, Yorkston, Goldberg, et al. (1972) performed an initial reliability study with three raters on 15 patients; they found excellent reliability on SSIAM factor scores (median ICC = .86, range from .78 to .97). As a test of cross-informant consistency, these researchers found moderate correlations with informant scores (median r = .48). Although not been widely used in clinical practice, the SSIAM may serve as a brief measure of overall functioning based on current evidence of interrater reliability and cross-informant consistency. Additional research is needed on the stability of SSIAM factors before specific conclusions about specific deficits in functioning are warranted.

Childhood Experience of Care and Abuse (CECA)

The CECA (Bifulco, Brown, & Harris, 1994) addresses parental issues (indifference, control, and antipathy), family conflict, and child abuse (physical and sexual). For its nine scales, the interrater reliabilities appear high (median kappa = .83). Convergent validity was sought by (1) sibling interviews about parenting after the death of a mother, and (2) relationship of CECA scores to adult depression. The key issue of physical and sexual abuse does not appear to be directly investigated. At present, the CECA appears useful as a research measure for determining parenting characteristics but not child abuse per se. For example, Marshall and Cooke (1999) evaluated the CECA with psychopaths and nonpsychopaths. They found that effects of familial factors appear to decrease as PCL-R scores increase.

Biographical Personality Interview (BPI)

The BPI (von Zerssen, Possl, et al., 1998) utilizes extensive clinical case notes to validate an interview for the categorization of personality types. This categorization reflects the authors' conceptualization and is not aligned with the DSM or ICD diagnoses. von Zerssen, Barthelmes, et al. (1998) report good interrater reliability for personality structures and moderate correlations with convergent measures. The BPI is intended as a research measure. At present, the practical applications of the BPI appear to be very limited.

Gender Role Assessment Schedule—Child (GRAS-C)

The GRAS-C (Meyer-Bahlburg, & Ehrhardt, 1988) queries children about their preferences regarding different aspects of gender roles and gender identity. Consentino, Meyer-Bahlburg, Alpert, and Gaines (1993) report satisfactory interrater reliability (85–95% agreement) but do not report kappa coefficients. They found that sexually abused girls appeared to have significantly more cross-gender behavior than clinical and nonclinical controls. Despite limited data on reliability, the GRAS-C is likely to be the best measure for evaluating gender roles and gender identity in children.

Derogatis Interview for Sexual Functioning (DISF)

The DISF (Derogatis, 1997) is a very brief, 25-item, semistructured interview for surveying sexual functioning and satisfaction. Normative data from non-patient community participants provide a basis for evaluating performance/satisfaction. Derogatis, Fagan, and Strand (2000) have reported excellent interrater reliability for domains (r's > .80), with comparable test–retest reliabilities at a 1-week interval. The DISF has moderate convergent validity when compared to a separate self-report measure, the Changes in Sexual Functioning Questionnaire (CSFQ; Clayton, McGarvey, & Clavet, 1997). As acknowledged by Derogatis et al. (2000), much of the validation research has been proprietary and is therefore unpublished and generally unavailable. While the items and domains appear to have face validity, most clinicians will likely await peer-reviewed research that rigorously assesses DISF concurrent and convergent validity.

Psychosocial Pain Inventory (PSPI)

The PSPI (Heaton, Lehman, & Getto, 1980) is a semistructured interview that assesses psychological and social factors in patients with chronic pain. As articulated by Getto and Heaton (1985), factors complicating treatment may include primary and secondary reinforcement (e.g., social or financial) for assuming the patient role, which interact with dimensions of personality, substance abuse, and iatrogenic influences. The PSPI addresses six general dimensions of pain and pain-related behavior: (1) environmental stresses,[2] (2) the family's awareness and response to the patient's pain, (3) past treatments, (4) prior work history and current disability status, (5) previous medical and psychological problems, and (6) substance abuse. For reliability, Getto and Heaton (1985) provided data on a small interrater reliability sample and report high overall agreement on PSPI scores ($r = .98$), but no data on individual items. Convergent validity with the MMPI and McGill Pain Questionnaire produced mostly modest correlations (r's $\leq .30$). Clinically, the PSPI offers a greater level of standardization than is typically found in pain evaluations. More recent research has been limited; examples include (1) studying selected scales of the PSPI in relationship to pain stages (Wade, Dougherty, Archer, & Price, 1996) and (2) evaluating the PSPI in relationship to the Beck Depression Inventory (Novy, Nelson, Berry, & Averill, 1995). In light of limited and dated research, the PSPI is not recommended for clinical practice.

[2]These ratings focus on how stress may affect pain. Therefore, life events caused by pain are supposed to be excluded. Given the multidimensionality of many stress events, this demarcation may sometimes be difficult to achieve.

V

Summary Chapters

14

Clinical Applications

Fundamental changes in the health care system have resulted in increased competition and accountability. More than ever, clinicians must avoid an insular approach to evaluations based on familiarity and tradition (see, e.g., Meyer & Deitsch, 1996). While not casting aside traditional methods, clinicians must keep current and competitive in both their application of innovative assessment methods and overall sophistication in diagnostic evaluations.

The judicious use of structured interviews is not a renouncement of traditional tests but an acknowledgment that other evaluative tools are also important to clinical assessments. As observed in the introductory chapter, the *either/or fallacy* unnecessarily polarizes both clinicians and their styles of evaluation. In the following sections, I discuss how structured interviews can play a crucial role in psychological assessments.

GOALS OF ASSESSMENT

The goals of an assessment depend on the type and quality of information needed to address the referral. Is the referral issue a matter of differential diagnosis? Alternatively, if the diagnosis has been firmly established, is the referral issue a comprehensive description of critical symptoms or syndromes? When considering treatment goals, systematic ratings of symptom severity often become the focal point. These differing goals of the evaluation have important implications for the use of structured interviews.

The goals of assessment must be considered in terms of how clinical constructs are validated. Toward this end, Table 14.1 summarizes the different clinical constructs used with structured interviews and their typical validation. For symptoms and associated features, practitioners are interested in a reliable description of both presence and severity. For syndromes and scales, practitioners are invested in whether a constellation of symptoms measures a single construct (internal consistency) and how that construct relates to similar (convergent validity) and possibly dissimilar (discriminant validity) con-

TABLE 14.1. Targeted Assessments: Symptoms, Syndromes/Scales, and Disorders

Type of assessment	Reliability	Validity
Symptoms	Interrater and test–retest	NA
Syndromes	Interrater, test–retest, and internal consistency	Convergent validity
Scales	Test–retest and internal consistency	Convergent, discriminant, or construct[a]
Disorders	Interrater, test–retest, and internal consistency	Concurrent, predictive, construct, and convergent

[a]Most scales are validated by clinical correlates (convergent validity), although others also employ (1) scales composed of items that differentiate between criterion groups (discriminant validity), or (2) scales that represent underlying and theoretically relevant dimensions (construct validity).

structs. For disorders and a few well-developed syndromes, validation is an exhaustive process. Beyond reliability, multiple measures of the same disorder (concurrent validity) are typically evaluated and often yield only moderate agreement. In validating disorders and extending their clinical usefulness, the relevance of specific disorders to future functioning (predictive validity) becomes paramount.

Articulation of general assessment goals takes into account the validation of clinical constructs. General examples are outlined as follows:

- *Treatment progress* focuses on the reduction of symptom severity and improved functioning. In addition to symptom severity, scales (e.g., the Global Assessment Functioning scale [GAF]) are typically used to measure functioning. Ideal measures (e.g., SADS, K-SADS, and CASH) include five or six gradations of symptom severity.
- *Clinical predictions* often rely on specific scales to refine the general predictions available for DSM-IV disorders. Examples include the SANS scale with schizophrenia and the PCL-R with antisocial personality disorder (APD).
- *Differential diagnoses* are mostly addressed by general Axis I and Axis II interviews that provide broad diagnostic coverage. Ideal measures include those diagnostic interviews that minimize diagnostic overlap, such as the SIDP-IV for personality disorders.
- *Response styles* address patients' styles of presentation and presumed motivations in approaching their assessments. Response styles can be evaluated either by use of specialized interviews (e.g., the SIRS) or by development of specialized scales for structured interviews (e.g., the SADS).

Referral sources are often inexplicit in defining assessment goals. Moreover, for some sources, referral questions are starting points rather than firm mandates. Clinicians bear the responsibility to clarify referral issues and to indicate possible alternatives. In some settings, the default referral question is about differential diagnosis. In a diagnostically clear case, the more relevant issues may involve treatment progress and clinical predictions. Practitioners should clarify and consult with referral sources in order to optimize the clinical usefulness of their consultations.

What structured interviews should be used for specific assessment goals with particular populations? Clinicians must contemplate many considerations in deciding about assessment measures. The next section provides a general framework to facilitate the selection of structured interviews.

SELECTION OF STRUCTURED INTERVIEWS

This section provides a synthesis of data on four general categories of structured interviews: Axis I interviews, child interviews, Axis II interviews, and focused interviews. Although varying across categories, Tables 14.2 through 14.5 distill key information about major interviews and summary ratings on their reliability, validity, and clinical applications. Review of these tables is an important first step in the selection of structured interviews; clinicians should refer to relevant chapters in making their final determinations.

Faced with dozens of structured interviews for assessing specific disorders and other clinical conditions, how should clinicians proceed with the assessment? One assessment paradigm is to progress from broad to specific diagnostic measures. This "narrowing down" process reduces the likelihood of missed diagnoses. For example, general Axis I and Axis II interviews would be administered prior to concentrating on focused interviews, such as the Anxiety Disorders Interview Schedule for DSM-IV (ADIS-IV) for generalized anxiety disorder (GAD) or the DIB for borderline personality disorder (BPD). Traditionally, evaluations have proceeded from Axis I to Axis II disorders. This approach seems reasonable because many referrals are precipitated by Axis I disorders. The only risk of this ordering is that clinicians may neglect personality disorders after establishing Axis I diagnoses.

Axis I Interviews

Clinicians face a solid array of well-established Axis I interviews (see Table 14.2). Six interviews are featured in this section: DIS, SADS, SCID, CASH, CIDI, and PSE/SCAN. These interviews differ substantially based on format (semistructured vs. structured), organization (grouping questions by diagnosis), evaluators (professionals vs. others), and diagnostic system (RDC, DSM, and ICD). Differences are also apparent in psychometric properties and clinical applications. In addition to these six interviews, I also review the MINI, an effective screen for Axis I disorders.

TABLE 14.2. Comparison of Axis I Structured Interviews: Characteristics and Psychometric Properties

Features	DIS	SADS	SCID	CASH	CIDI	PSE/SCAN
General characteristics						
Semistructured	No	Yes	Yes	Yes	No	Yes
Professional interviewer	No	Yes	Yes	Yes	No	No
Congruent with DSM criteria	Yes[a]	No[b]	Yes	Yes[c]	Yes[d]	No[e]
Present diagnosis	Yes	Yes	Yes	Yes	Yes	Yes
Lifetime diagnosis	Yes	Yes	Yes	Yes	Yes	Yes
Severity of symptoms	Lim[f]	Yes[g]	Yes[f]	Yes[h]	Lim[f]	Lim[f]
Etiology of symptoms	Yes	No	No	No	Yes	No
Questions grouped by diagnosis	Yes	Yes[i]	Yes	No[j]	Yes	No
Reliability						
Individual symptoms	?	+	?	+[k]	?	?
Diagnosis	=	+	+	?	+[l]	=
Lifetime diagnosis	=	=	=	?	=	=
Validity studies						
Clinical diagnosis	=	=	+[m]	?	=	−
Convergent validity	=	+	+	?	−	=[n]
Longitudinal dimensions						
Risk factors	=	=	=	?	=	=
Course of the disorder	+	+	+	?	=	+
Treatment outcome	?	+	+	?	?	=
Applications						
Inpatients	Yes	Yes	Yes	Lim	Yes	Yes
Outpatients	Yes	Yes	Yes	Yes	Yes	Yes
Epidemiological	Yes	Yes	No	No	Yes	Yes
Hispanic version	Yes[o]	No	No	No	No	No

Note. DIS = Diagnostic Interview Schedule; SADS = Schedule of Affective Disorders and Schizophrenia; SCID = Structured Clinical Interview for DSM-III-R Disorders; CASH = Comprehensive Assessment of Symptoms and History; CIDI = Composite International Diagnostic Interview; PSE/SCAN = Present State Examination/Schedules for Clinical Assessment of Neuropsychiatry; Lim = limited. Comparative data are coded in the following manner: ? for insufficient studies to make a comparison; − for poor or weaker than other measures; = for average or comparable to other measures; + for superior or stronger than other measures.

[a]Also Feighner and research diagnostic criteria (RDC).

[b]The correspondence between RDC and DSM often allows DSM diagnoses directly from the SADS.

[c]Also RDC.

[d]Also ICD criteria.

[e]Only ICD criteria.

[f]Limited range (no, subclinical, yes).

[g]Gradations for most symptoms (no, subclinical, mild, moderate, and severe); psychotic symptoms have limited range (no, suspected/likely, and yes).

[h]Gradations for all symptoms (no, subclinical, mild, moderate, and severe).

[i]Part I of the SADS is organized by syndromes and Part II, by diagnosis.

[j]Organized by syndromes.

[k]Based mostly on the SAPS and SANS (Scales for the Assessment of Positive/Negative Symptoms).

[l]Including some studies with CIDI–DIS comparisons.

[m]Several important studies use the Longitudinal Expert Evaluation using All Data (LEAD) model, which likely inflates agreement via criterion contamination.

[n]Most studies focus on overall impairment rather than specific disorders.

[o]The DIS has validated Mexican, Mexican American, and Puerto Rican translations.

Diagnostic Interview Schedule (DIS)

The DIS offers broad coverage of mental disorders and criteria that are direct-ly translatable into DSM-III-R and DSM-IV disorders. Because of its breadth, the DIS limits most of its questions directly to the DSM inclusion criteria. Originally intended as an epidemiological measure, the DIS is a structured in-terview that formally dictates clinical inquiries and their sequencing.

Its comparative strengths are as follows:

- The DIS is the only structured interview that has been adequately vali-dated for Hispanic populations (i.e., Puerto Rican, Mexican Ameri-can, and Mexican).
- The DIS can screen for suspected dementia via its inclusion of the MMSE.
- The DIS provides useful information about the course of Axis I disor-ders and factors likely to influence outcome.
- The DIS has been tested on diverse cultures outside North America.

Schedule of Affective Disorders and Schizophrenia (SADS)

The SADS is more concentrated that other Axis I interviews. Its primary em-phasis is on mood and psychotic disorders, with secondary emphasis on anxi-ety symptomatology. This concentration affords the SADS considerable depth in examining symptoms and features beyond those needed for diagnoses. De-spite close correspondence between RDC and DSM classifications, the SADS requires clinicians to ask additional questions when making a DSM-IV diag-nosis.

Comparative strengths of the SADS are as follows:

- The SADS is unparalleled in its reliable measurement of Axis I symp-toms and symptom severity. For measuring treatment progress, it is likely the best interview for mood and psychotic disorders.
- The SADS is excellent for establishing symptomatology and diagnoses at discrete time periods (e.g., worst time in current episode and cur-rent time). This focus on discrete periods is especially useful in foren-sic evaluations.
- The SADS has data on response styles, especially the screening of feigned presentations.
- The SADS is valuable in predicting treatment outcome.

Structured Clinical Interview for DSM-IV (SCID)

Remarkable progress has occurred in the validation of the SCID during the last decade. The SCID has largely achieved its primary objective of rendering reliable diagnoses for current episodes. In achieving this objective efficiently, the SCID applies screening questions to eliminate further evaluation of diagnostic sections. The trade-off for this efficiency is that symptoms and subdiagnostic manifestations of specific disorders are likely to be overlooked.

Its comparative strengths are as follows:

- The SCID's excellent reliability for establishing Axis I disorders appears to be maintained across diverse cultures and several translations.
- The SCID has extensive validation with anxiety disorders, especially panic disorders.
- The SCID comprehensively covers substance abuse disorders.

Comprehensive Assessment of Symptoms and History (CASH)

The CASH incorporates SADS inquiries into an extensive Axis I interview that focuses on psychotic and mood disorders. Its major contribution is its coverage of psychotic symptoms with gradational ratings. Unfortunately, research on the CASH itself have been very limited. Instead, studies have focused on two ancillary scales, the SAPS and the SANS.

Comparative strengths of the CASH are as follows:

- Clinicians may wish to use the severity ratings of psychotic symptoms to supplement other Axis I interviews, such as the SADS.
- The SAPS and SANS subscales are highly reliable measures of positive and negative psychotic symptoms. They are useful in evaluating the predicted course of schizophrenic disorders and their response to treatment.

Composite International Diagnostic Interview (CIDI)

The CIDI is a hybrid interview that combines the DIS and portions of the PSE. Its primary application is the examination of patients using multiple diagnostic systems (DSM, RDC, and ICD). The CIDI is distinguished by large-scale epidemiological and cross-cultural applications. Its routine clinical use is likely to be constrained by limited need to evaluate multiple diagnostic systems.

Its comparative advantage is as follows:

- Clinicians offering specialized treatment programs may find the CIDI useful in evaluating changes in symptomatology across both DSM and ICD systems.

Present State Examination–Schedules for Clinical Assessment of Neuropsychiatry (PSE–SCAN)

The PSE with its phenomenological emphasis, addresses the ICD classification, focusing primarily on symptoms rather than diagnoses. The SCAN incorporates both the PSE-10 and several ancillary measures. For clinical applications, the PSE and the SCAN are unparalleled in their research on diverse cultures and translations.

Comparative advantages of the PSE are as follows:

- The PSE is the interview of choice for evaluating ICD symptomatology and diagnoses.
- The PSE is likely to be valuable in evaluating cultural influences on the presentation of symptomatology.

Mini-International Neuropsychiatric Interview (MINI)

The MINI performs a very different function than the Axis I interviews included in Table 14.2. Unlike these diagnostic interviews, it is intended to be a comprehensive screen for common Axis I disorders. The MINI seeks to maximize diagnostic information within an average administration time of 15 minutes. It is intended to screen patients with mental disorders rapidly and efficiently. Positive findings on the MINI should then be fully evaluated with another Axis I interview.

Its comparative advantage is as follows:

- The MINI is a reliable and effective screen for 23 common mental disorders. For resource utilization, paraprofessionals can easily be trained in its administration.

In summary, clinicians will likely develop proficiency in administering several Axis I interviews that best match their professional practices. For those working with the DSM-IV, the SCID-CV and DIS-IV have respective strengths in evaluating a broad range of Axis I disorders. For the coverage of discrete episodes and symptom severity, the SADS is unmatched in its validation. In addition, many clinics and health care facilities desire rapid but effective screening for common mental disorders. In this regard, the MINI is the strongest candidate. Other considerations are likely to include the availability of (1) validated translations, (2) data on treatment response and treatment, and (3) parallel forms (adult and child) for systematic evaluations of families. Finally, clinicians must decide whether clinical needs extend beyond current diagnosis to the assessment of key symptomatology.

Child and Adolescent Structured Interviews

Five major diagnostic interviews (K-SADS, CAS, DISC, DICA, and CHIPS) that have been validated for children and adolescents are summarized in Table 14.3. Developed for comparable ages, they combine child interviews and parent-informant interviews, and yield current diagnoses. Beyond these

TABLE 14.3. Comparison of Child and Adolescent Structured Interviews: Characteristics and Psychometric Properties

Features	K-SADS	CAS	DISC	DICA	CHIPS
General characteristics					
Ages	6–18	7–17	8–17	6–17	6–18
Semistructured	Yes	Yes	No	No[a]	Yes[b]
Professional interviewer	Yes	Yes	No	Yes	No
Parallel forms (parent–child)	Yes	Yes	Yes	Yes	Yes
Parallel form with adult	Yes	No	Yes	No	No
Congruent with DSM criteria	Yes	Yes	Yes	Yes	Yes
Present diagnosis	Yes	Yes	Yes	Yes	Yes
Lifetime diagnosis	No	No	No	Yes	No
Severity of symptoms	Yes	No	No	No	No
Questions grouped by diagnosis	Yes	No	Yes	Yes	Yes
Reliability					
Individual symptoms	+	+	+	=	?
Diagnosis	+	=	=	=	?
Scales	+	+	=	NA	NA
Total score	NA	=	+	NA	NA
Parent–child agreement[c]	=	=	=	=	=
Validity studies					
Clinical diagnosis	=[d]	=[e]	–	=	=[f]
Convergent—CBCL and TRF	=	+	=	?	?
Convergent—other	=	=	=	?	?
Longitudinal dimensions					
Risk factors	?	?	+	+	?
Course of the disorder	=	?	+	=	?
Treatment outcome	=	?	=	?	?
Applications					
Inpatients	Yes	No[g]	Yes	Yes	Yes
Outpatients	Yes	Yes	Yes	Yes	Yes
Epidemiological	No[h]	No	Yes	Yes	No
Hispanic	No	No	Yes	No	Yes

Note. For more detailed comparisons, see Gutterman et al. (1987) and Hodges (1993). K-SADS = Schedule of Affective Disorders and Schizophrenia for School-Age Children; CAS = Child Assessment Schedule; DISC = Diagnostic Interview Schedule for Children; DICA = Diagnostic Interview for Children and Adolescents; CHIPS = Children's Interview for Psychiatric Syndromes; CBCL = Child Behavior Checklist; TRF = Teacher's Report Form. Comparative data are coded in the following manner: ? for insufficient studies to make a comparison; – for poor or weaker than other measures; = for average or comparable to other measures; + for superior or stronger than other measures.
[a]Although the DICA is described as "structured," clinicians are allowed to make some exceptions.
[b]Questions of clarification and requests for examples are allowed.
[c]It is not reliability per se, but cross-informant consistency. These are modest for all child interviews.
[d]Limited range of diagnoses represented.
[e]Limited research.
[f]Results are likely inflated by use of "rare kappa."
[g]Most studies have been of outpatients and excluded psychotic children.
[h]The K-SADS-E, developed for epidemiological studies, was only infrequently used.

common features, these child interviews have respective strengths in the diagnostic assessment of youth.

Schedule of Affective Disorders and Schizophrenia for School-Age Children (K-SADS)

The K-SADS parallels the SADS for the evaluation of mood and psychotic disorders but augments the coverage with the addition of childhood and developmental disorders. Like the SADS, the K-SADS distinguishes itself with respect to reliability and symptom severity. It is especially useful in evaluating youth with severe mental disorders; parents are interviewed first, so that potential discrepancies between parent and child reports can be addressed directly.

Its comparative advantages are as follows:

- The hallmark of the K-SADS is the reliability of its diagnoses and key symptoms; this strength distinguishes it from the other child interviews.
- Despite the complexity of its ratings, the K-SADS allows direct comparisons of symptom ratings (parent, child, and composite) that are likely to be beneficial in subsequent treatment interventions.

Child Assessment Schedule (CAS)

The CAS evaluates the child's functioning in important spheres (e.g., school, family, and friends) of his or her life. Although the CAS yields diagnostically relevant information, it is not a formal diagnostic interview. Rather, the CAS systematically appraises strengths and problems related to the child's functioning.

Its comparative strengths are as follows:

- The CAS provides dimensional ratings for evaluating psychological problems in several contexts: family, friends, activities, and school.
- The CAS aids treatment interventions by defining common ground (areas of agreement) and therapeutic goals (areas of disagreement).

Diagnostic Interview Schedule for Children (DISC)

The DISC, like the DIS, was developed as a structured interview for community/epidemiological studies. As a fully structured interview, the DISC may be especially useful in clinical settings where paraprofessionals contribute to the assessment process. Overall, the DISC is a well-validated child interview that is applicable to a range of clinical settings, particularly those with multicultural clientele.

Its comparative strengths are as follows:

- The DISC has good reliability and substantial evidence of convergent validity when used by either professionals or paraprofessionals.

- The DISC is the first choice among child interviews for Spanish-speaking children and English-speaking children from different cultures.
- The DISC is particularly useful in the early assessment of risk factors for mental disorders.

Diagnostic Interview for Children and Adolescents (DICA)

The DICA is the only child interview that pays close attention to the lifetime prevalence of mental disorders. For clinicians attempting to understand the etiology of disorders and/or to formulate early intervention programs, this feature is certainly attractive. In general, the DICA has demonstrated satisfactory reliability and validity.

Comparative strengths of the DICA are as follows:

- The DICA, which collects extensive data on the onset, duration and recency of specific symptoms, may be helpful in the evaluation of complex cases.
- The DICA, which seeks to protect the confidentiality of evaluated children, may encourage increased self-disclosure.
- The DICA's adolescent version contains items that focus on this age group.

Children's Interview for Psychiatric Syndromes (CHIPS)

Developed as a straightforward interview for evaluating 20 common disorders in children and adolescents, the CHIPS is intended to be administered by paraprofessionals as an extensive screen. Positive findings are then evaluated by mental health professionals. In comparison to other child interviews, the CHIPS has less validation. In particular, more data are needed to document its reliability.

A comparative advantage of the CHIPS is as follows:

- The CHIPS is time-efficient (30–50 minutes) in screening clinical samples.

In summary, clinicians conducting child interviews face daunting diagnostic challenges given (1) the array of diagnoses, complicated by those typically arising in childhood and adolescence, and (2) the divergence of perspectives among children, parents, and interested professionals (e.g., teachers, child care workers, and health care professionals). Although child interviews do not typically achieve the same reliabilities as adult Axis I interviews, they provide a standardized and generally reliable method of assessing diagnoses and dimensions of psychopathology.

Clinicians that specialize in child and adolescent populations are likely to develop proficiencies in several child interviews. The K-SADS and the DISC have the strongest evidence of reliability and validity. For family assessments, both interviews have the added advantage of parallel adult measures (SADS and DIS). In addition, the DISC has the broadest application to different cultures. The CAS must be seen as a top contender for evaluating psychological problems in different spheres and developing appropriate interventions. The DICA may be considered for specific populations (e.g., adolescents and substance abuses), while the CHIPS is likely to be valuable when local reliability has been demonstrated.

Major Axis II Interviews

The foremost Axis II interviews (SIDP-IV and IPDE) are not well known by the majority of mental health professionals. These measures provide a superb opportunity for clinicians to develop additional expertise in the assessment of personality disorders, with a relatively low investment in training and experience. Both interviews are supported by a wealth of studies on their reliability and validity. In addition, two other structured interviews, namely, the SCID-II and PDI-IV, show considerable promise. Table 14.4 summarizes the major Axis II interviews.

Structured Interview for DSM-IV Personality Disorders (SIDP)

The hallmark of the SIDP is that its organization and format elicit a broad range of clinical information with a natural flow. The SIDP uses general questions that are often low in transparency (i.e., evaluatees have trouble inferring specific psychopathology from particular questions). It has good reliability and excellent convergent validity, and has been validated with a wide range of inpatients and outpatients. Overall, the SIDP is an excellent Axis II interview that should be strongly considered in a wide range of clinical settings.

Its comparative advantages are as follows:

- An important feature of SIDP diagnostic validity is the low degree of overlap among personality disorders. Using the SIDP often results in the diagnosis of a single Axis II disorder, thereby facilitating the diagnostic understanding and treatment implications with a particular patient.
- The SIDP is the obvious interview of choice when considering how Axis I–Axis II interactions may affect treatment outcome.

Personality Disorder Examination (PDE)

The PDE and the IPDE-DSM have been extensively validated for use with Axis II disorders in predominantly outpatient settings. As such, the PDE should not be used with severe Axis I disorders (e.g., psychotic disorders or severe depression). It places a comparable emphasis on both categorical diag-

TABLE 14.4. Comparison of Major Axis II Structured Interviews: Characteristics and Psychometric Properties

Features	SIDP	PDE/IPDE	SCID-II	PDI
General characteristics				
Semistructured	Yes	Yes	Yes	Yes
Professional interviewer	Yes	Yes	Yes	No[a]
Use of an informant	Yes	opt	No	No
Congruent with DSM criteria	Yes	Yes	Yes	Yes
Present diagnosis	Yes	Yes	Yes	Yes
Past diagnosis	No	Yes	No	No
Dimensional scores	No	Yes	No	No
Severity of symptoms	Yes[b]	Yes[c]	Yes[d]	Yes[e]
Questions grouped by diagnosis	No	No	Yes	No[f]
Reliability				
Individual symptoms	=	+	+	?
Scales	NA	+	=[g]	NA
Diagnosis	+	+	+	=[h]
Validity studies				
Clinical diagnosis	=	+	=	?
Convergent validity	+	+	=[i]	=
Diagnostic overlap	+	=	=	=
Longitudinal dimensions				
Risk factors	=	=	?	?
Course of the disorder	=	+	=	?
Response to treatment	+	=	=	?
Applications				
Inpatients	Yes	Yes	Yes	Yes
Outpatients	Yes	Yes	Yes	Yes
Epidemiological	No	No	No	Yes
Multicultural	No	Yes[j]	No	No

Note. SIDP = Structured Interview for DSM-III Personality Disorders; PDE = Personality Disorder Examination; IPDE = International Personality Disorder Examination—DSM version; SCID-II = Structured Clinical Interview for DSM-III-R—Axis II Disorders; PDI = Personality Disorder Interview; opt = optional but recommended. Comparative data are coded in the following manner: ? for insufficient studies to make a comparison; − for poor or weaker than other measures; = for average or comparable to other measures; + for superior or stronger than other measures.

[a]Although designed for nonprofessionals, all the reliability data appear to have been collected by psychology staff.

[b]Four-point scale (0–3) with "1" subthreshold, "2" present, and "3" strongly present.

[c]Three-point scale (0–2) with "1" exaggerated and "2" meeting criterion.

[d]Three-point scale (1–3) with "2" subthreshold and "3" meeting criterion.

[e]Three-point (0–2) scale with "1" meeting criterion and "2" severe.

[f]A version organized by diagnosis is now available, although validity studies were carried out on the topical version.

[g]Axis II clusters.

[h]A single study appeared to produce high reliability estimates.

[i]Modest findings of convergent validity, but a large factor-analytic study offered good evidence of construct validity.

[j]The international version (IPDE) has been tested in 11 countries; unfortunately, a Hispanic version is not currently available.

noses and dimensional ratings. Importantly, reliabilities are very good for both approaches. In general, the PDE should be viewed as a first-rate interview, especially suited for multicultural settings.

PDE and IPDE comparative strengths are as follows:

- The PDE's dimensional ratings, in addition to diagnoses, are often useful in assessing changes in clinical status.
- The PDE systematically addresses past Axis II disorders instead of facilely assuming "once a personality disorder, always a personality disorder." Similarly, clinicians have the option of classifying early or late onset.
- The PDE and the IPDE stand out as closely related Axis II interviews that pay continued attention to multicultural and cross-cultural issues.

Structured Clinical Interview for DSM-IV—Axis II (SCID-II)

The SCID-II is a straightforward measure that considers DSM-IV criteria by diagnosis and by their order of presentation in DSM-IV (American Psychiatric Association, 2000). This organization, coupled with the SCID-II-Q screen, facilitates the rapid evaluation of personality disorders. The trade-off for this organization is that the flow is less natural than that of the SIDP or the PDE. Recent studies have demonstrated good reliability and validity for the SCID-II.

Comparative strengths of the SCID-II are as follows:

- The SCID-II, combined with the SCID-II-Q, is the most efficient method of evaluating current personality disorders. However, important personality traits are likely to be missed.
- The SCID-II has excellent reliability for both symptoms and diagnoses.
- The SCID-II has been used extensively with forensic populations.

Psychiatric Diagnostic Interview (PDI)

The PDI is limited as an Axis II interview since recent studies have not been forthcoming of its reliability and validity. Because existing validational studies were conducted on different versions of the PDI, current data are insufficient to recommend its use in clinical practice.

Its comparative advantage is as follows:

- The PDI manual is a valuable sourcebook of specific personality disorders and their clinical presentation.

In summary, clinicians have three excellent interviews for Axis II disorders. The SIDP and PDE have thematic presentations that facilitate the interview flow and patient rapport. Both interviews have excellent validation. In contrast, the SCID-II, which is highly efficient for rendering DSM-IV diagnoses, also has well-established validity. In conjunction with Axis II interviews, self-report screens are strongly recommended: (1) The PDQ-R has the most validation and appears to encourage endorsement of Axis II symptoms, and (2) the SCID-II-Q has satisfactory validation and matches the SCID-II.

Focused Interviews

A diverse group of focused interviews has been developed to address extensively single disorders and other clinical constructs (e.g., response styles and psychological impairment). Because of their specialized nature, these measures often have important yet circumscribed clinical applications. This section addresses focused interviews for (1) single diagnosis or syndrome and those for (2) specialized purpose.

Focused Interviews for a Single Diagnosis or Syndrome

Focused interviews often address a single disorder or cluster of disorders. Table 14.5 summarizes the major focused interviews used for this purpose. These focused interviews are often unique in their scope; therefore, this review does not include a summary of comparative strengths.

Diagnostic Interview for Borderline (DIB). The importance of the DIB to clinical practice lies less in its diagnostic validity and more in its theoretical formulations. In other words, general Axis II interviews provide sufficient reliability and validity for the diagnosis of BPD. What the DIB contributes is an operationalization of Gunderson's widely accepted conceptual model of borderlines. Psychologists providing specialized treatment consistent the Gunderson's formulations are likely to find the DIB extremely valuable. Moreover, the DIB extends beyond diagnosis and offers a relatively reliable measure of critical borderline dimensions. From this perspective, the DIB may be a valuable resource in systematically assessing these dimensions.

Psychopathy Checklist (PCL). Clinicians will likely choose between two closely related measures: the PCL-R and the PCL:SV. In noncorrectional settings, the PCL:SV has advantages in terms of its content and efficiency. Despite statements in DSM-IV, the clinical constructs of psychopathy and APD are very different; PCL measures cannot be substituted for DSM-IV diagnosis. Clearly, the PCL-R and the PCL:SV are the best available measures of adult psychopathy, encapsulating both core personality characteristics and antisocial behavior. Clinicians must decide whether to use the PCL-R and the PCL:SV as dimensional or categorical measures. Dimensionally, the PCL-R and PCL:SV have superb reliabilities for their total scores, with strong evidence of convergent validity. Categorically, these measures have several challenges: (1) Reliabilities are only moderate; (2) SE_M limits the interpretable

TABLE 14.5. An Overview of Structured Interviews for Specific Disorders: Characteristics and Psychometric Properties

Variables	DIB	PCL-R	ADIS	CAPS	ASI	EDE
		General characteristics				
Semistructured	Yes	Yes	Yes	No	Yes	Yes
Professional interviewer	Yes	Yes	Yes	No	No	Yes
Use of corroborative data	Yes	Yes	Yes	Yes	Yes	Yes
Congruent with DSM criteria	No	No	Yes	Yes	No	Yes
Present diagnosis	Yes	Yes	Yes	Yes	No	Yes
Past diagnosis	No	No	No	Yes	No	No
Dimensional scores	Yes	Yes	No	Yes	Yes	Yes
Severity of symptoms	No[a]	Yes[b]	Yes[c]	Yes	No	Yes
Questions grouped by scales or clusters	Yes	No	Yes	Yes	Yes	Yes
		Reliability				
Individual symptoms	+	+	?	?	=	=[d]
Scales	=[e]	+[f]	NA	+[g]	+	=[d]
Diagnosis	+	=	=	+	NA	?
		Validity studies				
Clinical diagnosis	=	=	=	+	NA	=[h]
Convergent validity	=	+	?	+	=	=
Longitudinal dimensions						
Risk factors	+	+[i]	?	?	?	?
Course of the disorder	+	+[i]	=	+	?	=
Response to treatment	=	=	=	=	–	=
		Applications				
Inpatients	Yes	Yes	No	Yes	Yes	Yes
Outpatients	Yes	Yes	Yes	Yes	Yes	Yes
Epidemiological	No	No	No	No	No	No
Multicultural	No	Lim[j]	No	No	No	Lim[k]

Note. DIB = Diagnostic Interview for Borderlines; PCL-R = Psychopathy Checklist—Revised; ADIS = Anxiety Disorders Interview Schedule for DSM-IV (adult version); CAPS = Clinician-Administered PTSD Scale for DSM-IV; ASI = Addiction Severity Index; EDE = Eating Disorder Examination; Lim = limited. Comparative data are coded in the following manner: ? for insufficient studies to make a comparison; – for poor or weaker than other measures; = for average or comparable to other measures; + for superior or stronger than other measures.

[a]Items are rated on a 3-point scale with respect to their certainty (no, probable, and definite).

[b]Items are rated on a 3-point scale that combines severity and certainty (no, maybe/in some respects, and yes).

[c]Many items are rated on a 5-point scale (none, mild, moderate, severe, very severe/grossly disabling).

[d]High reliabilities but based on only a modest sample.

[e]DIB sections.

[f]Total PCL-R score.

[g]Combat PTSD.

[h]Actually discriminant validity, with scale differences between eating disorder diagnoses.

[i]Risk factors and the course of the disorder are related to violence and adjustment.

[j]Little data are available on minorities with reference to external validation; moreover, Kosson, Smith, and Newman (1990) found a very different distribution between African American and white inmates.

[k]Limited studies from different countries.

range of psychopathy; and (3) studies use different cut scores. The advantage of the categorical approach is the extensive research on risk assessment.

Anxiety Disorders Interview Schedule (ADIS). The ADIS offers a very extensive outline of symptoms and situations for clinical intervention. Because of its specific information, the ADIS can easily be used as a template for treatment planning. Clinicians can individualize treatment priorities and specify treatment methods. The ADIS also provides a convenient framework for discussing treatment goals and priorities. Beyond anxiety disorders, the ADIS allows clinicians to consider both comorbidity and differential diagnoses.

Clinician-Administered PTSD Scale for DSM-IV (CAPS). Practitioners are becoming increasingly aware of the prevalence and importance of PTSD in clinical practice. The CAPS is a first-rate, focused interview for evaluating PTSD and assessing the frequency and intensity of symptoms. The CAPS is distinguished by its excellent concurrent and superb construct validity. In addition, it has important treatment implications for both baseline evaluations and subsequent follow-ups. While less data are available on nonveteran populations, the CAPS should still be strongly considered for general clinical practice.

Addiction Severity Index (ASI). A diagnostic challenge for clinicians is the assessment of substance abuse disorders and the resulting impairment. The ASI focuses on impairment rather than diagnoses. By examining different facets, the ASI provides an efficient method of evaluating with the client both strengths and weaknesses in his or her functioning. Ideally, the ASI serves as a template for mutually established treatment goals. When the issue is differential diagnosis, clinicians may wish to consider the SCID or possibly the CIDI. When the issue is forthrightness, the CDP is likely to be the interview of choice. However, the ASI has considerable merit for use with motivated patients with substance abuse in determining impairment and treatment needs.

Eating Disorder Examination (EDE). The EDE provides a useful, focused interview for assessing the attitudinal and behavioral aspects of eating disorders. While a useful adjunct, the EDE is not a substitute for DSM-IV diagnoses. Rather, the EDE adopts a dimensional approach to eating disorders. Problem areas, such as physical shape, are evaluated separately. This approach allows clinicians to develop treatment interventions in cooperation with their clients that focus on these dimensions. The primary limitation of the EDE is its limited reliability data. Despite this limitation, the EDE is still useful in the treatment of patients with eating disorders.

Focused Interviews for Specialized Purposes

Structured interviews have been developed for a broad range of specialized purposes, including evaluation of past experiences and symptoms (e.g.,

IRAOS, BPI, and CECA), general personality (SIFFM), sexual functioning (DISF), identity (GRAS-C), impairment (PRIME-ED), and response styles (SIRS). As summarized in Chapter 13, many of these interviews are in their early stages of development. Therefore, this subsection addresses the three major focused interviews for specialized purposes: SIRS, SIFFM, and IRAOS.

Structured Interview of Reported Symptoms (SIRS). The SIRS is a focused interview developed for the evaluation of feigning and related response styles. It has outstanding reliability and discriminant validity, with carefully cross-validated results with both simulation studies and known-groups comparisons. This focused interview is recommended for any evaluation in which there is substantial concern regarding the possibility of feigned mental disorders or overreported psychopathology. The SIRS was not designed to evaluate feigned cognitive impairment (e.g., mental retardation or memory loss) and should not be used for that purpose.

Structured Interview for the Five-Factor Model of Personality (SIFFM). The SIFFM was developed as a semi-structured interview to measure the five bipolar dimensions of personality: neuroticism versus emotional stability, extraversion versus introversion, openness to experience versus closedness to experience, agreeableness versus antagonism, and conscientousness versus negligence. Knowledge of these dimensions may be useful for a variety of professional contexts and issues (e.g., understanding marital conflict or defining career goals). The SIFFM has superb reliability for both its domains and their respective facets. It is likely to be useful for well-adjusted persons experiencing personal discomfort or interpersonal distress.

Interview for the Retrospective Assessment of the Onset of Schizophrenia (IRAOS). The IRAOS is a semistructured interview for assessing retrospective symptoms in patients with schizophrenia or other psychotic disorders. While serving primarily research purposes, the IRAOS achieves a moderate reliability in establishing the onset and chronicity of symptoms. Informants are often used, although cross-informant consistency is typically modest. Clinically, the IRAOS could be used to trace the emergence of symptoms. Such information may assist in plotting the course of the disorder and in identifying periods of good adjustment. Such periods may help to facilitate therapeutic and environmental changes in an effort to optimize adjustment.

INTEGRATED EVALUATIONS AND REPORTS

The overall purpose of most clinical evaluations is a well-integrated and coherent report that addresses the referral question and other critical issues.

How is this integration achieved? What happens to discordant information? Are all clinical findings treated as if they were equally valid? Is the logic, from clinical data to overall conclusions, explicit to the informed reader? This section provides a useful framework for examining how these issues affect professional practice.

Referrals and Reports

The content and organization of any evaluation are largely dependent on the referral source. Reports should differ in sophistication depending on whether they are written for (1) other mental health professionals, (2) professionals outside of mental health, and (3) nonprofessionals. Reports vary in their depth and coverage depending on the referral question. For some treatment consultations, the watchword is succinctness. Busy clinicians may desire highly targeted evaluations that emphasize key recommendations. Alternatively, clinicians may desire comprehensive reports with extensive differential diagnoses. Four basic issues should be considered in composing diagnostic reports:

1. In reviewing a handful of evaluations written for a single referral source, do these reports have a boilerplate quality to them? Use of the same outline and standard paragraphs may produce repetitive reports that collectively appear redundant, unoriginal, and imitative. "Time-saving" devices are likely to backfire if they devalue the report's genuine contributions.

2. In reviewing evaluations across referral sources, do clinicians subscribe to the notion of "one-size-fits-all?" Are reports for psychologists with extensive psychometric training similar to reports for educational specialists and clinical social workers? Diagnostic reports are often unhelpful because they presume too much or too little knowledge.

3. In asking others to review evaluations, do clinicians' reports achieve *clarity without condescension*? Professionals are often sensitive to reports that are patronizing and appear to "talk-down" to the referral source. Moreover, many clinicians become jargon-bound and do not appreciate how their esoteric terms are offensive to other professionals.

4. In asking others to review evaluations, do clinicians' reports treat clients with respect? Clients are likely to have the right to review their own diagnostic reports. In some instances, referral sources share the report with their clients. Clinicians may find it useful to assume that clients have access to the evaluations and write their reports based on this assumption.

A useful method of evaluating reports is to consider basic polarities that address important dimensions of report writing. Three bipolar dimensions are outlined in the following paragraphs.

Accuracy versus Simplicity

At the extremes, overly detailed reports may excruciatingly delineate each and every clinical finding, while overly distilled reports leave large gaps in clinical data. Clinicians must make judgments regarding major and minor findings, and treat the clinical data accordingly. Major findings should be verifiable based on the presented information. For minor findings, the inclusion of supporting data may simply overwhelm even knowledgeable readers.

Synthesis versus Syncretism

In both clinical and forensic practices, I frequently review evaluations in which all the pieces appear to fit together. While integration is the goal of evaluations, clinical data are often discordant and lack concinnity. To force disparate information to fit is syncretism, not synthesis. To ignore nonconvergent findings is likely to mislead referral sources. Assessments must openly acknowledge nonconvergent and discrepant findings about major issues. Such forthrightness does not detract from the report but adds to its credibility.

Certainty versus Fallibility

Several related issues emerge from this dimension. Many clinical reports are written with a degree of certitude that is totally unjustified by the data. On the other hand, wallowing in self-doubt, while much rarer among clinicians, provides more confusion than clarity. One alternative (Rogers, 1986) is to provide qualifying descriptors (e.g., these symptoms are "likely to be . . ." or this profile is "consistent with . . ."). The critical issue is whether the consumers of clinical assessments make any actual discriminations regarding the certainty of conclusions. How can clinicians clarify their lack of certitude in certain clinical findings?

- Clinicians may make explicit statements about the certitude of a conclusion (e.g., "While the test results *suggest* . . . , this finding should be viewed as *preliminary*.").
- Clinicians may offer explicit cautions about the accuracy of clinical methods (e.g., "While the best measure available, the PCL-R has not been sufficiently validated with Hispanic American women. Therefore, these results should be viewed as tentative.").
- Clinicians can offer several alternatives for a particular finding (e.g., "The elevations on the MMPI-2 Depression scale can reflect general dissatisfaction or depressed mood."). The presentation of alternatives minimizes the possibility that any one interpretation is accepted as conclusive.

- The final alternative is to omit the finding altogether, if it is peripheral to the referral issue and nonessential to understanding the patient. This alternative is typically selected when other options do not appear "worth the effort."

Structured Interviews in Clinical Assessments

The reporting of structured interviews is easily integrated into comprehensive evaluations. General guidelines for the incorporation of structured interviews are provided.

Description of Structured Interviews

Many mental health professionals lack familiarity with diagnostic and structured interviews. Clinicians need to educate their referral sources regarding the standardized measures. Professionals are unlikely to accord much weight to any procedure that they do not understand. This description may be accomplished in one or two sentences. For example, a personal injury consultation might include the following statements about the SADS: "I also administered the Schedule of Affective Disorders and Schizophrenia (SADS), an extensive, semistructured diagnostic interview. The SADS was an appropriate measure in this case because of its excellent reliability in assessing both current and past episodes, and its usefulness in estimating the severity of symptoms at different time periods." In this example, the emphasis is twofold: (1) standardization and (2) clinical relevance.

Sources of Data

Can a knowledgeable reader discern the source of a diagnostic statement or conclusions? No all data sources are equally validated. As an extreme example, should a self-serving denial of pedophilac behavior be given equal weight to findings from a criminal investigation? Ideally, data systematically derived from structured interviews should be identifiable. Likewise, data from collateral sources and past records should be clearly designated.

Diagnosis and Clinical Findings

For most clinical evaluations, three levels of abstraction are useful in providing a comprehensive delineation of the conclusions and the basis of the conclusions. The most common example of the three-tiered approach is found with diagnosis:

   1. *Diagnosis* represents a medium abstraction; clinicians must evaluate criteria against multiple disorders in achieving a differential diagnosis. Clinical findings should include a clear diagnosis of the mental disorder,

typically with accompanying information about its onset, duration, and course.

2. *Diagnostic criteria* represents a low abstraction; clinicians must integrate patients' reports and their own observations in deciding whether symptoms are sufficient to meet the diagnostic standard. Clinical findings should include an account of inclusion criteria (e.g., DSM-IV or ICD-10) met by the patient, typically with accompanying information about the frequency and severity of each criterion.

3. *Examples/description* are not an abstraction but a selective reporting of "raw data." Clinical descriptions often include quotes from the patient (e.g., actual words used in a suicide threat), a distillation of the patient's account (e.g., the specifics of a paranoid delusion, including the "perpetrators"), or specific ratings from a structured interview.

Clinical reports that provide these three levels of abstraction enable other professionals to evaluate both the data and the conclusions. Adherence to this format ensures that the logic/basis of the diagnosis is clearly presented. Moreover, this model allows clinicians to present multiple perspectives in especially complex cases. In summary, clinicians are much more likely to be convincing and credible in such cases when the conclusions, and the basis of those conclusions, are carefully delineated.

Predictive Statements

Referring professionals often desire clinical predictions on treatment effectiveness and risk assessment. Unfortunately, both structured interviewing and psychological testing rarely yield high-quality predictive information. Typically, the best predictions are rendered from extreme data (e.g., predicting suicide on the basis of dozens of nearly lethal and very recent attempts). In such extreme cases, is the prediction even necessary?[1]

Clinicians should be circumspect in making any predictions. Predictive statements should *always* be accompanied by both probability estimates and cautions. Clinicians must strive for general accuracy in making the prediction. If the probability is unknown, then the ensuing predictions are likely to be more harmful than helpful. With regard to probability estimates, a caution is almost always required, since even the best predictive data probably do not completely correspond to the patient in question and his or her circumstances. Substantive differences either in clinical setting or diagnosis/symptomatology of the patients are likely to affect the accuracy of prediction.

Risk assessments provide a valuable example of how predictive statements can go seriously awry (Rogers, 2000). Frequently, risk assessments are

[1]For example, a very high scorer on the PCL-R typically has extensive criminal history and considerable documentation of institutional problems within prisons and forensic hospitals. Could not the relevant authorities make these determinations without PCL-R data?

fundamentally biased by the methodology. Clinicians frequently (1) overemphasize the risk factors, (2) overlook the protective factors, and (3) neglect the moderator effects entirely. Despite highly variable rates of violence, some clinicians adopt a convenient but dangerous fiction in assuming both a known and a stable base rate for their risk predictions. The clinical applications for the PCL-R in Chapter 12 illustrates some of these serious problems with risk assessment.

It is useful to distinguish between negative and positive predictions. Negative predictions involve statements that are likely to curtail opportunities, coerce treatment, and deprive the patient of freedom. In contrast, positive predictions usually enable the patient through the selection of treatments or other services. When the "cost" of a positive prediction is relatively low (e.g., recommendation of cognitive-behavioral treatment for an anxiety disorder), clinicians are likely to be less concerned about probability estimates and cautions than when the cost is both large and experienced as negative by the patient (e.g., civil commitment). From this context, treatment recommendations for a motivated patient, while based on implicit predictions, are largely determined by comparative effectiveness and availability.

15

Research: Current Models and Future Directions

The previous chapters on structured and diagnostic interviews include scores of implicit research questions that merit further investigation. Moreover, the summary tables in Chapter 14 (i.e., Tables 14.2 to 14.5) offer an overview of structured interviews, both their current validation and, implicitly, their future research needs. Because of these resources, this chapter does not attempt to recapitulate the considerable array of specific research questions. Rather, this chapter focuses on a broad conceptualization of structured interviews and their roles, both current and potential, in clinical research.

This chapter is organized into five sections addressing research applications for clinical constructs, theory development, and specific issues. The first section begins with simple lessons learned about the development of structured interviews. The second section, which addresses the assessment of psychopathology, is subdivided into symptoms, scales, and diagnoses. The third section considers motivational concerns in clinical assessment. The fourth section offers examples of how structured interviewing may be used in testing theories. The fifth section summarizes other applications of structured interviewing in professional settings.

LESSONS ABOUT STRUCTURED INTERVIEWS

The development and validation of structured interviews could easily fill a substantial volume. This section has very modest goals in highlighting issues that are often overlooked in the creation of structured interviews. Such issues involve item and interview development.

Item development is not a simple process. Studies with the DISC (see Chapter 6) illustrate problems with interview questions that span both structure and content. For example, the length of interview questions is likely to affect comprehension (Breton et al., 1995). While this has been demonstrated with children, we cannot assume that adults are exempt from problems with question complexity. Other key issues need to be considered in the creation of structured inquiries:

- Diagnostic questions are often concerned about time, frequency, and duration. How these questions are worded may affect the quality of the responses (see, e.g., Fallon & Schwab-Stone, 1994).
- Affectively laden questions (e.g., "I am worried about . . .") likely assess emotional states more than specific content (Clark & Watson, 1995).
- Comparative questions (e.g., "compared to your usual self" or "compared to other children") require special scrutiny. Researchers need to know what metric is employed in responding to these complex questions. An alternative is to divide the question into two components, asking about the person and then inquiring about comparisons to others.
- The content of certain inquiries may be difficult to understand. Breslau (1987) found that both children and adults (i.e., their parents) had trouble understanding questions about certain symptoms (e.g., obsessions and compulsions). Persons with diverse cultural backgrounds may have substantial difficulty in understanding question content (Reinhardt, 2000).
- Interview questions are rarely evaluated to see how they may be influenced by social desirability or, perhaps more accurately, social pejorativeness.

The development of a structured interview involves important decisions, including the basic theme implicit in its format. A comparison of the SCID-II and SIDP is instructive. The theme of the SCID-II is "clinician convenience." Items (1) parallel the DSM-IV, (2) are presented in order, and (3) are scored unidirectionally. The theme of the SIDP is "patient rapport." Items (1) have a natural flow and (2) are not always indicative of psychopathology. The format of the structured interview is likely to affect patient reporting. This hypothesis could be tested directly by comparing alternative versions (i.e., thematic vs. diagnostic formats) of the SIDP and PDI.

Most structured interviews define the core features of relevant clinical constructs and then proceed to evaluate these features. This process is especially useful for establishing convergent validity but is often limited for demonstrating discriminant validity. As a hypothetical, assume that you want to develop a structured interview that differentiates between specific anxiety and mood disorders. Because these broad diagnostic categories have many symptoms in common, simply focusing on salient symptoms is likely to produce very poor discriminant validity. Instead, research could concentrate on *distinguishing features*. Structured interviews would include very different questions to address distinguishing features. As a concrete example, Cloninger et al. (1985; see Chapter 1) found that the "absence of buying sprees" was highly discriminating. This emphasis would have far-ranging effects on both structured interviews and diagnoses. As an example of the latter, Rogers and Cruise (2000) critiqued the DSM-IV classification of malingering and found that it lacked distinguishing features and, consequently, discriminant validity.

This book on structured interviews clearly stresses diagnostic over nondiagnostic measures. While diagnostic interviews are central to clinical practice, this focus is also necessitated by the lack of nondiagnostic structured interviews. Stated bluntly, little reason exists to develop another Axis I or Axis II interview. Researchers need to consider other clinical constructs that are critical to professional practice.

ASSESSMENT OF PSYCHOPATHOLOGY

A major thrust of clinical research is the accurate appraisal of psychopathology. The selection of measures in such research often appears to be dictated by brevity and familiarity. As an example of the former, many studies have employed the BDI as a measure of depression, when other, more comprehensive measures are readily available. As an example of the latter, the MCMI-II is sometimes used in research as a substitution for Axis II diagnosis, although its lack of correspondence with DSM disorders has been convincingly established (Rogers et al., 1999). Brevity and familiarity are not adequate criteria for the selection of measures. A small but appreciable improvement could be made throughout clinical research if each published study were required to justify explicitly through systematic comparisons its selection of interviews, tests, or scales.

A variation of brevity is the expediency of group administrations. While the measures themselves are often extensive (e.g., the MMPI-2), the expenditure of researchers' effort is typically minimal. In some cases, multiscale inventories are an optimal choice for clinical research. In most diagnostic studies, the selection of such inventories appears to be dictated by expediency rather than experimental rigor and diagnostic validity.

If "brevity," "familiarity," and "expediency" are not the watchwords of clinical research, on what basis should measures be selected? The overall validation of any measure is an obvious consideration. Equally important are decisions regarding the type of measurement for psychopathology and its specific validation. For examples, the SADS focuses on symptom severity, while the DIS attends to the etiology of symptoms. For any study addressing specific symptoms, clear preferences should be easily established between the SADS and the DIS based simply on the type of clinical data required. Measures also differ in the breadth of symptomatology. For instance, in descriptive studies of psychotic patients, clinical researchers may opt for the CASH or the RPMIP given their comprehensive review of relevant symptoms.

The assessment of psychopathology can be simply but effectively organized on a continuum of abstraction that is composed of symptoms, scales, and disorders. Depending on the purpose of the study, researchers must decide which of these three categories is their primary focus. In turn, this decision will inform the subsequent selection of psychological measures based on their comparative strengths.

Focus of Specific Symptoms

The primary focus of many longitudinal studies with clinical populations is changes in symptoms rather than disorders. As noted in Chapter 1, longitudinal research on schizophrenia might examine alterations in symptoms during prodromal, active, and residual phases. An interesting question is whether symptoms at each phase reflect discrete changes in psychopathology or simply represent observable changes in severity. Are overvalued ideas and delusions essentially the same symptom expressed at different levels?[1] Another question is whether negative symptoms constitute true inclusion criteria or whether they actually indicate the resulting impairment that often arises from the positive symptoms.

The answer to these questions would rely on the systematic assessment of schizophrenic symptoms across short intervals, which would allow for the investigation of symptom severity as well as the emergence of new symptoms. In other words, the primary focus is symptomatology and its concomitant severity. Structured interviews, such as the SADS and the CASH, might well be considered. In addition, similar questions could be posed for mood disorders in differentiating dysthymia and major depression based on symptomatic differences.

An alternative to longitudinal studies of symptomatology would be retrospective research on structured interviews. While most research has sought to corroborate retrospective reporting through collateral sources (e.g., the IRAOS), a time-lapse model offers a superior research design (Rogers, in press). With the time-lapse model, the structured interview is administered twice: (1) a current assessment (e.g., the present month), and (2) a retrospective assessment for the original time period (i.e., the same month as the first administration). Differences in consistent reporting could by evaluated systematically for specific symptoms and clinical populations. Variations of the time-lapse model have been successfully used with the SADS-C and the PDE

---

[1]One confound to understanding prodromal psychotic symptoms is that they are rarely diagnosed in the presence of active psychotic symptoms. In other words, overvalued ideas, superstitiousness, and recurrent illusions are typically not recorded in the presence of delusions, paranoid ideation, and hallucinations. Therefore, clinicians are at a serious disadvantage in attempting to assess whether active psychotic symptoms are an accentuation of prodromal symptoms or whether they represent new developments.

(see Rogers, in press). This approach could lead to exciting, cost-effective developments in longitudinal research.

Treatment studies typically address differences in symptoms. For example, psychopharmacological interventions are aimed at the reduction of targeted symptoms, not cure or even full remission of mental disorders. For instance, the primary focus of anxiolytic medication is the reduction and control of specific anxiety symptoms. Toward this end, structured interviews that emphasize diagnostic reliability, but not symptom reliability, may not be appropriate measures. In this case, use of the ADIS would not be appropriate unless researchers undertook to establish its reliability on a symptom level.

The importance of symptoms, in their own right, merits further study. Although delusions can be diagnosed in a diverse group of organic, schizophrenic, delusional, schizoaffective, and mood disorders, what about understanding the delusions themselves? Research on the content of delusions, their complexity, and their effects on behavior are all worthy of study. For example, what are the precursors to the emergence of a pseudocommunity? How does cultural relativism affect delusions (see Murphy, 1986) even among ethnic groups within the United States?[2] Do combinations of delusions (e.g., grandiose and paranoid) signal a difference in overall functioning or prognosis?

The severity of symptoms warrants further investigation. Structured interviews have often used a curious admixture of criteria in establishing the severity of symptoms. With mood symptoms, for example, severity is typically evaluated in terms of frequency and subjective distress. For personality disorders, common criteria are personal distress and negative effects on others. For psychotic and anxiety disorders, severity is commonly assessed with respect to its behavioral consequences (e.g., the patient obeyed the command hallucinations; see Rogers, Gillis, Turner, & Smith, 1990). The assessment of individual symptoms on multiple dimensions would represent a particularly interesting avenue of research. Table 15.1 presents multiple perspectives of symptom severity that could be incorporated into structured interviews and self-report measures.

Focus on Scales

The relationship between structured interviews and traditional psychological tests deserves a brief comment. Many structured interviews and psychological tests were designed for the same general purpose, namely, the assessment of psychopathology. The key difference is that many structured interviews were constructed specifically to measure DSM diagnoses. In contrast, psychological

---

[2]Cultural influences can affect both patients (i.e., the content and style of presentation of delusional material) and mental health professionals (i.e., assessment and interventions of similar delusions in patients from different subcultures).

TABLE 15.1. Assessment of Symptom Severity from Multiple Perspectives

Indicators of severity	Representative inquiries
Frequency	How often does it occur? How long do you typically go without experiencing it?
Duration	How long does it last?
Subjective distress	Does it bother (upset) you? How much? Can you ever ignore it?
Behavioral consequences	What do you usually do when it occurs? What is the worst thing you have done?
Effects on others	What do others do when it occurs?
Relative importance	How important is it for you to get help for this problem? Is this (problem or symptom) worse than others? How would your life be different if this did not occur?

tests often focus on alternative approaches. How are these divergent models of mental disorders reconciled?

Prior to DSM-III, psychological tests provided the optimal standardization of the assessment of psychopathology through systematic comparisons of psychometric data. Rorschach and MMPI data were clearly superior to idiosyncratic interviews and arduous history taking. Even when test data were compared to DSM diagnoses, the lack of strong relationships was often blamed, perhaps appropriately, on the frailties of DSM-II. With the emergence of DSM-III and the concomitant development of structured interviews, this historical advantage no longer exists.

Researchwise, structured interviews provide an ideal avenue for the validation of clinical scales on psychological tests. Researchers must grapple with these missed opportunities. For example, how many studies have compared MMPI-2 scales and 2-point codes to SADS or SCID diagnoses? Or compared the schizophrenic index of the Rorschach with diagnostic data that have established reliability? The common answer to both questions is "less than a handful." Moreover, recent studies with the MMPI-2 (e.g., Fantoni-Salvador & Rogers, 1997) and MMPI-A (e.g., Cashel et al., 1998) suggest that refinements are needed in scale interpretation. A rich opportunity exists for studies to make a substantial impact on psychological tests by applying the most rigorous standards to test validation.

Gynther et al. (1973) set the standard for MMPI validation when they employed systematic data from the MMS (see Chapter 2) in the validation of MMPI code types. They only accepted a clinical descriptor if its description could be cross-validated on very large psychiatric populations (> 10,000). A similarly rigorous standard could be set for multiscale inventories and employ more sophisticated structured interviews than the MMS. For example, Cashel et al. (1998) utilized only individual symptoms with high reliability (kappa ≥

.80) in validating MMPI-A scales. In summary, researchers need to validate traditional tests against the highest standards for the assessment of symptoms, syndromes, and disorders. The highest standards are often found in structured interviews.

Substantial progress has been made on the validation of self-report measures with structured interviews. Interestingly, the *Journal of Personality Disorders* has set a standard for the assessment of Axis II disorders with many studies that employ the SIDP, the PDE, and the SCID-II. These studies, along with clinical diagnosis, have typically found that the MCMI-II lacks any diagnostic equivalence, but have demonstrated the usefulness of the PDQ-R as an effective screening measure. These studies have also underscored the dangers of "descriptor fallacy" (Rogers & Ornduff, 1994) that occurs when similar clinical terms are erroneously equated despite their divergent operational definitions and nonconvergent research.

Researchers of the MMPI–MMPI-2 in particular should be aware of pervasive problems with the *lack of bidirectionality* of findings. For example, patients with schizophrenia often have certain profiles (e.g., 6–8 profiles, that is, the highest elevations are found on scales 6 and 8). But the obverse is not true. Most 6–8 profiles are not found among patients with schizophrenia. Problems with the lack of bidirectionality permeate both research and professional practice. Professionally, clinicians may couch their reports in such profiles (e.g., "The patient's profile is 'consistent with' a schizophrenic disorder."), which is likely misleading to most referral sources. From a research perspective, studies are urgently needed that define the sensitivity and specificity rates for commonly used clinical scales.

Projective methods frequently fall short in their validation of specific indices, which are sometimes more theory-based than empirically derived. Studies that are conducted often address only the degree of association between two methods. A much more sophisticated model would be the mulitrait–multimethod matrix proposed by Campbell and Fiske (1959). For example, components of the Rorschach Hypervigilance Index (Exner, 1991) could be compared to suspiciousness and paranoid symptoms as measured by structured interviews and other tests (i.e., convergent validity), with the inclusion of other Rorschach and clinical data that are predicted to be unrelated to the hypervigilance index (i.e., discriminant validity). Rorschach interpretation supported by the mulitrait–multimethod matrix would be easily defensible on both theoretical and empirical grounds.

This discussion of psychological tests and their validation may seem unduly critical, possibly even heretical. On the contrary, the most positive long-term perspective involves the rigorous testing and refinement of psychological tests. By insisting of the highest standards, clinicians ensure that psychological tests will continue to prosper. By acknowledging current problems (e.g., overinterpretation, descriptor fallacy, and lack of bidirectionality), research can develop empirically validated solutions.

Focus on Disorders

This section considers two major facets of diagnostic research, namely, the use of Syndeham's criteria and the comparison of dimensional, categorical, and synthesized models. Furthermore, additional observations concerning underinvestigated elements of diagnostic research are presented.

Syndeham's Criteria

What would happen if researchers truly invoked Syndeham's criteria for disorders? If only those disorders with clear inclusion and exclusion criteria were allowed to be diagnosed? If we insisted that disorders have identifiable outcome criteria that set them apart from other disorders?

The first step in this process, as described in Chapter 1, would be the refinement of inclusion and expansion of exclusion criteria to maximize differentiation among disorders. Inclusion criteria, which are common to many disorders (e.g., social withdrawal), are obviously not effective. By the same token, nonspecific exclusion criteria provide little assistance in the demarcation of specific disorders. The second, more challenging step would be the demonstration of outcome criteria. For example, are subtypes of schizophrenia justifiable in systematic examinations of their precursors, course, or response to treatment? Moreover, do familial and laboratory correlates support the specific etiology of these subtypes?

As a *gedanken*, or thought experiment, consider what might happen if Syndeham's criteria were strictly followed. Many Axis I disorders would become simplified. It is doubtful that psychotic disorders would manifest differential outcomes to such a degree as to warrant more than a few diagnoses. Even more, most Axis II disorders would cease to exist given their predicted chronicity and overlap with other disorders. Alternatively, certain personality disorders might flourish, with increased attention to differential outcomes and discriminative responses to treatment. At present, nonspecific treatments generally yield nonspecific results.

Large-scale, existing data sets on the SADS and the DIS could assist in the refinement of diagnosing mental disorders. In other words, longitudinal data currently exist to implement Syndeham's criteria with some Axis I disorders. This research would likely lead to hierarchical diagnoses, since differential outcome criteria would be next to impossible to establish with multiple disorders. Moreover, the whole focus of diagnostic research could be sharpened simply by insisting that we follow Syndeham's dicta. Genetic and familial studies would provide valuable ancillary data for more refined diagnoses.

Categorical and Dimensional Models

The debate over categorical and dimensional diagnosis is far from resolved. The advantages of the categorical model are well-known for clinician acceptance and straightforward communication of information (see Gunderson, Links, & Reich, 1991). In contrast, dimensional ratings provide both a continuum from normal to abnormal and diagnostic overlap. As noted by Clark, Livesley, and Morey (1997), dimensional ratings should be highly skewed in nonclinical populations but normally distributed in clinical populations. In general, dimensional models offer information that is superior to the nominal data of categorical diagnosis and allow for more sophisticated analysis (Widiger, 1991).

Widiger (1992), as a proponent of the dimensional approach, is strongly critical of the current categorical paradigm. He argues that the boundaries for establishing mental disorders are largely arbitrary. For example, the DSM-III-R Personality Disorder Advisory Committee had no empirical data to guide the establishment of cut scores for nine of the 11 personality disorders but was guided by pragmatism and consensus. He made the cogent observation that, often, the presence of one or two symptoms to an extreme degree may likely qualify as a personality disorder causing social impairment and distress. As a further example, research on the CAPS has clearly demonstrated that small shifts in cut scores for PTSD are likely have substantial effects on diagnoses (Weathers et al., 1999).

Widiger (1991) has proposed a synthesis of the categorical and dimensional model through an ordinal organization of symptoms divided into six groups: absent, traits, subthreshold, threshold, moderate, and prototypical. Gunderson et al. (1991) also suggested a synthesized model with dimensional ratings for certain psychotic processes and personality traits, and a categorical model for certain other disorders. I would like to propose two alternatives for further study:

1. The *polythetic–dimensional* approach utilizes a categorical model (i.e., a minimum number of inclusion criteria) to establish the disorder and then dimensional ratings to evaluate its severity. The IPDE is a current example of how this synthesized model could be used.
2. The *nested–polythetic* approach was described in Chapter 1. With PTSD as the prime example, patients must have symptoms from clusters (i.e., nested symptoms) of highly correlated symptoms. With the CAPS as a current example, these clusters could be measured both dimensionally and categorically.

The presence of symptoms should not be considered equal to the establishment of a mental disorder. For conduct disorder, running away from home overnight should not be equated with arson or sexual assault. Moreover, there needs to be some consideration for the severity of the behavior. Burning an isolated tool shed and torching a densely populated apartment building should not be equated. As an alternative to the pure polythetic model, a more sophisticated alternative would require both a minimum number of inclusion criteria and a minimum severity score (inclusion criteria multiplied by severity ratings). A more elaborate model might also incorporate prototyp-icality, so that frequent arson and frequent lying would be differentially scored.

Why this brief discussion of categorical, dimensional, and synthesized di-agnostic models? If researchers could agree on the fundamental criteria, for example, Syndeham's criteria, then the choice of the optimum organization and type of measurement would become obvious. The important lesson from structured interviews is that reliable dimensions for specific inclusion criteria can be established. We have also learned from prototypical analyses that core characteristics of particular mental disorders can be reliably established. These methodologies could be combined to study the most effective model for establishing distinctive outcome criteria. What we now need is systematic re-search to establish specific outcome criteria that are understandable in terms of current theory and defensible with respect to treatment outcomes. Meta-methodological research could have a very real impact on diagnosis if system-atic comparisons of different diagnostic models proved the superiority of one paradigm over others.

Other Considerations

A largely ignored facet of the diagnosis is symptom content. Does it matter whether paranoid ideation involves family/friends, governmental agencies, or extraterrestrial beings? Does it matter whether paranoid thoughts involve dif-ferent forms of killing or simply discrediting a person's standing in the com-munity? For example, research on hallucinations (Larkin, 1979; Rogers, Gillis, Turner, et al., 1990) has suggested that the content of hallucinations may be closely related to patients' adjustment. Likewise, mood and personali-ty disorders could be categorized by symptom content. Certainly, the excel-lent work accomplished on the treatment of specific types of anxiety symp-toms would recommend further examination of this approach. In other words, symptom content, such as that found with delusional disorders, may have merit in establishing diagnostic validity for other disorders.

Research (Chapter 9, see, e.g., Reich & Troughton, 1988b) demonstrat-ed the potential effect that Axis I diagnoses may have on the assessment of Axis II disorders. What remains unexplored is the reverse: the effect of Axis II disorders on the assessment of major mental disorders. For example, does the presence of a narcissistic personality disorder limit the disclosure of major de-pression? How does preexisting avoidant personality disorder affect the diag-nosis of GAD? Certainly, more research is needed to understand Axis I–Axis II interactions fully, as well as effects of substance abuse disorders on both. With respect to the latter, are functional disorders underdiagnosed because of attributions made by patients and clinicians about the presence of substance abuse?

Diagnostic research in general remains appallingly simplistic in its cross-cultural considerations. This research typically assumes that all African

Americans and Hispanic Americans are similar and will respond similarly to psychometric measures. This unfounded assumption entirely ignores within-minority differences in language and culture (Puente, 1990). Many studies of minorities naively assume that comparable norms justify the generalization of external validity data from one cultural group to another. Simply because Anglo Americans and African Americans may evidence similar scores on the PCL-R has no direct bearing on the *validity* of these scores when compared to external measures. As a further example, researchers should never conclude that self-referral to counseling centers represents similar levels of distress across cultural groups. For example, certain ethnic groups may have higher elevations on MMPI-2 profiles not necessarily because of cultural differences on the test itself but because of differences in their referral patterns.

A final consideration might be "diagnosis by treatment." If clinicians accepted that the overriding objective of assessment is the effective treatment of persons with mental disorders, then the logical conclusion would be to link diagnosis to treatment. This model would represent an adaptation of Syndeham's criteria, with treatment response considered a necessary component of diagnoses. What would be the implications of this radical departure from the current nosology? First and foremost, "untreatable" disorders would no longer be unnecessarily stigmatized. As noted by Rogers and Lynett (1991), the diagnosis of APD typically signals to the criminal justice system the presence of an untreatable person who is likely to receive very punitive criminal sanctions. Of course, the obvious limitation of this approach is that treatment methods might never be developed. An apparent solution would be the development of provisional disorders that would be "sunsetted" after a specified period of time, if effective treatment were not forthcoming. This solution provides clinicians with a common language and standard, though tentative, criteria for treatment research. If effective treatments are not forthcoming, the "sunsetting" of disorders would likely (1) reduce stigmatization and punitive sanctions for untreatable conditions, and (2) increase targeted treatment research on specific syndromes and potential disorders.

MOTIVATIONAL ISSUES IN PSYCHOLOGICAL ASSESSMENT

Nearly all psychological measures are based on three unballasted assumptions: that each patient (1) is psychologically engaged in the assessment process, (2) shares the same goals as the clinician, and (3) cooperates with the clinician's methods of achieving these goals. Research directly on these assumptions might offer valuable insights as to their viability in clinical assessments. For example, we could attempt to assess patients' motivations, their understanding of the clinician's motivations, and the level of consensus on how the assessment should proceed.

The first assumption, psychological engagement in the assessment process, has been systematically evaluated with several multiscale inventories (e.g., MMPI and PAI). With these measures, patient's responses are evaluated whether items are being read and responded to consistently. The response style inherent in this approach is "irrelevant responding" (see Rogers, 1997). Irrelevant responding has not been systematically explored with either structured interviewing or most types of psychological testing. Research that combines interview and self-report measures (e.g., the SCID-II and SCID-II-Q) might be particularly effective at assessing consistency of self-report, which is the underlying strategy to detect irrelevant responding.

The second assumption, shared goals, is likely to be instrumental in determining the extent and quality of reported data, thereby affecting the accurate appraisal of the diagnosis. The patient may be motivated to exaggerate/fabricate symptoms in light of an external goal (i.e., malingering and factitious disorders), minimize/deny symptoms (defensiveness), or acknowledge only symptoms that are less stigmatizing (social desirability). Two additional and largely unexplored response styles in clinical assessment include (1) "role assumption" (Kroger & Turnbull, 1975), in which the patient assumes the role of a different person as a method of foiling the evaluation, and (2) "impression management" (Tetlock & Manstead, 1985), in which the patient attempts to create the desired social image. In addition, patients may develop hybrid response styles in which they combine more than one of the aforementioned styles. A classic example of hybrid response style is the male pedophile who often self-discloses about most aspects of his life but is highly defensive about his sexual interest and arousal toward children.

Research on response styles has proceeded rather unevenly. Malingering has received concerted attention in the last decade, with a proliferation of studies (see Reynolds, 1998; Rogers, 1997). A smaller literature has been established on defensiveness and social desirability. In contrast, very little clinical research has been conducted on role assumption and impression management. Certainly, more systematic research is needed on all forms of response styles, particularly as they relate to structured interviews and projective techniques.

The third assumption is that patients agree with clinicians in the selection of assessment methods. Patients' willingness or unwillingness to engage in certain forms of assessment has yet to be systematically studied. Although "resistance" has been described in patients who give only minimal responses to projective techniques, perhaps the more basic issue is the agreement, explicitly or implicitly, between the clinician and the examinee. The effects of negotiated versus non-negotiated assessments have yet to be empirically investigated. In other words, how does coercion, whether acknowledged or not, affect participation and results?

Test conditions have long been known to affect motivation and performance, particularly on aptitude tests (Cronbach, 1970). How do situational characteristics affect patients' performance on clinical measures? For example, we could compare symptoms and diagnoses for children tested in both juvenile detention facilities with the same children tested in the community. By the same token, we could also compare diagnoses made from videotapes by mental health professionals who were blind to the location of the testing. In this way, we could test for "real" differences in motivation and self-reporting while simultaneously estimating the situational effects on the examining clinicians. My point is that much more sophisticated research is possible on the relationship between situational characteristics and reported psychopathology. Likewise, internal states (e.g., fatigue or tiredness) could be experimentally manipulated and rigorously tested.

Unfamiliarity with testing procedures may represent a related confound to psychological assessment. For example, some Mexicans and Mexican Americans may not be acquainted with multiple-choice questions and Likert-type ratings; such unfamiliarity is likely to be an impediment to their cooperation and compliance. Lack of enculturation in American-style schooling may have profound effects on performance, especially when the format of the assessment differs substantially from patients' past educational experiences.

THEORY TESTING

I, like many of my academic colleagues, have frequent occasions to review dissertations and am struck by how many are simply isolated empirical exercises proliferated in the absence of theory. Perhaps draconian, I would like to see an additional standard imposed by assessment journals: At a minimum, the results should be tied to theory. Atheoretical assessment studies are not accidental. Indeed, the DSM-III promulgated this stance in an attempt to reconcile differences between dynamic and biological schools (see Faust & Miner, 1986). Theory extends beyond etiology to diagnostic models (e.g., categorical vs. dimensional), diagnostic validity (e.g., Syndeham's criteria), response styles and motivation, and, of course, treatment methods.

The contemplation of new diagnoses underscores the importance of theory to assessment. The provisional diagnostic criteria for factitious disorder by proxy (American Psychiatric Association, 1994) highlight the role of theory in deciding which criteria and associated features characterize this proposed disorder. Researchers who winnow through dozens of potential indices for factitious disorder by proxy must take into account both theory and research (Rogers, 1998).

A resurgence of interest in the assessment of personality per se, especially in methodology, has been observed with greater sophistication (Jackson & Paunonen, 1980). The relationship of personality to Axis I and Axis II disorders has generated considerable theoretical interest (Schroeder, Wormworth, & Livesley, 1992; Trull & Widiger, 1997). The theoretical possibilities of integrating personality and disorders are exciting. Moreover, much assessment research with dimensional ratings provides a basis for theoretical exploration of normality versus abnormality.

Longitudinal research is the sine qua non of theory testing and building.

While systematic comparisons of measures may further our understanding of important theory-based relationships, only through repeated measures can these relationships be fully understood. Even the best-crafted cross-sectional study offers but a single time perspective, although this may be augmented by the use of structured interviews that gather data regarding previous episodes. For example, Meehl's (1990) theory of schizotaxia as the etiological basis of schizophrenia should be tested optimally through longitudinal research. Best efforts at theory testing require stable samples with longitudinal assessments. A laudable goal for nearly all researchers is the identification of a clinical sample that is likely to remain relatively accessible to research across time.

Some theoretically based research may not require exhaustive efforts, but simply waits to be conducted. For example, could the effects of social labeling theory on treatment outcome be empirically tested? In many mental health clinics, diagnosis is deemphasized. Research with diagnostic interviews could establish "true" diagnoses and compare these to the "working diagnoses" of the clinician and patients' self-descriptions. In examining predictive utility, differences between true and presumed diagnoses could be evaluated systematically. In a naturalistic design, the potential effects social labeling theory (both salutary and harmful) could be investigated.

Theory-based interventions represent a vibrant component of treatment outcome research. Beyond its obvious merits, the vitality of cognitive-behavioral treatment lies in systematic research that tests its relative efficacy with specific patient populations. Many other theoretical schools have languished, partly because of this inattention to theory-based research. Clinical researchers, searching to make important contributions, would do well to venture beyond the well-trodden ground of cognitive-behavioral therapy. They should consider other theory-based interventions and perform systematic investigations into their treatment potential.

OTHER APPLICATIONS

The use and application of structured interviews extends far beyond the reaches of general clinical practice. Standardized interview data have formed the basis of many endeavors to evaluate individual competencies. As reviewed in Chapter 13, structured interviews have been successfully employed in two circumscribed areas of forensic assessment: psychopathy and competency to stand trial. Both civil competencies (e.g., personal injury and child custody) and other criminal competencies (e.g., insanity and treatability of sex offenders) offer fertile opportunities to advance forensic assessment.

Research on structured interviews could easily be expanded beyond clinical issues to include educational and vocational applications. Standardization of interview and other data may improve predictive validity of important decisions, such as graduate students' success, even when less than elegant models are employed (Dawes, 1979). By the same token, standardized interviews could be tested for the measurement of interpersonal functioning and its underlying dimensions, which might lead to a more comprehensive understanding of different types of relationships. Even vague constructs such as "adjustment" or superior functioning could be operationalized and assessed.

Clinicians have emphasized scale development, sometimes to the exclusion of other potentially valuable methods. An expansion of assessment methods does not imply the jettisoning of inventories, scales, and ratings. By invoking a multimethod approach to assessment, researchers can evaluate important assessment domains while controlling for method variance. Robust multimethod approaches are likely to combine the best of written self-report measures and the dynamic possibilities of structured interviews.

CONCLUDING COMMENTS

We often experience the separability of clinical practice and applied research is in both our training and professional lives. This division in the mental health professions has profound implications for the unnecessary and often detrimental compartmentalization of practice and research. In their own small way, I hope that the structured interview methods embraced by this book may forge a common ground that is selectively employed by practitioners and vigorously tested by researchers.

References

Abel, J. L., & Borkovec, T. D. (1995). Generalizability of DSM-III-R generalized anxiety disorders to proposed DSM-IV criteria and cross-validation of proposed changes. *Journal of Anxiety Disorders, 9,* 303–315.

Abous-Saleh, M. T., Suhaili, A. R. A., Karim, L., Prais, V., & Hamdi, E. (1999). Single-photon emission tomography with 99M Tc-labelled hexamethyl propylene amine oxime in Arab patients with schizophrenia. *Nordic Journal of Psychiatry, 53,* 49–54.

Abrams, R. C., Alexopoulos, G. S., & Young, R. C. (1987). Geriatric depression and DSM-III-R personality disorder criteria. *Journal of the American Geriatrics Society, 35,* 383–386.

Achenbach, T. M. (1985). Clinical data systems: Rating scales and interviews. In R. Michels, J. O. Cavenar, A. M. Cooper, S. B. Guze, L. L. Judd, G. L. Klerman, & A. J. Solnit (Eds.), *Psychiatry* (Vol. 2, chap. 23). Philadephia: Lippincott.

Achenbach, T. M., & Edelbrock, C. S. (1979). The child behavior profile: II. Boys aged 12–16 and girls aged 6–11 and 12–16. *Journal of Consulting and Clinical Psychology, 47,* 223–233.

Achenbach, T. M., & Edelbrock, C. S. (1983). *Manual for the Child Behavior Checklist and Revised Child Behavior Profile.* Burlington: University of Vermont, Department of Psychiatry.

Achenbach, T. M., & Edelbrock, C. S. (1986). *Manual for the Teacher's Report Form and Teacher Version of the Child Behavior Profile.* Burlington: University of Vermont, Department of Psychiatry.

Achenbach, T. M., & Edelbrock, C. S. (1987). *Manual for the Youth Self-Report and profile.* Burlington, VT: University Associates in Psychiatry.

Achenbach, T. M., McConaughy, S. H., & Howell, C. T. (1987). Child/adolescent behavioral and emotional problems: Implications of cross-informant correlations for situational specificity. *Psychological Bulletin, 101,* 213–232.

Allen-Meares, P. (1991). A study of depressive characteristics in behaviorally disordered children and adolescents. *Children and Youth Services Review, 13,* 271–286.

Alnaes, R., & Torgersen, S. (1989). Personality and personality disorders among patients with major depression in combination with dysthymic and cyclothymic disorders. *Acta Psychiatrica Scandinavica, 79,* 363–369.

Alnaes, R., & Torgersen, S. (1997). Personality and personality disorders predict development and relapses of major depression. *Acta Psychiatrica Scandinavica, 95,* 336–342.

Alterman, A. I., Brown, L. S., Jr., Zaballero, A., & McKay, J. R. (1994). Interviewer severity ratings and composite scores on the ASI: A further look. *Drug and Alcohol Dependence, 34,* 201–209.

Alterman, A. I., Cacciola, J. S., & Rutherford, M. J. (1993). Reliability of the revised Psychopathy Checklist in substance abuse patients. *Psychological Assessment, 5,* 442–448.

Alterman, A. I., Snider, E. C., Cacciola, J. S., Brown, L. S., Jr., Zaballero, A., & Siddiqui, N. (1996). Evidence for response set effects in structured research interviews. *Journal of Nervous and Mental Disease, 184,* 403–410.

Altman, H., Angle, H. B., Brown, M. L., & Sletten, I. W. (1972). Prediction of hospital stay. *Comprehensive Psychiatry, 13,* 471–480.

Altman, H., Evenson, R. C., & Cho, D. W. (1976). New discriminant functions for computer diagnosis. *Multivariate Behavioral Research, 11,* 367–376.

Altman, H., Evenson, R. C., & Cho, D. W. (1977). *Predicting danger to self and others among psychiatric patients.* Unpublished technical report, Missouri Institute of Psychiatry, Mental Health Systems Research Unit, St. Louis.

Altman, H., Evenson, R. C., Hedlund, J. L., & Cho, D. W. (1978). Missouri Actuarial Report System (MARS). *Comprehensive Psychiatry, 19,* 185–192.

Altman, H., Evenson, R. C., & Sletten, I. W. (1973). Comparison of psychotropic drug assignment by psychiatrists and by a multivariate computer model. *International Research Communications System, 73,* 32–27–1.

Ambrosini, P. J. (1992). *Schedule for Affective Disorders and Schizophrenia for School-Age Children (6–18 years): Kiddie-SADS (K-SADS) (Present State version).* Philadelphia: Medical College of Pennsylvania.

Ambrosini, P. J., & Dixon, M. (1996). *Schedule for Affective Disorders and Schizophrenia, Childhood Version* (4th ed.). Philadelphia: Medical College of Pennsylvania.

Ambrosini, P. J., Metz, C., Prabucki, K., & Lee, J.-C. (1989). Videotape reliability of the third revised edition of the K-SADS. *Journal of the American Academy of Child and Adolescent Psychiatry, 28,* 723–728.

Ambrosini, P. J., Wagner, K. D., Biederman, J., Glick, I., Tan, C. Elia, J., Hebeler, J. R., Rabinovich, H., Lock, J., & Geller, D. (1999). Multicenter open-label sertraline study in adolescent outpatients with major depression. *Journal of the American Academy of Child and Adolescent Psychiatry, 38,* 566–572.

American Psychiatric Association. (1968). *Diagnostic and statistical manual of mental disorders* (2nd. ed.). Washington, DC: Author.

American Psychiatric Association. (1980). *Diagnostic and statistical manual of mental disorders* (3rd ed.). Washington, DC: Author.

American Psychiatric Association. (1987). *Diagnostic and statistical manual of mental disorders* (3rd ed., rev.). Washington, DC: Author.

American Psychiatric Association. (1991). *DSM-IV options book: Work in progress.* Washington, DC: Author.

American Psychiatric Association. (1993). *DSM-IV draft criteria.* Washington, DC: Author.

American Psychiatric Association. (1994). *Diagnostic and statistical manual of mental disorders* (4th ed.). Washington, DC: Author.

American Psychiatric Association. (1996). *Practice guidelines*. Washington, DC: Author.

American Psychiatric Association. (1997). *Practice guideline for the treatment of patients with schizophrenia*. Washington, DC: Author.

American Psychiatric Association. (2000). *Diagnostic and statistical manual of mental disorders: Text revision* (4th ed.). Washington, DC: Author.

American Psychological Association. (1992). Ethical principles of psychologists and code of conduct. *American Psychologist, 47,* 1597–1611.

Amorim, P., Lecrubier, Y., Weiller, E., Hergueta, T., & Sheehan, D. (1998). DSM-III-R psychotic disorders: Procedural validity of the Mini International Neuropsychiatric Interview (MINI), concordance and causes of discordance with the CIDI. *European Psychiatry, 13,* 26–34.

Anderson, G., Yasenik, L., & Ross, C. A. (1993). Dissociative experiences and disorders among women who identify themselves as sexual abuse survivors. *Child Abuse and Neglect, 17,* 677–686.

Anderson, H. S., Sestoft, D., Lillebaek, T., Mortensen, E. L., & Kramp, P. (1999). Psychopathy and psychopathological profiles in prisoners on remand. *Acta Psychiatrica Scandinavica, 99,* 33–39.

Anderson, J. C., Williams, S., McGee, R., & Silva, P. A. (1987). DSM-III disorders in preadolescent children. *Archives of General Psychiatry, 42,* 69–76.

Andrade, L., Eaton, W. W., & Chilcoat, H. D. (1996). Lifetime comorbidity of panic attacks and major depression in a population-based study: Age of onset. *Psychological Medicine, 26,* 991–996.

Andreasen, N. C. (1977). Reliability of proverbs: Interpretation to assess mental status. *Comprehensive Psychiatry, 18,* 465–473.

Andreasen, N. C. (1982). Negative symptoms in schizophrenia: Definition and reliability. *Archives of General Psychiatry, 39,* 784–788.

Andreasen, N. C. (1984a). *Scale for the Assessment of Negative Symptoms (SANS)*. Iowa City: University of Iowa College of Medicine.

Andreasen, N. C. (1984b). *Scale for the Assessment of Positive Symptoms (SAPS)*. Iowa City: University of Iowa College of Medicine.

Andreasen, N. C. (1987a). *Comprehensive Assessment of Symptoms and History*. Iowa City: University of Iowa College of Medicine.

Andreasen, N. C. (1987b). The concept of negative symptoms: Definition, specificity, and significance. *Psychiatry and Psychobiology, 2,* 240–251.

Andreasen, N. C. (1990). Methods for assessing positive and negative symptoms. In N. C. Andreasen (Ed.), *Modern problems of pharmacopsychiatry: Positive and negative symptoms and syndromes* (pp. 73–88). Basel, Switzerland: Karger.

Andreasen, N. C. (1997). Improvement of negative symptoms: Concepts, definition, and assessment. *International Clinical Psychopharmacology, 12*(Suppl. 2), S7–S10.

Andreasen, N. C., Arndt, S., Miller, D., Flaum, M., & Nopoulos, P. (1995). Correlational studies of the Scales of the Assessment of Ngative Symptoms and the Scale for the Assessment of Positive Symptoms: An overview and update. *Psychopathology, 28,* 7–17.

Andreasen, N. C., Flaum, M., & Arndt, S. (1992). The Comprehensive Assessment of Symptoms and History (CASH): An instrument for assessing diagnosis and psychopathology. *Archives of General Psychiatry, 49,* 615–623.

Andreasen, N. C., Flaum, M., Arndt, S., & Swayze, V. W. (1991). Positive and negative symptoms: Assessment and validity. In A. Marneros, N. C. Andreasen, & M. T. Tsuagn (Eds.), *Negative versus positive schizophrenia* (pp. 28–52). Berlin: Springer-Verlag.

Andreasen, N. C., Flaum, M., Swayze, V. W., Tyrrell, G., & Arndt, S. (1990). Positive and negative symptoms in schizophrenia: A critical reappraisal. *Archives of General Psychiatry, 47,* 615–621.

Andreasen, N. C., & Grove, W. M. (1986). Evaluation of positive and negative symptoms in schizophrenia. *Psychiatry and Psychobiology, 1,* 108–121.

Andreasen, N. C., Grove, W. M., Shapiro, R. W., Keller, M. B., Hirschfield, R. A., & McDonald-Scott, P. (1981). Reliability of lifetime diagnosis. *Archives of General Psychiatry, 35,* 400–405.

Andreasen, N. C., McDonald-Scott, P., Grove, W. M., Keller, M. B., Shapiro, R. W., & Hirschfeld, R. M. A. (1982). Assessment of reliability in multicenter collaborative research with a videotape approach. *American Journal of Psychiatry, 139,* 876–882.

Andreasen, N. C., Nopoulos, P., Schultz, S., Miller, D., Gupta, S. , Swayze, V., & Flaum, M. (1994). Positive and negative symptoms of schizophrenia: Past, present, and future. *Acta Psychiatrica Scandinavica, 90*(Suppl. 384), 51–59.

Andrews, G., Peters, L., Guzman, A. M., & Bird, K. (1995). A comparison of two structured diagnostic interviews: CIDI and SCAN. *Australian and New Zealand Journal of Psychiatry, 29,* 124–132.

Anduaga, J. C., Forteza, C. G., & Lira, L. R. (1991). Concurrent validity of the DIS: Experience with psychiatric patients in Mexico City. *Hispanic Journal of Behavioral Sciences, 13,* 63–77.

Angold, A., Cox, A., Prendergast, M., Rutter, M., & Simonoff, E. (1987). *The Child and Adolescent Psychiatric Assessment (CAPA).* Unpublished manuscript.

Angus, L. E., & Marziali, E. (1988). A comparison of three measures for the diagnosis of borderline personality disorder. *American Journal of Psychiatry, 145,* 1453–1454.

Anthony, J. C., Folstein, M., Romanoski, A. J., Von Korff, M. R., Nestadt, G. R., Chahal, R., Merchant, A., Brown, H., Shapiro, S., Kramer, M., & Gruenber, E. M. (1985). Comparison of the lay Diagnostic Interview Schedule and a standardized psychiatric diagnosis. *Archives of General Psychiatry, 42,* 667–675.

Anthony, J. C., LeResche, L., Niaz, U., Von Korff, M. R., & Folstein, M. F. (1982). Limits of the Mini-Mental State Examination as a screening test for dementia and delirium among hospital patients. *Psychological Medicine, 12,* 397–408.

Apter, A., Bleich, A., Plutchik, R., Mendelsohn, S., & Tyano, S. (1988). Suicidal behavior, depression, and conduct disorder in hospitalized adolescents. *Journal of the American Academy of Child and Adolescent Psychiatry, 27,* 696–699.

Apter, A., Orvaschel, H., Laseg, M., Moses, R., & Tyano, S. (1989). Psychometric properties of the K-SADS-P in an Israeli adolescent inpatient population. *Journal of the American Academy of Child and Adolescent Psychiatry, 28,* 61–65.

Arboleda-Florez, J. e., Lover, E. J., Fick, G., O'Brien, K., Hashman, K., & Aderibigbe, Y. (1995). An epidemiological study of mental illness in a remanded population. *International Medical Journal, 2,* 113–126.

Armelius, B. A., Kullgren, G., & Renberg, E. (1985). Borderline diagnosis from hospital records: Reliability and validity of Gunderson's Diagnostic Interview for Borderlines (DIB). *Journal of Nervous and Mental Diseases, 173,* 32–34.

Arntz, A., van Beijsterveldt, B., Hoesksta, R., Hofman, A., Eussen, M., & Saligerts,

S. (1992). The interrater reliability of a Dutch version of the structured interview for DSM-III-R personality disorders. *Acta Psychiatrica Scandinavica, 85,* 394–400.

Aronen, E. A., Noam, G. G., & Weinstein, S. R. (1993). Structured diagnostic interviews and clinicians' discharge diagnoses in hospitalized adolescents. *Journal of American Academy of Child and Adolescent Psychiatry, 32,* 674–681.

Bachneff, S. A., & Engelsmann, F. (1983). Correlates of cerebral event-related slow potentials and psychopathology. *Psychological Medicine, 13,* 763–770.

Bagby, R. M., Nicholson, R. A., Rogers, R., & Nussbaum, D. (1992). Domains of competency to stand trial. *Law and Human Behavior, 16,* 491–507.

Baer, L., Jenike, M. A., Black, D. W., Treece, C., Rosenfeld, R., & Griest, J. (1992). Effect of Axis II diagnosis on treatment outcome with clomipramine in 55 patients with obsessive–compulsive disorder. *Archives of General Psychiatry, 49,* 862–866.

Baer, R. A., Wetter, M. W., & Berry, D. T. R. (1992). Detection of underreporting of psychopathology on the MMPI: A meta-analysis. *Clinical Psychology Review, 12,* 509–525.

Bailey, B., West, K. Y., Widiger, T. A., & Freiman, K. (1993). The convergent and discriminant validity of the Chapman scales. *Journal of Personality Assessment, 61,* 121–135.

Baker, D. G., Diamnon, B. I., Gillette, G., Hamner, M., Katzelnick, D., Keller, T., Mellman, T. A., Pontius, E., Rosenthal, M., Tucker, P., Kolk, B. A., & Katz, R. (1995). A double-blind, randomized, placebo-controlled multicenter study of brofaromine in the treatment of posttraumatic stress disorder. *Psychopharmocology, 122,* 386–389.

Baldelli, M. V., Toschi, A., Motta, M., Marra, R., & Muratori, C. (1991). Cognitive assessment of the elderly patients: The choice of suitable assessment tools. *Archives of Gerontology and Geriatrics, 2,* 91–94.

Ballenger, J. C., Burrows, G. D., DuPont, R. L., Jr., Lesser, I. M., Noyes, R., Pecknold, J. C., Rifkin, A., & Swinson, R. P. (1988). Alprazolam in panic disorder and agoraphobias: Results from a multicenter trial: I. Efficacy in short-term treatment. *Archives of General Psychiatry, 45,* 413–422.

Banks, M. H. (1983). Validation of the general health questionnaire in a young community sample. *Psychological Medicine, 13,* 349–353.

Barbaree, H. E. (1999). Effect of treatment on risk for recidivism in sex offenders. In American Psychological Association (Ed.), *Psychological expertise and criminal justice* (pp. 217–220). Washington, DC: American Psychological Association.

Barber, J. P., & Morse, J. Q. (1994). Validation of the Wisconsin Personality Disorders Inventory and the SCID-II and PDE. *Journal of Personality Disorders, 8,* 307–319.

Barlow, D. H. (1991). Diagnoses, dimensions, and DSM-IV: The science of classification [Special issue]. *Journal of Abnormal Psychology, 100.*

Barlow, D. H., Blanchard, E. B., Vermilyea, J. A., Vermilyea, B. B., & DiNardo, P. A. (1986). Generalized anxiety and generalized anxiety disorders: Description and reconceptualization. *American Journal of Psychiatry, 143,* 40–44.

Barlow, D. H., DiNardo, P. A., Vermilyea, B. B., Vermilyea, J. A., & Blanchard, E. B. (1986). Comorbidity and depression among the anxiety disorders: Issues in classification and diagnosis. *Journal of Nervous and Mental Disease, 174,* 63–72.

Barrera, M., Jr., & Garrison-Jones, C. V. (1988). Properties of the Beck Depression

Inventory for adolescent depression. *Journal of Abnormal Child Psychology, 16,* 263–273.

Barrash, J., Kroll, J., Carey, K., & Sines, L. (1983). Discriminating borderline disorder from other personality disorders: Cluster analysis of the Diagnostic Interview for Borderlines. *Archives of General Psychiatry, 40,* 1297–1302.

Barrash, J., Pfohl, B., & Blum, N. (1993). "Unstable" personality disorders: Prognostic implications for major depression. *Journal of Personality Disorders, 7,* 155–167.

Bartlett, J. A., Schleifer, S. J., Johnson, R. L., & Keller, S. E. (1991). Depression in inner city adolescents attending an adolescent medicine clinic. *Journal of Adolescent Health, 12,* 316–318.

Bateman, A. W. (1989). Borderline personality in Britain: A preliminary study. *Comprehensive Psychiatry, 30,* 385–390.

Beaber, J. R., Marston, A., Michelli, J., & Mills, M. J. (1985). A brief test for measuring malingering in schizophrenic individuals. *American Journal of Psychiatry, 142,* 1478–1481.

Beals, J., Piasecki, J., Nelson, S., Jones, M., Keane, E., Dauphinais, P., Shirt, R. R., Sacke, W. H., & Manson, S. M. (1997). Psychiatric disorder among American Indian adolescents: Prevalence in northern Plains youth. *Journal of the American Academy of Child and Adolescent Psychiatry, 36,* 1252–1259.

Bebbington, P.E. (1992). Welcome to the ICD–10. *Social Psychiatry and Psychiatric Epidemiology, 27,* 255–257.

Bebbington, P. E., Brugha, T., Hill, T., Marsden, L., & Window, S. (1999). Validation of the Health of the Nation Outcome Scales. *British Journal of Psychiatry, 174,* 389–394.

Bebbington, P. E., & Nayani, T. (1995). Psychosis Screening Questionnaire. *International Journal of Methods in Psychiatric Research, 5,* 11–19.

Bebbington, P. E., Sturt, E., & Kumakura, N. (1983). The study of depressive disorders using the PSE-ID-CATEGO system. *Acta Psychiatrica Scandinavica, 72,* 55–64.

Beck, A. T., Ward, C. H., Mendelson, M., Mock, J. E., & Erbaugh, J. (1961). An inventory for measuring depression. *Archives of General Psychiatry, 4,* 561–571.

Beck, A. T., Weissman, A., Lester, D., & Trexler, L. (1974). The measurement of pessimism: The Hopelessness Scale. *Journal of Consulting and Clinical Psychology, 42,* 861–865.

Becker, D. F., Grilo, C. M., Morey, L. C., Walker, M. L., Edell, W. S., & McGlashan, T. H. (1999). Applicability of personality disorder criteria to hospitalized adolescents: Evaluation of internal consistency and criterion overlap. *Journal of American Academy of Child and Adolescent Psychiatry, 38,* 200–205.

Bell, R. C., & Jackson, H. J. (1992). The structure of personality disorders in DSM-III. *Acta Psychiatrica Scandinavica, 85,* 279–287.

Benjamin, R. S., Costello, E. J., & Warren, M. (1990). Anxiety disorders in a pediatric sample. *Journal of Anxiety Disorders, 4,* 293–316.

Bentler, P. M. (1995). *EQS structural equations program manual.* Encino, CA: Multivariate Software, Inc.

Berstein, D. P., Kasapis, C., Bergman, A., Weld, E., Mitropoulou, V., Horvath, T., Klar, H. M., Silverman, J., & Siever, L. J. (1997). Assessing Axis II disorders by informant interview. *Journal of Personality Disorders, 11,* 158–167.

Berwick, D. M., Murphy, J. M., Goldman, P. A., Ware, J. E., Jr., Barsky, A. J., & Weinstein, M. C. (1991). Performance of a five-item mental health screening test. *Medical Care, 29,* 169–176.

Bidaut-Russell, M., Reich, W., Cottler, L. B., Robins, L. N., Compton, W. M., & Mattison, R. E. (1995). The Diagnostic Interview Schedule for Children (PC-DISC v. 3.0): Parents and adolescents suggest reasons for expecting discrepant answers. *Journal of Abnormal Child Psychology, 23,* 641–659.

Biederman, J., Farone, S. V., Doyle, A., Lehman, B. K., Kraus, I., Perrin, J., & Tsuang, M. T. (1993). Convergence of the Child Behavior Checklist with a structured interview-based psychiatric diagnosis of ADHD children with and without comorbidity. *Journal of Child Psychology and Psychiatry, 34,* 1241–1251.

Biederman, J., Keenan, K., & Farone, S. V. (1990). Parent-based diagnosis of attention deficit disorder predicts a diagnosis based on teacher report. *Journal of the American Academy of Child and Adolescent Psychiatry, 29,* 698–701.

Biederman, J., Rosenbaum, J. F., Hirshfeld, D. R., Faraone, S. V., Bolduc, E. A., Gersten, M., Meminger, S. R., Kagan, J., Snidman, N., & Reznick, J. S. (1990). Psychiatric correlates of behavioral inhibition in young children of parents with and without psychiatric disorders. *Archives of General Psychiatry, 47,* 21–26.

Bien, T. H., Miller, W. R., & Boroughs, J. M. (1993). Motivational interviewing with alcohol outpatients. *Behavioral and Cognitive Psychotherapy, 21,* 347–356.

Bienvenu, O. J., & Eaton, W. W. (1998). The epidemiology of blood–injection–injury phobia. *Psychological Medicine, 28,* 1129–1136.

Bifulco, A., Brown, G. W., & Harris, T. O. (1994). Childhood Experience of Care and Abuse (CECA): A retrospective interview measure. *Journal of Child Psychology and Psychiatry, 35,* 1419–1435.

Bird, H. R., Canino, G., Gould, M. S., Ribera, J., Rubio-Stipec, M., Woodbury, M., Huertas-Goldman, S., & Sesman, M. (1987). Use of the Child Behavior Checklist as a screening instrument of epidemiological research in child psychiatry: Results of a pilot study. *Journal of the American Academy of Child and Adolescent Psychiatry, 26,* 207–213.

Bird, H. R., Canino, G., Rubio-Stipec, M. R., Gould, M. S., Ribera, J., Sesman, M., Woodbury, M., Huertas-Goldman, S., Pagan, A., Sanchez-Lacay, A., & Moscoso, M. (1988). Estimates of the prevalence of childhood maladjustment in a community survey in Puerto Rico. *Archives of General Psychiatry, 45,* 1120–1126.

Bird, H. R., Canino, G., Rubio-Stipec, M. R., & Shrout, P. (1987). Use of the Mini-Mental State Examination in a probability sample of a Hispanic population. *Journal of Nervous and Mental Disease, 175,* 731–737.

Bird, H. R., Gould, M. S., & Staghezza, B. (1992). Aggregating data from multiple informants in child psychiatry epidemiological research. *Journal of the American Academy of Child and Adolescent Psychiatry, 31,* 78–85.

Bird, H. R., Gould, M. S., Yager, T., Staghezza, B., & Canino, G. (1989). Risk factors for maladjustment in Puerto Rican children. *Journal of the American Academy of Child and Adolescent Psychiatry, 28,* 847–850.

Birt, A. R., Porter, S., & Woodworth, M. (2000, March). *Criminal career profiles as a function of psychopathy and sexual violence.* Paper presented at the American Psychology–Law Society, New Orleans.

Blackburn, R., & Coid, J. W. (1998). Psychopathy and dimensions of personality disorder in violent offenders. *Personality and Individual Differences, 25,* 129–145.

Blackburn, R., & Coid, J. W. (1999). Empirical clusters of DSM-III personality disorders in violent offenders. *Journal of Personality Disorders, 13,* 18–34.

Blake, D. D., Weathers, F., Nagy, L. M., Kaloupek, D. G., Charney, D. S., & Keane, T. M. (1998). *Clinician-Administered PTSD Scale for DSM-IV.* Boston: National Center for Posttraumatic Stress Disorder.

Blake, D. D., Weathers, F., Nagy, L. M., Kaloupek, D. G., Gusman, F. D., Charney, D. S., & Keane, T. M. (1995). Development of a Clinician-Administered PTSD Scale. *Journal of Traumatic Stress, 8,* 75–90.

Blake, D. D., Weathers, F., Nagy, L. M., Kaloupek, D. G., Klauminzer, G., Charney, D. S., & Keane, T. M. (1990). A clinician ratings scale for assessing clinical and lifetime PTSD: The CAPS–1. *Behavior Therapist, 13,* 187–188.

Blanchard, E. B., Gerardi, R. J., Kolb, L. C., & Barlow, D. H. (1986). The utility of the Anxiety Disorders Interview Schedule (ADIS) in the diagnosis of post-traumatic stress disorder (PTSD) in Vietnam veterans. *Behaviour Research and Therapy, 24,* 577–580.

Blanchard, E. B., Hickling, E. J., Taylor, A. E., Forneris, C. A., Loos, W., & Jaccard, J. (1995). Effects of varying scoring rules of the Clinician Administered PTSD (CAPS) for the diagnosis of posttraumatic stress disorder in motor vehicle accident victims. *Behaviour Research and Therapy, 33,* 471–475.

Blanchard, E. B., Jones-Alexander, J., Buckley, T. C., & Forneris, C. A. (1996). Psychometric properties of the PTSD Checklist (PCL). *Behaviour Research and Therapy, 34,* 669–673.

Bland, R. C., Newman, S. C., & Orn, H. (1997). Age and remission of psychatric disorders. *Canadian Journal of Psychiatry, 42,* 722–729.

Bland, R. C., Newman, S. C., Thompson, A. H., & Dyck, R. J. (1998). Psychiatric disorders in the population and in prisoners. *International Journal of Law and Psychiatry, 21,* 273–279.

Blashfield, R. K. (1992, August). *Are there any prototypical patients with personality disorders?* Paper presented at the American Psychological Association convention, Washington, DC.

Blashfield, R. K., Blum, N., & Pfohl, B. (1992). The effects of changing Axis II diagnostic criteria. *Comprehensive Psychiatry, 33,* 245–252.

Blashfield, R. K., & Livesley, W. J. (1991). Metaphorical analysis of psychiatric classification as a psychological test. *Journal of Abnormal Psychology, 100,* 262–270.

Bleecker, M. L., Bolla-Wilson, K., Kawas, C., & Agnew, J. (1988). Age-specific norms for the Mini-Mental State Exam. *Neurology, 38,* 1565–1568.

Blehar, M. C., DePaulo, J. R., Jr., Gershon, E. S., Reich, T., Simpson, S. G., & Nurnberger, J. I., Jr. (1998). Women with bipolar disorder: Findings from the NIMH genetics intiative sample. *Psychopharmocology, 34,* 239–243.

Blessed, G., Tomlinson, B. E., & Roth, M. (1968). The association between quantitative measures of dementia and senile change in the cerebral grey matter of elderly subjects. *British Journal of Psychiatry, 114,* 797–811.

Blouin, A. G., Perez, E. L., & Blouin, J. H. (1988). Computerized administration of the Diagnostic Interview Schedule. *Psychiatry Research, 23,* 335–344.

Bodholdt, R. H., Richards, H. R., & Gacono, C. B. (2000). Assessing psychopathy in adults: The Psychopathy Checklist—Revised and Screening Version. In C. B. Gacono (Ed.), *The clinical and forensic assessment of psychopathy* (pp. 55–86). Mahwah, NJ: Erlbaum.

Boer, J. A. D., & Dunner, D. L. (1999). Physician attitudes concerning diagnosis and treatment of social anxiety disorder in Europe and North America. *International Journal of Psychiatry in Clinical Practice, 3,* 513–519.

Bonnie, R. J. (1992). The competence of criminal defendants: A theoretical reformulation. *Behavioral Sciences and the Law, 10,* 291–316.

Boon, S., & Draijer, N. (1991). Diagnosing dissociative disorders in the Netherlands: A pilot study with the Structured Clinical Interview for DSM-III-R Dissociative Disorders. *American Journal of Psychiatry, 148,* 458–462.

Booth, B. M., Kirchner, J.-A. E., Hamilton, G., Harrell, R., & Smith, G. R. (1998). Diagnosing depression in the medically ill: Validity of lay-administered structured diagnostic interview. *Journal of Psychiatric Research, 32,* 353–360.

Booth, R. E., & Zhang, Y. (1996). Severe aggression and related conduct problems among runaway and homeless adolescents. *Psychiatric Services, 47,* 75–80.

Borst, S. R., Noam, S. G., & Bartok, J. A. (1991). Adolescent suicidality: A clinical-development approach. *Journal of the American Academy of Child and Adolescent Psychiatry, 30,* 796–803.

Borum, R., & Grisso, T. (1995). Psychological test use in criminal forensic evaluations. *Professional Psychology: Research and Practice, 26,* 465–473.

Borum, R., Otto, R., & Golding, S. (1993). Improving clinical judgment and decision making in forensic evaluation. *Journal of Psychiatry and Law, 21,* 35–76.

Boscarino, J. A. (1995). Post-traumatic stress and associated disorders among Vietnam veterans: The significance of combat exposure and social support. *Journal of Traumatic Stress, 8,* 317–336.

Boyd, J. H., Weissman, M. M., Thompson, W. D., & Myers, J. K. (1983). Different definitions of alcoholism: I. Impact of seven definitions on prevalence rates in a community sample. *American Journal of Psychiatry, 140,* 1309–1313.

Boyle, M. H., Offord, D. R., Hofmann, H. G., Catlin, G. P., Byles, J. A., Cadman, D. T., Crawford, J. W., Links, P. S., Rae-Grant, N. I., & Szatmari, P. (1987). Ontario child health study: Methodology. *Archives of General Psychiatry, 44,* 826–831.

Boyle, M. H., Offord, D. R., Racine, Y., Sanford, M., Szatmari, P., Fleming, J. E., & Price-Munn, N. (1993). Evaluation of the Diagnostic Interview for Children and Adolescents for use in general population samples. *Journal of Abnormal Child Psychology, 21,* 663–681.

Boyle, M. H., Offord, D. R., Racine, Y. A., Szatmari, P., Sanford, M., & Fleming, J. E. (1997). Adequacy of interviews vs. checklists for classifying childhood psychiatric disorder based on parent reports. *Archives of General Psychiatry, 54,* 793–799.

Brandt, J. R., Kennedy, W. A., Patrick, C. J., & Curtin, J. J. (1997). Assessment of psychopathy in a population of incarcerated adolescent offenders. *Psychological Assessment, 9,* 429–435.

Brawman-Mintzer, O., Lydiard, R. B., Emmanuel, N., Payeur, R., Johnson, M., Roberts, J., Jarrell, M. P., & Ballenger, J. C. (1993). Psychiatric comorbidity in patients with generalized anxiety disorder. *American Journal of Psychiatry, 150,* 1216–1218.

Bremmer, J. D., Steinberg, M., Southwick, S. M., Johnson, D. R., & Charney, D. S. (1993). Use of the Structured Clinical Interview for DMS-IV Dissociative Disorders for systematic assessment of dissociative symptoms in post-traumatic stress disorder. *American Journal of Psychiatry, 150,* 1011–1014.

Brent, D. A., Zelenak, J. P., Busstein, O., & Brown, R. V. (1990). Reliability and validity of the Structured Interview for Personality Disorders in adolescents. *Journal of the American Academy of Child and Adolescent Psychiatry, 29,* 349–354.

Breslau, N. (1987). Inquiring about the bizarre: False positives in Diagnostic Interview

Schedule for Children (DISC)—ascertainment of obsessions, compulsions, and psychotic symptoms. *Journal of the American Academy of Child and Adolescent Psychiatry, 26,* 639–644.

Breslau, N., Davis, G. C., Peterson, E. L., & Schultz, L. (1997). Psychiatric sequelae of post traumatic stress disorder in women. *Archives of General Psychiatry, 54,* 81–87.

Breslau, N., Davis, G. C., & Prabucki, K. (1987). Searching for evidence on the validity of generalized anxiety disorder: Psychopathology in children of anxious mothers. *Psychiatry Research, 20,* 285–297.

Breslau, N., Kessler, R. C., Chilcoat, H. D., Schultz, L. R., Davis, G. C., & Andreski, P. (1998). Trauma and post-traumatic stress disorder in the community. *Archives of General Psychiatry, 55,* 626–632.

Breton, J. J., Bergeron, L., Valla, J. P., Berthiaume, C., & St. Georges, M. (1998). Diagnostic Inteview Schedule for Children (DISC–2.25) in Quebec: Reliability findings in light of the MECA study. *Journal of the American Academy of Child and Adolescent Psychiatry, 37,* 1167–1174.

Breton, J. J., Bergeron, L., Valla, J. P., Lepine, S., Houde, L., & Gaudet, N. (1995). Do children aged 9–11 understand the DISC version 2.25 questions? *Journal of the American Academy of Child and Adolescent Psychiatry, 34,* 946–954.

Bromet, E. J., Bunn, L. O., Connell, M. M., Dew, M. A., & Schulberg, H. C. (1986). Long-term reliability of diagnosing lifetime major depression in a community sample. *Archives of General Psychiatry, 43,* 435–440.

Brooks, R. B., Baltazar, P. L., McDowell, D. E., Munjack, D. J., & Bruns, J. R. (1991). Personality disorders co-occurring with panic disorder with agoraphobia. *Journal of Personality Disorders, 5,* 328–336.

Brothwell, J., Casey, P. R., & Tyrer, P. (1992). Who gives the most reliable account of a psychiatric patient's personality? *British Journal of Psychological Medicine, 9,* 90–93.

Broughton, R. (1990). The prototype concept in personality assessment. *Canadian Psychology, 31,* 26–37.

Brown, G. W., & Moran, P. M. (1997). Single mothers, poverty, and depression. *Psychological Medicine, 27,* 21–33.

Brown, J. M., & Miller, W. R. (1993). Impact of motivational interviewing on participation and outcome in residential alcoholism treatment. *Psychology of Addictive Behaviors, 7,* 211–218.

Brown, T. A., Anthony, M. M., & Barlow, D. H. (1995). Diagnostic comorbidity in panic disorder: Effect on treatment outcome and course of comorbid diagnoses following treatment. *Journal of Consulting and Clinical Psychology, 63,* 408–418.

Brown, T. A., DiNardo, P. A. , & Barlow, D. H. (1995). *Anxiety Disorders Interview Schedule for DSM-IV (ADIS-IV).* Albany: Center for Stress and Anxiety Disorders, State University of New York.

Brown, T. A., Marten, P. A., & Barlow, D. H. (1995). Discriminant validity of symptoms constituting the DSM-III-R and DSM-IV associated symptom criterion of generalized anxiety disorders. *Journal of Anxiety Disorders, 9,* 317–328.

Brugha, T. S., Bebbinton, P. E., Jenkins, R., Meltzer, H., Taub, N. A., Janas, M., & Vernon, J. (1999). Cross validation of a general population survey diagnostic interview: A comparison of CIS-R with the SCAN ICD–10 diagnostic categories. *Psychological Medicine, 29,* 1029–1042.

Brugha, T. S., Kaul, A., Gignon, A., Teather, D., & Wills, K. M. (1996). Present State Examination by microcomputer: Objectives and experience of preliminary steps. *International Journal of Methods in Psychiatric Research, 6,* 143–151.

Brugha, T. S., Nienhuis, F., Bagchi, D., Smith, J., & Meltzer, H. (1999). The survey form of SCAN: The feasibility of using experienced lay survey interviewers to administer a semistructured systematic clinical assessment of psychotic and nonpsychotic disorders. *Psychological Medicine, 29,* 703–711.

Brunshaw, J. M., & Szatmari, P. (1988). The agreement between behavior checklists and structured psychiatric interviews for children. *Canadian Journal of Psychiatry, 33,* 474–481.

Bryant, R. A., Harvey, A. G., Dang, S. T., & Sackville, T. (1998). Assessing acute stress disorder: Psychometric properties of a structured interview. *Psychological Assessment, 10,* 215–220.

Bucholz, K. K., Marion, S. L., Shayka, J. J., Marcus, S. C., & Robins, L. N. (1996). A short computer interview for obtaining psychiatric diagnoses. *Psychiatric Services, 47,* 293–297.

Bucholz, K. K., Robins, L. N., Shayka, J. J., Przybeck, T. R., Helzer, J. E., Goldring, E., Klein, M. H., Griest, J. H., Erdman, H. P., & Skare, S. S. (1991). Performance of two forms of a computer psychiatric screening interview: Version I of the DIS-SI. *Journal of Psychiatric Research, 25,* 117–129.

Buckner, J. C., & Bassuk, E. L. (1997). Mental disorders and service utilization among youths from homeless and low-income housed families. *Journal of the American Academy of Child and Adolescent Psychiatry, 36,* 890–900.

Burnam, M. A., Hough, R. L., Karno, M., Escobar, J. I., & Telles, C. A. (1987). Acculturation and lifetime prevalence of psychiatric disorders among Mexican-Americans in Los Angeles. *Journal of Health and Social Behavior, 28,* 89–102.

Burnam, M. A., Karno, M., Hough, R. L., Escobar, J. I., & Forsythe, A. B. (1983). The Spanish Diagnostic Interview Schedule: Reliability and comparison with clinical diagnoses. *Archives of General Psychiatry, 40,* 1189–1196.

Burns, G. L., Formea, G. M., Keortge, S., & Sternberger, L. G. (1995). The utilization on nonpatient samples in the study of obsessive compulsive disorder. *Behaviour Research and Therapy, 33,* 133–144.

Bushnell, J. A., Wells, J. E., Hornblow, A. R., Oakley-Browne, M. A., & Joyce, P. (1990). Prevalence of three bulimia syndromes in the general population. *Psychological Medicine, 20,* 671–680.

Buss, A. H. (1966). *Psychopathology.* New York: Wiley.

Butler, S. F., Newman, F. L., Cacciola, J. S., Frank, A., Budman, S. H., McLellan, A. T., Ford, S., Blaine, J., Gastfriend, D., Moras, K., Salloum, I. M., & Barber, J. P. (1998). Predicting Addiction Severity Index (ASI) interviewer severity ratings for a computer-administered ASI. *Psychological Assessment, 10,* 399–407.

Buydens-Branchey, L., Branchey, M. H., & Noumair, D. (1989). Age of alcoholism onset: I. Relationship to psychopathology. *Archives of General Psychiatry, 46,* 225–230.

Cacciola, J. S., Alterman, A. I., Fureman, M. A., Parikh, G. A., & Rutherford, M. J. (1997). The use of vignettes for the Addiction Severity Index training. *Journal of Substance Abuse Treatment, 14,* 439–443.

Cacciola, J. S., Koppenhaver, J. M., McKay, J. R., & Alterman, A. I. (1999). Test–retest reliability of the lifetime items on the Addiction Severity Index. *Psychological Assessment, 11,* 86–93.

Cacciola, J. S., Rutherford, M. J., & Alterman, A. I. (1990, June). *Use of the Psychopathy Checklist with opiate addicts.* Paper presented to Committee on Problems in Drug Dependence, National Drug Administration, Richmond, VA.

Cacciola, J. S., Rutherford, M. J., Alterman, A. I. , & Snider, E. C. (1994). An examination of the diagnostic criteria for antisocial personality disorder in substance abusers. *Journal of Nervous and Mental Disease, 182,* 517–523.

Campbell, D. T., & Fiske, D. W. (1959). Convergent and discriminant validation by the multitrait–multimethod matrix. *Psychological Bulletin, 56,* 81–105.

Canals, J., Domenech, E., Carbajo, G., & Blade, J. (1997). Prevalence of DSM-III-R and ICD–10 psychiatric disorders in a Spanish population of 18 year-olds. *Acta Psychiatrica Scandinavica, 96,* 287–294.

Canino, G. J., Bird, H. R., Shrout, P. E., Rubio-Stipee, M., Bravo, M., Martinez, R., Sesman, M., Guzman, A., & Guevara, L. M. (1987a). The prevalence of specific psychiatric disorders in Puerto Rico. *Archives of General Psychiatry, 44,* 727–735.

Canino, G. J., Bird, H. R., Shrout, P. E., Rubio-Stipee, M., Bravo, M., Martinez, R., Sesman, M., Guzman, A., Guevara, L. M., & Costas, H. (1987b). The Spanish Diagnostic Interview Schedule: Reliability and concordance with clinical diagnoses in Puerto Rico. *Archives of General Psychiatry, 44,* 720–726.

Canive, J. M., Clark, R. D., Calais, L. A., Qualls, C., & Tauson, V. B. (1997). Bupropion treatment in veterns with posttraumatic stress disorder: An open study. *Journal of Clinical Psychopharmocology, 18,* 379–383.

Carlson, G. A., Kashani, J. H., Thomas, M. D. F., Vaidya, A., & Daniel, A. E. (1987). Comparison of the DISC and the K-SADS-P interviews in an epidemiological sample of children. *Journal of the American Academy of Child and Adolescent Psychiatry, 26,* 645–648.

Carlson, G. A., & Kelly, K. L. (1998). Manic symptoms in psychiatrically hospitalized children: What do they mean? *Journal of Affective Disorders, 51,* 123–135.

Carlson, G. A., Loney, J., Salisbury, H., & Volpe, R. J. (1998). Young referred boys with DICA-P manic symptoms vs. two comparison groups. *Journal of Affective Disorders, 121,* 113–121.

Carnes, M., Gunter-Hunt, G., & Rodgers, E. (1987). The effect of an interdisciplinary geriatrics clinic visit on mental status. *Journal of the American Geriatrics Society, 35,* 1035–1036.

Carpenter, W. T., Jr., & Gunderson, J. G. (1977). Five year follow-up comparison of borderline and schizophrenic patients. *Comprehensive Psychiatry, 18,* 567–571.

Carrion, V. G., & Steiner, H. (2000). Trauma and dissociation in delinquent adolescents. *Journal of the American Academy of Child and Adolescent Psychiatry, 39,* 353–359.

Carson, R. C. (1991). Dilemmas in the pathway of the DSM-IV. *Journal of Abnormal Psychology, 100,* 302–307.

Carter, J. D., Joyce, P. R., Mulder, R. T., Luty, S. E., & Sullivan, P. F. (1999). Early deficient parenting in depressed outpatients is associated with personality dysfunction and not with depression subtypes. *Journal of Affective Disorders, 54,* 29–37.

Cashel, M. L., Rogers, R., Sewell, K. W., & Holliman, N. (1998). Preliminary validation of the MMPI-A for a male delinquent sample: An investigation of clinical correlates and discriminant validity. *Journal of Personality Assessment, 71,* 49–69.

Cassano, G. B., Dell'Osso, L., Frank, E., Miniati, M., Fagiolini, A., Shear, K., Pini, S., & Maser, J. (1999). The bipolar spectrum: A clinical reality in search of diagnostic criteria and an assessment methodology. *Journal of Affective Disorders, 54,* 319–328.

Cassano, G. B., Pini, S., Saettoni, M., Rucci, P., & Dell'Osso, L. (1998). Occurrence and clinical correlates of psychiatric comorbidity in patients with psychotic disorders. *Journal of Clinical Psychiatry, 59,* 60–68.

Cavanaugh, S. V., & Wettstein, R. M. (1989). Emotional and cognitive dysfunction associated with medical disorders. *Journal of Psychosomatic Research, 33,* 505–514.

Chambers, W. J., Puig-Antich, J., Hirsch, M., Paez, P., Ambrosini, P. J., Tabrizi, M. A., & Davies, M. (1985). The assessment of affective disorders in children and adolescents by semistructured interview: Test–retest reliability of the Schedule for Affective Disorders and Schizophrenia for School-Age Children, present episode version. *Archives of General Psychiatry, 42,* 696–702.

Chapman, L. J., & Chapman, J. P. (1987). The search of symptoms predictive of schizophrenia. *Schizophrenia Bulletin, 13,* 497–503.

Chapman, T. F., Mannuzza, S., Klein, D. F., & Fyer, A. J. (1994). Effects of informant mental disorder on psychiatric family history. *American Journal of Psychiatry, 151,* 574–579.

Chilcoat, H. D., & Breslau, N. (1997). Does psychiatric history bias mothers' reports? An application on a new analytic approach. *Journal of the American Academy of Child and Adolescent Psychiatry, 36,* 971–979.

Chilcoat, H. D., & Breslau, N. (1998). Post traumatic stress disorder and drug disorders: Testing causal pathways. *Archives of General Psychiatry, 55,* 913–917.

Christensen, H., Hadzi-Pavlovic, D., & Jacomb, P. (1991). The psychometric differentiation of dementia from normal aging: A meta-analysis. *Psychological Assessment: A Journal of Clinical and Consulting Psychology, 3,* 147–155.

Clark, C. M., Sheppard, L., Fillenbaum, G. G., Galasko, D., Morris, J. C., Koss, E., Mohs, R., & Heyman, A. (1999). Variability in annual Mini-Mental State Examination score in patients with probable Alzheimer disease. *Archives of Neurology, 56,* 857–862.

Clark, L. A. (1996). *Schedule of Nonadaptive and Adaptive Personality: Manual for administration, scoring, and interpretation.* Minneapolis: University of Minnesota Press.

Clark, L. A., Livesley, W. J., & Morey, L. (1997). Personality disorder assessment: The challenge of construct validity. *Journal of Personality Disorders, 11,* 205–231.

Clark, L. A., & Watson, D. (1991). Tripartite model of anxiety and depression: Psychometric evidence and taxonomic implications. *Journal of Abnormal Psychology, 100,* 316–336.

Clark, L. A., & Watson, D. (1995). Constructing validity: Basic issues in objective scale development. *Psychological Assessment, 7,* 309–319.

Clark, R. D., Canive, J. M., Calais, L. A., Qualls, C. R., & Tauson, V. B. (1999). Divalproex in posttraumatic stress disorder: An open-label clinical trial. *Journal of Traumatic Stress, 12,* 395–401.

Clarkin, J. F., Hull, J. W., & Hurt, S. W. (1993). Factor structure of borderline personality disorder criteria. *Journal of Personality Disorders, 7,* 137–143.

Clayton, A. H., McGarvey, E. L., & Clavet, G. J. (1997). The Changes in Sexual Functioning Questionnaire (CSFQ): Development, reliability, and validity. *Psychopharmacology Bulletin, 33,* 731–745.

Cleckley, H. (1976). *The mask of insanity* (4th ed.). St. Louis: Mosby.

Cloninger, C. R., Martin, R. L., Guze, S. B., & Clayton, P. J. (1985). Diagnosis and prognosis in schizophrenia. *Archives of General Psychiatry, 42,* 15–25.

Coccaro, E. F., Silverman, J. M., Klar, H. M., Horvath, T. B., & Siever, L. J. (1994). Familial correlates of reduced central serotonergic system function in patients with personality disorders. *Archives of General Psychiatry, 51,* 318–324.

Cohen, J. (1960). A coefficient of agreement for nominal scales. *Educational and Psychological Measurement, 20,* 37–46.

Cohen, P., Kasen, S., Brook, J. S., & Struening, E. L. (1991). Diagnostic predictors of treatment patterns in a cohort of adolescents. *Journal of the American Academy of Child and Adolescent Psychiatry, 30,* 989–993.

Cohen, P., O'Conner, P., Lewis, S., Veliz, C. N., & Malachowski, B. (1987). Comparison of DISC and K-SADS-P interviews of an epidemiological sample of children. *Journal of American Academy of Child and Adolescent Psychiatry, 26,* 662–667.

Coie, J. D., Terry, R., Lenox, K., Lochman, J., & Hyman, C. (1995). Childhood peer rejection and aggression as predictors of stable patterns of adolescent disorder. *Development and Psychopathology, 7,* 697–713.

Coie, J. D., Watt, N. F., West, S. G., Hawkins, J. D., Asarnow, J. R., Markman, H. J., Ramey, S. L., Shure, M. B., & Long, B. (1993). The science of prevention: A conceptual framework and some directions for a national research program. *American Psychologist, 48,* 1013–1022.

Columbia DISC Development Group. (1999). *National Institute of Mental Health Diagnostic Interview Schedule for Children (NIMH-DISC).* Unpublished report, Columbia University/New York State Psychiatric Institute.

Compton, W. M., Cottler, L. B., Dorsey, K. B., Spitznagel, E. L., & Mager, D. E. (1996). Comparing assessments of the DSM-IV substance dependence disorders with the CIDI-SAM and the SCAN. *Drug and Alcohol Dependence, 41,* 179–187.

Connell, D. K. (1991). *The SIRS and the M test: The differential validity and utility of two instruments designed to detect malingered psychosis in a correctional sample.* Unpublished dissertation, University of Louisville, KY.

Conners, C. (1969). A teacher rating scale for use in drug studies in children. *American Journal of Psychiatry, 126,* 152–156.

Consentino, C. E., Meyer-Bahlburg, H. F. L., Alpert, J. L., & Gaines, R. (1993). Cross-gender behavior and gender conflict in sexually abused girls. *Journal of the American Academy of Child and Adolescent Psychiatry, 32,* 940–947.

Constans, J. I., Lenhoff, K., & McCarthy, M. (1997). Depression subtyping in PTSD patients. *Annals of Clinical Psychology, 9,* 235–240.

Cooke, D. J. (1998). Cross-cultural aspects of psychopathy. In T. Millon, E. Simonsen, M. Birket-Smith, & R. D. Davis (Eds.), *Psychopathy: Antisocial, criminal, and violent behavior* (pp. 260–276). New York: Guilford Press.

Cooke, D. J., & Michie, C. (1997). An item response theory analysis of the Hare Psychopathy Checklist—Revised. *Psychological Assessment, 9,* 3–14.

Cooke, D. J., & Michie, C. (in press). Refining the construct of psychopathy: Towards a hierarchical model. *Psychological Assessment.*

Cooke, D. J., Michie, C., Hart, S. D., & Hare, R. D. (1999). Evaluating the screening version of the Hare Psychopathy Checklist—Revised: An item response theory analysis. *Psychological Assessment, 11,* 3–13.

Cooney, N. L., Kadden, R. M., & Litt, M. D. (1990). A comparison of methods for assessing sociopathy in male and female alcoholics. *Journal of Studies of Alcohol, 51,* 42–48.

Cooper, J. E., Copeland, J. R. M., Brown, G. W., Harris, T., & Gourlay, A. J. (1977). Further studies on interviewer training and interrater reliability of the Present State Examination (PSE). *Psychological Medicine, 7,* 517–523.

Cooper, J. E., Kendell, R. E., Gurland, B. J., Sharpe, L., Copeland, J. R. M., & Simon, R. (1972). *Psychiatric diagnosis in New York and London.* London: Oxford University Press.

Cooper, P. J., Taylor, M. J., Cooper, Z., & Fairburn, C. G. (1987). The development and validation of the Body Shape Questionnaire. *International Journal of Eating Disorders, 6,* 1–8.

Cooper, Z., Cooper, P. J., & Fairburn, C. G. (1989). The validity of the Eating Disorder Examination. *British Journal of Psychiatry, 154,* 808–812.

Cooper, Z., & Fairburn, C. G. (1987). The Eating Disorder Examination: A semistructured interview for the assessment of the specific psychopathology of eating disorders. *International Journal of Eating Disorders, 6,* 1–8.

Cornell, D. G., Silk, K. R., Ludolph, P. S., & Lohr, N. E. (1983). Test–retest reliability of the Diagnostic Interview for Borderlines. *Archives of General Psychiatry, 40,* 1307–1310.

Cornell, D. G., Warren, J., Hawk, G., Stafford, E., Oram, G., & Pine, D. (1996). Psychopathy in instrumental and reactive violent offenders. *Journal of Consulting and Clinical Psychology, 64,* 783–790.

Coryell, W. H., Akiskal, H. S., Leon, A. C., Winokur, G., Maser, J. D., Mueller, T. I., & Keller, M. B. (1994). The time course of nonchronic major depressive disorder. *Archives of General Psychiatry, 51,* 405–410.

Coryell, W. H., & Noyes, R. (1988). Placebo response in panic disorder. *American Journal of Psychiatry, 145,* 1138–1140.

Coryell, W. H., & Zimmerman, M. (1989). Personality disorder in the families of depressed, schizophrenic, and never-ill probands. *American Journal of Psychiatry, 146,* 496–502.

Cosoff, S. J., & Hafner, R. J. (1998). The prevalence of comorbid anxiety in schizophrenia, schizoaffective disorder and bipolar disorder. *Australian and New Zealand Journal of Psychiatry, 32,* 67–72.

Costa, P. T., Jr., & McCrae, R. R. (1985). *The NEO Personality Inventory manual.* Tampa, FL: Psychological Assessment Resources.

Costa, P. T., Jr., & McCrae, R. R. (1992). *Revised NEO Personality Inventory (NEO-PI-R) and NEO Five-Factor Inventory (NEO-FFI).* Odessa, FL: Psychological Assessment Resources.

Costello, A. J., Edelbrock, C. S., Dulcan, M. K., Kalas, R., & Klaric, S. H. (1984). *Development and testing of the NIMH Diagnostic Interview Schedule for Children on a clinical population: Final report.* Rockville, MD: Center for Epidemiological Studies, National Institute of Mental Health.

Costello, E. J. (1989). Child psychiatric disorders and their correlates: A primary care pediatric sample. *Journal of the American Academy of Child and Adolescent Psychiatry, 28,* 851–855.

Costello, E. J., Angold, A., & Keeler, G. P. (1999). Adolescent outcomes of childhood disorders: The consequences of severity and impairment. *Journal of the American Academy of Child and Adolescent Psychiatry, 38,* 121–128.

Costello, E. J., Costello, A. J., Edelbrock, C., Burns, B. J., Dulcan, M. K., Brent, D., & Janiszewski, S. (1988). Psychiatric disorders in pediatric primary care: Prevalence and risk factors. *Archives of General Psychiatry, 45,* 1107–1116.

Costello, E. J., Edelbrock, C. S., & Costello, A. J. (1985). Validity of the NIMH Diagnostic Interview Schedule for Children: A comparison between psychiatric and pediatric referrals. *Journal of Abnormal and Child Psychology, 13,* 579–595.

Cottler, L. B., Compton, W. M., Ridenour, A., Abdallah, A. B., & Gallagher, T. (1998). Reliability of self-reported antisocial personality disorder symptoms among substance abusers. *Drug and Alcohol Dependence, 49,* 189–199.

Cottler, L. B., Grant, B. F., Blaine, J., Mavreas, V., Pull, C., Hasin, D., Compton, W. M., Rubio-Stipec, M., & Mager, D. (1997). Concordance of the DSM-IV alcohol and drug use disorder criteria and diagnoses as measured by the AUDADIS-ADR, CIDE, and SCAN. *Drug and Alcohol Dependence, 47,* 195–207.

Couch, A., & Keniston, K. (1960). Yeasayers and naysayers: Agreeing response set as a personality variable. *Journal of Abnormal and Social Psychology, 60,* 151–174.

Craft M. J. (1965). *Ten studies into psychopathic personality.* Bristol, UK: John Wright.

Cronbach, L. J. (1970). *Essentials of psychological testing* (3rd ed.). New York: Harper & Row.

Cronbach, L. J., & Meehl, P. E. (1955). Construct validity in psychological tests, *Psychological Bulletin, 52,* 281–302.

Cruise, K. R. (2000). *Multitrait-multimethod approach to adolescent psychopathy.* Unpublished doctoral dissertation, University of North Texas.

Cruise, K. R., & Rogers, R. (1998). An analysis of competency to stand trial: An integration of case law and clinical knowledge. *Behavioral Sciences and the Law, 16,* 35–50.

Cunnien, A. J. (1988). Psychiatric and medical syndromes associated with deception. In R. Rogers (Ed.), *Clinical assessment of malingering and deception* (pp. 13–33). New York: Guilford Press.

Dahl, A. A., & Bordahl, P. E. (1993). Obstetric complications as a risk factor for subsequent development of personality disorders. *Journal of Personality Disorders, 7,* 22–27.

Dalton, J. E., Pederson, S. L., Blom, B. E., & Holmes, N. R. (1987). Diagnostic errors using the Short Portable Mental Status Questionnaire with a mixed clinical population. *Journal of Gerontology, 42,* 512–514.

D'Angelo, E. J. (1991). Convergent and discriminant validity of the Borderline Syndrome Index. *Psychological Reports, 69,* 631–635.

Darke, S., Kaye, S., Finlay-Jones, J. R., & Hall, W. (1998). Factor structure of psychopathy among methadone maintenance patients. *Journal of Personality Disorders, 12,* 162–171.

Davidson, J. R. T., & Foa, E. B. (1991). Diagnostic issues in posttraumatic stress disorder: Considerations for DSM-IV. *Journal of Abnormal Psychology, 100,* 346–355.

Davies, W., & Feldman, P. (1981). The diagnosis of psychopathy by forensic specialists. *British Journal of Psychiatry, 138,* 329–331.

Davis, L. L., Nugent, A. L., Murray, J., Kramer, G. L., & Petty, F. (2000). Nefazone treatment for chronic posttraumatic stress disorder: An open trial. *Journal of Clinical Psychopharmocology, 20,* 159–164.

Dawes, R. M. (1979). Robust beauty of improper linear model in decision making. *American Psychologist, 34,* 571–582.

Dean, C., Surtees, P. G., & Sahsidharan, S. P. (1983). Comparison of research diagnostic systems in an Edinburgh community sample. *British Journal of Psychiatry, 142,* 247–256.

Deas-Nesmith, D., Brady, K. T., & Campbell, S. (1998). Comorbid substance abuse and anxiety disorders in adolescents. *Journal of Psychopathology and Behavioral Assessment, 20,* 139–148.

Deb, S., Lyons, I., Koutzoukis, C., Ali, I., & McCarthy, G. (1999). Rates of psychiatric illness 1 year after traumatic brain injury. *American Journal of Psychiatry, 156,* 374–378.

Demalle, D. A., Cottler, L. B., & Compton, W. M., III. (1995). Alcohol abuse and dependence: Consistency in reporting of symptoms over ten years. *Addiction, 90,* 615–625.

Denicoff, K. D., Joffe, R. T., Lakshmanan, M. C., Robbins, J., & Rubinow, D. R. (1990). Neuropsychiatric manifestations of altered thyroid state. *American Journal of Psychiatry, 147,* 94–99.

DePaulo, J. R., & Folstein, M. R. (1978). Psychiatric disturbances in neurological patients: Detection, recognition, and hospital course. *Annals of Neurology, 4,* 225–228.

Derksen, J. (1990). An exploratory study of borderline personality disorder in women with eating disorders and psychoactive substance abuse patients. *Journal of Personality Disorders, 4,* 372–380.

Derogatis, L. R. (1977). *The SCL-90, R version manual: Scoring administration and procedures for the SCL-90.* Baltimore: Johns Hopkins University, School of Medicine.

Derogatis, L. R. (1997). Derogatis Interview for Sexual Functioning (DISF/DISF-SR): A preliminary report. *Journal of Sex and Marital Therapy, 23,* 291–304.

Derogatis, L. R., Fagan, P. J., & Strand, J. G. (2000). Sexual disorders measures. In A. J. Rush, H. A. Pincus, M. B. First, D. Blacker, J. Endicott, S. J. Keith, K. A. Phillips, N. D., Ryan, G. R. Smith, M. T. Tsuang, T. A. Widiger, & D. A. Zarin (Eds.), *Handbook of psychiatric measures* (pp. 631–671). Washington, DC: American Psychiatric Press.

Derogatis, L. R., & Spencer, P. M. (1982). *The Brief Symptom Inventory (BSI): Administration, scoring and procedures manual.* Baltimore: Johns Hopkins University Press.

Deshpande, S. N., Mathur, M. N. L., Das, S. K., Bhatia, T., Sharma, S., & Nimgaonkar, V. L. (1998). A Hindi version of the Diagnostic Interview for Genetic Studies. *Schizophrenia Bulletin, 24,* 489–493.

Dick, J. P. R., Guiloff, R. J., Stewart, A., Blackstock, J., Bielawska, C., Paul, E. A., & Marsden, C. D. (1984). Mini-Mental State Examination in neurological patients. *Journal of Neurology, Neurosurgery, and Psychology, 47,* 496–499.

Dignon, A. M. (1996). Acceptability of a computer-administered psychiatric interview. *Computers in Human Behavior, 12,* 177–191.

DiNardo, P. A., Moras, K., Barlow, D. H., Rapee, R. M., & Brown, T. A. (1993). Reliability of DSM-III-R anxiety disorder categories: Using the Anxiety Disorders Interview Schedule—Revised (ADIS-R). *Archives of General Psychiatry, 50,* 251–256.

DiNardo, P. A., O'Brien, G. T., Barlow, D. H., Waddell, M. T., & Blanchard, E. B.

(1982). *Anxiety Disorders Interview Schedule (ADIS)*. Albany: Center for Stress and Anxiety Disorders, State University of New York at Albany.

DiNardo, P. A., O'Brien, G. T., Barlow, D. H., Waddell, M. T., & Blanchard, E. B. (1983). Reliability of DSM-III anxiety disorders using a new structured interview. *Archives of General Psychiatry, 40,* 1070–1074.

DiNardo, P. A., O'Brien, G. T., Barlow, D. H., Waddell, M. T., & Blanchard, E. B. (1985). *Anxiety Disorders Interview Schedule—Revised (ADIS-R)*. Albany: Center for Stress and Anxiety Disorders, State University of New York.

Divac-Jovanovic, M., Svrakic, D., & Lecic-Tosevski, D. (1993). Personality disorders: Model for conceptual approach and classification. *American Journal of Psychotherapy, 47,* 558–571.

Dodds, L. D. (2000, March). *Legislative exclusion statutues and psychopathy as predictors of violent crimes.* Paper presented the the American Psychology–Law Society conference, New Orleans.

Dooley, D., Catalano, R., & Wilson, G. (1994). Depression and unemployment: Panel findings from the Epidemiologic Catchment Area study. *American Journal of Community Psychology, 22,* 745–765.

Doraiswamy, P. M., & Kaiser, L. (2000). Variability of the Mini-Mental State Examination in dementia. *Neurology, 54,* 1538–1549.

Douglas, K. S., Ogloff, J. R. P., & Nicholls, T. L. (1997, June). *Personality disorders and violence in civil psychiatric patients.* Paper presented at the 5th International Congress on Disorders of Personality, Vancouver, BC.

Dreessen, L., & Arntz, A. (1998). Short-interval test–retest interrater reliability of the Structured Clinical Interview for DSM-III-R Personality disorder (SCID-II) in outpatients. *Journal of Personality Disorders, 12,* 138–148.

Dreessen, L., Hildebrand, M., & Arntz, A. (1998). Patient–informant concordance for Structured Clinical Interview for DSM-III-R Personality disorder (SCID-II). *Journal of Personality Disorders, 12,* 149–161.

Dreessen, L., Hoekstra, R., & Arntz, A. (1997). Personality disorders do not influence the results of cognitive and behavior therapy for obsessive–compulsive disorder. *Journal of Affective Disorders, 11,* 503–521.

Drope v. Missouri, 420 U.S. 162 (1974).

Duclos, C. W., Beals, J., Novins, D. K., Maritn, C., Jewett, C. S., & Manson, S. M. (1998). Prevalence of common psychiatric disorders among American Indian adolescent detainees. *Journal of the American Academy of Child and Adolescent Psychiatry, 37,* 866–873.

Duncan, D. K. (1987). A comparison of two structured diagnostic interviews (Doctoral dissertation, York University, 1987). *Dissertation Abstracts International, 48,* 3109B.

Duncan, J. (1995). *Medication compliance in schizophrenic patients.* Unpublished dissertation, University of North Texas, Denton, TX.

Duncan, J. C., & Rogers, R. (1998). Medication compliance in patients with chronic schizophrenia: Implications for the community management of mentally disordered offenders. *Journal of Forensic Sciences, 43,* 1143–1147.

Dusky v. United States, 362 U.S. 402 (1960).

Earls, F., Smith, E., Reich, W., & Jung, K. G. (1988). Investigating psychopathological consequences of a disaster in children: A pilot study incorporating a structured diagnostic interview. *Journal of the American Academy of Child and Adolescent Psychiatry, 27,* 90–95.

Earls, F., Reich, W., Jung, K. G., & Cloninger, C. R. (1988). Psychopathology in children of alcoholic and antisocial parents. *Alcoholism: Clinical and Experimental Research, 12,* 481–487.

Easton, C., Meza, E., Mager, D., Ulug, B., Kilic, C., Gogus, A., & Babor, T. F. (1997). Test–retest reliability of the alcohol and drug use disorder sections of the Schedules for Clinical Assessment of Neuropsychiatry (SCAN). *Drug and Alcohol Dependence, 47,* 187–194.

Eaton, W. W., Anthony, J. C., Gallo, J., Cai, G., Tien, A., Romanoski, A., Lyketsos, C., & Chen, L. S. (1997). Natural history of Diagnostic Interview Schedule/DSM-IV major depression. *Archives of General Psychiatry, 54,* 993–999.

Eaton, W. W., Kramer, M., Anthony, J. C., Dryman, A., Shapirokins, S., & Locke, B. Z. (1989). The incidence of specific DIS/DSM-III mental disorders: Data from the NIMH Epidemiologic Catchment Area program. *Acta Psychiatrica Scandanavica, 79,* 163–178.

Eaton, W. W., Romanoski, A., Anthony, J. C., Tien, A., Gallo, J., Cai, G., Neufeld, K., Schlaepfer, T., Laugharne, J., & Chen, L. S. (1998). Onset and recovery from panic disorder in the Baltimore Epidemiological Catchment Area follow-up. *British Journal of Psychiatry, 173,* 501–507.

Edelbrock, C., & Costello, A. J. (1988). Convergence between statistically derived behavior problem syndromes and child psychiatric diagnoses. *Journal of Abnormal Child Psychology, 16,* 219–231.

Edelbrock, C., Costello, A. J., Dulcan, M. K., Kalas, R., & Conover, N. C. (1985). Age differences in the reliability of the psychiatric interview of the child. *Child Development, 56,* 265–275.

Edell, W. S., Joy, S. P., & Yehuda, R. (1990). Discordance between self-report and observer-rated psychopathology in borderline patients. *Journal of Personality Disorders, 4,* 381–390.

Edwards, D. W., Stearns, K. A., Yarvis, R. M., Swanson, A. J., & Mirassou, M. M. (1997, October). *Varied strengths of the SIRS in a jail setting.* Paper presented as the American Academy of Psychiatry and Law conference, Denver, CO.

Edwards, J., McGorry, P. D., Waddell, F. M., & Harrigan, S. M. (1999). Enduring negative symptoms in first episode psychosis: Comparison of six methods using follow-up data. *Schizophrenia Research, 40,* 147–158.

Eggers, C., & Bunk, D. (1997). The long-term course of child-onset schizophrenia: A 42-year follow-up. *Schizophrenia Research, 23,* 105–117.

Ekselius, L., Lindstrom, E., von Knorring, L., Bodlund, O., & Kullgren, G. (1994). SCID-II interviews and the SCID screen questionnaire as diagnostic tools for personality disorders in DSM-III-R. *Acta Psychiatrica Scandinavica, 90,* 120–123.

Endicott, J., Cohen, J., Nee, J., Fleiss, J., & Sarantakos, S. (1981). Hamilton Depression Rating Scale: Extracted from regular and change versions of the Schedule for Affective Disorders and Schizophrenia. *Archives of General Psychiatry, 38,* 98–103.

Endicott, J., Nee, J., Cohen, J., Fleiss, J. L., & Simon, R. (1986). Diagnosis of schizophrenia: Prediction of short-term outcome. *Archives of General Psychiatry, 43,* 13–19.

Endicott, J., & Spitzer, R. L. (1972). Current and Past Psychopathology Scales (CAPPS): Rationale, reliability, and validity. *Archives of General Psychiatry, 27,* 678–687.

Endicott, J., & Spitzer, R. L. (1978). A diagnostic interview: The Schedule of Affective Disorders and Schizophrenia. *Archives of General Psychiatry, 35,* 837–844.

Endicott, J., & Spitzer, R. L. (1979). Use of the Research Diagnostic Criteria and the Schedule of Affective Disorders and Schizophrenia to study affective disorders. *American Journal of Psychiatry, 136,* 52–56.

Endicott, J., Spitzer, R. L., & Fleiss, J. L. (1975). The Mental Status Evaluation Record (MSER): Reliability and validity. *Comprehensive Psychiatry, 16,* 285–301.

Endicott, J., Spitzer, R. L., Fleiss, J. L., & Cohen, J. (1976). The Global Assessment Scale: A procedure for measuring overall severity of psychiatric disturbance. *Archives of General Psychiatry, 33,* 766–771.

Engdah, B. E., Speed, N., Eberly, R. E., & Schwartz, J. (1991). Comorbidity of psychiatric disorders and personality profiles of American World War II prisoners of war. *Journal of Nervous and Mental Disease, 179,* 181–187.

Engel, I. M. (1979). The Mental Status Examination in psychiatry: Origin, use, and content. *Journal of Psychiatric Education, 3,* 99–108.

Eppright, T. D., Kashani, J. H., Borison, B. D., & Reid, J. C. (1993). Comorbidity of conduct disorder and personality disorders in an incarcerated juvenile population. *American Journal of Psychiatry, 150,* 1233–1236.

Erdman, H. P., Klein, M. H., Greist, J. H., Bass, S. M., Bires, J. K., & Machtinger, P. E. (1987). A comparison of the Diagnostic Interview Schedule and clinical diagnosis. *American Journal of Psychiatry, 144,* 1477–1480.

Erdman, H. P., Klein, M. H., Greist, J. H., Skare, S. S., Husted, J. J., Robins, L. N., Helzer, J. E., Goldring, E., Hamburger, M., & Miller, J. P. (1992). A comparison of two computer-administered versions of the NIMH Diagnostic Interview Schedule. *Journal of Psychiatric Research, 26,* 85–95.

Escobar, J. I., Burnham, A., Karno, M., Forsythe, A., Landsverk, J., & Golding, J. M. (1986). Use of the Mini-Mental State Examination (MMSE) in a community population of mixed ethnicity: Cultural and linguistic artifacts. *Journal of Nervous and Mental Disease, 174,* 607–614.

Evenson, R. C., Altman, H., Cho, D. W., & Sletten, I. W. (1974a). The relationship of diagnosis and target symptoms to psychotropic drug assignment. *Comprehensive Psychiatry, 15,* 173–178.

Evenson, R. C., Altman, H., Cho, D. W., & Sletten, I. W. (1974b). Simple algorithms for predicting psychotropic drugs assigned to psychiatric inpatients. *Diseases of the Nervous System, 35,* 80–83.

Evenson, R. C., Altman, H., Sletten, I. W., & Cho, D. W. (1973). Clinical judgment versus multivariate formulae in assignment of psychotropic drugs. *Journal of Clinical Psychology, 29,* 332–337.

Everington, C. (1990). Competence Assessment for Standing Trial for Defendants with Mental Retardation (CAST-MR). *Criminal Justice and Behavior, 17,* 147–168.

Exner, J. E., Jr. (1991). *The Rorschach, a comprehensive system: Vol. 2. Interpretation* (2nd ed.). New York: Wiley.

Ezpeleta, L., Osa, N., Domenech, J. M., Navarro, J. B., Losilla, J. M., & Judez, J. (1997). Diagnostic agreement between clinicians and the Diagnostic Interview for Children and Adolescents—DICA-R—in an outpatient sample. *Journal of Child Psychology and Psychiatry, 38,* 431–440.

Fairburn, C. G. , & Cooper, Z. (1993). The Eating Disorder Examination (12th ed.).

In C. G. Fairburn & G. T. Wilson (Eds.), *Binge eating: Nature, assessment, and treatment* (pp. 317–360). New York: Guilford Press.

Fairburn, C. G., & Wilson, G. T. (Eds.). (1993). *Binge eating: Nature, assessment, and treatment.* New York: Guilford Press.

Fallon, T., Jr., & Schwab-Stone, M. (1994). Determinants of reliability in psychiatric surveys of children aged 6–12. *Journal of Psychology and Psychiatry, 35,* 1391–1408.

Famularo, R., Kinscherff, R., & Fenton, T. (1992). Psychiatric diagnoses of maltreated children: Preliminary findings. *Journal of the American Academy of Child and Adolescent Psychiatry, 31,* 863–867.

Fantoni-Salvador, P., & Rogers, R. (1997). Spanish versions of the MMPI-2 and PAI: An investigation of concurrent validity with Hispanic patients. *Assessment, 4,* 29–39.

Farber, J. F., Schmitt, F. A., & Logue, P. E. (1988). Predicting intellectual level from the Mini-Mental State Examination. *Journal of the American Geriatrics Society, 36,* 509–510.

Farmer, A. E., Chubb, H., Jones, I., Hillier, J., Smith, A., & Borysiewicz, L. (1996). Screening for psychiatric morbidity in subjects presenting with chronic fatigue syndrome. *British Journal of Psychiatry, 168,* 354–358.

Farmer, A. E., Cosyns, P., Leboyer, M., Maier, W., Mors, O., Sargeant, M., Bebbington, P. A., & McGuffin, P. (1993). A SCAN-SADS comparison study of psychotic subjects and their first-degree relatives. *European Archives of Psychiatry and Clinical Neurosciences, 242,* 352–356.

Farmer, A. E., Katz, R., McGuffin, P., & Bebbington, P. A. (1987). A comparison of the Present State Examination and the Composite International Diagnostic Interview. *Archives of General Psychiatry, 44,* 1064–1068.

Faust, D., & Miner, R. A. (1986). The empiricist and his new clothes: DSM-III in perspective. *American Journal of Psychiatry, 143,* 962–967.

Faustman, W. O., Moses, J. A., & Csernansky, J. G. (1990). Limitations of the Mini-Mental State Examination in predicting neuropsychological functioning in a psychiatric sample. *Acta Psychiatrica Scandinavica, 81,* 126–131.

Feighner, J. P., Robins, E., Guze, S. B., Woodruff, R. A., Jr., Winokur, G., & Munoz, R. (1972). Diagnostic criteria for use in psychiatric research. *Archives of General Psychiatry, 26,* 57–63.

Fendrich, M., Weissman, M. M., & Warner, V. (1991). Longitudinal assessment of major depression and anxiety disorders in children. *Journal of American Academy of Child and Adolescent Psychiatry, 30,* 38–42.

Fennig, S., Bromet, E. J., Jandorf, L., Schwartz, J. E., Lavelle, J., & Ram, R. (1994). Eliciting psychotic symptoms using a semistructured diagnostic interview. *Journal of Nervous and Mental Disease, 182,* 20–26.

Fillenbaum, G. G. (1980). Comparison of two brief tests of organic impairment, the MSQ and the Short Portable MSQ. *Journal of the American Geriatric Society, 28,* 381–384.

Fink, L. A., Bernstein, D., Handelsman, L., Foote, J., & Lovejoy, M. (1995). Initial reliability and validity of the Childhood Trauma Interview: A new multidimensional measure of childhood interpersonal trauma. *American Journal of Psychiatry, 152,* 1329–1335.

Fink, P., Ewald, H., Jensen, J., Sorensen, L., Engberg, M., Holm, M., & Munk-Jorgensen, P. (1999). Screening for somatization and hypochondriasis in primary care and neurological inpatients: A seven-item scale for hypochondriasis and somatization. *Journal of Psychosomatic Research, 46,* 261–273.

First, M. B., Gibbon, M., Spitzer, R. L., Williams, J. B. W., & Benjamin, L. (1997). *The Structured Clinical Interview for DSM-IV Axis II Personality Disorders (SCID-II).* Washington, DC: American Psychiatric Press.

First, M. B., Spitzer, R. L., Gibbon, M., Williams, J. B. W., & Benjamin, L. (1994). The Structured Clinical Interview for DSM-IV Axis II Personality Disorders (SCID-II) (Version 2.0). New York: Biometrics Research, New York State Psychiatric Institute.

First, M. B., Spitzer, R. L., Gibbon, M., & Williams, J. B. W. (1995a). The Structured Clinical Interview for DSM-III-R Personality Disorders (SCID-II). Part I: Description. *Journal of Personality Disorders, 9,* 83–91.

First, M. B., Spitzer, R. L., Gibbon, M., Williams, J. B. W., Davies, M., Borus, J., Howes, M. J., Kane, J., Pope, H. G., & Rounsaville, B. (1995b). The Structured Clinical Interview for DSM-III-R Personality Disorders (SCID-II). Part II: Multisite test–retest reliability study. *Journal of Personality Disorders, 9,* 92–104.

First, M. B., Spitzer, R. L., Williams, J. B. W., & Gibbon, M. (1997). *Structured Clinical Interview for DSM-IV Disorders (SCID).* Washington, DC: American Psychiatric Association.

Fisher, P. W., Lucas, C., Shaffer, D., Schwab-Stone, M., Graae, F., Lichtman, J., Willoughby, S., & Gerald, J. (1997). *Diagnostic Interview Schedule for Children, Version IV (DISC-IV): Test–retest reliability in a clinical sample.* Poster presentation at the 44th Annual Meeting of the American Academy of Child and Adolescent Psychiatry, Toronto.

Fisher, P. W., Shaffer, D., Piacentini, J. C., Lapkin, J., Kafantaris, V., Leonard, H., & Herzog, D. B. (1993). Sensitivity of the Diagnostic Interview Schedule for Children, 2nd edition (DISC-2.1) for specific diagnoses of children and adolescents. *Journal of American Academy of Child and Adolescent Psychiatry, 32,* 666–673.

Fisk, A. A., & Pannill, F. C., III. (1987). Assessment and care of the community-dwelling Alzheimer's disease patient. *Journal of the American Geriatrics Society, 35,* 307–311.

Fitcher, M. M., Elton, M., Engel, K., Meyer, A. E., Mall, H., & Poustka, F. (1991). Structured Interview for Anorexia and Bulimia Nervosa (SIAB): Development of a new instrument for the assessment of eating disorders. *International Journal of Eating Disorders, 10,* 571–592.

Fleiss, J. L., & Cohen, J. (1973). The equivalence of weighted kappa and the intraclass correlation coefficient as measures of reliability. *Educational and Psychological Measurement, 33,* 613–619.

Fleming, M. P., & Difede, J. A. (1999).Effects of varying scoring rules of the Clinician-Administered PTSD Scale (CAPS) for the diagnosis of PTSD after acute burn injury. *Journal of Traumatic Stress, 12,* 535–542.

Flisher, A. J., Kramer, R. A., Hoven, C. W., Greenwald, S., Alegria, M., Bird, H. R., Canino, G., Connell, R., & Moore, R. E. (1997). Psychosocial characteristics of physically abused children and adolescents. *Journal of the American Academy of Child and Adolescent Psychiatry, 36,* 123–131.

Fogelson, D. L., Nuechterlein, K. H., Asarnow, R. F., Subotnik, K. L., & Talovic, S. A. (1991). Interrater reliability of the Structured Clinical Interview for DSM-III-R, Axis II: Schizophrenia spectrum and affective spectrum disorders. *Psychiatric Research, 39,* 55–63.

Folstein, M. F., Anthony, J. C., Parhad, I., Duffy, B., & Gruenberg, E. M. (1985). The meaning of cognitive impairment in the elderly. *Journal of the American Geriatrics Society, 33,* 228–235.

Folstein, M. F., Folstein, S. E., & McHugh, P. R. (1975). Mini-mental state: A practical method of grading cognitive state of patients for the clinician. *Journal of Psychiatric Research, 12,* 189–198.

Ford, C. V., King, B. R., & Hollender, M. H. (1988). Lies and liars: Psychiatric aspects of prevarication. *American Journal of Psychiatry, 145,* 554–562.

Ford, J., Hillard, J. R., Giesler, L. J., Lassen, K. L., & Thomas, H. (1989). Substance abuse/mental illness: Diagnostic issues. *American Journal of Drug and Alcohol Abuse, 15,* 297–305.

Foreman, M. D. (1987). Reliability and validity of mental status questionnaires in elderly hospitalized patients. *Nursing Research, 36,* 216–220.

Forth, A. E., Brown, S. L., Hart, S. D., & Hare, R. D. (1996). The assessment of psychopathy in male and female noncriminals: Reliability and validity. *Personality and Individual Differences, 20,* 531–543.

Forth, A. E., Hart, S. D., & Hare, R. D. (1990). Assessment of psychopathy in male young offenders. *Psychological Assessment: A Journal of Consulting and Clinical Psychology, 2,* 342–344.

Forth, A. E., Kosson, D. S., & Hare, R. D. (in press). *The Psychopathy Checklist: Youth Version (PCL:YV).* Toronto: MultiHealth Systems.

Forth, A. E., & Mailloux, D. L. (2000). Psychopathy in youth: What do we know? In C. B. Gacono (Ed.), *The clinical and forensic assessment of psychopathy* (pp. 25–54). Mahwah, NJ: Erlbaum.

Fossati, A., Maffei, C., Bagnato, M., Bonati, D., Donini, M., Florilli, M., Novella, L., & Ansoldi, M. (1998). Brief communication: Criterion validity of the Personality Diagnostic Questionnaire—4+ (PDQ-4+) in a mixed psychiatric sample. *Journal of Personality Disorders, 12,* 172–178.

Foster, J. R., Sclan, S., Welkowitz, J., Boksay, I., & Seeland, I. (1988). Psychiatric assessment in medical long-term care facilities: Reliability of commonly used rating scales. *International Journal of Geriatric Psychiatry, 3,* 229–233.

Frances, A., Clarkin, J. F., Gilmore, M., Hurt, S. W., & Brown, R. (1984). Reliability of criteria for borderline personality disorder: A comparison of DSM-III and the Diagnostic Interview for Borderline Patients. *American Journal of Psychiatry, 141,* 1080–1084.

Frances, A. J. (1982). Categorical and dimensional systems of personality disorders: A comparison. *Comprehensive Psychiatry, 23,* 516–527.

Frances, A. J. (1985). Introduction to personality disorders. In R. Michels, J. O. Cavenar, A. M. Cooper, S. B. Guze, L. L. Judd, G. L. Klerman, & A. J. Solnit (Eds.), *Psychiatry* (Vol. 1, chap. 14). Philadephia: J. B. Lippincott.

Freeman, T. W., Clothier, J. L., Pazzaglia, P., Sesem, M. D., & Swann, A. C. (1992). A double-blind comparison of valproate and lithium in the treatment of acute mania. *American Journal of Psychiatry, 149,* 108–111.

Friedman, A. S., Glickman, N. W., & Morrissey, M. R. (1988). What mothers know about their adolescents' alcohol/drug use and problems, and how mothers react to finding out. *Journal of Drug Education, 18,* 155–167.

Fristad, M. A., Cummins, J., Verducci, J. S., Teare, M., Weller, E. B., & Weller, R. A. (1998a). Study IV: Concurrent validity of the DSM-IV revised Children's Interview for Psychiatric Syndromes (CHIPS). *Journal of Child and Adolescent Psychopharmocology, 8,* 227–236.

Fristad, M. A., Cummins, J., Glickman, A. R., Verducci, J. S., Teare, M., Weller, E. B.,

& Weller, R. A. (1998b). Study V: Children's Interview for Psychiatric Syndromes (CHIPS): Psychometrics in two community samples. *Journal of Child and Adolescent Psychopharmocology, 8,* 227–236.

Fristad, M. A., Teare, M., Weller, E. B., Weller, R. A., & Salmon, P. (1998). Study III: Development and concurrent validity of the Children's Interview for Psychiatric Syndromes—Parent's version (P-CHIPS). *Journal of Child and Adolescent Psychopharmocology, 8,* 213–219.

Fyer, A. J., Endicott, J., Manuzza, S., & Klein, D. F. (1985). *Schedule for Affective Disorders and Schizophrenia—Lifetime version (modified for the study of anxiety disorders).* New York: Anxiety Disorder Clinic, New York State Psychiatric Institute.

Fyer, A. J., Mannuzza, S., Martin, L. Y., Gallops, M. S., Endicott, J., Schleyer, B., Gorman, J. M., Liebowitz, M. R., & Klein, D. F. (1989). Reliability of anxiety assessment: II. Symptom agreement. *Archives of General Psychiatry, 46,* 1102–1110.

Gacono, C. B., & Hutton, H. E. (1994). Suggestions for the clinical and forensic use of the Hare Psychopathy Checklist—Revised (PCL-R). *International Journal of Psychiatry, 17,* 303–317

Gadow, K. D., & Sprafkin, J. (1987). *Stony Brook Child Psychiatric Checklist—3R.* Stony Brook: State University of New York at Stony Brook, Dept. of Psychiatry.

Gaffney, F. A., Fenton, B. J., Lane, L. D., & Lake, R. (1988). Hemodynamic, ventilatory, and biochemical responses of panic patients and normal controls with sodium lactate infusion and spontaneous panic attacks. *Archives of General Psychiatry, 45,* 53–60.

Galbaud du Fort, G., Bland, R. C., Newman, S. C., & Boothroyd, L. J. (1998). Spouse similarity for lifetime psychiatric history in the general population. *Psychological Medicine, 28,* 789–803.

Gallagher, D. E., & Thompson, L. W. (1983). Effectiveness of psychotherapy for both endogenous and nonendogenous depression in older adult outpatients. *Journal of Gerontology, 38,* 707–712.

Ganellen, R. J., Matuzas, W., Uhlenhuth, E. H., Glass, R., & Easton, C. R. (1986). Panic disorder, agoraphobia, and anxiety-relevant cognitive style. *Journal of Affective Disorders, 11,* 219–225.

Gartner, A. R., Marcus, R. N., Halmi, K., & Loranger, A. W. (1989). DSM-III-R personality disorders in patients with eating disorders. *American Journal of Psychiatry, 146,* 1585–1591.

Garyfallos, G., Karastergiou, A., Adamopoulou, A., Moutzoukis, C., Alagiozidou, E., Mala, D., & Garyfallos, A. (1991). Greek version of the General Health Questionnaire: Accuracy of translation and validity. *Acta Psychiatrica Scandinavica, 84,* 371–378.

Gavin, D. R., Ross, H. E., & Skinner, H. A. (1989). Diagnostic validity of the Drug Abuse Screening Test in the assessment of DSM-III drug disorders. *British Journal of Addictions, 84,* 301–307.

Geller, B., Fox, L. W., & Clark, K. A. (1994). Rate and predictors of prepubertal bipolarity during follow-up of 6 and 12 year-old depressed children. *Journal of the American Academy of Child and Adolescent Psychiatry, 33,* 461–468.

Getto, C. J., & Heaton, R. K. (1985). *Psychosocial Pain Inventory manual.* Odessa, FL: Psychological Assessment Resources.

Getto, C. J., Heaton, R. K., & Lehman, A. W. (1983). PSPI: A standardized approach to the evaluation of psychosocial factors in chronic pain. In J. J. Bonica (Ed.), *Advances in pain research and therapy* (Vol. 5, pp. 885–889). New York: Raven Press.

Gillis, J. J., Gilger, J. W., Pennington, B. F., & DeFries, J. C. (1992). Attention deficit disorder in reading-disabled twins: Evidence for a genetic etiology. *Journal of Abnormal Child Psychology, 20,* 303–315.

Gillis, L. S., Elk, R., Ben-Arie, O., & Teggin, A. (1982). The Present State Examination: Experiences with Xhosa-speaking psychiatric patients. *British Journal of Psychiatry, 141,* 143–147.

Goater, N., King, M., Cole, E., Leavey, G., Johnson-Sabine, E., Blizard, R., & Hoar, A. (1999). Ethnicity and outcome of psychosis. *British Journal of Psychiatry, 175,* 34–42.

Goff, D. C., Olin, J. A., Jenike, M. A., Baer, L., & Buttolph, M. L. (1992). Dissociative symptoms in patients with obsessive–compulsive disorder. *Journal of Nervous and Mental Disease, 180,* 332–337.

Goldberg, D. (1978). *Manual for the General Health Questionnaire.* Windsor, Great Britain: NFER.

Goldberg, P. A., & Miller, S. J. (1966). Structured personality tests and dissimulation. *Journal of Projective Techniques and Personality Assessment, 30,* 452–455.

Golding, S. L., Roesch, R., & Schreiber, J. (1984). Assessment and conceptualization of competency to stand trial: Preliminary data on the Interdisciplinary Fitness Interview. *Law and Human Behavior, 8,* 321–334.

Golomb, M., Fava, M., Abraham, M., & Rosenbaum, J. F. (1995). Gender differences in personality disorders. *American Journal of Psychiatry, 152,* 579–582.

Gomez-Beneyto, M., Villar, M., Renovell, M., Perez, F., Hernandez, M., Leal, C., Cuquerella, M. A., Slok, C., & Asencio, A. (1994). The diagnosis of personality disorder with a modified version of the SCID-II in a Spanish sample. *Journal of Personality Disorders, 8,* 104–110.

Goodman, G., Hull, J. W., Clarkin, J. F., & Yeomans, F. E. (1999). Childhood antisocial behaviors as predictors of psychotic symptoms and DSM-III-R criteria among inpatients with borderline personality disorder. *Journal of Personality Disorders, 13,* 35–46.

Goodman, W. K., Price, L. H., Rasmussen, S. A., Mazure, C., Delgado, P., Henigner, G. R., & Charney, D. S. (1989). The Yale–Brown Obsessive–Compulsive Scale (YBOCS): I. Development, use, and reliability. *Archives Of General Psychiatry, 46,* 1006–1011.

Goodness, K. (1999). *Retrospective assessment of the malingering: R-SIRS and CT-SIRS.* Unpublished doctoral dissertation, University of North Texas, Denton.

Gorenstein, C., Gentil, V., Melo, M., Lotufo-Neto, R., & Lauriano, V. (1998). Mood improvement in "normal" volunteers. *Journal of Psychopharmocology, 12,* 246–251.

Gormley, N., O'Leary, D. O., & Costello, F. (1999). First admissions for depression: Is the "no treatment interval" a critical predictor of time to remission? *Journal of Affective Disorders, 54,* 49–54.

Gothard, S. (1993). *Detection of malingering in mental competency evaluations.* Unpublished dissertation, California School of Professional Psychology, San Diego.

Gothard, S., Rogers, R., & Sewell, K. W. (1995). Feigning incompetency to stand trial: An investigation of the GCCT. *Law and Human Behavior, 19,* 363–373.

Gould, M. S., King, R., Greenwald, S., Fisher, P., Schwab-Stone, M., Kramer, R.,

Flisher, A. J., Goodman, S., Canino, G., & Shaffer, D. (1998). Psychopathology associated with suicidal ideation and attempts among children and adolescents. *Journal of the American Academy of Child and Adolescent Psychiatry, 37,* 915–923.

Graber, R. A., & Miller, W. R. (1988). Abstinence or controlled drinking goals for problem drinkers: A randomized clinical trial. *Psychology of Addictive Behaviors, 2,* 20–33.

Graham, P., & Rutter, M. (1968). The reliability and validity of psychiatric assessment of the child: II. Interview with the parent. *British Journal of Psychiatry, 114,* 581–592.

Grann, M., Langstrom, N., Tengstrom, A., & Stalenheim, E. G. (1998). Reliability of file-based retrospective ratings of psychopathy with the PCL-R. *Journal of Personality Assessment, 70,* 416–426.

Gray, K. C., & Hutchinson, H. C. (1964). The psychopathic personality: A survey of Canadian psychiatrists' opinions. *Canadian Psychiatric Association Journal, 9,* 452–461.

Grayson, P., & Carlson, G. A. (1991). The utility of a DSM-III-R based checklist in screening child psychiatric patients. *Journal of the American Academy of Child and Adolescent Psychiatry, 30,* 669–673.

Green, C. J. (1989). The Personality Disorder Examination. *Journal of Personality Disorders, 3,* 352–354.

Green, M. L., Foster, M. A., Morris, M. A., Muir, J. J., & Morris, R. D. (1998). Patient assessment of psychological and behavioral functioning following pediatric acquired brain injury. *Journal of Pediatric Psychology, 23,* 289–299.

Green, R. L., & Price, T. R. P. (1986). Procedural validity of an abbreviated version of the SADS/RDC diagnostic process. *Psychiatry Research, 18,* 379–391.

Greenbaum, P. E., Prange, M. E., Friedman, R. M., & Silver, S. E. (1991). Substance abuse prevalence and comorbidity with other psychiatric disorders among adolescents with severe emotional disturbances. *Journal of the American Academy of Child and Adolescent Psychiatry, 30,* 575–583.

Greene, R. L. (2000). *The MMPI-2: An interpretive manual* (2nd ed.). Boston: Allyn and Bacon.

Greenhill, L. L., & Malcolm, J. (2000). Child and adolescent measures for diagnosis and screening. In A. J. Rush, H. A. Pincus, M. B. First, D. Blacker, J. Endicott, S. J. Keith, K. A. Phillips, N. D., Ryan, G. R. Smith, M. T. Tsuang, T. A. Widiger, & D. A. Zarin (Eds.), *Handbook of psychiatric measures* (pp. 277–324). Washington, DC: American Psychiatric Press.

Greenwald, J., & Satow, Y. (1978). A short social desirability scale. *Psychological Reports, 27,* 131–135.

Griest, J. H., Klein, M. H., Erdman, H. P., Bires, J., Bass, S., Machtinger, P., & Kresge, D. (1987). Psychiatric diagnosis via direct patient–computer interview. *Hospital and Community Psychiatry, 38,* 1305–1311.

Griest, J. H., Mathisen, K. S., Klein, M. H., Benjamin, L. S., Erdman, H. P., & Evans, F. J. (1984). Psychiatric diagnosis: What role for the computer? *Hospital and Community Psychiatry, 35,* 1089–1093.

Griffin, M. L., Weiss, R. D., Mirin, S. M., Wilson, H., & Bouchard-Voelk, B. (1987). The use of the Diagnostic Interview Schedule in drug-dependent patients. *American Journal of Drug and Alcohol Abuse, 13,* 281–291.

Grinker, R. R., Werble, B., & Drye, R. (1968). *The borderline syndrome: A behavioral study of ego functions*. New York: Basic Books.

Grove, W. M., Andreasen, N. C., McDonald-Scott, P., Keller, M. B., & Shapiro, R. W. (1981). Reliability studies of psychiatric diagnoses. *Archives of General Psychiatry, 38,* 408–413.

Gunderson, J. G. (1982). *Diagnostic Interview for Borderline Patients* (2nd ed.). New York: Roerig-Pfizer.

Gunderson, J. G., Carpenter, W. T., Jr., & Strauss, J. S. (1975). Borderline and schizophrenic patients: A comparative study. *American Journal of Psychiatry, 132,* 1257–1264.

Gunderson, J. G., & Kolb, J. E. (1976, May). *Diagnosing borderlines: A semi-structured interview.* Paper presented at the American Psychiatric Association Convention, Miami Beach, FL.

Gunderson, J. G., & Kolb, J. E. (1978). Discriminating features of borderline patients. *American Journal of Psychiatry, 135,* 792–796.

Gunderson, J. G., Kolb, J. E., & Austin, V. (1981). The Diagnostic Interview for Borderline Patients. *American Journal of Psychiatry, 138,* 896–903.

Gunderson, J. G., Links, P. S., & Reich, J. H. (1991). Competing models of personality disorders. *Journal of Personality Disorders, 5,* 60–68.

Gunderson, J. G., & Singer, J. T. (1975). Defining borderline patients. *American Journal of Psychiatry, 132,* 1–10.

Gunderson, J. G., & Zanarini, M. C. (1992). *Revised Diagnostic Interview for Borderlines (DIB-R).* Boston: Harvard Medical School.

Gurland, B. J., Yorkston, N. J., Goldberg, K., Fleiss, J. L., Sloane, R. B., & Cristol, A. H. (1972). The Structured and Scaled Interview to Assess Maladjustment (SSI-AM): II. Factor analysis, reliability, and validity. *Archives of General Psychiatry, 27,* 264–267.

Gurland, B. J., Yorkston, N. J., Stone, A. R., Frank, J. D., & Fleiss, J. L. (1972). The Structured and Scaled Interview to Assess Maladjustment (SSIAM): I. Description, rationale and development. *Archives of General Psychiatry, 27,* 259–264.

Gutterman, E. M., O'Brien, J. D., & Young, J. G. (1987). Structured diagnostic interviews for children and adolescents: Current status and future directions. *Journal of American Academy of Child and Adolescent Psychiatry, 26,* 621–630.

Guzder, J., Paris, J., Zelkowitz, P., & Feldman, R. (1999). Psychological risk factors for borderline pathology in school-aged children. *Journal of the American Academy of Child and Adolescent Psychiatry, 38,* 206–212.

Guzder, J., Paris, J., Zelkowitz, P., & Marchessault, K. (1996). Risk factors for borderline pathology in children. *Journal of the American Academy of Child and Adolescent Psychiatry, 35,* 26–33.

Gynther, M. D., Altman, H., & Sletten, I. W. (1973). Replicated correlates of MMPI two-point code types: The Missouri Actuarial System (monograph). *Journal of Clinical Psychology, 29,* 363–289.

Haddad, L. B., & Coffman, T. L. (1987). A brief neuropsychological screening exam for psychiatric–geriatric patients. *Clinical Gerontologist, 6,* 3–10.

Hafner, H., Riecher-Rossler, A., Hambrecht, M., Loffler, W., Maurer, K., Meissner, S., Schmidtke, A., Munk-Jorgensen, P., Fatkenheuer, B., Loffler, W., & Van der Heiden, W. (1992). IRAOS: An instrument for the assessment of onset and early course of schizophrenia. *Schizophrenic Research, 6,* 209–223.

Haley, G. M. T., Fine, S., & Marriage, K. (1988). Psychotic features in adolescents with major depression. *Journal of the American Academy of Child and Adolescent Psychiatry, 27,* 489–493.

Halikas, J. A., Crosby, R. D., Pearson, V. L., Nugent, S. M., & Carlson, G. A. (1994).

Psychiatric comorbidity in treatment-seeking cocaine abusers. *American Journal of Addictions, 3,* 25–35.

Hambrecht, M., & Hafner, H. (1996). Substance abuse and the onset of schizophrenia. *Biological Psychiatry, 40,* 1155–1163.

Hambrecht, M., Hafner, H., & Loffler, W. (1994). Beginning schizophrenia observed by significant others. *Social Psychiatry and Psychiatric Epidemiology, 29,* 53–60.

Hamilton, M. (1960). A rating scale for depression. Journal of *Neurology, Neurosurgery, and Psychiatry, 23,* 56–62.

Hammen, C. (1988). Self-cognitions, stressful events, and the prediction of depression in children of depressed mothers. *Journal of Abnormal Child Psychology, 16,* 347–360.

Hammen, C., Gordon, D., Burge, D., Adrian, C., Jaenicke, C., & Hiroto, D. (1987). Maternal affective disorders, illness, and stress: Risk for children's psychopathology. *American Journal of Psychiatry, 144,* 736–741.

Hapke, U., Rumpf, H. J., & John, U. (1998). Differences between hospital patients with alcohol problems referred for counseling by physicians' routine clinical practice versus screening questionnaire. *Addiction, 93,* 1777–1785.

Hare, R. D. (1980). A research scale for the assessment of psychopathy in criminal populations. *Personality and Individual Differences, 1,* 111–119.

Hare, R. D. (1985a). Comparison of procedures for the assessment of psychopathy. *Journal of Consulting and Clinical Psychology, 53,* 7–16.

Hare, R. D. (1985b). *The Psychopathy Checklist.* Unpublished manuscript, University of British Columbia, Vancouver, BC.

Hare, R. D. (1991). *Manual for the revised Psychopathy Checklist.* Toronto: Multi-Health Systems.

Hare, R. D. (1998a). The Hare PCL-R: Some issues concerning its use and misuse. *Legal and Criminological Psychology, 3,* 99–119.

Hare, R. D. (1998b). Psychopaths and their nature: Implications for the mental health and criminal justice system. In T. Millon, E. Simonsen, M. Birket-Smith, & R. D. Davis (Eds.), *Psychopathy: Antisocial, criminal and violent behavior* (pp. 188–212). New York: Guilford Press.

Hare, R. D., & Cox, D. N. (1978). Clinical and empirical conceptions of psychopathy, and the selection of subjects for research. In R. D. Hare & S. Schalling (Eds.), *Psychopathic behavior: Approaches to research* (pp. 1–21). Chichester, UK: Wiley.

Hare, R. D., Cox, D. N., & Hart, S. D. (1989). *Preliminary manual for the Psychopathy Checklist: Clinical Version (PCL:CV).* Unpublished manuscript, University of British Columbia, Vancouver.

Hare, R. D., & Hart, S. D. (1993). Psychopathy, mental disorder and crime. In S. Hodgins (Ed.), Mental disorder and crime (pp. 104–115). Newbury Park, CA: Sage.

Hare, R. D., & Hart, S. D. (1995). Commentary on antisocial personality disorder: The DSM-IV field trial. In W. J. Livesley (Ed.), *The DSM-IV personality disorders* (pp. 127–140). New York: Guilford Press.

Hare, R. D., Hart, S. D., & Harpur, T. J. (1991). Psychopathy and the DSM-IV criteria for antisocial personality disorder. *Journal of Abnormal Psychology, 100,* 391–398.

Hare, R. D., McPherson, L. M., & Forth, A. E. (1988). Male psychopaths and their criminal careers. *Journal of Clinical and Consulting Psychology, 56,* 710–714.

Harkness, A. R. (1992, August). *Multiply diagnosable patient: Hierarchical personality models and clinical judgment.* Paper presented at the American Psychological Association convention, Washington, DC.

Harpur, T. J., & Hare, R. D. (1994). Assessment of psychopathy as a function of age. *Journal of Abnormal Psychology, 103,* 604–609.

Harris, K. B., & Miller, W. R. (1990). Behavioral self-control training for problem drinkers: Components of efficacy. *Psychology of Addictive Behavior, 4,* 82–90.

Hart, S. D., Cox, D. N., & Hare, R. D. (1997). *Manual for the Screening Version of Psychopathy Checklist Revised (PCL-SV).* Toronto: Multi-Health Systems.

Hart, S. D., Dutton, D. G., & Newlove, T. (1993). The prevalence of personality disorder among wife assaulters. *Journal of Personality Disorders, 7,* 329–341.

Hart, S. D., Forth, A. E., & Hare, R. D. (1991). The MCMI-II and psychopathy. *Journal of Personality Disorders, 5,* 318–327.

Hart, S. D., Hare, R. D., & Harpur, T. J. (1992). The Psychopathy Checklist—Revised (PCL-R): An overview for researchers and clinicians. In J. C. Rosen, & P. McReynold (Eds.), *Advances in Psychological Assessment* (Vol. 8, pp. 103–130). New York: Plenum.

Hasin, D. S., & Grant, B. F. (1987a). Assessment of specific drug disorders in a sample of substance abuse patients: A comparison of the DIS and the SADS-L procedures. *Drugs and Alcohol Dependence, 19,* 165–176.

Hasin, D. S., & Grant, B. F. (1987b). Diagnosing depressive disorders in patients with alcohol and drug problems: A comparison of the SADS-L and the DIS. *Journal of Psychiatric Research, 21,* 301–311.

Hasin, D. S., & Grant, B. F. (1987c). Psychiatric diagnosis of patients with substance abuse problems: A comparison of two procedures, the DIS and the SADS-L. *Journal of Psychiatric Research, 21,* 7–22.

Hassiotis, A., Tyrer, P., & Cicchetti, D. (1997). Detection of personality disorders by a community mental health team: A study of diagnostic accuracy. *Irish Journal of Medicine, 14,* 85–88.

Hayes, J. S., Hale, D. R., & Gouvier, W. D. (1998). Malingering detection in a mentally retarded forensic population. *Applied Neuropsychology, 5,* 33–36.

Hayward, C., Killen, J. D., Hammer, L. D., Litt, I. F., Wilson, D. M., Simmonds, B., & Taylor, C. B. (1992). Pubertal stage and panic attack history in sixth- and seventh-grade girls. *American Journal of Psychiatry, 149,* 1239–1243.

Heaton, R. Q., Lehman, R. A. W., & Getto, C. J. (1980). *Psychosocial Pain Inventory.* Odessa, FL: Psychological Assessment Resources.

Hedlund, J. L., Evenson, R. C., Sletten, I. W., & Cho, D. W. (1980). The computer and clinical prediction. In J. B. Sidowski, J. Johnson, & T. A. Williams (Eds.), *Technology in mental health care delivery systems* (pp. 201–235). Norwood, NJ: Ablex.

Hedlund, J. L., Sletten, I. W., Altman, H., & Evenson, R. C. (1973). Prediction of patients who are dangerous to others. *Journal of Clinical Psychology, 29,* 443–447.

Heilbrun, K., Hart, S., Hare, R., Gustafson, D., Nunez, C., & White, A. (1998). Inpatient and postdischarge aggression in mentally disordered offenders: The role of psychopathy. *Journal of Interpersonal Violence, 13,* 514–527.

Heilbrun, K., Rogers, R., & Otto, R. K. (2000). *Forensic assessment: Current status and future directions.* Manuscript submitted for publication.

Helzer, J. E., Brockington, I. F., & Kendell, R. E. (1981). Predictive validity of the

DSM-III and Feighner definitions of schizophrenia. *Archives of General Psychiatry, 38,* 791–797.

Helzer, J. E., Clayton, P. J., Pambakian, R., Reich, T., Woodruff, R. A., & Reveley, M. A. (1977). Reliability of psychiatric diagnosis. *Archives of General Psychiatry, 34,* 136–141.

Helzer, J. E., & Robins, L. N. (1988). The Diagnostic Interview Schedule: Its development, evolution, and use. *Social Psychiatry and Psychiatric Epidemiology, 23,* 6–16.

Helzer, J. E., Robins, L. N., McEnvoy, L. T., Spitznagel, E. L., Stoltzman, R. K., Farmer, A., & Brockington, I. F. (1985). A comparison of clinical and Diagnostic Interview Schedule diagnoses. *Archives of General Psychiatry, 42,* 657–666.

Hemphill, J. F., Hare, R. D., & Wong, S. (1998). Psychopathy and recidivism: A review. *Legal and Criminological Psychology, 3,* 139–170.

Henderson, S. Duncan-Jones, P., Byrne, D. G., Scott, R., & Adcock, S. (1979). Psychiatric disorder in Canberra: A standardized study of prevalence. *Acta Psychiatrica Scandinavica, 60,* 355–374.

Hendrie, H. C., Hall, K. S., Brittain, H. M., Austrom, M. G., Farlow, M., Parker, J., & Kane, M. (1988). The CAMDEX: A standardized instrument for the diagnosis of mental disorder in the elderly—a replication with a US sample. *Journal of the American Geriatrics Society, 36,* 402–408.

Herjanic, B., & Campbell, W. (1977). Differentiating psychiatrically disturbed children of the basis of a structured interview. *Journal of Abnormal Child Psychology, 5,* 127–134.

Herjanic, B., Herjanic, M., Brown, F., & Wheatt, T. (1975). Are children reliable reporters? *Journal of Abnormal and Child Psychology, 3,* 41–48.

Herjanic, B., & Reich, W. (1982). Development of a structured psychiatric interview for children: Agreement between child and parent on individual symptoms. *Journal of Abnormal Child Psychology, 10,* 307–324.

Herjanic, B., & Reich, W. (1983a). *Diagnostic Interview for Children and Adolescents (DICA-C): Child version.* St. Louis: Washington University School of Medicine.

Herjanic, B., & Reich, W. (1983b). *Diagnostic Interview for Children and Adolescents (DICA-P): Parent version.* St. Louis: Washington University School of Medicine.

Herrmann, D. J. (1982). Know thy memory: The use of questionnaires to assess and study memory. *Psychological Bulletin, 92,* 434–452.

Hersch, E. L., Kral, V. A., & Palmer, R. B. (1978). Clinical value of the London Psychogeriatric Rating Scale. *Journal of the American Geriatrics Society, 26,* 348–354.

Hershey, L. A., Jaffe, D. F., Greenough, P. G., & Yang, S. L. (1987). Validation of cognitive and functional assessment instruments in vascular dementia. *International Journal of Psychiatry in Medicine, 17,* 183–192.

Herst, L. D., Voss, C. B., & Waldman, J. (1990). Cortical function assessment in the elderly. *Journal of Neuropsychiatry and Clinical Neurosciences, 2,* 385–390.

Herz, M. I., Spitzer, R. L., Gibbon, M., Greenspan, K., & Reibel, S. (1974). Individual versus group aftercare treatment. *American Journal of Psychiatry, 131,* 808–812.

Herzog, D. B., Keller, M. B., Sacks, N. R., Yeh, C. J., & Lavori, P. W. (1992). Psychiatric comorbidity in treatment-seeking anxorexics and bulimics. *Journal of the American Academy of Child and Adolescent Psychiatry, 31,* 810–818.

Hesselbrock, V., Stabenau, J., Hesselbrock, M., Mirkin, P., & Meyer, R. (1982). A comparison of two interview schedules: The Schedule for Affective Disorders and Schizophrenia—Lifetime and the National Institute of Mental Health Diagnostic Interview Schedule. *Archives of General Psychiatry, 39,* 674–677.

Heun, R. , Muller, H., Freyberger, H. J., & Maier, W. (1998). Reliability of interview information in a family study in the elderly. *Social Psychiatry and Psychiatric Epidemiology, 33,* 140–144.

Hicks, M. M., Rogers, R., & Cashel, M. L. (2000). Predictions of violent and total infractions among institutionalized male juvenile offenders. *Journal of the American Academy of Psychiatry and Law, 28,* 183–190.

Hill, A., Rumpf, H. J., Hapke, U., Driessen, M., & Ulrich, J. (1998). Prevalence of alcohol dependence and abuse in general practice. *Alcoholism: Clinical and Experimental Research, 22,* 935–940.

Hill, C., Rogers, R., & Bickford, M. (1996). Predicting aggressive and socially disruptive behavior in a maximum security hospital. *Journal of Forensic Sciences, 41,* 56–59.

Hill, R. D., Gallagher, D., Thompson, L. W., & Ishida, T. (1988). Hopelessness as a measure of suicidal intent in the depressed elderly. *Psychology and Aging, 3,* 230–232.

Hindley, P. A., Hill, P. D., McGuigan, S., & Kitson, N. (1994). Psychiatric disorder in deaf and hearing impaired children and young people: A prevalence study. *Journal of Child Psychology and Psychiatry, 35,* 917–934.

Hodges, K. (1990). Depression and anxiety in children: A comparison of self-report questionnaires to clinical interview. *Psychological Assessment: A Journal of Clinical and Consulting Psychology, 2,* 376–381.

Hodges, K. (1993). Structured interviews for assessing children. *Journal of Child Psychology and Psychiatry, 34,* 49–68.

Hodges, K., Cools, J., & McKnew, D. (1989). Test–retest reliability of a clinical research interview for children: The Child Assessment Schedule (CAS). *Psychological Assessment: A Journal of Consulting and Clinical Psychology, 1,* 317–322.

Hodges, K., Gordon, Y., & Lennon, M. P. (1990). Parent–child agreement on symptoms assess via a clinical research interview for children: The Child Assessment Schedule (CAS). *Journal of Child Psychology and Psychiatry, 31,* 427–436.

Hodges, K., Kline, J., Fitch, P., McKnew, D., & Cytryn, L. (1981). The Child Assessment Schedule: A diagnostic interview for research and clinical use. *Catalog of Selected Documents in Psychology, 17,* 56.

Hodges, K., Kline, J., Stern, L., Cytryn, L., & McKnew, D. (1982). The development of a Child Assessment Interview for research and clinical use. *Journal of Abnormal and Child Psychology, 10,* 173–189.

Hodges, K., McKnew, D., Burbach, D. J., & Roebuck, L. (1987). Diagnostic concordance between the Child Assessment Schedule (CAS) and the Schedule for Affective Disorders and Schizophrenia for School-Age children (K-SADS) in an outpatient sample using lay interviewers. *Journal of American Academy of Child and Adolescent Psychiatry, 26,* 654–661.

Hodges, K., McKnew, D., Cytryn, L., Stern, L., & Kline, J. (1982). The Child Assessment Schedule (CAS) diagnostic interview: A report on reliability and validity. *Journal of the American Academy of Child Psychiatry, 21,* 468–473.

Hodges, K., & Saunders, W. (1989). Internal consistency of a diagnostic interview for children: The Child Assessment Schedule. *Journal of Abnormal Child Psychology, 17,* 691–701.

Hodges, K., Saunders, W., Kashani, J., Hamlett, K., & Thompson, R. J., Jr. (1990). Internal consistency of DSM-III diagnoses using the symptom scales of the Child Assessment Schedule. *Journal of American Academy of Child and Adolescent Psychiatry, 29,* 635–641.

Hodgins, D. C., & El-Guebaly, N. (1992). More data on the Addiction Severity Index: Reliability and validity with the mentally ill substance abuser. *Journal of Nervous and Mental Disease, 180,* 197–201.

Hodiamont, P., Peer, N., & Sybern, N. (1987). Epidemiological aspects of psychiatric disorder in Dutch health area. *Psychological Medicine, 17,* 495–505.

Hoge, S. K., Bonnie, R. J., Poythress, N., Monahan, J., Eisenberg, M., & Feucht-Haviar, T. (1997). The MacArthur Adjudicative Competence Study: Development and validation of a research instrument. *Law and Human Behavior, 21,* 141–182.

Hogg, B., Jackson, H. J., Rudd, R. P., & Edwards, J. (1990). Diagnosing personality disorders in recent-onset schizophrenia. *Journal of Nervous and Mental Disease, 178,* 194–199.

Hokanson, J. E., Rubert, M. P., Welker, R. A., Hollander, G. R., & Hedeen, C. (1989). Interpersonal concomitants and antecedents of depression among college students. *Journal of Abnormal Psychology, 98,* 209–217.

Hon, J., Huppert, F. A., Holland, A. J., & Watson, P. (1999). Neuropsychological assessment of older adults with Down's syndrome: An epidemiological study using Cambridge Cognitive Examination (CAMCOG). *British Journal of Clinical Psychology, 38,* 155–165.

Hoppe, S. K., Leon, R. L., & Realini, J. P. (1989). Depression and anxiety among Mexican Americans in a family health center. *Social Psychiatry and Psychiatric Epidemiology, 24,* 63–68.

Horowitz, M., Wilner, N., & Alvarez, W. (1979). Impact of Event Scale: A measure of subjective distress. *Psychological Medicine, 21,* 209–218.

Horton, J., Compton, W. M., & Cottler, L. (1998). *Assessing psychiatric disorders among drug users: Reliability of the DIS-IV.* Unpublished manuscript, Washington University School of Medicine, St. Louis, MO.

Horvath, P., & Jonsdottir-Baldursson, T. (1990). Methodological variations in the use of the MMPI for diagnosis of borderline personality disorder among alcoholics. *Journal of Clinical Psychology, 46,* 238–243.

Horwath, E., Wolk, S. I., Goldstein, R. B., Wickramaratne, P., Sobin, C., Adams, P., Lish, J. D., & Weissman, M. M. (1995). Is the comorbidity between social phobia and panic disorder due to familial cotransmission or other factors? *Archives of General Psychiatry, 52,* 574–582.

Hotopf, M., Mayou, R., Wadsworth, M., & Wessely, S. (1998). Temporal relationships between physical symptoms and psychiatric disorder. *British Journal of Psychiatry, 173,* 255–261.

Hout, M. A., & Griez, E. (1984). Validity and utility of the Present State Examination in assessing neurosis: Empirical findings and critical considerations. *Journal of Psychiatric Research, 18,* 161–172.

Hughes, M., Denney, R. L., & Cannedy, R. (2000, March). *Competency of juvenile to stand trial in criminal court.* Paper presented at the biennial convention of the American Psychology–Law Society, New Orleans.

Hunt, C., & Andrews, A. (1992). Measuring personality disorder: The use of self-report questionnaires. *Journal of Personality Disorders, 6,* 125–133.

Hurt, S. W., Clarkin, J. F., Frances, A., Abrams, R., & Hunt, H. (1985). Discriminant validity of the MMPI for borderline personality disorder. *Journal of Personality Assessment, 49,* 56–61.

Hurt, S. W., Clarkin, J. F., Koenigsberg, H. W., Frances, A., & Nurnberg, H. G. (1986). Diagnostic interview for borderlines: Psychometric properties and validity. *Journal of Consulting and Clinical Psychology, 54,* 256–260.

Hurt, S. W., Friedman, R. C., Clarkin, J., Corn, R., & Aronoff, M. S. (1982). Rating the severity of depressive symptoms in adolescents and young adults. *Comprehensive Psychiatry, 23,* 263–270.

Hurt, S. W., Hyler, S. E., Frances, A., Clarkin, J. F., & Brent, R. (1984). Assessing borderline personality disorder with self-report, clinical interview, or semistructured interview. *American Journal of Psychiatry, 141,* 1228–1231.

Huxley, P., Korer, J., & Tolley, S. (1987). The psychiatric "caseness" of clients referred to an urban social services department. *British Journal of Sociology, 17,* 507–520.

Hwu, H. G., Yeh, E. K., & Chang, L. Y. (1986). Chinese Diagnostic Interview Schedule: Agreement with psychiatrist's diagnosis. *Acta Psychiatrica Scandinavica, 73,* 225–233.

Hwu, H. G., Yeh, E. K., & Chang, L. Y. (1989). Prevalence of psychiatric disorders in Taiwan defined by the Chinese Diagnostic Interview Schedule. *Acta Psychiatrica Scandinavica, 79,* 136–147.

Hwu, H. G., Yeh, E. K., Chang, L. Y., & Yeh, Y. L. (1986). Chinese Diagnostic Interview Schedule: A validity study on estimation of lifetime prevalence. *Acta Psychiatrica Scandinavica, 73,* 348–357.

Hwu, H. G., Yeh, E. K., Yeh, Y. L., & Chang, L. Y. (1988). Alcoholism by Chinese Diagnostic Interview Schedule: A prevalence and the validity study. *Acta Psyhiatrica Scandinavia, 77,* 7–13.

Hyer, L., Summers, M. N., Boyd, S., Litaker, M., & Boudewyns, P. (1996). Assessment of older combat veterans with the Clinician-Administered PTSD Scale. *Journal of Traumatic Stress, 9,* 587–593.

Hyler, S. E., & Rieder, R. O. (1987). *PDQ-R: Personality diagnostic questionnaire-revised.* New York: New York State Psychiatric Institute.

Hyler, S. E., Skodol, A. E., Kellman, H. D., Oldham, J. M., & Rosnick, L. (1990). Validity of the Personality Diagnostic Questionnaire—Revised: Comparison with two structured interviews. *American Journal of Psychiatry, 147,* 1043–1048.

Hyler, S. E., Skodol, A. E., Oldham, J. M., Kellman, H. D., & Doidge, N. (1992). Validity of the Personality Diagnostic Questionnaire—Revised: A replication in an outpatient sample. *Comprehensive Psychiatry, 33,* 73–77.

Ikuta, N., Zanarini, M. C., Minakawa, K., Miyake, Y., Moriya, N., & Nishizono-Maher, A. (1994). Comparison of American and Japanese outpatients with borderline personality disorder. *Comprehensive Psychiatry, 35,* 382–385.

Jackson, D. N., & Paunonen, S. V. (1980). Personality structure and assessment. *Annual Review of Psychology, 31,* 503–551.

Jackson, H. J., Grazis, J., Rudd, R. P., & Edwards, J. (1991). Concordance between two personality disorder instruments. *Comprehensive Psychiatry, 32,* 252–260.

Jackson, H. J., McGorry, P. D., & Dudgeon, P. (1995). Prodromal symptoms of schizophrenia in first-episode psychosis: Prevalence and specificity. *Comprehensive Psychiatry, 36,* 241–250.

Jackson, R. L., Rogers, R., Neumann, C. E., & Lambert, P. L. (2001). *Psychopathy in women: An investigation of its underlying dimensions.* Manuscript submitted for publication.

Jackson, H. J., Whiteside, H. L., Bates, G. W., Bell, R., Rudd, R. P., Edwards, J. (1991). Diagnosing personality disorders in psychiatric inpatients. *Acta Psychiatrica Scandanavica, 83,* 206–213.

Jackson, J. E., & Ramsell, J. W. (1988). Use of the Mini-Mental State Examination (MMSE) to screen for dementia in elderly outpatients. *Journal of the American Geriatrics Society, 36,* 662.

Jacobs, J. W., Bernhard, M. R., Delgado, A., & Strain, J. J. (1977). Screening for organic mental syndromes in the medically ill. *Annals of Internal Medicine, 107,* 481–485.

Janca, A., Robins, L. N., Bucholz, K. K., Early, T. S., & Shayka, J. J. (1992). Comparison of the Composite International Diagnostic Interview and clinical DSM-III-R criteria checklist diagnoses. *Acta Psychiatrica Scandinavica, 85,* 440–443.

Janca, A., Robins, L. N., Cottler, L. B., & Early, T. S. (1992). Clinical observation of assessment using the Composite International Diagnostic Interview (CIDI): Analysis of the CIDI field trials—Wave II at the St. Louis site. *British Journal of Psychiatry, 160,* 815–818.

Janca, A., Ustun, T. B., & Sartorius, N. (1994). New versions of the World Health Organization instruments for the assessment of mental disorders. *Acta Psychiatrica Scandinavica, 90,* 73–83.

Jastak, J., Bijou, S., & Jastak, S. (1978). *Wide Range Achievement Test.* Wilmington, DE: Jastak Assessment Systems.

Jenkins, R., Lewis, G., Bebbington, P., Brugha, T., Farrell, M., Gill, B., & Meltzer, H. (1997a). The national psychiatric morbidity surveys of Great Britain: Initial findings from the household survey. *Psychological Medicine, 27,* 775–789.

Jenkins, R., Lewis, G., Bebbington, P., Brugha, T., Farrell, M., Gill, B., Meltzer, H., & Petticrew, M. (1997b). The national psychiatric morbidity surveys of Great Britain: Strategy and methods. *Psychological Medicine, 27,* 765–774.

Jensen, P. S., Roper, M., Fisher, P., Piacentini, J., Canino, G., Richters, J., Rubio-Stipec, M., Dulcan, M., Goodman, S., Davies, M., Rae, D., Shaffer, D., Bird, H., Lahey, B., & Schwab-Stone, M. (1995). Test–retest reliability for the Diagnostic Interview Schedule for Children (DISC 2.1). *Archives of General Psychiatry, 52,* 61–71.

Jensen, P. S., & Wantanabe, H., H. (1999). Sherlock Holmes and child psychopathology assessment approaches: The case of the false-positive. *Journal of the American Academy of Child and Adolescent Psychiatry, 38,* 138–146.

Jensen, P. S., Wantanabe, H., H., Richters, J. E., Cortes, R., Roper, M., & Liu, S. (1995). Prevalence of mental disorder in military children and adolescents: Findings from a two-stage community survey. *Journal of the American Academy of Child and Adolescent Psychiatry, 34,* 1514–1524.

Jensen, P. S., Wantanabe, H., H., Richters, J. E., Roper, M., Hibbs, E. D., Salzberg, A. D., & Liu, S. (1996). Scale, diagnoses, and child psychopathology: II. Comparing the CBCL and the DISC against external validators. *Journal of Abnormal Child Psychology, 24,* 151–168.

Johnson, J., Williams, T., Klingler, D., & Gianetti, R. (1988). Interventional relevance and retrofit programming: Concepts for the improvement of clinical acceptance of computer-generated assessment reports. *Behavioral Research Methods and Instrumentation, 9,* 123–132.

Johnson, M. H., Magaro, P. A., & Stern, S. L. (1986). Use of the SADS-C as a diagnostic and symptom severity measure. *Journal of Consulting and Clinical Psychology, 54,* 546–551.

Jones, L. R., Badger, L. W. , Ficken, R. P., Leeper, J. D., & Anderson, R. L. (1988). Mental health training of primary care physicians: An outcome study. *International Journal of Psychiatry in Medicine, 18,* 107–121.

Jones, M. C., Dauphinais, P., Sack, W. H., & Somervell, P. D. (1997). Trauma-related symptomatology among American Indian adolescents. *Journal of Traumatic Stress, 10,* 163–173.

Jonsdottir-Baldursson, T., & Horvath, P. (1987). Borderline personality-disordered alcoholics in Iceland: Descriptions on demographic, clinical, and MMPI variables. *Psychological Assessment, 55,* 738–741.

Kahn, R. L., Goldfarb, A. I., Pollack, M., & Peck, A. (1960). Brief objective measures for the determination of mental status in the aged. *American Journal of Psychiatry, 117,* 326–328.

Kaplan, C. A., & Kolvin, I. (1994). The assessment of personality in young adulthood: Data on a normative sample. *European Child and Adolescent Psychiatry, 3,* 37–45.

Kaplan, H. I., & Sadock, B. J. (1988). *Synopsis of psychiatry, behavioral sciences, clinical psychiatry* (5th ed.). Baltimore: Williams & Wilkins.

Kaplan, L. M., & Reich, W. (1991). *Manual for Diagnostic Interview for Children and Adolescents—Revised (DICA-R).* St. Louis: Washington University.

Karayiorgou, M., Sobin, C., Blundell, M. L., Galke, B. L., Malinova, L., Goldberg, P., Ott, J., & Gogos, J. A. (1999). Family-based association studies support a sexually dimorphic effect of COMT and MAOA on genetic susceptibility to obsessive–compulsive disorder. *Biological Psychiatry, 45,* 1178–1189.

Karno, M., Burnam, A., Escobar, J. L., Hough, R. L., & Eaton, W. W. (1983). Development of the Spanish-language version of the National Institute of Mental Health Diagnostic Interview Schedule. *Archives of General Psychiatry, 40,* 1183–1188.

Karpman, B. (1961). The structure of neurosis: With special differentials between neurosis, psychosis, homosexuality, alcoholism, psychopathy, and criminality. *Archives of Criminal Psychodynamics, 4,* 599–646.

Kashani, J. H., Orvaschel, H., Rosenberg, T. K., & Reid, J. C. (1989). Psychopathology in a community sample of child and adolescents: A developmental perspective. *Journal of the American Academy of Child and Adolescent Psychiatry, 28,* 701–706.

Kashani, J. H., Reid, J. C., & Rosenberg, T. K. (1989). Levels of hopelessness in children and adolescents: A development perspective. *Journal of Consulting and Clinical Psychology, 57,* 496–499.

Kashani, J. H., Sherman, A. D., Parker, D. P., & Reid, J. C. (1990). Utility of the Beck Depression Inventory with clinic-referred adolescents. *Journal of the American Academy of Child and Adolescent Psychiatry, 29,* 278–282.

Kashani, J. H., Strober, M., Rosenberg, T. K., & Reid, J. C. (1988). Correlates of psychopathology in adolescents. *Psychiatry Research, 26,* 141–148.

Katon, W., Lin, E., Von Korff, M., Russo, J., Lipscomb, P., & Bush, T. (1991). Somatization: A spectrum of severity. *American Journal of Psychiatry, 148,* 34–40.

Katz, M. M., Marsella, A., Dube, K. C., Olatawura, M., Takahashi, R., Nakane, Y., Wynne, L. C., Gift, T., Brennan, J., Sartorius, N., & Jablensky, A. (1988). On the expression of psychosis in different cultures: Schizophrenia in an Indian and in a Nigerian community. *Culture, Medicine, and Psychiatry, 12,* 331–355.

Kaufman, D. M., Weinberger, M., Strain, J. J., & Jacobs, J. W. (1979). Detection of cognitive deficits by a brief mental status examination. *General Hospital Psychiatry, 1,* 247–255.

Kaufman, J., Birmaher, B., Brent, D., Rao, U., Flynn, C., Moreci, P., Williamson, D., & Ryan, N. (1997). Schedule for Affective Disorders and Schizophrenia for School-Age Children—Present and Lifetime Version (K-SADS-PL): Initial reliability and validity data. *Journal of the American Academy of Child and Adolescent Psychiatry, 36,* 980–988.

Kavoussi, R. J., Coccaro, E. F., Klar, H. M., Berstein, D., & Siever, L. J. (1990). Structured interviews for borderline personality disorder. *American Journal of Psychiatry, 147,* 1522–1525.

Kaye, A. L., & Shea, M. T. (2000). Personality disorders, personality traits, and defense mechanism measures. In A. J. Rush, H. A. Pincus, M. B. First, D. Blacker, J. Endicott, S. J. Keith, K. A. Phillips, N. D. Ryan, G. R. Smith, M. T. Tsuang, T. A. Widiger, & D. A. Zarin (Eds.), *Handbook of psychiatric measures* (pp. 713–750). Washington, DC: American Psychiatric Press.

Keane, T. M., Caddell, J. M., & Taylor, K. L. (1988). Mississippi Scale for Combat-Related Posttraumatic Stress Disorder: Three studies in reliability and validity. *Journal of Consulting and Clinical Psychology, 56,* 85–90.

Keller, M. B., Lavori, P. W., McDonald-Scott, P., Scheftner, W. A., Andreason, N. C., Shapiro, R. W., & Croughan, J. (1981). Reliability of lifetime diagnoses and symptoms in patients with a current psychiatric disorder. *Journal of Psychiatric Research, 16,* 229–240.

Keller, M. B., & Manschreck, T. C. (1981). The bedside mental status examination—reliability and validity. *Comprehensive Psychiatry, 22,* 500–511.

Kelly, T., Soloff, P. H., Cornelius, J., George, A., Lis, J. A., & Ulrich, R. (1992). Can we study (treat) borderline patients? Attrition from research and open treatment. *Journal of Personality Disorders, 6,* 417–433.

Kendell, R. E. (1985). Schizophrenia: Clinical features. In R. Michels, J. O. Cavenar, A. M. Cooper, S. B. Guze, L. L. Judd, G. L. Klerman, & A. J. Solnit (Eds.), *Psychiatry* (Vol. 1, Chapt. 53). Philadephia: Lippincott.

Kendell, R. E., Everitt, B., Cooper, J. E., Sartorius, N., & David, M. E. (1968). Reliability of the Present State Examination. *Social Psychiatry, 3,* 123–129.

Kendler, K. S., Gruenberg, A. M., & Kinney, D. K. (1994). Independent diagnoses of adoptees and relatives as defined by DSM-III in the provincial and national samples of the Danish adoption study of schizophrenia. *Archives of General Psychiatry, 51,* 456–468.

Kendler, K. S., Walters, E. E., Neale, M. C., Kessler, R. C., Heath, A. C., & Eaves, L. J. (1995). The structure of the genetic and environmental risk factors for six major psychiatric disorders in women. *Archives of General Psychiatry, 52,* 374–383.

Kernberg, O. F. (1967). Borderline personality organization. *Journal of the American Psychoanalytic Association, 15,* 641–685.

Kernberg, O. F. (1981). Structural interviewing. *Psychiatric Clinics of North America, 4,* 169–195.

Kessler, L. G., Cleary, P. D., & Burke, J. D., Jr. (1985). Psychiatric disorders in primary care: Results of a follow-up study. *Archives of General Psychiatry, 42,* 583–587.

Kessler, R. C., McGonagle, K. A., Zhao, S., Nelson, C. B., Hughes, M., Eshleman, S., Wittchen, H. U., & Kendler, K. S. (1994). Lifetime and 12-month prevalence of DSM-III-R psychiatric disorders in the United States. *Archives of General Psychiatry, 51,* 8–19.

Kidorf, M., Brooner, R. K., King, V. L., Chutuape, M. A., & Stitzer, M. L. (1996). Concurrent validity of cocaine and sedative dependence diagnoses in opioid-dependent outpatients. *Drug and Alcohol Dependence, 42,* 117–123.

Kiernan, R. J., Mueller, J., Langston, J. W., & Van Dyke, C. (1987). The Neurobehavioral Cognitive Screening Examination: A brief but quantitative approach to cognitive assessment. *Annals of Internal Medicine, 107,* 481–485.

Kiesler, D. J. (1983). The 1982 interpersonal circle: A taxonomy for complementarity in human transactions. *Psychological Review, 90,* 185–214.

Kiesler, D. J. (1986). Interpersonal methods of diagnosis and treatment. In E. Michels, J. O. Cavenar, & A. M. Cooper (Eds.), *Psychiatry* (Vol. 1, chap. 4). Philadelphia: Lippincott.

King, C. A., Katz, S. H., Ghaziuddin, N., Brand, E., Hill, E., & McGovern, L. (1997). Diagnosis and assessment of depression and suicidality using the NIMH Diagnostic Interview Schedule for Children (DISC–2.3). *Journal of Child Abnormal Psychology, 25,* 173–181.

King, D. W., Leskin, G. A., King, L. A., & Weathers, F. W. (1998). Confirmatory factor analysis of the Clinician-Administered PTSD Scale: Evidence for the dimensionality of the posttraumatic stress disorder. *Psychological Assessment, 10,* 90–96.

Klein, M. H., Benjamin, L. S., Rosenfeld, R., Treece, C., Husted, J., & Griest, J. H. (1993). The Wisconsin Personality Disorders Inventory: Development, reliability, and validity. *Journal of Personality Disorders, 7,* 285–303.

Knight, R. (1953). Borderline states. *Bulletin of the Menninger Clinic, 17,* 1–12.

Knopman, D. S., Kitto, J., Deinar, S., & Heiring, J. (1988). Longitudinal study of death and institutionalization in patients with primary degenerative dementia. *Journal of the American Geriatrics Society, 36,* 108–112.

Kobak, K. A., Taylor, L. H., Dottl, S. L., Greist, J. H., Jefferson, J. W., Burroughs, D., Katzelnick, D. J., & Mandell, M. (1997). Computerized screening for psychiatric disorders in an outpatient community mental health clinic. *Psychiatric Services, 48,* 1048–1057.

Koenig, H. G., Johnson, S., Bellard, J., Denker, M., & Fenlon, R. (1995). Depression and anxiety disorder among older male inmates at a federal correctional facility. *Psychiatric Services, 46,* 399–401.

Koenigsberg, H. W., Kernberg, O. F., & Schomer, J. (1983). Diagnosing borderline conditions in an outpatient setting. *Archives of General Psychiatry, 40,* 49–53.

Kolb, J. E., & Gunderson, J. G. (1980). Diagnosing borderline patients with a semistructured interview. *Archives of General Psychiatry, 37,* 37–41.

Korenblum, M., Marton, P., Golombek, H., & Stein, B. (1990). Personality status: Changes through adolescence. *Adolescence: Psychiatric Clinics of North America, 13,* 389–399.

Kosson, D. S., Smith, S. S., & Newman, J. P. (1990). Evaluating the construct validity of psychopathy on black and white male inmates: Three preliminary studies. *Journal of Abnormal Psychology, 99,* 250–259.

Kosson, D. S., Steuerwald, B. L., Forth, A. E., & Kirkhart, K. J. (1997). A new method for assessing the interpersonal behavior of psychopathic individuals: Preliminary validation studies. *Psychological Assessment, 9,* 89–101.

Kosten, T. R., Rounsaville, B. J., & Kleber, H. D. (1986). A 2.5-year follow-up of depression, life crises, and treatment effects on abstinence among opioid addicts. *Archives of General Psychiatry, 43,* 733–738.

Kovacs, M. (1978). *Children's Depression Inventory (CDI).* Pittsburgh: University of Pittsburgh, Pittsburgh, PA.

Kovacs, M. (1983). *Interview Schedule for Children (ISC): Form C and follow-up form.* Unpublished manuscript, University of Pittsburgh.

Kovacs, M., Akiskal, H. S., Gatsonis, C., & Parrone, P. L. (1994). Childhood-onset dysthymic disorder. *Archives of General Psychiatry, 41,* 365–374.

Kovacs, M., Feinberg, T. L., Crouse-Novak, M., Paulauskas, S. L., & Finkelstein, R. (1984a). Depressive disorders in childhood: I. A longitudinal prospective study of characteristics and recovery. *Archives of General Psychiatry, 41,* 229–237.

Kovacs, M., Feinberg, T. L., Crouse-Novak, M., Paulauskas, S. L., Pollock, M., & Finkelstein, R. (1984b). Depressive disorders in childhood: II. A longitudinal study of the risk for subsequent major depression. *Archives of General Psychiatry, 41,* 643–649.

Kovess, V., & Fournier, L. (1990). The DISSA: An abridged self-administered version of the DIS. *Social Psychiatry and Psychiatric Epidemiology, 25,* 179–186.

Kranzler, H. R., Kadden, R. M., Babor, T. F., Tennen, H., & Rounsaville, B. J. (1996). Validity of the SCID in substance abuse patients. *Addiction, 91,* 859–868.

Kroger, R. O., & Turnbull, W. (1975). Invalidity of validity scales: The case of the MMPI. *Journal of Consulting and Clinical Psychology, 43,* 48–55.

Kroll, J., Pyle, R., & Zander, J. (1981). Borderline personality disorder: Interrater reliability of the Gunderson Diagnostic Interview for Borderlines (DIB). *Schizophrenia Bulletin, 7,* 269–272.

Kroll, J., Sines, L., Martin, K., Lari, S., Pyle, R., & Zander, J. (1981). Borderline personality disorder: Construct validity of the concept. *Archives of General Psychiatry, 38,* 1021–1026.

Kropp P. R. (1992). *Antisocial personality disorder and malingering.* Unpublished doctoral dissertation, Simon Fraser University, Burnaby, BC, Canada.

Kruedelbach, N., McCormick, R. A., Schulz, S. C., & Grueneich, R. (1993). Impulsivity, coping styles, and triggers for craving in substance abusers with borderline personality disorders. *Journal of Personality Disorders, 7,* 214–222.

Kullgren, G. (1987). An empirical comparison of three different borderline concepts. *Acta Psychiatrica Scandinavica, 76,* 246–255.

Kullgren, G. (1988). Factors associated with completed suicide in borderline personality disorder. *Journal of Nervous and Mental Disease, 176,* 40–44.

Kullgren, G., & Armelius, B.-A. (1990). The concept of personality organization: A long-term comparative follow-up study with special reference to borderline personality organization. *Journal of Personality Disorders, 4,* 203–212.

Kullgren, G., Renberg, E., & Jacobsson, L. (1986). An empirical study of borderline personality disorder and psychiatric suicides. *Journal of Nervous and Mental Disease, 174,* 328–331.

Kupersmidt, J. B., & Martin, S. L. (1997). Mental health problems of children of migrant and seasonal farm workers: A pilot study. *Journal of the American Academy of Child and Adolescent Psychiatry, 36,* 224–232.

Kurtz, R., & Meyer, R. G. (1994, March). *Vulnerability of the MMPI-2, M test, and*

SIRS to different strategies of malingering psychosis. Paper presented at the American Psychology–Law Society, Santa Fe, NM.

Kutcher, S. P., Yanchyshyn, G., & Cohen, C. (1985). Diagnosing affective disorder in adolescents: The use of the Schedule for Affective Disorders and Schizophrenia. *Canadian Journal of Psychiatry, 30,* 605–608.

Kutlesic, V., Williamson, D. A., Gleaves, D. H., Barbin, J. M., & Murphy-Eberenz, K. P. (1998). The Interview for the Diagnosis of Eating Disorders-IV: Application to DSM-IV diagnostic criteria. *Psychological Assessment, 10,* 41–48.

Kye, C. H., Waterman, G. S., Ryan, N. D., Birmaher, B., Williamson, D. E., Iyengar, S., & Dachille, S. (1996). A randomized, controlled trial of amitriptyline in acute treatment of adolescent major depression. *Journal of the American Academy of Child and Adolescent Psychiatry, 35,* 1139–1144.

Laboratory of Community Psychiatry. (1973). *Competency to stand trial and mental illness.* Rockville, MD: U.S. Department of Health, Education, and Welfare.

Lachar, D., & Gdowski, C. L. (1979). *Actuarial assessment of child and adolescent personality: An interpretive guide for the Personality Inventory for Children profile.* Los Angeles: Western Psychological Services.

Lahey, B. B., Loeber, R., Hart, E. L., Frick, P. J., Applegate, B., Zhang, Q., Green, S. M., & Russo, M. F. (1995). Four-year longitudinal study of conduct disorder in boys: Patterns and predictors of persistence. *Journal of Abnormal Psychology, 104,* 83–93.

Lahey, B. B., Loeber, R., Stouthamer-Loeber, M., Christ, M. A. G., Green, S., Russo, M. R., Frick, P. J., & Duncan, M. (1990). Comparison of DSM-III and DSM-III-R diagnoses for prepubertal children: Changes in prevalence and validity. *Journal of the American Academy of Child and Adolescent Psychiatry, 29,* 620–626.

Lahey, B. B., Piacentini, J. C., McBurnett, K., Stone, P., Hartdagen, S., & Hynd, G. (1988). Psychopathology in the parents of children with conduct disorder and hyperactivity. *Journal of the American Academy of Child and Adolescent Psychiatry, 27,* 163–170.

Lahmeyer, H. W., Val, E., Gaviria, F. M., Prasad, R. B., Pandey, G. N., Rodgers, P., Weiler, M., & Altman, E. G. (1988). EEG sleep, lithium transport, dexamethasone suppression, and mononamine oxidase activity in borderline peronality disorder. *Psychiatry Research, 25,* 19–30.

Lancker, D. V. (1990). The neurology of proverbs. *Behavioral Neurology, 3,* 169–187.

Larkin, A. R. (1979). The form and content of schizophrenic hallucinations. *American Journal of Psychiatry, 136,* 940–943.

Larson, L. M., & Heppner, P. P. (1989). Problem-solving appraisal in an alcoholic population. *Journal of Counseling Psychology, 36,* 73–78.

LaRue, A., Spar, J., & Hill, C. D., (1986). Cognitive impairment in late-life depression: Clinical correlates and treatment implications. *Journal of Affective Disorders, 11,* 179–184.

Last, C. G., Strauss, C. C., & Francis, G. (1987). Comorbidity among childhood anxiety disorders. *Journal of Nervous and Mental Disease, 175,* 726–730.

Lautenschlaeger, E., Meier, H. M. R., & Donnelly, M. (1986). Folstein vs. Goldfarb mental status exams. *Clinical Gerontologist, 4,* 40–42.

LaVesser, P. D., Smith, E. M., & Bradford, S. (1997). Characteristics of homeless women and dependent children: A controlled study. *Journal of Prevention and Intervention in the Community, 15,* 37–52.

Lavoro, S. A., Geddings, V. J., & Patrick, C. J. (1994, March). *Temperamental variables in the criminal psychopath.* Paper presented at the American Psychology–Law Society Convention, Santa Fe, NM.

Leboyer, M., Maier, W., Teherani, M., Lichtermann, D., D'Amato, T., Franke, P., Lepine, J.-P., Minges, J., & McGuffin, P. (1991). The reliability of the SADS-LA in a family study setting. *European Archives of Psychiatry and Clinical Neuroscience, 241,* 165–169.

Leckman, J. F., Sholomsaks, D., Thompson, W. D., Belanger, A., & Weissman, M. M. (1982). Best estimates of lifetime psychiatric diagnoses. *Archives of General Psychiatry, 39,* 879–883.

Le Couteur, A., Rutter, M., Lord, C., Rios, P., Robertson, S., Holdgrafer, M., & McLennan, F. (1989). Autism Diagnostic Interview: A standardized investigator-based instrument. *Journal of Autism and Developmental Disorders, 19,* 363–387.

Lecrubier, Y., Sheehan, D. V., Weiller, E., Amorim, P., Bonora, I., Sheehan, K. H., Janavs, J., & Dunbar, G. C. (1997). The Mini-International Neuropsychiatric Interview (MINI): Reliability and validity according to the CIDI. *European Psychiatry, 12,* 224–231.

Leenstra, A. S., Ormel, J., & Giel, R. (1995). Positive life change and recovery from depression and anxiety. *British Journal of Psychiatry, 166,* 333–343.

Lees-Haley, P. R., English, L. T., & Glenn, W. J. (1991). A fake bad scale on the MMPI-2 for personal-injury claimants. *Psychological Reports, 68,* 203–210.

Lehtinen, V., Lindholm, T., Veijola, J., & Vaisanen, E. (1990). The prevalence of PSE-CATEGO disorders in a Finnish adult population cohort. *Social Psychiatry and Psychiatric Epidemiology, 25,* 187–192.

Lejoyeux, M., Feuche, N., Loi, S., Solomon, J., & Ades, J. (1999). Study of impulse-control disorders among alcohol-dependent patients. *Journal of Clinical Psychiatry, 60,* 302–305.

Lenzenweger, M. F., Loranger, A. W., Kofine, L., & Neff, C. (1997). Detecting personality disorders in a nonclinical population: Application of a two-stage procedure for case identification. *Archives of General Psychiatry, 54,* 345–351.

Lerner, V., Bergman, J., Liberman, M., & Polyakova, I. (1999). A longitudinal study of positive symptoms in schizoaffective and paranoid schizophrenia. *International Journal of Psychiatry in Clinical Practice, 3,* 181–188.

Lesage, A. D., Cyr, M., & Toupin, J. (1991). Reliable use of the Present State Examination by psychiatric nurses for clinical studies of psychotic and nonpsychotic patients. *Acta Psychiatrica Scandinavia, 83,* 121–124.

Lesher, E. L., & Whelihan, W. M. (1986). Reliability of mental status instruments administered to nursing home residents. *Journal of Consulting and Clinical Psychology, 54,* 726–727.

Lesser, I. M., Rubin, R. T., Lydiard, R. B., Swinson, R., & Pecknold, J. (1987). Past and current thyroid function in subjects with panic disorder. *Journal of Clinical Psychiatry, 48,* 473–476.

Lesser, I. M., Rubin, R. T., Pecknold, J. C., Rifkin, A., Swinson, R. P., Lydiard, R. B., Burrows, G. D., Noyes, R., & DuPont, R. L., Jr. (1988). Secondary depression in panic disorder and agoraphobia: II. Frequency, severity and response to treatment. *Archives of General Psychiatry, 45,* 437–443.

Levin, F. R., Evans, S. M., & Kleber, H. D. (1998). Prevalence of adult attention deficit hyperactivity disorder among cocaine abusers seeking treatment. *Drug and Alcohol Dependence, 52,* 15–25.

Lewis, G., Pelosi, A. J., Araya, R., & Dunn, G. (1992). Measuring psychiatric disorder in the community: A standardized assessment for use by lay interviewers. *Psychological Medicine, 22,* 465–486.

Lezak, M. D. (1983). *Neuropsychological assessment.* New York: Oxford University Press.

Liberty, P. G., Jr., Lunneborg, C. E., & Atkinson, G. C. (1964). Perceptual defense, dissimulation, and response styles. *Journal of Consulting Psychology, 28,* 529–537.

Lin, E., Goering, P. N., Lesage, A., & Streiner, D. L. (1997). Epidemiologic assessment of overmet need in mental health care. *Social Psychiatry and Psychiatric Epidemiology, 32,* 355–362.

Linblad, A. D. (1993). *Detection of malingered mental illness with a forensic population: An analogue study.* Unpublished doctoral dissertation, University of Saskatchewan, Saskatoon, Canada.

Links, P. S., Heselgrave, R. J., Mitton, J. E., Van Reekum, R., & Patrick, J. (1995). Borderline psychopathology and recurrences of clinical disorders. *Journal of Nervous and Mental Diseases, 183,* 583–586.

Links, P. S., Heselgrave, R. J., & Van Reekum, R. (1999). Impulsivity: Core aspect of borderline personality disorder. *Journal of Personality Disorders, 13,* 1–9.

Links, P. S., Mitton, J. E., & Steiner, M. (1990). Predicting outcome for borderline personality disorder. *Comprehensive Psychiatry, 31,* 490–498.

Links, P. S., Steiner, M., Boiago, I., & Irwin, D. (1990). Lithium therapy for borderline patients: Preliminary findings. *Journal of Personality Disorders, 4,* 173–181.

Links, P. S., Steiner, M., & Mitton, J. (1989). Characteristics of psychosis in borderline personality disorder. *Psychopathology, 22,* 188–193.

Links, P. S., Steiner, M., Offord, D. R., & Eppel, A. (1985). Stability of the Diagnostic Interview for Borderlines diagnosis. *American Journal of Psychiatry, 142,* 1525.

Linszen, D. H., Dingemans, P. M., Lenior, M. E., Nugter, M. A., Scholte, W. F., & Van der Does, A. J. W. (1994). Relapse criteria in schizophrenic disorders: Different perspectives. *Psychiatry Research, 54,* 273–281.

Lipsitt, P. D., Lelos, D., & McGarry, A. L. (1971). Competency for trial: A screening instrument. *American Journal of Psychiatry, 128,* 105–109.

Liss, J. L., Welner, A., & Robins, E. (1972). Undiagnosed psychiatric patients. Part II: Follow-up study. *British Journal of Psychiatry, 121,* 647–651.

Livesley, W. J. (1985a). The classification of personality disorder: I. The choice of category concept. *Canadian Journal of Psychiatry, 30,* 353–358.

Livesley, W. J. (1985b). The classification of personality disorder: II. The problem of diagnostic criteria. *Canadian Journal of Psychiatry, 30,* 359–362.

Livesley, W. J. (1986). Trait and behavioral prototypes of personality disorder. *American Journal of Psychiatry, 143,* 728–732.

Livesley, W. J., & Jackson, D. N. (1986). The internal consistency and factorial structure of behaviors judged to be associated with DSM-III personality disorders. *American Journal of Psychiatry, 143,* 1473–1474.

Livesley, W. J., Reiffer, L. I., Sheldon, A. E. R., & West, M. (1987). Prototypicality ratings of DSM-III criteria for personality disorders. *Journal of Nervous and Mental Disease, 175,* 395–401.

Livingston, R. L., Dykman, R. A., & Ackerman, P. T. (1990). The frequency and significance of additional self-reported psychiatric diagnoses in children with attention deficit disorder. *Journal of Abnormal Child Psychology, 18,* 465–478.

Livingston, R. L., Dykman, R. A., & Ackerman, P. T. (1992). Psychiatric comorbidity and response to two doses of methylphenidate in children with attention deficit disorder. *Journal of Child and Adolescent Psychopharmacology, 2,* 115–122.

Loebel, A. D., Lieberman, J. A., Alvir, J. M. J., Mayerhoff, D. I., Geisler, S. H., & Szymanski, S. R. (1992). Duration of psychosis and outcome in first-episode schizophrenia. *American Journal of Psychiatry, 149,* 1183–1188.

Loebel, C. M. (1992). Relationship between childhood sexual abuse and borderline personality disorder in women psychiatric inpatients. *Journal of Child Sexual Abuse, 1,* 63–80.

Loranger, A. W. (1988). *Personality Disorder Examination (PDE) manual.* Yonkers, NY: DV Communications.

Loranger, A. W. (1990). The impact of DSM-III on diagnostic practice in a university hospital. *Archives of General Psychiatry, 47,* 672–675.

Loranger, A. W. (1992). Are current self-report and interview measures adequate for epidemiological studies of personality disorders? *Journal of Personality Disorders, 6,* 313–325.

Loranger, A. W. (1999a). *International Personality Disorder Examination (IPDE) manual.* Odessa, FL: Psychological Assessment Resources.

Loranger, A. W. (1999b). *International Personality Disorder Examination (IPDE) Screening Questionnaire.* Odessa, FL: Psychological Assessment Resources.

Loranger, A. W., Hirschfeld, R. M. A., Sartorius, N., & Regier, D. A. (1991). The WHO/ADAMHA international pilot study of personality disorders: Background and purpose. *Journal of Personality Disorders, 5,* 296–306.

Loranger, A. W., Lenzenweger, M. F., Gartner, A. F., Susman, V. L., Herzig, J., Zammit, G. K., Gartner, J. D., Abrams, R. C., & Young, R. C. (1991). Trait–state artifacts and the diagnosis of personality disorders. *Archives of General Psychiatry, 48,* 720–728.

Loranger, A. W., Oldham, J. M., Russakoff, L. M., & Susman, V. (1984). Structured interviews and borderline personality disorder. *Archives of General Psychiatry, 41,* 565–568.

Loranger, A. W., Sartorius, N., Andreoli, A., Berger, P., Buchheim, P., Channabasavanna, S. M., Coid, B., Dahl, A., Diekstra, R. F. W., Ferguson, B., Jacobsberg, L. B., Mombour, W., Pull, C., Ono, Y., & Regier, D. A. (1994). The International Personality Disorder Examination: The World Health Organization and Alcohol, Drug Abuse and Mental Health Administration international pilot study of personality disorders. *Archives of General Psychiatry, 51,* 215–224.

Loranger, A. W., Susman, V. L., Oldham, J. M., & Russakoff, L. M. (1985). *The Personality Disorder Examination (PDE): A structured interview for DSM-III-R personality disorders.* Unpublished manuscript, New York Hospital—Cornell Medical Center, White Plains, NY.

Loranger, A. W., Susman, V. L., Oldham, J. M., & Russakoff, L. M. (1987). The Personality Disorder Examination: A preliminary report. *Journal of Personality Disorders, 1,* 1–13.

Loving, J. L., Jr., & Russell, W. F. (2000). Selected Rorschach variables of psychopathic juvenile offenders. *Journal of Personality Assessment, 75,* 126–142.

Luce, K. H., & Crowther, J. H. (1999). The reliability of the Eating Disorder Examination—Self-Report Questionnaire Version (EDE-Q). *International Journal of Eating Disorders, 25,* 349–351.

Lukeoff, D., Nuechterlein, K. H., & Ventura, J. (1986). Manual for the expanded Brief Psychiatric Rating Scale (BPRS). *Schizophrenia Bulletin, 12,* 594–602.

Luria, R. E., & Guziec, R. J. (1981). Comparative description of the SADS and the PSE. *Schizophrenia Bulletin, 8,* 248–257.

Luria, R. E., & McHugh, P. R. (1974). Reliability and clinical utility of the "Wing" Present State Examination. *Archives of General Psychiatry, 30,* 866–871.

Lyketsos, C. G., Aritzi, S., & Lyketsos, G. C. (1994). Effectiveness of office-based practice using a structured diagnostic interview to guide treatment. *Journal of Nervous and Mental Disease, 182,* 720–723.

Lynam, D. R. (1996). Early identification of chronic offenders: Who is the fledgling psychopath? *Psychological Bulletin, 120,* 209–234.

Lynam, D. R. (1998). Early identification of the fledging psychopath: Locating the psychopathic child in the current nomenclature. *Journal of Abnormal Psychology, 107,* 566–575.

Lyon, M. J., True, W. R., Eisen, S. A., Goldberg, J., Meyer, J. M., Fararone, S. V., Eaves, L. J., & Tsuang, M. T. (1995). Differential heritability of adult and juvenile antisocial traits. *Archives of General Psychiatry, 52,* 906–915.

Maffei, C., Fossati, A., Agostoni, I., Barraco, A., Bagnato, M., Donati, D., Namia, C., Novella, L., & Petrachi, M. (1997). Interrater reliability and internal consistency of the Structured Clinical Interview for DSM-IV Axis II Personality Disorders (SCID-II), Version 2.0. *Journal of Personality Disorders, 11,* 279–284.

Maier, W., Buller, R., Sonntag, A., & Heuser, I. (1986). Subtypes of panic attacks and ICD–9 classification. *European Archives of Psychiatry and Neurological Sciences, 235,* 361–366.

Maier, W., Lichertermann, D., Klingler, T., Heun, R., & Hallmayer, J. (1992). Prevalences of personality disorders (DSM-III-R) in the community. *Journal of Personality Disorders, 6,* 187–196.

Malekzai, A. S. B., Niazi, J. M., Paige, S. R., Hendricks, S. E., Fitzpatrick, D., Leuschen, M. P., & Millimet, C. R. (1996). Modification of the CAPS–1 for diagnosis of PTSD in Afghan refugees. *Journal of Traumatic Stress, 9,* 891–898.

Malow, R. M., West, J. A., Williams, J. L., & Sutker, P. B. (1989). Personality disorder classification and symptoms in cocaine and opioid addicts. *Journal of Consulting and Clinical Psychology, 57,* 765–767.

Mann, A. H., Jenkins, R., & Belsey, E. (1981). The twelve-month outcome of patients with neurotic illness in general practice. *Psychological Medicine, 11,* 535–550.

Mann, A. H., Jenkins, R., Cutting, J. C., & Cowen, P. J. (1981). The development and use of a standardized assessment of abnormal personality. *Psychological Medicine, 11,* 839–847.

Mann, A. H., & Pilgrim, J. A. (1992). *Standardized Assessment of Personality: ICD–10 version.* London: University of London, Institute of Psychiatry.

Mann, A. H., Raven, P., Pilgraim, J., Khanna, S., Velayudham, A., Suresh, K. P., Channabasavanna, S. M., Janca, A., & Sartorius, N. (1999). An assessment of the Standardized Assessment of Personality as a screening instrument for the International Personality Disorder Examination: A comparison of informant and patient assessment for personality disorder. *Psychological Medicine, 29,* 985–989.

Manuzza, S., Fyer, A. J., Klein, D. F., & Endicott, J. (1986). Schedule for Affective Disorders and Schizophrenia—Lifetime Version modified for the study of anxiety disorders (SADS-LA): Rationale and conceptual development. *Journal of Psychiatric Research, 20,* 317–325.

Manuzza, S., Fyer, A. J., Martin, L. Y., Gallops, M. S., Endicott, J., Gorman, J., Liebowitz, M. R., & Klein, D. F. (1989). Reliability of anxiety assessment: I. Diagnostic agreement. *Archives of General Psychiatry, 46,* 1093–1101.

Marcotte, T. D., van Gorp, W., Hinkin, C. H., & Osato, S. (1997). Concurrent validity of the Neurobehavioral Cognitive Status Examination subtests. *Journal of Clinical and Experimental Neuropsychology, 19,* 386–395.

Marin, D. B., Kocsis, J. H., Frances, A. J., & Klerman, G. L. (1993). Personality disorders in dysthymia. *Journal of Personality Disorders, 7,* 223–231.

Marlatt, G. A., & Miller, W. R. (1984). *Comprehensive drinker profile.* Odessa, FL: Psychological Assessment Resources.

Marlowe, D. B., Husband, S. D., Bonieskie, L. M., Kirby, K. C., & Platt, J. J. (1997). Structured interview versus self-report test vantages for the assessment of personality pathology in cocaine dependence. *Journal of Personality Disorders, 11,* 177–190.

Marshall, L. A., & Cooke, D. J. (1999). The childhood experiences of psychopaths: A retrospective study of familial and societal factors. *Journal of Personality Disorders, 13,* 211–225.

Marton, P., Churchard, M., Kutcher, S., & Korenblum, M. (1991). Diagnostic utility of the Beck Depression Inventory with adolescent psychiatric outpatients and inpatients. *Canadian Journal of Psychiatry, 36,* 428–431.

Marziali, E., Munroe-Blum, H., & Links, P. (1994). Severity as a diagnostic dimension of borderline personality disorder. *Canadian Journal of Psychiatry, 39,* 540–544.

Maser, J. D., Kaelber, C., & Weise, R. E. (1991). International use and attitudes toward DSM-III and DSM-III-R: Growing consensus in psychiatric classification. *Journal of Abnormal Psychology, 100,* 271–279.

Masi, G., Mucci, M., Favilla, L., & Poli, P. (1999). Dysthymic disorder in adolescents with intellectual disability. *Journal of Intellectual Disability Research, 43,* 80–87.

Matarazzo, J. D. (1983). The reliability of psychiatric and psychological diagnosis. *Clinical Psychology Review, 3,* 103–145.

Mathisen, K. S., Evans, F. J., & Meyers, K. (1987). Evaluation of a computerized version of the Diagnostic Interview Schedule. *Hospital and Community Psychiatry, 38,* 1311–1315.

Mattanah, J. J. F., Becker, D. R., Levy, K. N., Edell, W. S., & McGlashan, T. H. (1995). Diagnostic stability in adolescents followed up 2 years after hospitalizations. *American Journal of Psychiatry, 152,* 889–894.

Maurer, K., Biehl, H., Kuhner, C., & Loffler, W. (1989). On the way to expert systems: Comparing DSM-III computer diagnosis with CATEGO (ICD) diagnoses in depressive and schizophrenic patients. *European Archives of Psychiatry and Neurological Sciences, 239,* 127–132.

Maurer, K., & Hafner, H. (1995). Methodological aspects on onset assessment in schizophrenia. *Schizophrenia Research, 15,* 265–276.

Mauri, M. Sarno, N., Rossi, V. M., Armani, A., Zambotto, S., Cassano, G. B., & Akiskal, H. S. (1992). Personality disorders associated with generalized anxiety, panic, and recurrent depressive disorders. *Journal of Personality Disorders, 6,* 162–167.

Mavreas, V. G., Beis, A., Mouyias, S., Rigoni, F., & Lyketsos, G. C. (1986). Prevalence of psychiatric disorders in Athens. *Social Psychiatry, 21,* 172–181.

Maziade, M., Roy, A.-A., Fournier, J.-P., Cliche, D., Merette, C., Caron, C., Garneau, Y., Montgrain, N., Shriqui, C., Dion, C., Nicole, L., Potvin, A., Lavallee, J.-C.,

Pires, A., & Raymond, V. (1992). Reliability of best-estimate diagnosis in genetic linkage studies of major psychoses. *American Journal of Psychiatry, 149,* 1674–1686.

Mazure, C., & Gershon, E. S. (1979). Blindness and reliability in lifetime psychiatric diagnosis. *Archives of General Psychiatry, 36,* 521–525.

McBride-Houtz, P. (1993). *Detecting cognitive impairment in older adults: A validation study of selected screening instruments.* Unpublished dissertation, University of North Texas, Denton.

McCaskill, P. A., Toro, P. A., & Wolfe, S. M. (1998). Homeless and matched housed adolescents: A comparative study of psychopathology. *Journal of Clinical Child Psychology, 27,* 306–319.

McCord, W. M., & McCord, J. (1964). *The psychopath: An essay on the criminal mind.* Princeton, NJ: Van Nostrand Reinhold.

McDermott, P. A., Alterman, A. I., Cacciola, J. S., Rutherford, M. J., Newman, J. P., & Mulholland, E. M. (2000). Generality of Psychopathy Checklist—Revised factors over prisoners and substance dependent patients. *Journal of Consulting and Clinical Psychology, 68,* 181–186.

McDonald, D. A., Nussbaum, D. N., & Bagby, R. M. (1991). Reliability, validity, and utility of the Fitness Interview Test. *Canadian Journal of Psychiatry, 36,* 480–484.

McDonald-Scott, P., & Endicott, J. (1984). Informed versus blind: The reliability of cross-sectional ratings of psychopathology. *Psychiatry Research, 12,* 207–217.

McGee, R., & Stanton, W. (1990). Parent reports of disability among 13-year-olds with DSM-III disorders. *Journal of Child Psychology and Psychiatry, 31,* 793–801.

McGorry, P., Bell, R. C., Dugeon, P. L., & Jackson, H. J. (1998). The dimensional structure of first episode psychosis: An exploratory factor analysis. *Psychological Medicine, 28,* 935–941.

McGorry, P., Copolov, D., & Singh, B. (1990). The Royal Park Multidiagnostic Instrument for Psychosis: Part I. Rationale and review. *Schizophrenia Bulletin, 16,* 501–515.

McGorry, P., Kaplan, I., Dossetor, C., Copolov, D., & Singh, B. (1988). *The Royal Park Multidiagnostic Instrument for Psychosis: A comprehensive assessment procedure for the acute psychotic episode (RPMIP).* Melbourne, Australia: Department of Psychological Medicine, Monash University.

McGorry, P. D., Mihalopoulos, C., Henry, L., Dakis, J., Jackson, H. J., Flaum, M., Harrigan, S., McKenzie, D., Kulkarni, J., & Karoly, R. (1995). Spurious precision: Procedural validity of diagnostic assessment in psychotic disorders. *American Journal of Psychiatry, 152,* 220–223.

McGorry, P., Singh, B., Copolov, D. L., Kaplan, I., Dossetor, C. R., & van Riel, R. J. (1990). The Royal Park Multidiagnostic Instrument for Psychosis: Part II. Development, reliability, and validity. *Schizophrenia Bulletin, 16,* 501–515.

McGorry, P., Singh, B., Connell, S., McKenzie, D., van Riel, R. J., & Copolov, D. L. (1992). Diagnostic concordance in functional psychosis revisited: A study of the inter-relationships between alternative concepts of psychotic disorder. *Psychological Medicine, 22,* 367–378.

McHugh, P. R., & Folstein, M. F. (1988). Organic mental disorders. In R. Michels, J. O. Cavenar, A. M. Cooper, S. B. Guze, L. L. Judd, G. L. Klerman, & A. J. Solnit (Eds.), *Psychiatry* (Vol. 1, Chap. 73). Philadelphia: Lippincott.

McKeon, J., Roa, B., & Mann, A. (1984). Life events and personality traits in obsessive–compulsive neurosis. *British Journal of Psychiatry, 144,* 185–189.

McLellan, A. T., Kushner, H., Metzger, D., Peters, R. Smith, I., Grissom, G., Pettinati, H., & Argeriou, M. (1992). The fifth edition of the Addiction Severity Index. *Journal of Substance Abuse Treatment, 9,* 199–213.

McLellan, A. T., Luborsky, L., Cacciola, J., & Griffith, J. E. (1985). New data on the Addiction Severity Index: Reliability and validity at three centers. *Journal of Nervous and Mental Disease, 173,* 412–423.

McLellan, A. T., Luborsky, L., Woody, G. E., & O'Brien, C. P. (1980). An improved diagnostic evaluation instrument for substance abuse patients: The Addiction Severity Index. *Journal of Nervous and Mental Disease, 168,* 26–33.

McManus, M., Brickman, A., Alessi, N. E., & Grapetine, W. L. (1984). Borderline personality in serious delinquents. *Comprehensive Psychiatry, 25,* 446–454.

McManus, M., Lerner, H., Robbins, D., & Barbour, C. (1984). Assessment of borderline symptomatology in hospitalized adolescents. *Journal of the American Academy of Child Psychiatry, 23,* 685–694.

Medin, D. L., Altom, M. W., Edelson, S. M., & Freko, D. (1982). Correlated symptoms and simulated medical classification. *Journal of Experimental Psychology: Learning, Memory, and Cognition, 8,* 37–50.

Meehl, P. E. (1990). Toward an integrated theory of schizotaxia, schizotypy, and schizophrenia. *Journal of Personality Disorders, 4,* 1–99.

Meek, P. S., Clark, H. W., & Solana, B. L. (1989). Neurocognitive impairment: The unrecognized component of dual diagnosis in substance abuse treatment. *Journal of Psychoactive Drugs, 21,* 153–160.

Mellman, T. A., Leverich, G. S., Hauser, P., Kramlinger, K., Post, R. M., & Uhde, T. W. (1992). Axis II pathology in panic and affective disorders: Relationship to diagnosis, course of illness, and treatment response. *Journal of Personality Disorders, 6,* 53–63.

Melton, G. B., Petrila, J., Poythress, N. G., & Slobogin C. (1997). *Psychological evaluations for the courts* (2nd ed.). New York: Guilford.

Melzack, R. (1975). The McGill Pain Questionnaire: Major properties and scoring methods. *Pain, 1,* 277–299.

Menezes, P. R., Rodrigues, L. C., & Mann, A. H. (1997). Predictors of clinical and social outcomes after hospitalization in schizophrenia. *European Archives of Psychiatry and Clinical Neurosciences, 247,* 137–145.

Merikangas, K. R. (1981). *The reliability of assortative mating to social adjustment and course of illness in primary affective disorder.* Unpublished doctoral dissertation, University of Pittsburgh, Pittsburgh, PA.

Merritt, K. A., Thompson, R. J., Jr., Keith, B. R., Johndrow, D. A., & Murphy, L. B. (1993). Screening for behavior and emotional problems in primary care pediatrics. *Developmental and Behavioral Pediatrics, 14,* 340–343.

Messer, S. C., & Beidel, D. C. (1994). Psychosocial correlates of childhood anxiety disorders. *Journal of the American Academy of Child and Adolescent Psychiatry, 33,* 975–983.

Meyer, R. G., & Deitsch, S. E. (1996). *The clinician's handbook: Integrated diagnostics, assessment, and intervention in adult and adolescent psychopathology* (4th ed.). Boston: Allyn & Bacon.

Meyer-Bahlburg, H. F. L., & Ehrhardt, A. A. (1988). *Gender Role Assessment Sched-*

ule—Child (GRAS-C). Unpublished interview schedule, New York State Psychiatric Institute, New York.

Mignolli, G., Faccinicani, C., Turit, L., Gavioli, I., & Micciolo, R. (1988). Interrater reliability of the PSE–9 (full version): An Italian study. *Social Psychiatry and Psychiatric Epidemiology, 23,* 30–35.

Miller, D. D., Flaum, M., Arndt, S., Fleming, F., & Andreasen, N. C. (1994). Effect of antipsychotic withdrawal on negative symptoms in schizophrenia. *Neuropsychopharmocology, 11,* 11–20.

Miller, D. D., Perry, P. J., Cadoret, R. J., & Andreasen, N. C. (1994). Clozapine's effect on negative symptoms in treatment refractory schizophrenics. *Comprehensive Psychiatry, 35,* 8–15.

Miller, L. S., & Kamboukos, D. (2000). Symptom-specific measures for disorder usually first diagnosed in infancy, childhood, or adolescence. In A. J. Rush, H. A. Pincus, M. B. First, D. Blacker, J. Endicott, S. J. Keith, K. A. Phillips, N. D. Ryan, G. R. Smith, M. T. Tsuang, T. A. Widiger, & D. A. Zarin (Eds.), *Handbook of psychiatric measures* (pp. 325–356). Washington, DC: American Psychiatric Press.

Miller, M. W., Geddings, V. J., Levenston, G. K., & Patrick, C. J. (1994, March). *The personality characteristics of psychopathic and nonpsychopathic sex offenders.* Paper presented at the American Psychology–Law Society Biannual Conference, Sante Fe, NM.

Miller, W. R. (1978). Behavior treatment of problem drinkers: A comparative outcome study of three controlled drinking therapies. *Journal of Consulting and Clinical Psychology, 46,* 74–86.

Miller, W. R., Benefield, R. G., & Tonigan, J. S. (1992). Enhancing motivation for change in problem drinking: A controlled comparison of two therapist styles. *Journal of Consulting and Clinical Psychology, 61,* 455–461.

Miller, W. R., Crawford, V. L., & Taylor, C. A. (1979). Significant others as corroborative sources for problem drinkers. *Addictive Behaviors, 4,* 67–70.

Miller, W. R., & Dougher, M. J. (1989). Covert sensitization: Alternative treatment procedures for alcoholism. *Behavioral Psychotherapy, 17,* 203–220.

Miller, W. R., Gribskow, C. J., & Mortell, R. L. (1981). Effectiveness of a self-control manual for problem drinkers with and without therapist contact. *International Journal of the Addictions, 16,* 1247–1254.

Miller, W. R., Hedrick, K. E., & Taylor, C. A. (1983). Addictive behaviors and life problems before and after behavioral treatment of problem drinkers. *Addictive Behaviors, 8,* 403–412.

Miller, W. R., Leckman, A. L., Delaney, H. D., & Tinkcom, M. (1992). Long-term follow-up of behavioral self-control training. *Journal of Studies on Alcohol, 53,* 249–261.

Miller, W. R., & Marlatt, G. A. (1984). *Manual for the Comprehensive Drinker Profile.* Odessa, FL: Psychological Assessment Resources.

Miller, W. R., & Marlatt, G. A. (1987). *Comprehensive Drinker Profile: Manual supplement.* Odessa, FL: Psychological Assessment Resources.

Miller, W. R., Sovereign, R. G., & Krege, B. (1988). Motivational interviewing with problem drinkers: II. The drinker's check-up as a preventive intervention. *Behavioral Psychotherapy, 16,* 251–268.

Miller, W. R., & Taylor, C. A. (1980). Relative effectiveness of bibliotherapy, individual and group self-control training in the treatment of problem drinkers. *Addictive Behaviors, 5,* 13–24.

Miller, W. R., Taylor, C. A., & West, J. C. (1980). Focused versus broad-spectrum behavior therapy for problem drinkers. *Journal of Consulting and Clinical Psychology, 48,* 590–601.

Miller-Johnson, S., Winn, D. M., Coie, J., Maumary-Gremaud, A., Hyman, C., Terry, R., & Lochman, J. (1999). Motherhood during the teen years: A developmental perspective on the risk factors of childbearing. *Development and Psychopathology, 11,* 85–100.

Millon, T. (1982). *Millon Clinical Multiaxial Inventory—II.* Minneapolis: National Computer Systems.

Millon, T. (1991). Classification in psychopathology: Rationale, alternatives, and standards. *Journal of Abnormal Psychology, 100,* 245–261.

Millon, T., Simonsen, E., Birket-Smith, M., & Davis, R. D. (Eds.). (1998). *Psychopathy: Antisocial, criminal and violent behaviors.* New York: Guilford Press.

Mirin, S. M., & Weiss, R. D. (1983). Substance abuse. In E. L. Bassuk, S. C. Schoonover, & A. J. Gelenberg (Eds.), *The practitioner's guide to psychoactive drugs* (pp. 221–291). New York: Plenum Medical.

Mitrushina, M., Abara, J., & Blumenfeld, A. (1994). Aspects of validity and reliability on the Neurobehavioral Cognitive Status Examination (NCSE) in the assessment of psychiatric patients. *Journal of Psychiatric Research, 28,* 85–95.

Modestin, J., Erni, T., & Oberson, B. (1998). Comparison of self-report and interview diagnoses of DSM-III-R personality disorders. *European Journal of Personality, 12,* 445–455.

Modestin, J., Oberson, B., & Erni, T. (1997). Possible correlates with DSM-III-R personality disorders. *Acta Psychiatrica Scandinavica, 96,* 424–430.

Moffitt, T. E. (1993). Adolescence-limited and life-course-persistent antisocial behavior: A developmental taxonomy. *Psychological Review, 100,* 674–701.

Molto, J., Poy, R., & Torrubia, R. (2000). Standardization of the Hare Psychopathy Checklist—Revised in a Spanish prison sample. *Journal of Personality Disorders, 14,* 84–96 .

Monsen, J. T., Odland, T, Faugli, A., Daae, E., & Eilertsen, D. E. (1995). Personality disorders: Changes and stability after intensive psychotherapy focusing on affect consciousness. *Psychotherapy Research, 5,* 33–48.

Morey, L. C. (1991a). Classification of mental disorder as a collection of hypothetical constructs. *Journal of Abnormal Psychology, 100,* 289–293.

Morey, L. C. (1991b). *Personality Assessment Inventory: Professional manual.* Tampa, FL: Psychological Assessment Resources.

Morey, L. C., Waugh, M. H., & Blashfield, R. K. (1985). MMPI scores for the DSM-III personality disorders: Their derivation and correlates. *Journal of Personality Assessment, 49,* 245–251.

Morgan, J. F., Lacey, J. H., & Sedgwick, P. M. (1999). Impact of pregnancy on bulimia nervosa. *British Journal of Psychiatry, 174,* 135–140.

Morika, N., Miyake, Y., Minakawa, K., Ikuta, N., & Nishizono-Maher, A. (1993). Diagnosis and clinical features of borderline personality disorder in the East and West: A preliminary report. *Comprehensive Psychiatry, 34,* 418–423.

Mueller, J. (1988). A new test for dementia syndromes. *Diagnosis, 10,* 33–40.

Mungas, D., Reed, B. R., Marshall, S. C., & Gonzalez, H. M. (2000). Development of psychometrically matched English and Spanish language neuropsychological tests for older persons. *Neuropsychology, 14,* 209–223.

Murphy, G. E., Woodruff, M., & Herjanic, M. (1974). Primary affective disorder: Selection efficiency of two sets of diagnostic criteria. *Archives of General Psychiatry, 31,* 182–184.

Murphy, G. E., Woodruff, M., Herjanic, M., & Fischer, J. R. (1974). Validity of clinical course of a primary affective disorder. *Archives of General Psychiatry, 30,* 757–761.

Murphy, G. L., & Medlin, D. L. (1985). The role of theories in conceptual coherence. *Psychological Review, 92,* 289–316.

Murphy, J. L. (1986). Cross-cultural psychiatry. In R. Michels, J. O. Cavenar, A. M. Cooper, S. B. Guze, L. L. Judd, G. L. Klerman, & A. J. Solnit (Eds.) *Psychiatry* (Vol. 3, Chapt. 2). Philadephia: Lippincott.

Murphy, J. M., & Helzer, J. E. (1985). Epidemiology of schizophrenia in adulthood. In R. Michels, J. O. Cavenar, A. M. Cooper, S. B. Guze, L. L. Judd, G. L. Klerman, & A. J. Solnit (Eds.), *Psychiatry* (Vol. 3, Chapt. 15). Philadephia: Lippincott.

Murray, R. M., Oon, M. C. H., Rodnight, R., Bireley, J. L. T., & Smith, A. (1979). Increased excretion of dimethyltryptamine and certain features of psychosis: A possible association. *Archives of General Psychiatry, 36,* 644–649.

Murrie, D. C., & Cornell, D. G. (2000). The Millon Adolescent Clinical Inventory and psychopathy. *Journal of Personality Assessment, 75,* 110–125.

Myers, J. K., & Weissman, M. M. (1980). Use of a self-report symptom scale to detect depression in a community sample. *American Journal of Psychiatry, 137,* 1081–1084.

Myers, J. K., Weissman, M. M., Tischler, G. L., Holzer, C. E., III, Leaf, P. J., Orvaschel, H., Anthony, J. C., Boyd, J. H., Burke, J. D., Kramer, M., & Stoltzman, R. (1984). Six-month prevalence of psychiatric disorders in three communities: 1980–1982. *Archives of General Psychiatry, 41,* 959–967.

Myers, W. C., Burket, R. C., Lyles, B., Stone, L., & Kemph, J. P. (1990). DSM-III diagnoses and offenses in committed female juvenile delinquents. *Bulletin of the American Academy of Psychiatry and Law, 18,* 47–54.

Myers, W. C., & Kemph, J. P. (1990). DSM-III-R classification of murderous youth: Help or hindrance? *Journal of Clinical Psychiatry, 51,* 239–242.

National Institute of Mental Health. (1991). *NIMH Diagnostic Interview for Children, Version 2.3.* Rockville, MD: Author.

Nazikian, H., Rudd, R. P., Edwards, J., & Jackson, H. J. (1990). Personality disorder assessment for psychiatric inpatients. *Australian and New Zealand Journal of Psychiatry, 24,* 37–46.

Nazroo, J. Y., Edwards, A. C., & Brown, G. W. (1997). Gender differences in the onset of depression following a shared life event: A study of couples. *Psychological Medicine, 27,* 9–19.

Neal, L. A., Busuttil, W., Herapath, R., & Strike, P. W. (1994). Development and validation of the computerized Clinician-Administered Posttraumatic Stress Disorder Scale-1—Revised. *Psychological Medicine, 24,* 701–706.

Nelson, A., Fogel, B. S., & Faust, D. (1986). Bedside cognitive screening instruments: A critical assessment. *Journal of Nervous and Mental Disease, 174,* 73–83.

Nelson, C. B., Rehm, J., Ustun, T. B., Grant, B., & Chatterji, S. (1999). Factor structure for DSM-IV substance disorder criteria endorsed by alcohol, cannabis, cocaine, and opiate users: Results from the WHO reliability and validity study. *Addictions, 94,* 843–855.

Nelson, E., & Rice, J. (1997). Stability of diagnosis of obsessive–compulsive disorder in the Epidemiologic Catchment Area study. *American Journal of Psychiatry, 154,* 826–831.

Nelson, H. F., Tennen, H., Tasman, A., Borton, M., Kubeck, M., & Stone, M. (1985). Comparison of three systems for diagnosing borderline personality disorder. *American Journal of Psychiatry, 142,* 855–858.

Nelson-Gray, R. O., Johnson, D., Foyle, L. W., Daniel, S. S., & Harmon, R., Jr. (1996). The effectiveness of cognitive therapy tailored to depressives with personality disorders. *Journal of Personality Disorders, 10,* 132–152.

Nestadt, G., Bienvenu, O. J., Cai, G., Samuels, J., & Eaton, W. W. (1998). Incidence of obsessive–compulsive disorder in adults. *Journal of Nervous and Mental Disease, 186,* 401–406.

Neufeld, K. J., Swartz, K. L., Bienvenu, O. J., Eaton, W. W., & Cai, G. (1999). Incidence of DIS/DSM-IV social phobia in adults. *Acta Psychiatrica Scandinavica, 100,* 186–192.

Newman, J. P., & Schmitt, W. A. (1998). Passive avoidance in psychopathic offenders: A replication and extension. *Journal of Abnormal Psychology, 107,* 527–532.

Newman, S. C., & Bland, R. C. (1998). Incidence of mental disorders in Edmonton: Estimates of rates and methodological issues. *Journal of Psychiatric Research, 32,* 273–282.

Nicholson, R. A. (1992, August). *Defining and assessing competency to stand trial.* Paper presented at the American Psychological Association annual convention, Washington, DC.

Nicholson, R. A., Briggs, S. R., & Robertson, H. C. (1988). Instruments for assessing competency to stand trial: How do they work? *Professional Psychology: Research and Practice, 19,* 383–394.

Nicholson, R. A., & Kugler, K. E. (1991). Competent and incompetent criminal defendants: A quantitative review of comparative research. *Psychological Bulletin, 109,* 357–370.

Nicholson, R. A., Robertson, H. C., Johnson, W. G., & Jensen, G. (1988). A comparison of instruments for assessing competency to stand trial. *Law and Human Behavior, 12,* 313–321.

Ni Nuallain, M., O'Hare, A., & Walsh, D. (1990). The prevalence of schizophrenia in three counties in Ireland. *Acta Psychiatrica Scandinavica, 82,* 136–140.

Norris, M. P., & May, M. C. (1998). Screening for malingering in a correctional setting. *Law and Human Behavior, 22,* 315–323.

North, C. S., Pollio, D. E., Thompson, S. J., Ricci, A. A., Smith, E. M., & Spitznagel, E. L. (1997). A comparison of clinical and structured interview diagnoses in a homeless mental health clinic. *Community Mental Health Journal, 35,* 531–543.

North, C. S., Smith, E. M., Pollio, D. E., & Spitznagel, E. L. (1996). Are the mentally ill homeless a distinct homeless group? *Annals of Clinical Psychiatry, 8,* 117–128.

North, C. S., Smith, E. M., & Spitznagel, E. L. (1997). One-year follow-up of survivors of a mass shooting. *American Journal of Psychiatry, 154,* 1696–1702.

Novy, D. M., Nelson, D. V., Berry, L. A., & Averill, P. M. (1995). What does the Beck Depression Inventory measure in chronic pain?: A reappraisal. *Pain, 61,* 261–270.

Noyes, R., Reich, J., Christiansen, J., Suelzer, M., Pfohl, B., & Coryell, W. A. (1990). Outcome of panic disorder: Relationship of diagnostic subtypes and comorbidity. *Archives of General Psychiatry, 47,* 809–818.

Nunes, E. V., Goehl, L., Seracini, A., Deliyannides, D., Donovan, S., Koegniz, T.,

Quitkin, F. M., & Williams, J. B. W. (1996). A modification of the Structured Clinical Interview for DSM-III-R to evaluate methadone patients. *American Journal on Addictions, 5,* 241–248.

Nurnberger, J. I., Blehar, M. C., Kaufmann, C. A., York-Cooler, C., Simpson, G., Harkavy-Friedman, J., Sever, J. B., Malaspina, D., Reich, T., Miller, M., Bowman, E. S., DePaulo, J. R., Cloninger, C. R., Robinson, G., Moldin, S., Gershon, E. S., Maxwell, E., Guroff, J., Kirch, D., Wynne, D., Berg, K., Tsuang, M., Pepple, J. R., Faraone, S., & Ritz, A. L. (1994). Diagnostic Interviews for Genetic Studies: Rationale, unique features, and training. *Archives of General Psychiatry, 51,* 849–859.

Nussbaum, D. N., & Rogers, R. (1992). Screening psychiatric patients for Axis II disorders. *Canadian Journal of Psychiatry, 37,* 658–660.

O'Boyle, M., & Self, D. (1990). A comparison of two interviews for DSM-III-R personality disorders. *Psychiatry Research, 32,* 85–92.

O'Conner, D. W. (1990). The contribution of CAMDEX to the diagnosis of mild dementia in community surveys. *Psychiatric Journal of the University of Ottawa, 15,* 216–220.

Ogloff, J. R. P., Wong, S., & Greenwood, A. (1990). Treating criminal psychopaths in a therapeutic community program. *Behavioral Sciences and the Law, 8,* 181–190.

Ohta, T., Okazaki, Y., & Anzai, N. (1985). Reliability of the Japanese version of the Scale for the Assessment of Negative Symptoms (SANS). *Japanese Journal of Psychiatry, 13,* 999–1010.

Okasha, A., & Ashour, A. (1981). Psycho-demographic study of anxiety in Egypt: The PSE in its Arabic version. *British Journal of Psychiatry, 139,* 70–73.

Oldham, J. M., Skodol, A. E., Kellman, H. D., Hyler, S. E., Rosnick, L., & Davies, M. (1992). Diagnosis of DSM-III-R personality disorders by two structured interviews: Patterns of comorbidity. *American Journal of Psychiatry, 149,* 213–220.

Olin, J. T., & Zelinski, E. M. (1991). The 12-month reliability of the Mini-Mental State Examination. *Psychological Assessment: A Journal of Clinical and Consulting Psychology, 3,* 427–432.

Oltmanns, T. F. (1998). [Unpublished data on the SIDP-IV reliability with Air Force recruits]. University of Virginia, Charlottesville.

Omer, H., Foldes, J., Toby, M., & Menczel, J. (1983). Screening for cognitive deficits in a sample of hospitalized geriatric patients. *Journal of American Geriatrics Society, 31,* 266–268.

Orley, J. H., & Wing, J. K. (1979). Psychiatric disorders in two African villages. *Archives of General Psychiatry, 36,* 513–520.

Ormel, J., Koeter, M. W. J., Van Den Brink, W., & Giel, R. (1989). Concurrent validity of GHQ–28 and PSE as measures of change. *Psychological Medicine, 19,* 1007–1013.

Orvaschel, H. (1990). Early onset psychiatric disorder in high risk children and increased familial morbidity. *Journal of the American Academy of Child and Adolescent Psychiatry, 29,* 184–188.

Orvaschel, H., Puig-Antich, J., Chambers, W., Tabrizi, M. A., & Johnson, R. (1982). Retrospective assessment of child psychopathology with the Kiddie-SADS-E. *Journal of the American Academy of Child Psychiatry, 21,* 392–397.

Osherson, D. N., & Smith, E. E. (1981). On the adequacy of prototype theory as a theory of concepts. *Cognition, 9,* 35–58.

Othmer, E., Penick, E. C., & Powell, B. J. (1981). *The Psychiatric Diagnostic Interview.* Los Angeles: Western Psychological Services.

Othmer, E., Penick, E. C., Powell, B. J., Othmer, S., & Read, M. R. (1989). *The Psychiatric Diagnostic Interview—Revised.* Los Angeles: Western Psychological Services.

Otto, R. K., Poythress, N. G., Nicholson, R. A., Edens, J. F., Monahan, J., Bonnie, R. J., Hoge, S. K., & Eisenberg, M. (1998). Psychometric properties of the MacArthur Competence Assessment Tool-Criminal Adjudication. *Psychological Assessment, 10,* 435–443.

Palmer, R. L., Christie, M., Cordle, C., Davis, D., & Kedrick, J. (1987). The Clinical Eating Disorders Rating Instrument (CEDRI): A preliminary description. *International Journal of Eating Disorders, 6,* 9–14.

Panzetta, A. F. (1974). Toward a scientific psychiatric nosology: Conceptual and pragmatic issues. *Archives of General Psychiatry, 30,* 154–161.

Paradis, C. M., Friedman, S., Lazar, R. M., Grubea, J., & Kesselman, M. (1992). Use of a structured interview to diagnose anxiety disorders in a minority population. *Hospital and Community Psychiatry, 43,* 61–64.

Paris, J., Zelkowitz, P., Guzder, J., Joseph, S., & Feldman, R. (1999). Neuropsychological factors associated with borderline pathology in children. *Journal of the American Academy of Child and Adolescent Psychiatry, 38,* 770–774.

Paulhus, D. L. (1998). *Paulhus deception scales.* Toronto: Multi-Health Systems.

Pecknold, J. C., Chang, H., Fleury, D., Koszychi, D., Quirion, R., Nair, N. P. V., & Suranyi-Cadotte, B. E. (1987). Platelet imipramine binding in patients with panic disorder and major familial depression. *Psychiatry Research, 21,* 319–326.

Pellegrino, J. F., Singh, N. N., & Carmanico, S. J. (1999). Concordance among three diagnostic procedures for identifying depression in children and adolescents with EBD. *Journal of Emotional and Behavioral Disorders, 7,* 118–127.

Penick, E. C., Powell, B. J., Nickel, E. J., Bingham, S. F., Riesenmy, K. R., Read, M. R., & Campbell, J. (1994). Co-morbidity of lifetime psychiatric disorder among male alcoholic patients. *Alcoholism: Clinical and Experimental Research, 18,* 1289–1293.

Perez, R. G., Ascaso, L. E., Massons, J. M. D., & Chaparro, N. O. (1998). Characteristics of the subject and the interview influencing the test–retest reliability of the Diagnostic Interview for Children and Adolescents—Revised. *Journal of Child Psychology and Psychiatry, 39,* 963–972.

Perry, J. C., & Klerman, G. L. (1978). The borderline patient: A comparative analysis of four sets of diagnostic criteria. *Archives of General Psychiatry, 35,* 141–150.

Perry, J. C., & Klerman, G. L. (1980). Clinical features of the borderline personality disorder. *American Journal of Psychiatry, 137,* 165–173.

Perry, J. C., Lavori, P. W., Cooper, S. H., Hoke, L., & O'Connell, M. E. (1987). The Diagnostic Interview Schedule and DSM-III antisocial personality disorder. *Journal of Personality Disorders, 1,* 121–131.

Peters, L., & Andrews, G. (1995). Procedural validity of the computerized version of the Composite International Diagnostic Interview (CIDI-Auto) in the anxiety disorders. *Psychological Medicine, 25,* 1269–1280.

Peters, L., Clark, D., & Carroll, F. (1998). Are computerized interviews equivalent to human interviews? CIDI-Auto versus CIDI in anxiety and depressive disorders. *Psychological Medicine, 28,* 893–901.

Peveler, R. C., & Fairburn, C. G. (1990). Measurement of neurotic symptoms by self-report questionnaire: Validity of the SCL-90-R. *Psychological Medicine, 20,* 873–879.

Pfeffer, C. R. (1986). *The suicidal child.* New York: Guilford Press.

Pfeiffer, E. (1975). A Short Portable Mental Status Questionnaire for the assessment of organic brain deficit in elderly patients. *Journal of the American Geriatrics Society, 23,* 433–441.

Pfohl, B., Barrash, J., True, B., & Alexander, B. (1989). Failure of two Axis II measures to predict medication noncompliance among hypertensive outpatients. *Journal of Personality Disorders, 3,* 45–52.

Pfohl, B., Blum, N., & Zimmerman, M. (1995). *The Structured Interview for DSM-IV Personality: SIDP-IV.* Iowa City: University of Iowa.

Pfohl, B., Blum, N., Zimmerman, M., & Stangl, D. (1989). *The Structured Interview for DSM-III Personality Disorders: SIDP-R.* Iowa City: University of Iowa.

Pfohl, B., Coryell, W., Zimmerman, M., & Stangl, D. (1986). DSM-III personality disorders: Diagnostic overlap and internal consistency of individual DSM-III criteria. *Comprehensive Psychiatry, 27,* 21–34.

Pfohl, B., Coryell, W., Zimmerman, M., & Stangl, D. (1987). Prognostic validity of self-report and interview measures of personality disorder in depressed inpatients. *Journal of Clinical Psychiatry, 48,* 468–472.

Pfohl, B., Stangl, D., & Zimmerman, M. (1982). *The Structured Interview for DSM-III Personality Disorders (SIDP).* Iowa City: University of Iowa.

Pfohl, B., Stangl, D., & Zimmerman, M. (1984). The implications of DSM-III personality disorders for patients with major depression. *Journal of Affective Disorders, 7,* 309–319.

Philipp, M., & Maier, W. (1986). The Polydiagnostic Interview: A structured interview for the polydiagnostic classification of psychiatric patients. *Psychopathology, 19,* 175–185.

Phillips, K. A., & Fallon, B. (2000). Somatoform and factitious disorders and malingering measures. In A. J. Rush, H. A. Pincus, M. B. First, D. Blacker, J. Endicott, S. J. Keith, K. A. Phillips, N. D. Ryan, G. R. Smith, M. T. Tsuang, T. A. Widiger, & D. A. Zarin (Eds.), *Handbook of psychiatric measures* (pp. 591–616). Washington, DC: American Psychiatric Press.

Piacentini, J., Shaffer, D., Fisher, P., Schwab-Stone, M., Davies, M., & Gioia, P. (1993). The Diagnostic Interview Schedule for Children—Revised version (DISC-R): III. Concurrent criterion validity. *Journal of American Academy of Child and Adolescent Psychiatry, 32,* 658–665.

Pica, S., Edwards, J., Jackson, H. J., Bell, R. C., Bates, G. W., & Rudd, R. P. (1990). Personality disorders in recent-onset bipolar disorder. *Comprehensive Psychiatry, 31,* 499–510.

Pike, K. M., Wolk, M. A., Gluck, M., & Walsh, B. T. (2000). Eating disorders measures. In A. J. Rush, H. A. Pincus, M. B. First, D. Blacker, J. Endicott, S. J., Keith, K. A. Phillips, N. D., Ryan, G. R. Smith, M. T. Tsuang, T. A. Widiger, & D. A. Zarin (Eds.), *Handbook of psychiatric measures* (pp. 647–672). Washington, DC: American Psychiatric Press.

Pilgrim, J. A., & Mann, A. H. (1990). Use of the ICD–10 version of the Standardized Assessment of Personality to determine the prevalence of personality disorder in psychiatric inpatients. *Psychological Medicine, 20,* 985–992.

Pilgrim, J. A., Mellers, J. D., Boothby, H. A., & Mann, A. H. (1993). Interrater and temporal reliability of the Standardized Assessment of Personality and the influence of informant characteristics. *Psychological Medicine, 23,* 779–786.

Pilkonis, P. A., & Frank, E. (1988). Personality pathology in recurrent depression: Nature prevalence, and relationship to treatment response. *American Journal of Psychiatry, 145,* 435–441.

Pilkonis, P. A., Heape, C. L., Proietti, J. M., Clark, S. W., McDavid, J. D., & Pitts, T. E. (1995). The reliability and validity of two structured diagnostic interviews for personality disorders. *Archives of General Psychiatry, 52,* 1025–1033.

Pilkonis, P. A., Heape, C. L., Ruddy, J., & Serrao, P. (1991). Validity in the diagnosis of personality disorders: The use of the LEAD standard. *Psychological Assessment: A Journal of Consulting and Clinical Psychology, 3,* 46–54.

Pincus, A. L., & Wiggins, J. S. (1990). Interpersonal problems and conceptions of personality disorders. *Journal of Personality Disorders, 4,* 342–352.

Pini, S., Cassano, G. B., Simonimi, E., Savino, M., Russo, A., & Montgomery, S. A. (1997). Prevalence of anxiety disorders comorbidity in bipolar depression, unipolar depression, and dysthymia. *Journal of Affective Disorders, 42,* 145–153.

Pitman, R. K., Altman, B., & Macklin, M. L. (1989). Prevalence of posttraumatic stress disorder in wounded Vietnam veterans. *American Journal of Psychiatry, 146,* 667–669.

Pollock, P. H. (1996). A cautionary note on the determination of malingering in offenders. *Psychology, Crime, and Law, 3,* 97–110.

Pope, H. G., Jr., Jonas, J. M., Hudson, J. I., Cohen, B. M., & Gunderson, J. G. (1983). The validity of DSM-III borderline personality disorder: A phenomenologic, family history, treatment response and long-term follow-up study. *Archives of General Psychiatry, 40,* 23–30.

Pope, H. G., Jr., Jonas, J. M., Hudson, J. I., Cohen, B. M., & Tohen, M. (1985). An empirical study of borderline personality disorder. *American Journal of Psychiatry, 142,* 1285–1290 .

Powell, B. J., Penick, E. C., & Othmer, E. (1985). The discriminant validity of the Psychiatric Diagnostic Interview. *Journal of Clinical Psychiatry, 46,* 320–322.

Poythress, N., G., Nicholson, R., Otto, R. K., Edens, J. F., Bonnie, R. J., Monahan, J., & Hoge, S. K. (1999). *Professional manual for the MacArthur Competence Assessment Tool—Criminal Adjudication.* Odessa, FL: Psychological Assessment Resources.

Poznanski, E. O., Grossman, J. A., Buchsbaum, Y., Banegas, M., Freeman, L., & Gibbons, R. (1984). Preliminary studies of the reliability and validity of the Children's Depression Rating Scales. *Journal of the American Academy of Child and Adolescent Psychiatry, 23,* 191–197.

Prange, M. E., Greenbaum, P. E., Silver, S. E., Friedman, R. M., Kutash, K., & Duchnowski, A. J. (1992). Family functioning and psychopathology among adolescents with severe emotional disturbances. *Journal of Abnormal Child Psychology, 20,* 83–102.

Preisig, M., Fenton, B. T., Matthey, M. L., Berney, A., & Ferrero, F. (1999). Diagnostic Interview for Genetic Studies (DIGS): Interrater and test–retest reliability of the French version. *European Archives of Psychiatry and Clinical Neurosciences, 249,* 174–179.

Prohovnik, I., Smith, G., Sackeim, H. A., Mayeux, R., & Stern, Y. (1989). Gray-matter degeneration in presenile Alzheimer's disease. *Annals of Neurology, 25,* 117–124.

Puente, A. E. (1990). Psychological assessment with minority group members. In G. Goldstein & M. Hersen (Eds.), *Handbook of psychological assessment* (2nd ed.) (pp. 505–520). New York: Pergamon Press.

Puig-Antich, J., & Chambers, W. J. (1978). *Schedule for Affective Disorders and Schizophrenia for School-Age Children: Kiddie SADS (K-SADS).* New York: Department of Child and Adolescent Psychiatry, New York State Psychiatric Institute.

Putnam, F. W., Noll, J., & Steinberg, M. (2000). Dissociative disorders measures. In A. J. Rush, H. A. Pincus, M. B. First, D. Blacker, J. Endicott, S. J. Keith, K. A. Phillips, N. D. Ryan, G. R. Smith, M. T. Tsuang, T. A. Widiger, & D. A. Zarin (Eds.), *Handbook of psychiatric measures* (pp. 617–630). Washington, DC: American Psychiatric Press.

Raczek, S. W. (1992). Childhood abuse and personality disorders. *Journal of Personality Disorders, 6,* 109–116.

Radloff, L. S. (1977). The CES-D scale: A self-report depression scale for research in the general population. *Applied Psychological Measurement, 3,* 385–401.

Rangel, L., Garralda, E., Levin, M., & Roberts, H. (2000). Personality in adolescents with chronic fatigue syndrome. *European Child and Adolescent Psychiatry, 9,* 39–45.

Rapee, R. M., Barrett, P. M., Dadds, M., & Evans, L. (1994). Reliability of the DSM-III-R childhood anxiety disorders using a structured interview: Interrater and parent–child agreement. *Journal of the American Academy of Child Psychiatry, 33,* 984–992.

Rapp, S. R., Parisi, S. A., & Walsh, D. A. (1988). Psychological dysfunction and physical health among elderly medical inpatients. *Journal of Consulting and Clinical Psychology, 56,* 851–855.

Rapp, S. R., Parisi, S. A., Walsh, D. A., & Wallace, C. E. (1988). Detecting depression in elderly medical inpatients. *Journal of Consulting and Clinical Psychology, 56,* 509–513.

Rees, A., Hardy, G. E., & Barkham, M. (1997). Covariance in the measurement of depression/anxiety and three cluster C personality disorders (avoidant, dependent, obsessive-compulsive). *Journal of Affective Disorders, 45,* 143–153.

Regier, D. A., Myers, J. K., Kramer, M., Robins, L. N., Blazer, D. G., Hough, R. L., Eaton, W. W., & Locke, B. Z. (1984). The NIMH Epidemiologic Catchment Area Program: Historical context, major objectives and study population characteristics. *Archives of General Psychiatry, 41,* 934–941.

Reich, J. (1986). The relationship between early life events and DSM-III personality disorders. *Hillsdale Journal of Clinical Psychiatry, 8,* 164–173.

Reich, J. (1988). DSM-III personality disorders and the outcome of treated panic disorder. *American Journal of Psychiatry, 145,* 1149–1152.

Reich, J. (1990). The effect of personality on placebo response in panic patients. *Journal of Nervous and Mental Disease, 178,* 699–702.

Reich, J., & Troughton, E. (1988a). Comparison of DSM-III personality disorders in recovered depressed and panic disorder patients. *Journal of Nervous and Mental Disease, 176,* 300–304.

Reich, J., & Troughton, E. (1988b). Frequency of DSM-III personality disorders in patients with panic disorder: Comparison with psychiatric and normal control subjects. *Psychiatry Research, 26,* 89–100.

Reich, W. (1992). Structured and semi-structured interviews. In L. K. G. Hsu & M.

Hersen (Eds.), *Research in psychiatry: Issues, strategies, and methods* (pp. 175–193). New York: Plenum.

Reich, W., & Earls, F. (1984). *Home Environment Interview for Children (HEIC)*. St. Louis: Washington University.

Reich, W., & Earls, F. (1987). Rules for making psychiatric diagnoses in children on the basis of multiple sources of information: Preliminary strategies. *Journal of Abnormal Child Psychology, 15,* 601–606.

Reich, W., & Earls, F. (1990). Interviewing adolescents by telephone: Is it a useful methodological strategy? *Comprehensive Psychiatry, 31,* 211–215.

Reich, W., Earls, F., Frankel, O., & Shayka, J. J. (1993). Psychopathology in children of alcoholics. *Journal of the American Academy of Child Psychiatry, 32,* 995–1002.

Reich, W., Earls, F., & Powell, J. (1988). A comparison of the home and social environments of children of alcoholic and non-alcoholic parents. *British Journal of Addiction, 83,* 831–839.

Reich, W., Herjanic, B., Welner, Z., & Gandhy, P. R. (1982). Development of a structured psychiatric interview for children: Agreement on diagnosis comparing child and parent interviews. *Journal of Abnormal Child Psychology, 10,* 325–336.

Reich, W., & Kaplan, L. (1994). The effects of psychiatric and psychosocial interviews on children. *Comprehensive Psychiatry, 35,* 50–53.

Reich, W., Shayka, J. J., & Taibleson, C. (1991a). *Diagnostic Interview for Children and Adolescents (DICA-R-A): Adolescent version.* St. Louis: Washington University.

Reich, W., Shayka, J. J., & Taibleson, C. (1991b). Diagnostic Interview for Children and Adolescents (DICA-R-C): Child version. St. Louis: Washington University.

Reich, W., Shayka, J. J., & Taibleson, C. (1991c). *Diagnostic Interview for Children and Adolescents (DICA-R-P): Parent version.* St. Louis: Washington University.

Reid, D. W., Tierney, M. C., Zorzitto, M. S., Snow, W. G., & Fisher, R. H. (1991). On the clinical value of the London Psychogeriatric Rating Scale. *Journal of the American Geriatric Society, 39,* 368–371.

Reinhardt, V. (2000). [Understanding of Axis I symptoms by Hispanic patients]. Unpublished raw data.

Reisberg, B., Ferris, S. H., De Leon, M. J., & Crook, T. (1982). The Global Deterioration Scale for assessment of primary degenerative dementia. *American Journal of Psychiatry, 139,* 1136–1139.

Reitan, R. M., & Wolfson, D. (1988). *Traumatic brain injury: Vol. 2. Recovery and rehabilitation.* Tucson, AZ: Neuropsychology Press.

Remington, M., Tyrer, P. J., Newson-Smith, J., & Cicchetti, D. V. (1979). Comparative reliability of categorical and analogue rating scales in the assessment of psychiatric symptomatology. *Psychological Medicine, 9,* 765–770.

Renneberg, B., Chambless, D. L., Dowdall, D. J., Fauerbach, J. A., & Gracely, E. J. (1992). The Structured Clinical Interview for DSM-III-R, Axis II and the Millon Clinical Multiaxial Inventory: A concurrent validity study of personality disorders among anxious outpatients. *Journal of Personality Disorders, 6,* 117–124.

Reynolds, C. R. (Ed.). (1998). *Detection of malingering during head injury litigation.* New York: Plenum.

Reynolds, C. F., III, Soloff, P. H., Kupfer, D. J., Taska, L. S., Fresifo, K., Coble, P. A., & McNamara, M. E. (1985). Depression in borderline patients: A prospective EEG sleep study. *Psychiatry Research, 22,* 1–15.

Reynolds, W. M. (1987). *Reynolds Adolescent Depression Scale: Professional manual.* Odessa, FL: Psychological Assessment Resources.

Ribera, J. C., Canino, G., Rubio-Stipec, M., Bravo, M., Bauermeister, J. J., Alegria, M., Woodbury, M., Huertas, S., Guevera, L. M., Bird, H. R., Freeman, D., & Shrout, P. E. (1996). The Diagnostic Interview Schedule for Children (DISC–2.1) in Spanish: Reliability in a Hispanic population. *Journal of Child Psychology and Psychiatry, 37,* 195–204.

Rice, M. E., & Harris, G. T. (1995). Psychopathy, schizophrenia, alcohol abuse, and violent recidivism. *International Journal of Law and Psychiatry, 18,* 333–342.

Richman, H., & Nelson-Gray, R. (1994). Nonclinical panicker personality: Profile and discriminative ability. *Journal of Anxiety Disorders, 8,* 33–47.

Riley, K. (1988). Measurement of dissociation. *Journal of Nervous and Mental Disease, 176,* 449–450.

Rippetoe, P. A., Alarcon, R. D., & Walter-Ryan, W. G. (1986). Interactions between depression and borderline personality disorder. *Psychopathology, 19,* 340–346.

Riskland, J. H., Beck, A. T., Berchick, R. J., Brown, G., & Steer, R. A. (1987). Reliability of DSM-III diagnoses for major depression and generalized anxiety disorder using the Structured Clinical Interview for DSM-III. *Archives of General Psychiatry, 44,* 817–820.

Riso, L. P., Klein, D. N., Anderson, R. L., Ouimette, P. C., & Lizardi, H. (1994). Concordance between patients and informants on the Personality Disorder Examination. *American Journal of Psychiatry, 151,* 568–573.

Roberts, R. E., Chen, Y. W., & Solovitz, B. L. (1995). Symptoms of DSM-III-R major depression among Anglo, African and Mexican American adolescents. *Journal of Affective Disorders, 36,* 1–9.

Robins, E., & Guze, S. B. (1970). Establishment of diagnostic validity in psychiatric illness: Its application of schizophrenia. *American Journal of Psychiatry, 126,* 107–111.

Robins, L. N. (1966). *Deviant children grow up.* Baltimore: Williams & Wilkins.

Robins, L. N. (1985). Epidemiology: Reflections on testing the validity of psychiatric interviews. *Archives of General Psychiatry, 42,* 918–924.

Robins, L. N. (1987). The assessment of psychiatric diagnosis in epidemiological studies. In M. M. Weissman (Ed.), *Psychiatric epidemiology: APA Annual Review* (pp. 592–607). Washington, DC: American Psychiatric Press.

Robins, L. N., Cottler, L. Bucholz, K., & Compton, W. (1995). *Diagnostic Interview Schedule, Version IV.* St. Louis: Washington School of Medicine.

Robins, L. N., Cottler, L. B., & Keating, S. (1991). *NIMH Diagnostic Interview Schedule, Version III—Revised (DIS-III-R): Question by question specifications.* St. Louis: Washington University School of Medicine.

Robins, L. N., & Helzer, J. E. (1991, December). *The half-life of a structured interview—the NIMH Diagnostic Interview Schedule (DIS).* Paper presented at the Annual Meeting of the American Public Health Association, Atlanta, GA.

Robins, L. N., Helzer, J. E., Cottler, L. B., Works, J., Goldring, E., McEvoy, L., & Stoltzman, R. (1985). *The DIS version III-A, training manual.* St. Louis: Washington University School of Medicine.

Robins, L. N., Helzer, J. E., Cottler, L. B., & Goldring, E. (1989). *NIMH Diagnostic Interview Schedule, Version III—Revised.* St. Louis: Washington University School of Medicine.

Robins, L. N., Helzer, J. E., Croughan, J., & Ratcliff, J. S. (1981). National Institute of Mental Health Diagnostic Interview Schedule. *Archives of General Psychiatry,* *38,* 381–389.

Robins, L. N., Helzer, J. E., Orvaschel, H., Anthony, J. C., Blazer, D., Burnam, M. A., Burke, J. D., Jr., & Eaton, W. W. (1982). Validity of the Diagnostic Interview Schedule, Version II: DSM-III diagnoses. *Psychological Medicine, 12,* 855–870.

Robins, L. N., Helzer, J. E., Weissman, M. M., Orvaschel, H., Gruenberg, E., Burke, J. D., Jr., & Regier, D. A. (1984). Lifetime prevalence of specific psychiatric disorders in three sites. *Archives of General Psychiatry, 41,* 949–958.

Robins, L. N., & Marcus, S. C. (1987). The Diagnostic Screening Procedure Writer: A tool to develop individualized screening procedures. *Medical Care, 25*(12), 106–122.

Robins, L. N., Wing, J. K., Wittchen, H. U., Helzer, J. E., Babor, T. R., Burke, J., Farmer, A., Jablenski, A., Pickens, R., Regier, D. A., Sartorius, N., & Towle, L. H. (1988). The Composite International Diagnostic Interview: An epidemiologic instrument suitable for use in conjunction with different diagnostic systems and in different cultures. *Archives of General Psychiatry, 45,* 1069–1077.

Rodgers, B., & Mann, S. A. (1986). The reliability and validity of PSE assessments by lay interviewers: A national population survey. *Psychological Medicine, 16,* 689–700.

Roemer, L., Borkovec, M., Posa, S., & Borkovec, T. D. (1995). A self-report diagnostic measure of generalized anxiety disorder. *Journal of Behavioral Therapy and Experimental Psychiatry, 26,* 345–350.

Roesch, R., Jackson, M. A., Sollner, R., Eaves, D., Glackman, W., & Webster, C. D. (1984). The fitness to stand trial interview test: How four professions rate videotaped fitness interviews. *International Journal of Law and Psychiatry, 7,* 115–131.

Roesch, R., Webster, C. D., & Eaves, D. (1984). *The Fitness Interview Test: A method for examining fitness to stand trial.* Toronto: Research Report, Center of Criminology, University of Toronto.

Roesch, R., Webster, C. D., & Eaves, D. (1994). *The Fitness Interview Test* (rev. ed.). Burnaby, BC: Mental Health, Law and Policy Institute.

Roesch, R., Zapf, P. A., Eaves, D., & Webster, C. D. (1998). *The Fitness Interview Test* (rev. ed.). Burnaby, BC: Mental Health, Law and Policy Institute.

Rogers, R. (1984). Towards an empirical model of malingering and deception. *Behavioral Sciences and the Law, 2,* 93–112.

Rogers, R. (1986). *Conducting insanity evaluations.* New York: Van Nostrand Reinhold.

Rogers, R. (1988). Structured interviews and dissimulation. In R. Rogers (Ed.), *Clinical assessment of malingering and deception* (pp. 250–268). New York: Guilford Press.

Rogers, R. (1990a). Development of a new classificatory model of malingering. *Bulletin of the American Academy of Psychiatry and Law, 18,* 323–333.

Rogers, R. (1990b). Models of feigned mental illness. *Professional Psychology: Research and Practice, 21,* 182–188.

Rogers, R. (1992). *Structured Interview of Reported Symptoms.* Tampa, FL: Psychological Assessment Resources.

Rogers, R. (1995). *Evaluation of Competency to Stand Trial (ECST): Professional manual.* Unpublished manuscript, University of North Texas, Denton.

Rogers, R. (Ed.) (1997). *Clinical assessment of malingering and deception* (2nd ed.). New York: Guilford.

Rogers, R. (1998, August). *Munchausen by proxy: Extrapolations from malingering and deception.* NIH Research Conference on Munchausen by Proxy, Stockholm, Sweden.

Rogers, R. (2000). The uncritical acceptance of risk assessment in forensic practice. *Law and Human Behavior, 24,* 595–605.

Rogers, R. (in press). Validating retrospective assessments: An overview of research models. In R. I. Simon & D. W. Shuman (Eds.), *Predicting the past: The retrospective assessment of mental states in civil and criminal litigation.* Washington, DC: American Psychiatric Press.

Rogers, R. & Bagby, M. (1994). Dimensions of psychopathy: A factor analytic study of the MMPI antisocial personality scale. *International Journal of Offender Therapy and Comparative Criminology, 38,* 297–308.

Rogers, R., Bagby, R. M., & Dickens, S. E. (1992). *Structured Interview of Reported Symptoms (SIRS) and professional manual.* Odessa, FL: Psychological Assessment Resources.

Rogers, R., Bagby, R. M., & Prendergast, P. (1993). *Vulnerability of the Structured Interview of DSM-III-R (SCID) to dissimulation and distortion.* Unpublished manuscript, University of North Texas, Denton, TX.

Rogers, R., Bagby, R. M., & Rector, N. (1989). Diagnostic legitimacy of factitious disorder with psychological symptoms. *American Journal of Psychiatry, 146,* 1312–1314.

Rogers, R., Bagby, R. M., Vincent, A. (1994). Factitious disorders with predominantly psychological signs and symptoms: A conundrum for forensic experts. *Journal of Psychiatry and Law, 22,* 99–106.

Rogers, R., & Cavanaugh, J. L., Jr. (1981). Application of the SADS diagnostic interview to forensic psychiatry. *Journal of Psychiatry and Law, 9,* 329–344.

Rogers, R., Cavanaugh, J. L., Jr., & Dolmetsch, R. (1981). Schedule of Affective Disorders and Schizophrenia, a diagnostic interview in evaluations of insanity: An exploratory study. *Psychological Reports, 49,* 135–138.

Rogers, R., & Cruise, K. R. (2000). Malingering and deception among psychopaths. In C. B. Gacono (Ed.), *The clinical and forensic assessment of psychopathy: A practitioner's guide* (pp. 269–284). New York: Erlbaum.

Rogers, R., & Cunnien, A. J. (1986). Multiple SADS evaluation in the assessment of criminal defendants. *Journal of Forensic Sciences, 30,* 222–230.

Rogers, R., & Dion, K. L. (1991). Rethinking the DSM-III-R diagnosis of antisocial personality disorder. *Bulletin of the American Academy of Psychiatry and Law, 19,* 21–31.

Rogers, R., Dion, K. L., & Lynett, E. (1992). Diagnostic validity of antisocial personality disorder: A prototypical analysis. *Law and Human Behavior, 16,* 677–689.

Rogers, R., Duncan, J. C., & Sewell, K. W. (1994). Prototypical analysis of antisocial personality disorder: DSM-IV and beyond. *Law and Human Behavior, 18,* 471–484.

Rogers, R., Gillis, J. R., & Bagby, R. M. (1990). Cross validation of the SIRS with a correctional sample. *Behavioral Sciences and the Law, 8,* 85–92.

Rogers, R., Gillis, J. R., Bagby, R. M., & Monteiro, E. (1991). Detection of malingering on the SIRS: A study of coached and uncoached simulators. *Psychological Assessment: A Journal of Consulting and Clinical Psychology, 3,* 673–677.

Rogers, R., Gillis, J. R., Dickens, S. E., & Bagby, R. M. (1991). Standardized assessment of malingering: Validation of the SIRS. *Psychological Assessment: A Journal of Clinical and Consulting Psychology, 3,* 89–96.

Rogers, R., Gillis, J. R., Turner, R. E., & Smith, T. (1990). The clinical presentation of command hallucinations. *American Journal of Psychiatry, 147,* 1304–1307.

Rogers, R., & Grandjean, N. (2000, March). *Competency measures and the Dusky standard: A conceptual mismatch?* Paper presented at the biennial convention of the American Psychology–Law Society, New Orleans.

Rogers, R., Grandjean, N., Tillbrook, C. E., Vitacco, M. J., & Sewell, K. W. (2001). *Recent interview-based measures of competency to stand trial: A critical review augmented with research data.* Manuscript submitted for publication.

Rogers, R., Harrell, E. H., & Liff. C. D. (1993). Feigning neuropsychological impairment: A critical review of methodological and clinical considerations. *Clinical Psychology Review, 13,* 255–274.

Rogers, R., Harris, M., & Wasyliw, O. E. (1983). Observed and self-reported psychopathology in NGRI acquittees in court mandated outpatient treatment. *International Journal of Offender Therapy and Comparative Criminology, 27,* 143–149.

Rogers, R., Hinds, J. D., & Sewell, K. W. (1996). Feigning psychopathology among adolescent offenders: Validation of the SIRS, MMPI-A, and SIMS. *Journal of Personality Assessment, 67,* 244–257.

Rogers, R., Johansen, J., Chang, J. J., & Salekin, R. T. (1997). Predictors of adolescent psychopathy: Oppositional and conduct-disordered symptoms. *Journal of the American Academy of Psychiatry and Law, 25,* 261–271.

Rogers, R., & Kelly, K. S. (1997). Denial and misreporting of substance abuse. In R. Rogers (Ed.), *Clinical assessment of malingering and deception* (2nd ed., pp. 108–129). New York: Guilford.

Rogers, R., Kropp, R., & Bagby, R. M. (1993). Faking specific disorders: A study of the Structured Interview of Reported Symptoms. *Journal of Clinical Psychology, 48,* 643–647.

Rogers, R., & Lynett, E. (1991). Role of Canadian psychiatry in dangerous offender testimony. *Canadian Journal of Psychiatry, 36,* 79–84.

Rogers, R., & Mitchell, C. N. (1991). *Mental health experts and the criminal courts: A handbook for lawyers and clinicians.* Toronto: Carswell.

Rogers, R., & Ornduff, S. R. (1994). Psychological measures in forensic assessments. In R. Rosner (Ed.), *Forensic psychiatry: A comprehensive textbook* (pp. 370–376). New York: Chapman and Hill.

Rogers, R., & Resnick, P. J. (1988). *Malingering and deception: Audiotape and guide.* New York: Guilford Publications.

Rogers, R., Salekin, R. T., Hill, C., Sewell, K. W., Murdock, M. E., & Neumann, C. E. (2000). The Psychopathy Checklist—Screening Version: An examination of criteria and subcriteria in three forensic samples. *Assessment, 7,* 1–15.

Rogers, R., Salekin, R. T., & Sewell, K. W. (1999). Validation of the Millon Multiaxial Inventory for Axis II disorders: Does it meet the Daubert standard? *Law and Human Behavior, 23,* 425–443.

Rogers, R., Salekin, R. T., & Sewell, K. W. (2000). The Millon Multiaxial Inventory: Separating rhetoric from reality. *Law and Human Behavior, 24,* 501–506.

Rogers, R., Salekin, R. T., Sewell, K. W., & Cruise, K. R. (2000). Prototypical analysis of antisocial personality disorder: A study of inmate samples. *Criminal Justice and Behavior, 27,* 216–233.

Rogers, R., Salekin, R. T., Sewell, K. W., Goldstein, A., & Leonard, K. (1998). A comparison of forensic and nonforensic malingerers: A prototypical analysis of explanatory models. *Law and Human Behavior, 22,* 353–367.

Rogers, R., Sewell, K. W., & Goldstein, A. (1994). Explanatory models of malingering: A prototypical analysis. *Law and Human Behavior, 18,* 543–552.

Rogers, R., Sewell, K. W., & Salekin, R. (1994). A meta-analysis of malingering on the MMPI-2. *Assessment, 1,* 227–237.

Rogers, R., Sewell, K. W., Ustad, K. L., Reinhardt, V., & Edwards, W. (1995). The Referral Decision Scale in a jail sample of disordered offenders. *Law and Human Behavior, 19,* 481–492.

Rogers, R., & Shuman, D. W. (2000). *Conducting insanity evaluations.* New York: Guilford Publications.

Rogers, R., Thatcher, A. A., & Cavanaugh, J. L., Jr. (1984). Use of the SADS diagnostic interview in evaluating legal insanity. *Journal of Clinical Psychology, 40,* 1538–1541.

Rogers, R., & Tillbrook, C. E. (1998). *Evaluation of Competency to Stand Trial-Revised (ECST-R): Professional manual.* Unpublished manuscript, University of North Texas, Denton.

Rogers, R., Ustad, K. L., & Salekin, R. T. (1998). Forensic applications of the PAI: A study of convergent validity. *Assessment, 5,* 3–12.

Rogers, R., Ustad, K. L., Sewell, K. W., & Reinhart, V. (1996). Dimensions of incompetency: A factor-analytic study of the Georgia Court Competency Test. *Behavioral Sciences and the Law, 14,* 323–330.

Rogers, R., & Vitacco, M. J. (in press). Forensic assessment of malingering and related response styles. In B. Van Dorsten (Ed.), *Forensic psychology: From classroom to courtroom.* Boston: Kluwer Academic/Plenum Publishers.

Rogers, R., Vitacco, M. J., Jackson, R. L., Martin, M., Collins, M., & Sewell, K. W. (2001, March). *Faking psychopathy? Response styles with antisocial youth.* Paper presentation for the Midwinter Conference of the Society for Personality Assessment, Philadelphia.

Rogers, R., & Wettstein, R. E. (1985). Relapse in NGRI patients: An empirical study. *International Journal of Offender Therapy and Comparative Criminology, 29,* 227–236.

Rogers, R., & Zinbarg, R. (1987). Bad or mad? Antisocial backgrounds of defendants evaluated for insanity. *International Journal of Law and Psychiatry, 10,* 75–80.

Romans-Clarkson, S. E., Walton, V. A., Herbison, G. P., & Mullen, P. E. (1990). Psychiatric morbidity among women in urban and rural New Zealand: Psychosocial correlates. *British Journal of Psychiatry, 156,* 84–91.

Rooney, M. T., Fristad, M. A., Weller, E. M., & Weller, R. A. (1999). *Administration manual for Children's Interview for Psychiatric Syndromes.* Washington, DC: American Psychiatric Press.

Rosch, E. (1973). On the internal structure of perceptual and semantic categories. In T. E. Moore (Ed.), *Cognitive development and the acquisition of language* (pp. 111–144). New York: Academic Press.

Rosch, E. (1978). Principles of categorization. In E. Rosch & B. B. Lloyd (Eds.), *Cognition and categorization* (pp. 27–48). Hillsdale, NJ: Erlbaum.

Rosen, A. M., & Fox, H. A. (1986). Tests of cognition and their relationship to psychiatric diagnosis and demographic variables. *Journal of Clinical Psychiatry, 47,* 495–498.

Rosen, J. C., Vara, L., Wendt, S., & Leitenberg, H. (1990). Validity studies of the Eating Disorder Examination. *International Journal of Eating Disorders, 9,* 519–528.

Rosen, W. G., Mohs, R. C., Johns, C. A., Small, N. S., Kendler, K. S., Horvath, T. B., & Davis, K. L. (1984). Positive and negative symptoms in schizophrenia. *Psychiatry Research, 13,* 277–284.

Rosenman, S. J., Korten, A. E., & Levings, C. T. (1997). Computerized diagnoses in acute psychiatry: Validity of the CIDI-Auto against routine clinical diagnoses. *Journal of Psychiatric Research, 31,* 581–592.

Rosowsky, E., & Gurian, B. (1991). Borderline personality disorder in late life. *International Psychogeriatrics, 3,* 39–52.

Ross, C. A. (1997). *Dissociative identity disorder: Diagnosis, clinical features, and treatment of multiple personality.* New York: Wiley.

Ross, C. A., Heber, S., Norton, G. R., Anderson, G., Anderson, D., & Barchet, P. (1989). The Dissociative Disorders Interview Schedule: A structured interview. *Dissociation, 2,* 169–189.

Ross, H. E., Gavin, D. R., & Skinner, H. A. (1990). Diagnostic validity of the MAST and the Alcohol Dependence Scale in the assessment of DSM-III alcohol disorders. *Journal of Studies on Alcohol, 51,* 506–513.

Ross, H. E., Swinson, R., Larkin, E. J., & Doumani, S. (1994). Diagnosing comorbidity in substance abusers. *Journal of Nervous and Mental Disease, 182,* 556–563.

Roth, M., Tym, E., Montjoy, C. Q., Huppert, F. A., Hendrie, H., Verma, S., & Goddard, R. (1986). CAMDEX: A standardized instrument for the diagnosis of mental disorders in the elderly with special reference to the early detection of dementia. *British Journal of Psychiatry, 149,* 698–709.

Rounsaville, B. J., Cacciola, J., Weissman, M. M., & Kleber, H. D. (1981). Diagnostic concordance in a follow-up study of opiate addicts. *Journal of Psychiatric Research, 16,* 191–201.

Rounsaville, B. J., & Poling, J. (2000). Substance abuse measures. In A. J. Rush, H. A. Pincus, M. B. First, D. Blacker, J. Endicott, S. J. Keith, K. A. Phillips, N. D. Ryan, G. R. Smith, M. T. Tsuang, T. A. Widiger, & D. A. Zarin (Eds.), *Handbook of psychiatric measures* (pp. 457–484). Washington, DC: American Psychiatric Press.

Rovner, B. W., & Folstein, M. F. (1987). Mini-Mental State Exam in clinical practice. *Hospital Practice, 22,* 99–110.

Rubio-Stipec, M., Bird, H., Canino, G., Bravo, M., & Alegria, M. (1991). Children of alcoholic parents in the community. *Journal of Studies on Alcohol, 52,* 78–88.

Rubio-Stipec, M., Shrout, P. E., Bird, H., Canino, G., & Bravo, M. (1989). Symptom scales of the Diagnostic Interview Schedule: Factor results in Hispanic and Anglo samples. *Psychological Assessment: A Journal of Consulting and Clinical Psychology, 1,* 30–34.

Ruegg R. G., Ekstrom, D. E., Dwight, L., & Golden, R. N. (1990). Introduction of a standardized report form improves the quality of Mental Status Examination reports by psychiatric residents. *Academic Psychiatry, 14,* 157–163.

Rutherford, M. J., Alterman, A. I., Cacciola, J. S., & McKay, J. R. (1998). Gender differences in the relationship of antisocial personality disorder criteria to Psychopathy Checklist—Revised scores. *Journal of Personality Disorders, 12,* 69–76.

Rutherford, M., Cacciola, J. S., Alterman, A. I., McKay, J. R., & Cook, T. G. (1999). The 2-year test–retest reliability of the Psychopathy Checklist—Revised in methadone patients. *Assessment, 6,* 285–291.

Rutter, M., & Graham, P. (1968). The reliability and validity of the Psychiatric Assessment of the Child: I. Interview with the child. *British Journal of Psychiatry, 114,* 563–579.

Ryan, N. D., Puig-Antich, J., Ambrosini, P., Rabinovich, H., Robinson, D., Nelson, B., Iyengar, S., & Twomey, J. (1987). The clinical picture of major depression in children and adolescents. *Archives of General Psychiatry, 44,* 854–861.

Salekin, R. T., Rogers, R., & Sewell, K. W. (1996). A review and meta-analysis of the Psychopathy Checklist and the Psychopathy Checklist—Revised: Predictive validity of dangerousness. *Clinical Psychology: Science and Practice, 3,* 203–215.

Salekin, R. T., Rogers, R., & Sewell, K. W. (1997). Construct validity of psychopathy in a female offender sample: A multitrait–multimethod evaluation. *Journal of Abnormal Psychology, 106,* 576–585.

Salekin, R. T., Rogers, R., Ustad, K. L., & Sewell, K. W. (1998). Psychopathy and recidivism among female inmates. *Law and Human Behavior, 22,* 109–128.

Salmon, D. P. (2000). Neuropsychiatric measures for cognitive measures. In A. J. Rush, H. A. Pincus, M. B. First, D. Blacker, J. Endicott, S. J. Keith, K. A. Phillips, N. D. Ryan, G. R. Smith, M. T. Tsuang, T. A. Widiger, & D. A. Zarin (Eds.), *Handbook of psychiatric measures* (pp. 417–456). Washington, DC: American Psychiatric Press.

Sanderson, W. C., DiNardo, P. A., Rapee, R. M., & Barlow, D. H. (1990). Syndrome comorbidity in patients diagnosed with a DSM-III-R anxiety disorder. *Journal of Abnormal Psychology, 98,* 308–312.

Sansone, R. A., & Fine, M. A. (1992). Borderline personality as a predictor of outcome in women with eating disorders. *Journal of Personality Disorders, 6,* 176–186.

Sansone, R. A., Fine, M. A., Seuferer, S., & Bovenzi, J. (1989). The prevalence of borderline personality symptomatology among women with eating disorders. *Journal of Clinical Psychology, 45,* 603–610.

Sansone, R. A., Sansone, L. A., & Fine, M. A. (1992). The relationship of obesity to borderline personality symptomatology, self-harm behaviors, and sexual abuse in female subjects in a primary care medical setting. *Journal of Personality Disorders, 9,* 254–265.

Sartorius, N., Ustun, T. B., Siva, J. A. C., Goldberg, D., Lecrubier, Y., Ormel, J., Von Korff, M., & Wittchen, H. U. (1993). International study of psychological problems in primary care. *Archives of General Psychiatry, 50,* 819–824.

Sato, T., Sakado, K., & Sato, S. (1993). Is there any specific personality disorder or personality disorder cluster that worsens the short-term treatment outcome of major depression? *Acta Psychiatrica Scandinavica, 88,* 342–349.

Schmidt, N. B., & Telch, M. J. (1990). Prevalence of personality disorders among bulimics, nonbulimic binge eaters, and normal controls. *Journal of Psychopathology and Behavioral Assessment, 12,* 169–185.

Schmidtt, F. A., Ranseen, J. D., & DeKosky, S. T. (1989). Cognitive mental status examinations. *Clinics of Geriatric Medicine, 5,* 545–564.

Schramke, C. J., Stow, R. M., Ratcliff, G., Goldstein, G., & Condray, R. (1998). Poststroke depression and anxiety: Different assessment methods result in variations in incidence and severity estimates. *Journal of Clinical and Experimental Neuropsychology, 20*, 723–737.

Schramm, E., Hohagen, F., Grasshoff, U., Riemann, D., Hajak, G., Hans-Gunther, W., & Berger, M. (1993). Test–retest reliability and validity of the Structured Interview for Sleep Disorders according to DSM-III-R. *American Journal of Psychiatry, 150*, 867–872.

Schroeder, M. L., Wormworth, J. A., & Livesley, W. J. (1992). Dimensions of personality disorder and their relationships to the Big Five dimensions of personality. *Psychological Assessment, 4*, 47–53.

Schwab-Stone, M., Fisher, P., Piacentini, J., Shaffer, D., Davies, M., & Briggs, M. (1993). The Diagnostic Interview Schedule for Children—Revised version (DISC-R): II. Test–retest reliability. *Journal of American Academy of Child and Adolescent Psychiatry, 32*, 651–657.

Schwab-Stone, M., Shaffer, D., Davies, M., Dulcan, M. K., Jensen, P. S., Fisher, P., Bird, H. R., Goodman, S. H., Lahey, B. B., Lichtman, J. H., Canino, G., Rubio-Stipec, M., & Rae, D. S. (1995). The Diagnostic Interview Schedule for Children—Version 2.3 (DISC-2.3). *Journal of American Academy of Child and Adolescent Psychiatry, 35*, 878–888.

Schwamm, L. H., VanDyke, C., Kiernan, R. J., Merrin, E. L., & Mueller, J. (1987). The Neurobehavioral Cognitive Status Examination: Comparison with Cognitive Capacity Screening Examination and the Mini-Mental State Examination in a neurosurgical population. *Annals of Internal Medicine, 107*, 486–491.

Schwartz, J. M., Aylward, E., Barta, P., Tune, L. E., & Pearlson, G. D. (1992). Sylvian fissure size in schizophrenia measured with the magnetic resonance imaging rating protocol of the consortium to establish a registry for Alzheimer's disease. *American Journal of Psychiatry, 149*, 1195–1198.

Schwenk, T. L., Coyne, J. C., & Fechner-Bates, S. (1996). Differences between detected and undetected patients in primary care and depressed psychiatric inpatients. *General Hospital Psychiatry, 18*, 407–415.

Secunda, S. K., Katz, M. M., Swann, A., Koslow, S. H., Maas, J. W., Chaung, S., & Croughan, J. (1985). Mania: Diagnosis, state measurement, and prediction of treatment response. *Journal of Affective Disorders, 8*, 113–121.

Segal, D. L., Hersen, M., & Van Hasselt, V. B. (1994). Reliability of the Structured Clinical Interview for DSM-III-R: An evaluative review. *Comprehensive Psychiatry, 35*, 316–327.

Segal, D. L., Kabacoff, R. I., Hersen, M., Van Hasselt, V. B., & Ryan, C. F. (1995). Update on the reliability of diagnosis in older psychiatric outpatients using the Structured Clinical Interview for DSM-III-R. *Journal of Clinical Geropsychology, 1*, 313–321.

Selzer, M. L. (1971). Michigan Alcoholism Screening Test: The quest for a new diagnostic instrument. *American Journal of Psychiatry, 127*, 1653–1658.

Selzer, M. L., Vinokur, A., & Van Rooijen, L. (1975). A self-administered Short Michigan Alcoholism Screening Test (SMAST). *Journal of Studies on Alcohol, 36*, 117–126.

Semler, G., Wittchen, H.-U., Joschke, K., Zaudig, M., von Geiso, T., Kaiser, S., von Cranach, M., & Pfister, H. (1987). Test–retest reliability of a standardized psychiatric interview (DIS/CIDI). *European Archives of Psychiatry and Neurological Sciences, 236*, 214–222.

Serin, R. C. (1993). Diagnosis of psychopathology with and without an interview. *Journal of Clinical Psychology, 49,* 367 372.

Serper, M. R., Bernstein, D. P., Maurer, G., Harvey, P. D., Horvath, T., Klar, H., Coccaro, E. F., & Siever, L. J. (1993). Psychological test profiles of patients with borderline and schizotypal personality disorders: Implications for DSM-IV. *Journal of Personality Disorders, 7,* 144–154.

Shadish, W. R., Jr., & Sweeney, R. B. (1991). Mediators and moderators in meta-analysis: There's a reason we don't let dodo birds tell us which psychotherapies should have prizes. *Journal of Consulting and Clinical Psychology, 59,* 883–893.

Shaffer, D., Schwab-Stone, M., Fisher, P., Cohen, P., Piacentini, J., Davies, M., Conners, C. K., & Regier, D. (1993). The Diagnostic Interview Schedule for Children—Revised version (DISC-R): I. Preparation, field testing, interrater reliability, and acceptability. *Journal of American Academy of Child and Adolescent Psychiatry, 32,* 643–650.

Shaffer, D., Schwab-Stone, M., Fisher, P., Davies, M., Piacentini, J., & Gioia, P. (1988). *A revised version of the Diagnostic Interview Schedule for Children (DISC-R): Results of a field trial and proposals for a new instrument (DISC-R).* Rockville, MD: Epidemiology and Psychopathology Research Branch, National Institute of Mental Health.

Shalev, A. Y., Freedman, S., Peri, T., Brandes, D., & Sahar, T. (1997). Predicting PTSD in traum survivors: Prospective evaluations of self-report and clinician-administered instruments. *British Journal of Psychiatry, 170,* 558–564.

Shaner, A., Roberts, L. J., Eckman, T. A., Racenstein, J. M., Tucker, D. E., Tsuang, J. W., & Mintz, J. (1998). Sources of diagnostic uncertainty for chronically psychotic cocaine abusers. *Psychiatric Services, 49,* 684–690.

Shapiro, M. B., Post, F., Lofving, B., & Inglis, J. (1956). "Memory function" in psychiatric patients over sixty: Some methodological and diagnostic implications. *Journal of Mental Sciences, 102,* 233–246.

Shapiro, S. K., & Garfinkel, B. D. (1986). The occurrence of behavior disorders in children: The interdependence of attention deficit disorder and conduct disorder. *Journal of the American Academy of Child Psychiatry, 25,* 809–819.

Shea, M. T., Glass, D. R., Pilkonis, P. A., Watkins, J., & Docherty, J. P. (1987). Frequency and implications of personality disorders in a sample of depressed outpatients. *Journal of Personality Disorders, 1,* 27–42.

Shear, M. K., Feske, U., Brown, C., Clark, D. B., Mammen, O., & Scotti, J. (2000). Anxiety disorder measures. In A. J. Rush, H. A. Pincus, M. B. First, D. Blacker, J. Endicott, S. J. Keith, K. A. Phillips, N. D. Ryan, G. R. Smith, M. T. Tsuang, T. A. Widiger, & D. A. Zarin (Eds.), *Handbook of psychiatric measures* (pp. 549–590). Washington, DC: American Psychiatric Press.

Sheehan, D. V., Lecrubier, Y., Sheehan, K. H., Amorim, P., Janavs, J., Weiller, E., Hergueta, T., Baker, R., & Dunbar, G. C. (1998). The Mini International Neuropsychiatric Interview (MINI): The development and validation of a structured diagnostic psychiatric interview for DSM-IV and ICD–10. *Journal of Clinical Psychiatry, 59*(Suppl. 20), 22–33.

Sheehan, D. V., Lecrubier, Y., Sheehan, K. H., Janavs, J., Weiller, E., Keskiner, A., Schinka, J., Knapp, E., Sheehan, M. R., & Dunbar, G. C. (1997). The validity of the Mini International Neuropsychiatric Interview (MINI) according to the SCID-P and its reliability. *European Psychiatry, 12,* 232–241.

Shelton, R. C., Davidson, J., Yonkers, K. A., Koran, L., Thase, M. E., Pearlstein, T., &

Halbreich, U. (1997). The undertreatment of dysthymia. *Journal of Clinical Psychiatry, 58,* 59–65.

Shrout, P. E., Spitzer, R. L., & Fleiss, J. L. (1987). Quantification of agreement in psychiatric diagnosis revisited. *Archives of General Psychiatry, 44,* 172–177.

Silk, K. R., Lohr, N. E., Ogata, S. N., & Westen, D. (1990). Borderline inpatients with affective disorder: Preliminary follow-up data. *Journal of Personality Disorders, 4,* 213–224.

Silverman, W. K., & Albano, A. M. (1996). *Anxiety Disorders Interview Schedule for DSM-IV Child Version (ADIS-IV-Child).* San Antonio, TX: Psychological Corporation.

Silverman, W. K., & Eisen, A. R. (1992). Age differences in the reliability of parent and child reports of child anxious symptomatology using a structured interview. *Journal of the American Academy of Child Psychiatry, 31,* 117–124.

Silverman, W. K., & Nelles, W. R. (1988). Anxiety Disorders Interview Schedule for Children. *Journal of the American Academy of Child Psychiatry, 27,* 772–778.

Silverstone, P. H. (1993). SCAN accurately gives diagnoses according to DSM-III-R criteria: Validation in psychiatric patients using SADS. *International Journal of Methods in Psychiatric Research, 3,* 209–213.

Silverthorn, P., & Frick, P. J. (1999). Developmental pathways to antisocial behavior: The delayed-onset pathway in girls. *Development and Psychopathology, 11,* 101–126.

Simon, R., Endicott, J., & Nee, J. (1987). Intake diagnoses: How representative? *Comprehensive Psychiatry, 28,* 389–396.

Singer, M. T., & Larson, D. G. (1981). Borderline personality and the Rorschach test. *Archives of General Psychiatry, 38,* 693–698.

Sinoff, G., Ore, L., Zlotogorsky, D., & Tamir, A. (1999). Short Anxiety Screening Test: A brief instrument for detecting anxiety in the elderly. *International Journal of Geriatric Psychiatry, 14,* 1062–1071.

Siris, S. G., Bermanzohn, P. C., Gonzalez, A., Mason, S. E., White, C. V., & Shuwall, M. A. (1991). The use of antidepressants for negative symptoms in a subset of schizophrenic patients. *Psychopharmacology Bulletin, 27,* 331–335.

Skeem, J. L., Golding, S. L., Cohn, N. B., & Berge, G. (1998). Logic and reliability of evaluations of competence to stand trial. *Law and Human Behavior, 22,* 519–547.

Skinner, H. A. (1982). The Drug Abuse Screening Test. *Addictive Behaviors, 7,* 363–371.

Skinner, H. A., & Blashfield, R. K. (1982). Increasing the impact of cluster analysis research: The case of psychiatric classification. *Journal of Consulting and Clinical Psychology, 50,* 727–735.

Skinner, H. A., & Horn, J. L. (1984). *Alcohol Dependence Scale (ADS): User's guide.* Toronto: Addiction Research Foundation.

Skodol, A. E., & Border, D. S. (2000). Diagnostic interviews for adults. In A. J. Rush, H. A. Pincus, M. B. First, D. Blacker, J. Endicott, S. J. Keith, K. A. Phillips, N. D. Ryan, G. R. Smith, M. T. Tsuang, T. A. Widiger, & D. A. Zarin (Eds.), *Handbook of psychiatric measures* (pp. 45–70). Washington, DC: American Psychiatric Press.

Skre, I., Onstad, S., Torgersen, S., & Kringlen, E. (1991). High interrater reliability for the Structured Clinical Interview for DSM-III-R Axis I (SCID-I). *Acta Psychiatrica Scandinavica, 84,* 167–173.

Skurla, E., Rogers, J. C., & Sunderland, T. (1988). Direct assessment of activities of daily living in Alzheimer's disease: A controlled study. *Journal of the American Geriatrics Society, 36,* 97–103.

Sletten, I. W., Altman, H., Evenson, R. C., & Cho, D. W. (1973). Computer assignment of psychotropic drugs. *American Journal of Psychiatry, 130,* 595–598.

Sletten, I. W., Ernhart, C. B., & Ulett, G. A. (1970). The Missouri Automated Mental Status Examination: Development, use and reliability. *Comprehensive Psychiatry, 11,* 315–327.

Sletten, I. W., & Evenson, R. C. (1972). The Missouri Automated Standard System of Psychiatry (SSOP): An overview. *Computer Medicine, 2,* 1–4.

Smith, A. (1967). The serial sevens subtraction test. *Archives of Neurology, 17,* 78–80.

Smith, D. E., Marcus, M. D., & Kaye, W. (1992). Cognitive-behavioral treatment of obese binge eaters. *International Journal of Eating Disorders, 12,* 257–262.

Smith, J., Carr, V., Morris, H., & Gilliland, J. (1988). The dexamethasone suppression test in relation to symptomatology: Preliminary findings controlling for serum dexamethasone concentrations. *Psychiatry Research, 25,* 123–133.

Soldz, S., Budman, S., Demby, A., & Merry, J. (1993a). Diagnostic agreement between the Personality Disorder Examination and the MCMI-II. *Journal of Personality Assessment, 60,* 486–499.

Soldz, S., Budman, S., Demby, A., & Merry, J. (1993b). Representation of personality disorders in circumplex and five-factor space: Explorations with a clinical sample. *Psychological Assessment, 5,* 41–52.

Soloff, P. H., George, A., Cornelius, J., Nathan, S., & Schulz, P. (1991). Pharmacotherapy and borderline subtypes. In J. M. Oldham (Ed.), *Personality disorders: New perspectives on diagnostic validity* (pp. 89–103). Washington, DC: American Psychiatric Press.

Soloff, P. H., & Ulrich, R. F. (1981). Diagnostic interview for borderline patients: A replication study. *Archives of General Psychiatry, 38,* 686–692.

Speltz, M. L., McClellan, J., DeKlyen, M., & Jones, K. (1999). Preschool boys with oppositional defiant disorder: Clinical presentation and diagnostic change. *Journal of the American Academy of Child and Adolescent Psychiatry, 38,* 838–845.

Spengler, P. A., & Wittchen, H. U. (1988). Procedural validity of standardized symptom questions for the assessment of psychotic symptoms: A comparison of the DIS with two clinical methods. *Comprehensive Psychiatry, 29,* 309–322.

Spielberger, C. D. (1973). *Preliminary manual for the State–Trait Anxiety Inventory for Children.* Palo Alto, CA: Consulting Psychologists Press.

Spiker, D. G., & Ehler, J. G. (1984). Structured psychiatric interviews for adults. In G. Goldstein & M. Hersen (Eds.), *Handbook of psychological assessment* (pp. 291–304). New York: Pergemon.

Spitzer, R. L. (1983). Psychiatric diagnosis: Are clinicians still necessary? *Comprehensive Psychiatry, 24,* 399–411.

Spitzer, R. L., & Endicott, J. (1970). *The Mental Status Evaluation Record (MSER).* New York: Biometrics Research.

Spitzer, R. L., & Endicott, J. (1975a). Psychiatric rating forms in the evaluation of psychiatric treatment. In A. M. Freedman, H. I. Kaplan, & B. J. Sadock (Eds.), *Comprehensive textbook in psychiatry* (Vol. 2, 2nd ed., pp. 2015–2031). Baltimore: Williams & Wilkins.

Spitzer, R. L., & Endicott, J. (1975b). *Schedule for Affective Disorders and Schizo-phrenia (SADS)* (2nd ed.). New York: Columbia University.

Spitzer, R. L., & Endicott, J. (1978a). *Schedule for Affective Disorders and Schizo-phrenia* (3rd ed.). New York: Biometrics Research.

Spitzer, R. L., & Endicott, J. (1978b). *Schedule for Affective Disorders and Schizo-phrenia—Change Version.* New York: Biometrics Research.

Spitzer, R. L., Endicott, J., Cohen, J., & Fleiss, J. L. (1974). Constraints on the validity of computer diagnosis. *Archives of General Psychiatry, 31,* 197–203.

Spitzer, R. L., Endicott, J., Fleiss, J. L., & Cohen, J. (1970). The Psychiatric Status Schedule: A technique of evaluating psychopathology and impairment in social role functioning. *Archives of General Psychiatry, 23,* 41–55.

Spitzer, R. L., Endicott, J., & Gibbon, M. (1979). Crossing the border into borderline personality and borderline schizophrenia. *Archives of General Psychiatry, 36,* 17–24.

Spitzer, R. L., Endicott, J., & Robins, E. (1975a). Clinical criteria for psychiatric diagnosis and DSM-III. *American Journal of Psychiatry, 132,* 1187–1192.

Spitzer, R. L., Endicott, J., & Robins, E. (1975b). *Research diagnostic criteria.* New York: New York State Psychiatric Institute, Biometrics Research.

Spitzer, R. L., Endicott, J., & Robins, E. (1978). Research diagnostic criteria for use in psychiatric research. *Archives of General Psychiatry, 35,* 773–782.

Spitzer, R. L., & Fleiss, J. L. (1974). A re-analysis of the reliability of psychiatric diagnosis. *British Journal of Psychiatry, 125,* 341–347.

Spitzer, R. L., Williams, J. B. W., & Gibbon, M. (1987a). *SCID personality question-naire.* New York: Biometrics Research.

Spitzer, R. L., Williams, J. B. W., & Gibbon, M. (1987b). *Structured Clinical Inter-view for DSM-III-R (SCID).* New York: Biometrics Research.

Spitzer, R. L., Williams, J. B. W., & Gibbon, M. (1987c). *Structured Clinical Inter-view for DSM-III-R personality disorders (SCID-II).* New York: Biometrics Re-search.

Spitzer, R. L., Williams, J. B. W., Gibbon, M., & First, M. B. (1989). *Instruction man-ual for the Structured Clinical Interview for DSM-III-R (SCID).* Washington, DC: American Psychiatric Press.

Spitzer, R. L., Williams, J. B. W., Gibbon, M., & First, M. B. (1990a). *SCID-II ques-tionnaire.* Washington, DC: American Psychiatric Press.

Spitzer, R. L., Williams, J. B. W., Gibbon, M., & First, M. B. (1990b). *Structured Clinical Interview for DSM-III-R (SCID).* Washington, DC: American Psychiatric Press.

Spitzer, R. L., Williams, J. B. W., Gibbon, M., & First, M. B. (1990c). *Structured Clin-ical Interview for DSM-III-R personality disorders (SCID-II).* Washington, DC: American Psychiatric Press.

Spitzer, R. L., Williams, J. B. W., Kroenke, K., Linzer, M., de Gruy, F. V., Hahn, S. R., Brody, D., & Johnson, J. G. (1994). Utility of a new procedure for diagnosing mental disorders in primary care: The PRIME-MD 1000 study. *Journal of the American Medical Association, 272,* 1749–1756.

Spitznagel, E. L., & Helzer, J. E. (1985). A proposed solution to the base rate problem in the kappa statistic. *Archives of General Psychiatry, 42,* 725–728.

Stalenheim, E. G., & von Knorring, L. (1996). Psychopathy and Axis I and Axis II psychiatric disorders in a forensic psychiatric population in Sweden. *Acta Psychi-atrica Scandinavica, 94,* 217–223.

Standage, K., & Ladha, N. (1988). An examination of the reliability of the Personality Disorder Examination and a comparison with other methods of identifying personality disorders in a clinical sample. *Journal of Personality Disorders, 2,* 267–271.

Stangl, D., Pfohl, B., Zimmerman, M., Bowers, W., & Corenthal, C. (1985). A structured interview for DSM-III personality disorders: A preliminary report. *Archives of General Psychiatry, 42,* 591–596.

Stavrakaki, C., Williams, E. C., Walker, S., Roberts, N., & Kotsopoulos, S. (1991). Pilot study of anxiety and depression in prepubertal children. *Canadian Journal of Psychiatry, 36,* 332–338.

Stefannson, J. G., Lindal, E., Bjornsson, J. K., & Guomundsdottir, A. (1991). Lifetime prevalence of specific mental disorders among people born in Iceland in 1931. *Acta Psychiatrica Scandinavica, 84,* 142–149.

Stein, S. J. (1987). Computer-assisted diagnosis in children's mental health. *Applied Psychology: An International Review, 36,* 343–355.

Steinberg, M. (1994). *Interviewer's guide to the Structured Clinical Interview for DSM-IV Dissociative Disorders (SCID-D).* Washington, DC: American Psychiatric Press.

Steinberg, M. (1996a). Diagnostic tools for assessing dissociation in children and adolescents. *Child and Adolescent Psychiatric Clinics of North America, 5,* 333–349.

Steinberg, M. (1996b). *Tips and techniques for assessing and planning treatment with dissociative disorder patients: A practical guide to the SCID-D.* Toronto: Multi-Health Systems.

Steinberg, M., Bancroft, J., & Buchanan, J. (1993). Multiple personality disorder in criminal law. *Bulletin of the American Academy of Psychiatry and the Law, 21,* 345–356.

Steinberg, M., & Hall, P. (1997). The SCID-D diagnostic interview and treatment planning for dissociative disorders. *Bulletin of the Menninger Clinic, 61,* 108–120.

Steinberg, M., Rounsaville, B., & Cicchetti, D. V. (1990). The Structured Clinical Interview for DSM-III-R Dissociative Disorders: Preliminary report on a new diagnostic instrument. *American Journal of Psychiatry, 147,* 76–82.

Stephens, J. H., Astrup, C., & Carpenter, W. T. (1982). A comparison of nine systems to diagnose schizophrenia. *Psychiatry Research, 6,* 127–143.

Stone, M. H. (1985). Borderline personality disorder. In R. Michels, J. O. Cavenar, A. M. Cooper, S. B. Guze, L. L. Judd, G. L. Klerman, & A. J. Solnit (Eds.), *Psychiatry* (Vol. 1, chap. 17). Philadephia: Lippincott.

Stonier, P. D. (1974). Score changes following repeated administration of Mental Status Questionnaire. *Age and Aging, 3,* 91–96.

Stout, A. L., Steege, J. F., Blazer, D. G., & George, L. K. (1986). Comparison of lifetime psychiatric diagnoses in premenstrual syndrome clinic and community samples. *Journal of Nervous and Mental Disease, 174,* 517–522.

Strain, J. J., Fulop, G., Lebovits, A., Ginsberg, B., Robinson, M., Stern, A., Charap, P., & Gany, F. (1988). Screening devices for diminished cognitive capacity. *General Hospital Psychiatry, 10,* 16–23.

Strakowski, S. M., Thohen, M., Stoll, A. L., Faedda, G. L., Mayer, P. V., Kolbrener, M. L., & Goodwin, D. C. (1993). Comorbidity in psychosis at first hospitalization. *American Journal of Psychiatry, 150,* 752–757.

Strober, M., Green, J., & Carlson, G. (1981). Reliability of psychiatric diagnosis in hospitalized adolescents. *Archives of General Psychiatry, 38,* 141–145.

Stuckenberg, K. W., Dura, J. R., & Kiecolt-Glaser, J. K. (1990). Depression screening scale validation in an elderly, community-dwelling population. *Psychological Assessment: A Journal of Clinical and Consulting Psychology, 2,* 134–138.

Sturt, E. (1981). Hierarchical patterns in the distribution of psychiatric symptoms. *Psychological Medicine, 11,* 783–794.

Sturt, E., & Wykes, T. (1987). Assessment schedules for chronic psychiatric patients. *Psychological Medicine, 17,* 485–493.

Sugawara, M., Mukai, T., Kitmura, T., Toda, M. A., Shima, S., Tomoda, A., Koizumi, T., Watanabe, K., & Ando, A. (1999). Psychiatric disorders among Japanese children. *Journal of the American Academy of Child and Adolescent Psychiatry, 38,* 444–452.

Sullivan, L. D., & Gretton, H. (1996, March). *Concurrent validity of the MMPI-A and the PCL-R in an adolescent forensic population.* Paper presented at the American Psychology–Law Society Convention, Hilton Head, SC.

Susser, E., & Wanderling, J. (1994). Epidemiology of nonaffective acute remitting psychosis vs. schizophrenia. *Archives of General Psychiatry, 51,* 294–301.

Svrakic, D. M., Whitehead, C., Przybeck, T. R., & Cloninger, C. R. (1993). Differential diagnosis of personality disorders by the seven-factor model of temperament and character. *Archives of General Psychiatry, 50,* 991–999.

Swanson, J. W., Borum, R., Swartz, M. S., & Monahan, J. (1996). Psychotic symptoms and disorders and the risk of violent behavior in the community. *Criminal Behavior and Mental Health, 6,* 309–329.

Swartz, L., Ben-Arie, O., & Teggin, A. F. (1985). Subcultural delusions and hallucinations: Comments on the Present State Examination in a multicultural context. *British Journal of Psychiatry, 146,* 391–394.

Swartz, M. S., Blazer, D. G., George, L. K., & Winfield, I. (1990). Estimating the prevalence of borderline personality disorder in the community. *Journal of Personality Disorders, 4,* 257–272.

Swartz, M. S., Blazer, D. G., George, L. K., Winfield, I., Zakris, J., & Dye, E. (1989). Identification of borderline personality disorder with the NIMH Diagnostic Interview Schedule. *American Journal of Psychiatry, 146,* 200–205.

Sylvester, C. E., Hyde, T. S., & Reichler, R. J. (1987). The Diagnostic Interview for Children and the Personality Inventory for Children in studies of children at risk for anxiety disorders or depression. *Journal of the American Academy of Child and Adolescent Psychiatry, 26,* 668–675.

Szadoczky, E., Papp, Z., Vitrai, J., Rihmer, Z., & Furedi, J. (1998). The prevalence of major depressive and bipolar disorder in Hungary. *Journal of Affective Disorders, 50,* 153–162.

Szasz, T. S. (1960). The myth of mental illness. *American Psychologist, 15,* 113–118.

Tancredi, L. R. (1987). The mental status examination. *Generations, 11,* 24–31.

Taylor, M. A. (1981). *The neuropsychiatric mental status examination.* New York: Spectrum.

Taylor, M. A., Abrams, R., Raber, R., & Almy G. (1980). Cognitive tasks in the mental status examination. *Journal of Nervous and Mental Disease, 168,* 167–170.

Taylor, R. E., Creed, F., & Hughes, D. (1997). Relation between psychiatric disorder and abnormal illness behavior in patients undergoing operations for cervical discectomy. *Journal of Neurology, Neurosurgery, and Psychiatry, 63,* 169–174.

Taylor, R. R., & Jason, L. A. (1998). Comparing the DIS with the SCID: Chronic fatigue syndrome and psychiatric comorbidity. *Psychology and Health, 13,* 1087–1104.

Teare, M., Fristad, M. A., Weller, E. B., Weller, R. A., & Salmon, P. (1998a). Study I: Development and critierion validity of the Children's Interview for Psychiatric Syndromes (CHIPS). *Journal of Child and Adolescent Psychopharmocology, 8,* 205–211.

Teare, M., Fristad, M. A., Weller, E. B., Weller, R. A., & Salmon, P. (1998b). Study II: Concurrent validity of the DSM-III-R Children's Interview for Psychiatric Syndromes (CHIPS). *Journal of Child and Adolescent Psychopharmocology, 8,* 213–219.

Tengstrom, A., Grann, M., Langstrom, N., & Kullgren, G. (2000). Psychopathy (PCL-R) as a predictor of violent recidivism among criminal offenders with schizophrenia. *Law and Human Behavior, 24,* 45–58.

Teplin, L. A. (1990). Detecting disorder: The treatment of mental illness among jail detainees. *Journal of Clinical and Consulting Psychology, 58,* 233–236.

Teplin, L. A., & Voit, E. S. (1996). Criminalizing the seriously mentally ill: Putting the problem into perspective. In B. D. Sales & S. A. Shah (Eds.), *Mental health and law: Research, policy and services* (pp. 283–318). Durham, NC: Carolina Academic Press.

Tesser, A., & Paulhus, D. (1983). The definition of self: Private and public self-evaluation management strategies. *Journal of Personality and Social Psychology, 44,* 672–682.

Tetlock, P. E., & Manstead, A. S. R. (1985). Impression management versus intrapsychic explanations in social psychology: A useful dichotomy? *Psychological Review, 92,* 59–77.

Thal, L. J., Salmon, D. P., Lasker, B., Bower, D., & Klauber, M. R. (1989). The safety and lack of efficacy of vinpocetine in Alzheimer's disease. *Journal of the American Geriatrics Society, 37,* 515–520.

Thevos, A. K., Brady, K. T., Grice, D., Dustan, L., & Malcolm, R. (1993). A comparison of psychopathology in cocaine and alcohol dependence. *American Journal of Addictions, 2,* 279–286.

Thompson, R. J., Jr., Hodges, K., & Hamlett, K. W. (1990). A matched comparison of adjustment in children with cystic fibrosis and psychiatrically referred and nonreferred children. *Journal of Pediatric Psychology, 15,* 745–759.

Thompson, R. J., Jr., Merritt, K. A., Keith, B. R., Murphy, L. B., & Johndrow, D. A. (1993). Mother-child agreement on the Child Assessment Schedule for nonreferred children: A research note. *Journal of Child Psychiatry and Psychology, 34,* 813–820.

Tillbrook, C. E. (1997). *Evaluation of Competency to Stand Trial (ECST) instrument: A preliminary assessment.* Unpublished master's thesis, University of Alabama, Tuscaloosa.

Tillbrook, C. E. (2000). *Competency to proceed. A comparative appraisal of approaches to assessment.* Unpublished doctoral dissertation, University of Alabama, Tuscaloosa.

Tilley, D. H., & Hoffman, J. A. (1981). Mental Status Examination: Myth or method. *Comprehensive Psychiatry, 22,* 562–564.

Timmons-Mitchell, J., Brown, C., Schulz, C., Webster, S. E., Underwood, L. A., & Semple, W. E. (1997). Comparing the mental health needs of female and male incarcerated juvenile delinquents. *Behavioral Sciences and the Law, 15,* 195–202.

Torgersen, S. (1980). Hereditary–environmental differentiation of general neurotic obsessive and impulsive hysterical personality traits. *Acta Genetica Medicae Gemellologiae, 29,* 193–207.

Torgersen, S., & Alnaes, R. (1989). Localizing DSM-III personality disorders in a three-dimensional structural space. *Journal of Personality Disorders, 3,* 274–281.

Torgersen, S., & Alnaes, R. (1990). The relationship between the MCMI personality scales and DSM-III, Axis II. *Journal of Personality Assessment, 55,* 698–707.

Torgersen, S., Skre, I., Onstad, S., Edvardsen, J., & Kringlen, E. (1993). The psychometric–genetic structure of DSM-III-R personality criteria. *Journal of Personality Disorders, 7,* 196–213.

Toupin, J., Mercier, H., Dery, M., Cote, G., & Hodgins, S. (1995). Validity of the PCL-R for adolescents. *Issues in Criminological and Legal Psychology, 24,* 143–145.

Trull, T. J. (1992). DSM-III-R personality disorders and the five-factor model of personality: An empirical comparison. *Journal of Abnormal Psychology, 101,* 553–560.

Trull, T. J., & Larson, S. L. (1994). External validity of two personality disorder inventories. *Journal of Personality Disorders, 8,* 96–103.

Trull, T. J., & Widiger, T. A. (1997). *Structured Interview for the Five-Factor Model of Personality (SIFFM): Professional manual.* Odessa, FL: Psychological Assessment Resources.

Trull, T. J., Widiger, T. A., & Frances, A. (1987). Covariation of criteria sets for avoidant, schizoid, and dependent personality disorders. *American Journal of Psychiatry, 144,* 767–771.

Trull, T. J., Widiger, T. A., Useda, J. D., Holcomb, J., Doan, B. T., Axelrod, S. R., Stern, B. L., & Gershuny, B. S. (1998). A structured interview for the assessment of the five-factor model of personality. *Psychological Assessment, 10,* 229–240.

Tsai, L., & Tsuang, M. T. (1979). The mini-mental state test and computerized tomography. *American Journal of Psychiatry, 136,* 436–439.

Tsao, J. C. I., Lewin, M. R., & Craske, M. G. (1998). The effects of cognitive-behavior treatment for panic disorder with comorbid conditions. *Journal of Anxiety Disorders, 12,* 357–371.

Tsuang, M. T., & Loyd, D. W. (1985). Other psychotic disorders. In R. Michels, J. O. Cavenar, A. M. Cooper, S. B. Guze, L. L. Judd, G. L. Klerman, & A. J. Solnit (Eds.), *Psychiatry* (Vol. 1, Chapt. 70). Philadephia: Lippincott.

Turner, J., Batik, M., Palmer, L. J., Forbes, D., & McDermott, B. M. (2000). Detection and importance of laxative use in adolescents with anorexia nervosa. *Journal of the American Academy of Child and Adolescent Psychiatry, 39,* 378–385.

Tyrer, P. J., & Alexander, J. (1979). Classification of personality disorder. *British Journal of Psychiatry, 135,* 163–167.

Tyrer, P. J., Alexander, J., Cicchetti, D., Cohen, M., & Remington, M. (1979). Reliability of a schedule for rating personality disorders. *British Journal of Psychiatry, 135,* 168–174.

Tyrer, P. J., Fowler-Dixon, R., Ferguson, B., & Kelemen, A. (1990). A plea for the diagnosis of hypochondriacal personality disorder. *Journal of Psychosomatic Research, 34,* 637–642.

Tyrer, P. J., Seivewright, N., & Seivewright, H. (1999). Long-term outcome of hypochondriacal personality disorder. *Journal of Psychosomatic Research, 46,* 177–185.

Tyrer, P. J., Strauss, J., & Cicchetti, D. (1983). Temporal reliability in psychiatric practice. *Psychological Medicine, 13,* 393–398.

Uhlmann, R. R., & Larson, E. B. (1991). Effect of education on the Mini-Mental State Examination as a screening test for dementia. *Journal of the American Geriatrics Society, 39,* 876–880.

Uhlmann, R. R., Larson, E. B., & Buchner, D. M. (1987). Correlations of the minimental state and modified dementia rating scale to measures of transitional health status in dementia. *Journal of Gerontology, 42,* 33–36.

Ustad, K. L., Rogers, R., & Salekin, R. T. (1998, March). *Effectiveness of the SADS and SADS-C in detecting malingering: An evaluation of the Rogers's models of malingering utilizing a known-groups design.* American Psychology-Law Society Biennial Conference, Redondo Beach, CA.

Ustad, K. L., Rogers, R., Sewell, K. W., & Guarnaccia, C. A. (1996). Restoration of competency to stand trial: Assessment with the GCCT-MSH and the CST. *Law and Human Behavior, 20,* 131–146.

Ustun, B., Compton, W., Mager, D., Babor, T., Baiyewu, O., Chatterji, S., Cottler, L., Gogus, A., Mavreas, V., Peters, L., Pull, C., Saunders, J., Smeets, R., Stipec, M. R., Vrasti, R., Hasin, D., Room, R., van den Brink, W., Regier, D., Blaine, J., Grant, B. F., & Sartorius, N. (1997). WHO study on the reliability and validity of the alcohol and drug use disorder instruments: Overview of methods and results. *Drug and Alcohol Dependence, 47,* 161–169.

Vaglum, P., Friis, S., Karterud, S., Mehlum, L., & Vaglum, S. (1993). Stability of the server personality disorder diagnosis: A 2- and 5-year prospective study. *Journal of Personality Disorders, 7,* 348–353.

van de Loo, K., Derksen, J., Dassel, Y., & Becking, J. (1987). A structural approach to anorexia nervosa. In J. Derksen (Ed.), *A structural approach in psychodiagnostics and psychopathology* (pp. 13–19). Leiden, Netherlands: Leiden University.

van der Kolk, B. A., Dreyfuss, D., Michaels, M., Shera, D., Berkowitz, R., Fisher, R., & Saxe, G. (1994). Fluoxetine in posttraumatic stress disorder. *Journal of Clinical Psychiatry, 55,* 517–522.

Vandiver, T., & Sheer, K. J. (1991). Temporal stability of the Diagnostic Interview Schedule. *Psychological Assessment: A Journal of Consulting and Clinical Psychology, 3,* 277–281.

Vandvik, I. H. (1990). Mental health and psychosocial functioning in children with recent onset rheumatic disease. *Journal of Child Psychology and Psychiatry, 31,* 961–971.

van Gorp, W. G., Marcotte, T. D., Sultzer, D., Hinkin, C., Mahler, M., & Cummings, J. L. (1999). Screening for dementia: Comparison of three commonly used instruments. *Journal of Clinical and Experimental Neuropsychology, 21,* 29–38.

Vazquez-Barquero, J. L., Diez-Manrique, J. F., Pena, C., Aldama, J., Samaniego, R. C., Menendez, A. J., & Mirapeix, C. (1987). A community mental health survey in Cantabria: A general description of morbidity. *Psychological Medicine, 17,* 227–241.

Vazquez-Barquero, J. L., Garcia, J. Simon, J. A., Iglesias, C., Montejo, J., Herran, A., & Dunn, G. (1997). Mental health in primary care: An epidemiological study of morbidity and the use of health resources. *British Journal of Psychiatry, 170,* 529–535.

Vazquez-Barquero, J. L., Nunez, M. J. C., Castanedo, S. H., Manrique, J. R. D., Pardo, G., & Dunn, G. (1996). Sociodemographic and clinical variables as predictors of diagnostic characteristics of first episodes of schizophrenia. *Acta Psychiatrica Scandinavica, 94,* 149–155.

Velez, C. N., Johnson, J., & Cohen, P. (1989). A longitudinal analysis of selected risk factors for childhood psychopathology. *Journal of the American Academy of Child and Adolescent Psychiatry, 28,* 861–864.

Ventura, J., Liberman, R. P., Green, M. F., Shaner, A., & Mintz, J. (1998). Training and quality assurances with the Structured Clinical Interview for DSM-IV (SCID-I/P). *Psychiatry Research, 79,* 163–173.

Verducci, J. S., Mack, M. E., & DeGroot, M. H. (1988). Estimating multiple rater agreement for a rare diagnosis. *Journal of Multivariate Analysis, 27,* 512–535.

Verheul, R., Hartgers, C., van den Brink, W., & Koeter, M. W. J. (1998). The effect of sampling, diagnostic criteria, and assessment procedures on the observed prevalence of DSM-III-R personality disorders among treated alcoholics. *Journal of Studies on Alcohol, 59,* 227–236.

Verhulst, F. C., Althaus, M., & Berden, G. F. M. G. (1987). The Child Assessment Schedule: Parent–child agreement and validity measures. *Journal of Child Psychology and Psychiatry, 28,* 455–466.

Verhulst, F. C., Ende, J., Ferdinand, R. F., & Kasius, M. C. (1997). The prevalence of DSM-III-R diagnoses in a national sample of Dutch adolescents. *Archives of General Psychiatry, 54,* 329–336.

Vernon, S. W., & Roberts, R. E. (1982). Use of the SADS-RDC in a tri-ethnic community survey. *Archives of General Psychiatry, 39,* 47–52.

Viatori, M. S. (1985). A review of the Psychiatric Diagnostic Interview. *Journal of Counseling and Development, 63,* 531.

Vitacco, M. J., Rogers, R., Neumann, C., Durant, S. & Collins, M. (2000, March). *Adolescent psychopathy: Contributions of sensation seeking, impulsivity and ADHD.* Biennial convention of the American Psychology-Law Society, New Orleans.

Vitiello, B., Malone, R., Buschle, P. M., Delaney, M. A., & Behar, D. (1990). Reliability of DSM-III diagnoses in hospitalized children. *Hospital and Community Psychiatry, 41,* 63–67.

von Zerssen, D., Barthelmes, H., Possl, J., Black, C., Garczynski, E., Wesse, E., & Hecht, H. (1998). The Biographical Personality Interview (BPI)—a new approach to the assessment of premorbid personality in psychiatric research: Part II. Psychometric properties. *Journal of Psychiatric Research, 32,* 25–35.

von Zerssen, D., Possl, J., Hecht, H., Black, C., Garczynski, E., & Barthelmes, H. (1998). The Biographical Personality Interview (BPI)—a new approach to the assessment of premorbid personality in psychiatric research: Part I. Development of the instrument. *Journal of Psychiatric Research, 32,* 19–25.

Wade, J. B., Dougherty, L. M., Archer, C. R., & Price, D. D. (1996). Assessing the stages of pain processing: A multivariate analytical approach. *Pain, 68,* 157–167.

Wade, T., Martin, N. G., Neale, M. C., Tiggemann, M., Treloar, S. A., Bucholz, K. K., Madden, P. A. F., & Heath, A. C. (1999). The structure of genetic and evironmental risk factors for three measures of disordered eating. *Psychological Medicine, 29,* 925–934.

Walters, G. D., Chlumsky, M. L., & Hemphill, L. L. (1988). Reliability and stability of a structured diagnostic interview in a group of incarcerated offenders. *International Journal of Offender Therapy and Comparative Criminology, 32,* 87–94.

Walters, G. D., Mann, M. F., Miller, M. P., Hemphill, L. L., & Chlumsky, M. L. (1988). Emotional disorders among offenders: Inter- and intra-setting comparisons. *Criminal Justice and Behavior, 15,* 433–453.

Wang, E. W., Rogers, R., Giles, C. L., Diamond, P. M., Herrington-Wang, L. E., & Taylor, E. R. (1997). A pilot study of the Personality Assessment Inventory (PAI) in Corrections: Assessment of malingering, suicide risk, and aggression in male inmates. *Behavioral Sciences and the Law, 15,* 469–482.

Ward, C. H., Beck, A. T., Mendelson, M., Mock, J. E., & Erbaugh, J. K. (1962). The psychiatric nomenclature. *Archives of General Psychiatry, 7,* 198–205.

Watt, D. C., Katz, K., & Shepherd, M. (1983). The natural history of schizophrenia: A 5-year prospective follow-up of a representative sample of schizophrenics by means of a standardized clinical and social assessment. *Psychological Medicine, 13,* 663–670.

Weathers, F. W., Blake, D. D., Krinsley, K., Haddad, W., Huka, J., & Keane, T. M. (November, 1992). *The Clinician-Administered PTSD Scale (CAPS): Reliability and construct validity.* Paper presented at the meeting of the Association for the Advancement of Behavior Therapy, Boston, MA.

Weathers, F. W., Litz, B. T., Herman, D. S., Huska, J. A., & Keane, T. M., (1993, October). *The PTSD Checklist (PCL): Reliability, validity and diagnostic utility.* Paper presented at the annual meeting of the International Society of Traumatic Stress Studies, San Antonio, TX.

Weathers, F. W., Ruscio, A. M., & Keane, T. M. (1999). Psychometric properties of nine scoring rules for the Clinician-Administered Posttraumatic Stress Disorder Scale. *Psychological Assessment, 11,* 124–133.

Weaver, T. L. (1998). Method variance and sensitivity of screening for traumatic stressors. *Journal of Traumatic Stress, 11,* 181–185.

Webster, J. S., Scott, R. R., Nunn, B., McNeer, M. R., & Varnell, N. (1984). A brief neuropsychological screening procedure that assesses left and right hemispheric function. *Journal of Clinical Psychology, 40,* 237–240.

Wechsler, D. (1997). *Wechsler Adult Intelligence Scale—Third edition.* San Antonio, TX: Psychological Corporation.

Weddington, W. W., Segraves, K. B., & Simon, M. A. (1986). Current and lifetime incidence of psychiatric disorders among a group of extremity sarcoma survivors. *Journal of Psychosomatic Research, 30,* 121–125.

Weinstein, S. R., Stone, K., Noam, G. G., Grimes, K., & Schwab-Stone, M. (1989). Comparison of the DISC and clinicians' DSM-III diagnoses in psychiatric patients. *Journal of the American Academy of Child and Adolescent Psychiatry, 28,* 53–60.

Weiss, G., Hechtman, L., Milroy, T., & Perlman, T. (1985). Psychiatric status of hyperactives as adults: A controlled prospective 15-year follow-up of 63 hyperactive children. *Journal of the American Academy of Child and Adolescent Psychiatry, 24,* 211–220.

Weiss, M. G., Raguram, R., & Channiabasavanna, S. M. (1995). Cultural dimensions of psychiatric diagnoses: A comparison of DSM-III-R and illness explanatory models in south India. *British Journal of Psychiatry, 166,* 353–359.

Weiss, M. G., Zelkowitz, P., Feldman, R. B., Vegel, J., Heyman, M., & Paris, J.

(1996). Psychopathology in offspring of methods with borderline personality disorder: A pilot study. *Canadian Journal of Psychiatry, 41,* 285–290.

Weiss, R. D., Griffin, M. L., & Hufford, C. (1992). Severity of cocaine dependence as a predictor of relapse to cocaine use. *American Journal of Psychiatry, 149,* 1595–1596.

Weiss, R. D., Mirin, S. M., Griffin, M. L., Gunderson, J. G., & Hufford, C. (1993). Personality disorders in cocaine dependence. *Comprehensive Psychiatry, 34,* 145–149.

Weiss, R. D., Najavits, L. M., Muenz, L. R., & Hufford, C. (1995). Twelve-month test–retest reliability of the Structured Clinical Interview for DSM-III-R Disorders in cocaine-dependent patients. *Comprehensive Psychiatry, 36,* 384–389.

Weissman, M. M., Bland, R. C., Canino, G. J., Faravelli, C., Greenwald, S., Hwu, H. G., Joyce, P. R., Karam, E. G., Lee, C. K., Lellouch, J., Lepine, J. P., Newman, S. C., Oakley-Browne, M. A., Rubio-Stipec, M., Wells, J. E., Wickramaratne, P. J., Wittchen, H. U., & Yeh, E. K. (1997). The cross-national epidemiology of panic disorder. *Archives of General Psychiatry, 54,* 305–309.

Weissman, M. M., & Myers, J. K. (1980). Psychiatric disorders in a US community: The application of the Research Diagnostic Criteria to a resurveyed community sample. *Acta Psychiatrica Scandinavica, 62,* 99–111.

Weissman, M. M., Myers, J. K., & Harding, P. S. (1978). Psychiatric disorders in a US urban community, 1975–1976. *American Journal of Psychiatry, 135,* 459–462.

Weissman, M. M., Wickarmaratne, P., & Warner, V. (1987). Assessing psychiatric disorders in children: Discrepancies between mothers' and children's reports. *Archives of General Psychiatry, 44,* 747–753.

Weller, E. B., Weller, R. A., Fristad, M. A., & Rooney, M. T. (1999). *Children's Interview for Psychiatric Syndromes.* Washington, DC: American Psychiatric Press.

Weller, R. A., Penick, E. C., Powell, B. J., Othmer, E., Rice, A. S., & Kent, T. A. (1985). Agreement between two structured interviews: DIS and the PDI. *Comprehensive Psychiatry, 26,* 157–163.

Wells, K. B., Burnam, A., Leake, B., & Robins, L. N. (1988). Agreement between face-to-face and telephone-administered versions of the depression section of the NIMH Diagnostic Interview Schedule. *Journal of Psychiatric Research, 22,* 207–220.

Welner, A., Liss, J. L., & Robins, E. (1972). Undiagnosed psychiatric patients: Part I. Record study. *British Journal of Psychiatry, 120,* 315–319.

Welner, A., Liss, J. L., & Robins, E. (1973). Undiagnosed psychiatric patients: Part III. The undiagnosable patient. *British Journal of Psychiatry, 123,* 91–98.

Welner, Z., Reich, W., Herjanic, B., Jung, K. G., & Amado, H. (1987). Reliability, validity, and parent–child agreement studies of the Diagnostic Interview for Children and Adolescents (DICA). *Journal of American Academy of Child and Adolescent Psychiatry, 26,* 649–653.

West, S. G., Sandler, I., Pillow, D. R., Baca, L., & Gersten, J. C. (1991). The use of structural equation modeling in generative research: Toward the design of preventive intervention with bereaved children. *American Journal of Community Psychology, 19,* 459–480.

Westen, D., Moses, M. J., Silk, K. R., Lohr, N. E., Cohen, R., & Segal, H. (1992). Quality of depressive experience in borderline personality disorder and major depression: When depression is not just depression. *Journal of Personality Disorders, 6,* 382–393.

Westenberg, P. M., Siebelink, B. M., Warmenhoven, N. J. C., & Treffers, P. D. A. (1999). Separation anxiety and overanxious disorders: Relations to age and level of psychosocial maturity. *Journal of American Academy of Child and Adolescent Psychiatry, 38,* 1000–1007.

Whisman, M. A., Strosahl, K., Fruzzetti, A. E., Schmaling, K. B., Jacobson, N. S., & Miller, D. M. (1989). A structured interview version of the Hamilton Rating Scale for Depression: Reliability and validity. *Psychological Assessment, 1,* 238–241.

Whittemore, K. E., Ogloff, J. R. P., & Roesch, R. (1997). An investigation of competency to participate in legal proceedings in Canada. *Canadian Journal of Psychiatry, 42,* 869–875.

Wickramaratne, P. J., & Weissman, M. M. (1998). Onset of psychopathology in offspring by developmental phase and parental depression. *Journal of American Academy of Child and Adolescent Psychiatry, 37,* 933–942.

Widiger, T. A. (1985). *Personality Interview Questions (PIQ).* Unpublished manuscript, University of Kentucky, Lexington.

Widiger, T. A. (1987). *Personality Interview Questions—II (PIQ-II).* Unpublished manuscript, University of Kentucky, Lexington.

Widiger, T. A. (1991). Personality disorder dimensional models proposed for DSM-IV. *Journal of Personality Disorders, 5,* 386–398.

Widiger, T. A. (1992). Categorical versus dimensional classification: Implications from and for research. *Journal of Personality Disorders, 6,* 287–300.

Widiger, T. A., & Corbitt, E. M. (1993). Antisocial personality disorder: Proposals for DSM-IV. *Journal of Personality Disorders, 7,* 63–77.

Widiger, T. A., & Corbitt, E. M. (1995). The DSM-IV antisocial personality disorder. In W. J. Livesley (Ed.), *The DSM-IV personality disorders* (pp. 103–126). New York: Guilford Press.

Widiger, T. A., Corbitt, E. M., Ellis, C. G., & Thomas, G. V. (1992). *Personality Interview Questions—III (PIQ-III).* Unpublished manuscript, University of Kentucky, Lexington.

Widiger, T. A., & Frances, A. (1985). The DSM-III personality disorders: Perspectives from psychology. *Archives of General Psychiatry, 42,* 615–623.

Widiger, T. A., & Frances, A. (1987). Interviews and inventories for the measurement of personality disorders. *Clinical Psychology Review, 7,* 49–75.

Widiger, T. A., Frances, A. J., Pincus, H. A., & Davis, W. W. (1990). DSM-IV literature reviews: Rationale, process and limitations. *Journal of Psychopathology and Behavioral Assessment, 12,* 189–202.

Widiger, T. A., Frances, A. J., Pincus, H. A., Davis, W. W., & First, M. B. (1991). Towards an empirical classification for the DSM-IV. *Journal of Abnormal Psychology, 100,* 280–288.

Widiger, T. A., Frances, A., Warner, L., & Bluhm, C. (1986). Diagnostic criteria for the borderline and schizoptypal personality disorders. *Journal of Abnormal Psychology, 95,* 43–51.

Widiger, T. A., Freiman, K., & Bailey, B. (1990). Convergent and discriminant validity of personality disorder prototypic acts. *Psychological Assessment: A Journal of Clinical and Consulting Psychology, 3,* 418–423.

Widiger, T. A., Mangine, S., Corbitt, E. M., Ellis, C. G., & Thomas, G. V. (1994). *Personality Disorder Interview–IV.* Unpublished manuscript, University of Kentucky, Lexington.

Widiger, T. A., Mangine, S., Corbitt, E. M., Ellis, C. G., & Thomas, G. V. (1995). *Personality Disorder Interview—IV*. Odessa, FL: Psychological Assessment Resources.

Widiger, T. A., Trull, T. J., Hurt, S., Clarkin, J. F., & Frances, A. (1987). A multidimensional scaling of the DSM-III personality disorders. *Archives of General Psychiatry, 44*, 557–563.

Widom, C. S. (1999). Posttraumatic stress disorder in abused and neglected children grown up. *American Journal of Psychiatry, 156*, 1223–1229.

Wiens, A. N. (1990). Structured clinical interviews for adults. In G. Goldstein & M. Hersen (Eds.), *Handbook of psychological assessment* (2nd ed., 324–341). New York: Pergamon Press.

Wierson, M., & Forehand, R. (1995). Predicting recidivism in juvenile deliquents: The role of mental health diagnoses and the qualifications of conclusions by race. *Behavioural Research and Therapy, 33*, 63–67.

Wiggins, J. S. (1962). Strategic, method, and stylistic variance in the MMPI. *Psychological Bulletin, 59*, 224–242.

Wiggins, J. S., & Broughton, R. (1985). The interpersonal circle: A structural model for the integration of personality research. In R. Hogan & W. Jones (Eds.), *Perspectives in personality* (Vol. 1; pp. 1–47). Greenwich, CT: JAI Press.

Wilcox, H., Field, T., Prodromidis, M., & Scafidi, F. (1998). Correlations between the BDI and CES-D in a sample of adolescent mothers. *Adolescence, 33*, 565–574.

Wildman, R., Batchelor, E., Thompson, L., Nelson, F., Moore, J., Patterson, M., & de Laosa, M. (1979). The Georgia Court Competency Test. *Newsletter of the American Association of Correctional Psychologists, 2*, 4 (abstract).

Wildman, R., Batchelor, E., Thompson, L., Nelson, F., Moore, J., Patterson, M., & de Laosa, M. (1980). *The Georgia Court Competency Test: An attempt to develop a rapid, qualitative measure for fitness for trial*. Unpublished manuscript, Forensic Services Division, Central State Hospital, Milledgeville, GA.

Wilfley, D. E., Schwartz, M. B., Spurrell, E. B., & Fairburn, C. G. (2000). Using the Eating Disorder Examination to identify the specific psychopathology of binge eating disorder. *International Journal of Eating Disorders, 27*, 259–269.

Williams, J. B. W., Gibbon, M., First, M. B., Spitzer, R. L., Davies, M., Borus, J., Howes, M. J., Kane, J., Pope, H. G., Jr., Rounsaville, B., & Wittchen, H. U. (1992). The structured clinical interview for DSM-III-R (SCID): II. Multisite test–retest reliability. *Archives of General Psychiatry, 49*, 630–636.

Williams, J. B. W., Spitzer, R. L., & Gibbon, M. (1992). International reliability of a diagnostic intake procedure for panic disorder. *American Journal of Psychiatry, 149*, 560–562.

Williams, S., McGee, R., Anderson, J., & Silva, P. A. (1989). The structure and correlates of self-reported symptoms in 11-year-old children. *Journal of Abnormal Child Psychology, 17*, 55–71.

Wilmink, F. W., & Snijders, T. A. B. (1989). Polytomous logistic regression analysis of the General Health Questionnaire and the Present State Examination. *Psychological Medicine, 19*, 755–764.

Wilson, G. T., & Eldredge, K. L. (1991). Frequency of binge eating in bulimic patients: Diagnostic validity. *International Journal of Eating Disorders, 5*, 557–561.

Wilson, G. T., Nonas, C. A., & Rosenblum, G. D. (1993). Assessment of binge eating in obese patients. *International Journal of Eating Disorders, 13*, 25–33.

Wing, J. K. (1976). A technique for studying psychiatric morbidity in inpatient and outpatient series and in general population samples. *Psychological Medicine, 6,* 665–671.

Wing, J. K. (1996). Scan and PSE tradition. *Social Psychiatry and Psychiatric Epidemiology, 31,* 50–54.

Wing, J. K., Babor, T., Brugha, T., Burke, F., Cooper, J. E., Giel, R., Jablenski, F., Regier, D., & Sartorius, N. (1990). SCAN: Schedules for clinical assessment in neuropsychiatry. *Archives of General Psychiatry, 47,* 589–593.

Wing, J. K., Birely, J. L. T., Cooper, J. E., Graham, P., & Isaacs, A. (1967). Reliability of a procedure for measuring and classifying present psychiatric state. *British Journal of Psychiatry, 113,* 499–515.

Wing, J. K., Cooper, J. E., & Sartorius, N. (1974). *The measurement and classification of psychiatric symptoms.* Cambridge, UK: Cambridge University Press.

Wing, J. K., Nixon, J. N., Mann, S. A., & Leff, J. P. (1977). Reliability of the PSE (9th edition) used in a population survey. *Psychological Medicine, 7,* 505–516.

Wing, J. K., Sartorius, N., & Ustun, T. B. (1998). *Diagnosis and clinical measurement in psychiatry: A reference manual for SCAN/PSE-10.* Cambridge, UK: Cambridge University Press.

Wittchen, H. U., (1994). Reliability and validity studies of the WHO Composite International Diagnostic Interview: A critical review. *Journal of Psychiatric Research, 28,* 57–84.

Wittchen, H. U., Burke, J. D., Semler, G., Pfister, H., Von Cranach, M., & Zaudig, M. (1989). Recall and dating of psychiatric symptoms: Test–retest reliability of time-related symptom questions in a standardized psychiatric interview. *Archives of General Psychiatry, 46,* 437–443.

Wittchen, H. U., Zhao, S., Kessler, R. C., & Eaton, W. W. (1994). DSM-III-R generalized anxiety disorder in the national comorbidity study. *Archives of General Psychiatry, 51,* 355–364.

Wong, S., & Elek, D. (1989, August). *The treatment of psychopathy: A review.* Paper presented at the American Psychological Association convention, New Orleans, LA.

Wood, I. K., Parmelee, D. X., & Arents, M. P. (1992). Factors associated with borderline pathology in school-age children. *Journal of Child and Family Studies, 1,* 167–181.

World Health Organization. (1979). *Schizophrenia: An international follow-up study.* New York: Wiley.

World Health Organization. (1993). *The Composite International Diagnostic Interview (CIDI), Core Version 1.1.* Washington, DC: American Psychiatric Association.

World Health Organization. (1994). *Schedules for Clinical Assessment of Neuropsychiatry (SCAN).* Geneva: Author.

World Health Organization. (1997). *The Composite International Diagnostic Interview (Version 2, 12 month).* Geneva: Author.

World Health Organization—Alcohol, Drug, and Mental Health Administration. (1987). *Composite International Diagnostic Interview (CIDI).* Geneva: Author.

Wu, P., Hoven, C. W., Bird, H. R., Moore, R. E., Cohen, P., Alegria, M., Dulcan, M. K., Goodman, S. H., Horwitz, S. M., Lichtman, J. H., Narrow, W. E., Rae, D. S., Regier, D. A., & Roper, M. T. (1999). Depressive and disruptive disorder and mental health service utilization in children and adolescents. *Journal of the American Academy of Child and Adolescent Psychiatry, 38,* 1081–1090.

Wyndrowe, J. (1987). The microcomputerized Diagnostic Interview Schedule: Clinical use in an outpatient setting. *Canadian Journal of Psychiatry, 32,* 93–99.

Wynkoop, T. F., Frederick, R. I., & Hoy, M. (2000, February). *Factor structure of the Structured Interview of Reported Symptoms (SIRS) psychiatric and cognitive components.* Paper presented at the Annual Meeting of the International Neuropsychological Society, Denver, CO.

Yesage, J. A., Brink, T. L., Rose, T. L., Lum, O., Huang, V., Adey, M., & Leirer, O. (1983). Development and validation of a geriatric depression screening scale: A preliminary report. *Journal of Psychiatric Research, 17,* 37–49.

Zahner, G. E. P. (1991). The feasibility of conducting structured diagnostic interviews with preadolescents: A community field trial of the DISC. *Journal of American Academy of Child and Adolescent Psychiatry, 30,* 659–668.

Zanarini, M. C., Frankenburg, F. R., Chauncey, D. L., & Gunderson, J. G. (1987). The Diagnostic Interview for Personality Disorders: Interrater and test–retest reliability. *Comprehensive Psychiatry, 28,* 467–480.

Zanarini, M. C., Frankenburg, F. R., & Gunderson, J. G. (1988). Psychopharmocology for borderline outpatients. *Comprehensive Psychiatry, 29,* 372–378.

Zanarini, M. C., Gunderson, J. G., & Frankenburg, F. R. (1989). Axis I phenomenology of borderline personality disorder. *Comprehensive Psychiatry, 30,* 149–156.

Zanarini, M. C., Gunderson, J. G., Frankenburg, F. R., & Chauncey, D. L. (1989). The revised Diagnostic Interview for Borderlines: Discriminating BPD from other Axis II disorders. *Journal of Personality Disorders, 3,* 10–18.

Zelinski, E. M., Gilewski, M. J., & Anthony-Berstone, C. R. (1990). Memory Functioning Questionnaire: Concurrent validity with memory performance and self-reported memory failures. *Psychology and Aging, 5,* 388–399.

Zimmerman, M., & Coryell, W. (1987). The Inventory to Diagnose Depression (IDD): A self-report scale to diagnose major depressive disorder. *Journal of Consulting and Clinical Psychology, 55,* 55–59.

Zimmerman, M., & Coryell, W. (1988). The validity of a self-report questionnaire for diagnosing major depressive disorder. *Archives of General Psychiatry, 45,* 738–740.

Zimmerman, M., & Coryell, W. (1989). DSM-III personality disorder diagnoses in a nonpatient sample: Demographic correlates and comorbidity. *Archives of General Psychiatry, 46,* 682–689.

Zimmerman, M., & Coryell, W. (1990). Diagnosing personality disorders in the community: A comparison of self-report and interview measures. *Archives of General Psychiatry, 47,* 527–531.

Zimmerman, M., Coryell, W., Pfohl, B., Corenthal, C., & Stangl, D. (1986). ECT response in depressed patients with and without a DSM-III personality disorder. *American Journal of Psychiatry, 143,* 1030–1032.

Zimmerman, M., & Mattia, J. I. (1998a). Body dysmorphic disorder in psychiatric outpatients: Recognition, prevalence, comorbidity, demographic and clinical correlates. *Comprehensive Psychiatry, 39,* 265–270.

Zimmerman, M., & Mattia, J. I. (1998b). Psychiatric diagnosis in clinical practice: Is comorbidity being missed? *Comprehensive Psychiatry, 40,* 182–191.

Zimmerman, M., Pfohl, B., Coryell, W., Stangl, D., & Corenthal, C. (1986). Assessment of DSM-III personality disorders: The importance of interviewing an informant. *Journal of Clinical Psychiatry, 47,* 261–263.

Zung, W. (1965). A self-rating depression scale. *Archives of General Psychiatry, 12,* 63–70.

Zwick, R. (1983). Assessing the psychometric properties of psychodiagnostic systems: How do the research diagnostic criteria measure up? *Journal of Consulting and Clinical Psychology, 51,* 117–131.

Author Index

Subject Index

Note: "b" indicates a box; "t" indicates a table.

506